Physician's Field Guide to Neuropsychology

Karen M. Sanders
Editor

Physician's Field Guide to Neuropsychology

Collaboration through Case Example

Springer

Editor
Karen M. Sanders
Department of Psychiatry and Behavioral Sciences
University of Washington School of Medicine
Seattle, WA, USA

ISBN 978-1-4939-8720-7 ISBN 978-1-4939-8722-1 (eBook)
https://doi.org/10.1007/978-1-4939-8722-1

Library of Congress Control Number: 2018962740

This Springer imprint is published by the registered company Springer Science+Business Media, LLC part of Springer Nature.
The registered company address is: 233 Spring Street, New York, NY 10013, U.S.A.

To my parents
Robert and Teresa Sanders

Foreword

Cognitive Neurologist Perspective

Proper care of patients has always required cross-disciplinary knowledge. One domain where such knowledge has become even more important is the realm of higher mental functions *across the life-span*—from our early stages of development in infancy and childhood to preserving quality of life in our later years. As people live longer, including those with chronic conditions that affect cognition, more and more individuals are striving to maintain optimal cognitive performance. Thus, there is an increasing need for physicians to understand laboratory tests for mental functions and the science behind this testing. Given that virtually all medical, neurological, and psychiatric conditions can have neurocognitive symptoms, an understanding of neuropsychology is important, even for physicians. Neuropsychology traditionally overlapped with neurology (especially behavioral and cognitive neurology) and with psychiatry (particularly neuropsychiatry). However, physicians in other fields cannot necessarily count on subspecialists in these fields to collaborate in the care of their patients. Availability, time, and economics all conspire against such collaboration in the current healthcare environment.

Conversely, physicians who are not specialists in behavioral neurology or neuropsychiatry can make themselves more competitive in the current healthcare environment by understanding the basics of neuropsychology and how it can contribute to the assessment and care of patients with disorders or suspected disorders of memory, language, executive functioning, mood, and other mental functions. *Physician's Field Guide to Neuropsychology* provides an excellent foundation for both students and practitioners to gain this understanding. It will help all of us to work better as partners in identifying and treating the emotional and cognitive disorders that are becoming more widely recognized and more treatable.

Barry Gordon, MD

Department of Neurology,
The Johns Hopkins Medical Institutions,
Baltimore, MD, USA

Neuropsychologist Perspective

Physicians are traditionally taught four vital signs: body temperature, blood pressure, pulse, and heart rate. More recent efforts at quality have promoted pain as the fifth vital sign, but if pain is the fifth vital sign, then cognition should be the sixth. Assessing cognitive function should be considered a critical component of marking normal development and wellness. At best, cognitive screening is a straightforward process that can identify gross disturbances, akin to finding a significantly elevated body temperature. Just like elevated temperature, cognitive screening can only reveal that there is a problem needing further investigation. Moreover, screening is often insensitive, and healthcare providers must frequently evaluate patients for whom there is concern for cognition in spite of normal cognitive screening. For these reasons and more, it is highly valuable for frontline healthcare providers to have neuropsychologists included in the integrated care team.

The National Academy of Medicine's (NAM, previously the Institute of Medicine) *Crossing the Quality Chasm* (NAM, 2001) is perhaps the single most influential publication in healthcare service delivery in the past 25 years. Among its many important recommendations is the need for more organized healthcare teams. *Physician's Field Guide to Neuropsychology* includes an outstanding group of authors who are themselves integrated into successful healthcare teams. These authors demonstrate the value of neuropsychology in the integrated healthcare team on a case-by-case basis. Their case examples cover the life-span from evaluation of the consequences of premature birth and developmental disorders through the adult issues of schizophrenia, epilepsy, and multiple sclerosis and into the range of later-life disorders (stroke, Alzheimer's, Lewy body disease). This book makes a strong "case" for the need to integrate the efforts of physicians and clinical neuropsychologists in serving patients that present with anomalies of the sixth vital sign, cognition.

Glenn Smith, PhD, ABPP
Department of Clinical and Health Psychology
University of Florida
Gainesville, FL, USA
Mayo Clinic College of Medicine
Rochester, MN, USA

Integrative Care Psychologist Perspective

Healthcare costs in the United States are the highest in the world, but our outcomes are not the best. Public health and health economists have, in recent years, turned their attention to the relatively small number of patients, estimated to be 5% of the population, who account for over half of all healthcare costs. Describing that population has been difficult, but a recent volume from the National Academy of Medicine (Long et al., 2017) has reviewed the literature and identified both the patient groups and the specific behavioral variables that determine those who have the most difficulty responding to care and who generate the highest costs. The clinical groups with the highest needs are children with complex needs, non-elderly disabled, those with multiple chronic illnesses, frail elderly, and those with advancing terminal illness. As a society, we have tended to focus on the end-of-life care of the elderly and those with terminal illness as the highest cost groups, but the other groups of patients with long-term disability have the worst outcomes and the longest duration of need. Social and economic variables play a key role in higher costs and poor outcome, but it is behavioral variables that have the highest impact, including substance abuse, serious mental illness, cognitive decline, and toxic chronic stress.

We know the clinical groups identified are at risk for disorders of memory, mood, and executive functioning that have a direct impact on patient function at home and health outcomes. In addition, for those patients with substance abuse, serious mental illness, cognitive decline, and exposure to toxic stress, neuropsychological dysfunction can enormously complicate their care. An understanding of neuropsychology by attending physicians and other care providers can assist in the formulation of realistic care plans and allow healthcare systems to use services wisely for the patients who need assistance to function at home.

Understanding the basics of neuropsychology and the evaluation of memory, language, mood, and executive function are essential to the design of achievable care plans for these complex patients. *Physician's Field Guide to Neuropsychology* provides the background and foundation for practitioners to gain this level of understanding of neuropsychological functioning which is essential for effective care implementation.

Center for Psychology and Health, APA
Washington, DC, USA

Doug Tynan, PhD, ABPP

Long, P., Abrams, M.K., Milstein, A., Anderson, G., Apton, K.L., Dahlberg, M.L. & Whicher, D., (Eds). (2017) *Effective Care for High Needs Patients: Opportunities for Improving Outcomes, Value and Health.* Washington DC: National Academy of Medicine.

Preface

Neurocognitive functioning is essential to quality of life. It has been called the "sixth vital sign." Neurocognitive health is a sensitive indicator of overall health. Both acute and chronic changes in cognitive function, routine daily living, illness, and/or injury can inform patients and care providers about wellness, prevention, and cure.

Accurate assessment is key to this vital information. In many cases, however, clinical knowledge is limited, tools are blunt and insensitive, and treatment is non-existent. Comprehensive neuropsychological assessment fills this gap in medical care.

Despite decades of development in the field, neuropsychology is little known to most medical practitioners. In addition, the powerful clinical knowledge and highly researched assessment tools of the clinical neuropsychologist are only minimally understood. Neurocognitive health is critical to day-to-day functioning, overall health, and quality of life. Neuropsychology has addressed this topic from a scientific and clinical standpoint for over 50 years. The scientific discipline of neuropsychology is recognized as integral to comprehensive care in many medical settings including surgical, inpatient, and outpatient medical rehabilitation as well as memory diagnostic centers. Neuropsychologists work closely with physicians and medical experts to accurately diagnose and treat neurocognitive functioning, such as traumatic brain injury, dementia, multiple sclerosis, stroke, epilepsy, childhood disorders, oncology, and movement disorders.

This book is designed to teach medical residents and non-neuropsychologist physicians through case examples about the utility of neuropsychology (NP) in a collaborative medical setting. Major medical schools are beginning to realize the need to teach medical residents the appropriate use of neuropsychology in medical settings—a specific pedagogy would be valuable for this purpose. This book will outline a method for teaching this vital material through case examples and collaboration. The purpose of this manual is not to teach neuropsychology to the medical resident, but rather to inform about the utility of neuropsychology in a collaborative setting.

There are three main goals for this manual:

Goal One: **Emphasize that neuropsychological testing is completely different from cognitive screens and requires extensive training.**

(a) Cognitive screens are not diagnostic endpoints when assessing neurocognitive functioning—a misdiagnosis can often occur in these cases (false positive/false negative). Undiagnosed or misdiagnosed complex neurocognitive functioning can significantly impact many aspects of a patient's life.
(b) Interpretation of neuropsychological tests requires comprehensive testing and in-depth training. Many disciplines use the principles of neuropsychology; however, the clinical neuropsychological evaluation is different. The trained clinical neuropsychologist has a doctorate in psychology and extensive post-doctoral training in medical neuropsychology (see theaacnorg/position_papers/Houston_Conference.pdf). Board certification in clinical neuropsychology is now sought after in major medical centers (see Braun chapter in this book).

Goal Two: **Clearly demonstrate the utility of neuropsychology through case examples in medical settings.**

Case examples are powerful teaching tools and clearly illustrate the difference between cognitive screens and neuropsychological evaluation. There is clear benefit in using neuropsychological knowledge from the beginning to the end of diagnosis and treatment in patient care. This workbook format will guide the learner through each case example and demonstrate through the support of evidenced-based literature the clear scientific benefit of a comprehensive assessment in the hands of a well-trained neuropsychologist.

Goal Three: **Foster collaboration between neuropsychology and medical cultures to increase coordinated care.**

A neuropsychologist and a physician who discuss a case from referral question through diagnosis will cowrite each chapter and present the recommended treatment, outlining the unique thought processes and diagnostic approaches of each discipline.

Goals Two and Three were informed by the work of Irby[1], who has written expansively about a pedagogy for medical resident training using case examples, Socratic, and iterative approaches and collaboration.

The book is divided into three sections:

Part I: The Distinct Worlds of Neuropsychology and Medicine

Braun, Lanca, and Schoenberg write about the foundation of neuropsychological theory, the statistical strength of the instruments, and the unique contribution of neuropsychological data in a collaborative workup.

1. The world of neuropsychology—a functional science focused on brain-behavior outcomes of neurological injury and illness (training, culture, thinking process, research, etc.).

[1] Irby, D. Three Exemplary Models of Case-Based Training. Academic Medicine. Volume 69 (12), December 1994.

2. The world of the medical practitioner—an anatomical and biological science focused on symptoms and clinical signs.
3. The difference between the approaches of neurology and neuropsychology to basic mental status.
4. The use of existing models of collaboration between medicine and psychology.

Part II: Medical Areas of Need: Case Examples

Each chapter in this section is written by at least one neuropsychologist and one physician to demonstrate collaboration by case example and to provide a teaching format for residents. Topics include dementia, childhood/developmental issues, TBI/sports concussion, cancer, cognition, cerebrovascular issues, LD/ADD, epilepsy, neuroimaging and NP, movement disorders, and more.

Part III: Treatment Issues

This part of the book will include chapters on rehabilitation, vocational rehabilitation, feedback, and forensic and multicultural issues. Neuropsychology informs treatment and rehabilitation on many levels. Each chapter in this section focuses on key topics of treatment.

It is essential to foster integration of neuropsychology into multidisciplinary medical settings. The goal of this book is to guide and inform medical residents early in their training to ensure that neuropsychology is utilized as standard of care in clinical, academic, and research settings. The authors in this volume are dedicated to the use of neuropsychology and offer rich information to this end. I am grateful for their contributions and devotion to the welfare of their patients.

Department of Psychiatry and Behavioral Sciences, University of Washington School of Medicine, Seattle, WA

Karen M. Sanders, PhD, ABPP

Acknowledgments

This book was a true collaboration. With gratitude, I list but a few:

First, to Janice Stern, senior editor of *Health and Behavior* and original Springer editor from 2014 to 2017, who was patient and supportive and professional. Thank you for believing in this project.

Katie Chabalko, senior editor of *Health and Behavior* and Springer editor from November 2017 to the completion of the book.

Christina Tuballes—assistant editor at Springer; Cathrine Selvaraj—project manager at Springer.

A warm thank-you to my faithful text editor, Carolyn MacGregor (texttunered-iting.com), who has been with me in this project since the first idea until the last and final track change. Heaven will reward your patient soul.

Karen Postal, PhD, ABPP—who set me on the way with author suggestions and contacts.

Margaret Lanca, PhD, for coordination of the integration ideas.

For numerous readers, reviewers, and medical residents:

Royce Morrison, MD
Kirsten Nestler, MD
Deborah Cowley, MD
Kate Grossman, MD
Robin Kang, MD
Suzanne Murray, MD
Bernice Marcopulos, PhD, ABBP
Robert Fallows, PhD, ABPP
Ernest Fung, PhD, ABPP
Marcie Hays, MD
Jamie Champion, PhD
Kira Armstrong, PhD, ABPP
Steven Rostad, MD-Radia
Daniel Susanto, MD-Radia

Brendan McCullough, MD, PhD-Radia
Charles Cobbs, MD
Sandra Vermeulen, MD
Kathleen Haaland, PhD, ABPP
Mark Vega, BA, Maria Vega, BA, and Matteo Vega—technical and emotional support, always with a smile.
Numerous supportive friends who kept me on my toes with a smile on their face.

Contents

Part I The Distinct Worlds of Neuropsychology and Medicine

1 **The Value of Neuropsychological Evaluation in Medical Practice** 3
Michelle M. Braun

2 **The Integration of Neuropsychology in Pediatric Care Teams** 17
Jennifer Queally and Tanya Diver

3 **A Model of Collaboration between Primary Care and Neuropsychology** 31
Margaret Lanca and Kirsten Meisinger

4 **Psychometrics of Assessment: Understanding What Neuropsychology Adds to the Physician's Understanding of the Patient** 45
Mike R. Schoenberg, Jason R. Soble, and Katie E. Osborn

Part II Case Examples

5 **Pediatric Case of Sickle Cell Disease** 63
Melissa Gerstle, Katherine Baum, Charles T. Quinn, and Dean W. Beebe

6 **Pediatric Traumatic Brain Injury: Collaboration through Case Example** 83
Paul C. Lebby and Jennifer V. Crocker

7 **Autism Spectrum Disorder with Seizures: Collaboration through Case Example** 115
Amy V. Davis, Emma Cole, and Gaurav Yadava

8 **Paediatric Neuro-Oncology: Medulloblastoma** 133
Laura Janzen and Ute Bartels

9 **Pediatric Stroke** ... 147
Robyn Westmacott, Jordana Waxman, and Nomazulu Dlamini

10 **Neuropsychological Assessment of Extremely Preterm Children** ... 169
Tricia Williams, Samantha Roberts, and Vann Chau

11 **Neuropsychology's Contributions to a Pediatric Epilepsy Surgery Team** ... 189
Molly Warner, Hillary Shurtleff, Catherine Amlie-Lefond, Russell Saneto, Edward Novotny, Jonathan Lopez, Sandra Poliachik, Andrew Poliakov, Dennis Shaw, and Jeffrey Ojemann

12 **Alzheimer's Disease and Overview of Dementia** ... 209
Emily H. Trittschuh and Lucy Wang

13 **Posterior Cortical Atrophy** ... 223
Ernest Y. S. Fung and Mark O. Herring

14 **Dementia with Lewy Bodies** ... 239
Jacqueline Phillips-Sabol and Dimitrios A. Nacopoulos

15 **Amyotrophic Lateral Sclerosis** ... 255
Jonathan S. Katz and Susan C. Woolley

16 **Vascular Cognitive Impairment** ... 267
Felicia C. Goldstein and Ihab Hajjar

17 **Right Middle Cerebral Artery Stroke in a Male of Prime Working Age** ... 277
Karen M. Sanders and William Likosky

18 **Deep Brain Stimulation for Parkinson's Disease** ... 291
Cynthia S. Kubu, Michal Gostkowski, Joseph Rudolph, and Sean Nagel

19 **Huntington's Disease Case Study** ... 305
Karen M. Sanders and Daniel J. Burdick

20 **Traumatic Brain Injury: Sports Concussion** ... 327
David B. Coppel and Stanley A. Herring

21 **Neurosurgery for Meningiomas** ... 363
Michael W. Parsons, Paramita Das, and Pablo Recinos

22 **Adult Epilepsy** ... 379
Erica M. Brandling-Bennett and David G. Vossler

23 **Multiple Sclerosis** ... 399
Kevin N. Alschuler and Annette Wundes

24 Schizophrenia Case Study: Residual Thought Disorder versus Emerging Dementia 409
Bernice A. Marcopulos and Robert Gardella

25 Neuroimaging and Neuropsychology 421
Erin D. Bigler

26 Traumatic Brain Injury Rehabilitation Case Study 435
Samantha L. Backhaus and Ana Durand-Sanchez

27 Neuropsychological Assessment of Adult Attention Deficit/Hyperactivity Disorder 457
Margaret Lanca, Flannery Geier, and Lenna Finger

Part III Related Issues in Collaboration: Specialties and Essential Considerations

28 Neuropsychology in the Twenty-First Century: The Rise of Multicultural Assessments 479
Margaret Lanca and Emily K. Wilner

29 Forensic Challenges in Medical Settings for Physicians and Neuropsychologists 495
Bernice A. Marcopulos, Michael Welner, and Kristen T. Campbell

30 Neuropsychological Interventions for Individuals with Brain Injury 507
Samantha L. Backhaus and Summer L. Ibarra

31 A Perspective on Vocational Rehabilitation for the Physician 531
Robert T. Fraser, Erica K. Johnson, and David Strand

32 Psychotherapy and Neuropsychotherapy 543
Michael B. Warren and Tedd Judd

33 Medication Effects on Cognition 561
Jeffrey A. Sordahl, Jessica Litke, Jennifer Lewis, and Megan Dunay

34 Effective Feedback Conversations 575
Karen Postal

Answers for Chapter Review Questions 587

Glossary of Neuropsychological and Medical Terms 591

Index 597

Contributors

Kevin N. Alschuler, PhD Department of Neurology, University of Washington School of Medicine, UW Medicine Multiple Sclerosis Center, Seattle, WA, USA

Department of Rehabilitation Medicine, University of Washington School of Medicine, UW Medicine Multiple Sclerosis Center, Seattle, WA, USA

Catherine Amlie-Lefond, MD Department of Neurology, Seattle Children's Hospital, Department of Neurology, University of Washington School of Medicine, Seattle, WA, USA

Samantha L. Backhaus, PhD Department of Physical Medicine and Rehabilitation, Rehabilitation Hospital of Indiana—Indiana University, Indianapolis, IN, USA

Ute Bartels, MD Division of Haematology/Oncology, The Hospital for Sick Children, Toronto, ON, Canada

Department of Pediatrics, University of Toronto, Toronto, ON, Canada

Katherine Baum, PhD Division of Behavioral Medicine and Clinical Psychology, Cincinnati Children's Hospital Medical Center, Department of Pediatrics, University of Cincinnati College of Medicine, Cincinnati, OH, USA

Dean W. Beebe, PhD, ABPP, ABPN Division of Behavioral Medicine and Clinical Psychology, Cincinnati Children's Hospital Medical Center, Department of Pediatrics, University of Cincinnati College of Medicine, Cincinnati, OH, USA

Erin D. Bigler, PhD, ABPP Department of Psychology, Brigham Young University, Provo, UT, USA

Neuroscience Center, Brigham Young University, Provo, UT, USA

Magnetic Resonance Imaging Research Facility, Brigham Young University, Provo, UT, USA

Department of Psychiatry, University of Utah, Salt Lake City, UT, USA

Erica M. Brandling-Bennett, PhD, ABPP UW Medicine—Valley Medical Center Neuroscience Institute, Renton, WA, USA

Michelle M. Braun, PhD, ABPP Department of Neurology and Neurosurgery, Ascension|Wheaton Franciscan Healthcare, Racine, WI, USA

Daniel J. Burdick, MD Evergreen Health Neurosciences Institute, Kirkland, WA, USA

Department of Neurology, University of Washington School of Medicine, Seattle, WA, USA

Booth Gardner Parkinson's Care Center, Evergreen Medical Center (EMC), Kirkland, WA, USA

Kristen T. Campbell, MA Department of Graduate Psychology, James Madison University, Harrisonburg, VA, USA

Vann Chau, MD, FRCPC Division of Neurology, Department of Pediatrics, SickKids Research Institute, The Hospital for Sick Children and University of Toronto, Toronto, ON, Canada

Neuroscience & Mental Health, SickKids Research Institute, The Hospital for Sick Children and University of Toronto, Toronto, ON, Canada

Emma Cole, PhD, NCSP Amita Health—Women and Children's Hospital, Center for Pediatric Brain, Hoffman Estates, IL, USA

Department of Neuropsychology, Kennedy Krieger Schools, Kennedy Krieger Institute, Baltimore, MD, USA

David B. Coppel, PhD Department of Neurological Surgery, UW Medicine Sports Concussion Program, University of Washington School of Medicine, Seattle, WA, USA

Jennifer V. Crocker, MD, ABPMR Valley Children's Hospital, Madera, CA, USA

Paramita Das, MD Cleveland Clinic, Cleveland Ohio, USA

Amy V. Davis, PhD, ABPP, ABPN Amita Health—Women and Children's Hospital, Center for Pediatric Brain, Hoffman Estates, IL, USA

Tanya Diver, PhD Boston Children's Hospital, Boston, MA, USA

Nomazulu Dlamini, MBBS, PhD Children's Stroke Program, Division of Neurology, Department of Pediatrics, The Hospital for Sick Children, Toronto, ON, Canada

Megan Dunay, MD, MPH Geriatrics and Palliative Care Division, Boise VA Medical Center, Medical Service, Boise, ID, USA

University of Washington Internal Medicine Residency, Seattle, WA, USA

Ana Durand-Sanchez, MD Department of Physical Medicine and Rehabilitation, Indiana University School of Medicine, Indianapolis, IN, USA

Lenna Finger, MD Harvard Medical School, Cambridge Health Alliance, Cambridge, MA, USA

Robert T. Fraser, PhD, CRC Neurological Vocational Services Unit, Harborview Medical Center, Rehabilitation Medicine, University of Washington School of Medicine, Seattle, WA, USA

Ernest Y. S. Fung, PsyD, ABPP Atlanta Neuropsychology, LLC, NP Neuropsychology, LLC, Atlanta, GA, USA

Robert Gardella, MD Department of Psychiatry and Neurobehavioral Sciences, University of Virginia Health Sciences Center, Charlottesville, VA, USA

Western State Hospital, Staunton, VA, USA

Flannery Geier, PsyD Harvard Medical Center/Cambridge Health Alliance, Cambridge, MA, USA

Melissa Gerstle, PhD, ABPP Division of Behavioral Medicine and Clinical Psychology, Cincinnati Children's Hospital Medical Center, Department of Pediatrics, University of Cincinnati College of Medicine, Cincinnati, Ohio, USA

Felicia C. Goldstein, PhD, ABPP Department of Neurology, Emory University School of Medicine, Atlanta, GA, USA

Barry Gordon, MD Department of Neurology, The Johns Hopkins Medical Institutions, Baltimore, MD, USA

Michal Gostkowski, DO Center for Neurological Restoration, Cleveland Clinic, Cleveland, OH, USA

Ihab Hajjar, MD, MS Department of Neurology, Emory University School of Medicine, Atlanta, GA, USA

Mark O. Herring, MD Oregon Neurology Associates, Springfield, OR, USA

Stanley A. Herring, MD Department of Rehabilitation Medicine, University of Washington School of Medicine, Seattle, WA, USA

Summer L. Ibarra, PhD Rehabilitation Hospital of Indiana, Indianapolis, IN, USA

Laura Janzen, PhD, ABPP, ABPN Division of Hematology/Oncology, Department of Psychology, The Hospital for Sick Children, Toronto, ON, Canada

Erica K. Johnson, PhD, CRC Health Promotion Research Center, University of Washington, Lynnwood, WA, USA

Independent Practice, Bellevue, WA, USA

Tedd Judd, PhD, ABPP Independent Practice, Bellingham, WA, USA

Jonathan S. Katz, MD Forbes Norris Center, California Pacific Medical Center, Sutter Pacific Medical Foundation, San Francisco, CA, USA

Cynthia S. Kubu, PhD, ABPP Center for Neurological Restoration, Cleveland Clinic, Cleveland, OH, USA

Margaret Lanca, PhD Harvard Medical School, Cambridge Health Alliance, Cambridge, MA, USA

Paul C. Lebby, PhD, ABPS, FNAN Valley Children's Hospital, Madera, CA, USA

Jennifer Lewis, MD Family Medicine Residency of Idaho, Geriatric Medicine, Boise, ID, USA

William Likosky, MD Department of Neurology, University of California at San Francisco/Fresno, Fresno, CA, USA

Jessica Litke, PharmD, BCPS Boise VA Medical Center—V-IMPACT TeleHub, Boise, ID, USA

Jonathan Lopez, MD Department of Neurology, Seattle Children's Hospital, Seattle, WA, USA

Department of Neurology, University of Washington, Seattle, WA, USA

Bernice A. Marcopulos, PhD, ABPP Department of Graduate Psychology, James Madison University, Harrisonburg, VA, USA

Department of Psychiatry and Neurobehavioral Sciences, University of Virginia Health Sciences Center, Charlottesville, VA, USA

Kirsten Meisinger, MD Department of Public Health, Harvard University/Cambridge Health Alliance, Cambridge, MA, USA

Dimitrios A. Nacopoulos, MD Department of Neurology, UPMC School of Medicine, Pittsburgh, PA, USA

Sean Nagel, MD Center for Neurological Restoration, Neurologic Institute, Cleveland Clinic, Cleveland, OH, USA

Edward Novotny, MD Department of Neurology, Seattle Children's Hospital, Seattle, WA, USA

Department of Neurology, University of Washington, Seattle, WA, USA

Jeffrey Ojemann, MD Department of Neurological Surgery, Seattle Children's Hospital, Seattle, WA, USA

Department of Neurological Surgery, University of Washington, Seattle, WA, USA

Katie E. Osborn, PsyD Vanderbilt University Medical Center, Nashville, TN, USA

Michael W. Parsons, PhD, ABPP Massachusetts General Hospital, Boston, Massachusetts, USA

Jacqueline Phillips-Sabol, PhD, ABPP Neuropsychology Speciality and Consultants, Erie, PA, USA

Sandra Poliachik, PhD Department of Neurology, Seattle Children's Hospital, Seattle, WA, USA

Center for Clinical and Translational Research, Seattle Children's Research Institute, Seattle, WA, USA

Applied Physics Laboratory, University of Washington, Seattle, WA, USA

Andrew Poliakov, PhD Department of Radiology, Seattle Children's Hospital, Seattle, WA, USA

Karen Postal, PhD, ABPP Harvard Medical School, Cambridge, MA, USA

Independent Practice, Andover, MA, USA

Jennifer Queally, PhD, ABPP Boston Children's Hospital, Boston, MA, USA

Charles T. Quinn, MD, MS Division of Hematology, Cincinnati Children's Hospital Medical Center, Department of Pediatrics, University of Cincinnati College of Medicine, Cincinnati, OH, USA

Pablo Recinos, MD Cleveland Clinic, Cleveland, Ohio, USA

Samantha D. Roberts, BA Division of Neurology, Department of Psychology, The Hospital for Sick Children, Toronto, ON, Canada

Joseph Rudolph, MD Center for Neurological Restoration, Neurologic Institute, Cleveland Clinic, Cleveland, OH, USA

Karen M. Sanders, PhD, ABPP Department of Psychiatry and Behavioral Sciences, University of Washington School of Medicine, Seattle, WA, USA

Russell Saneto, DO, PhD Department of Neurology, Seattle Children's Hospital, Seattle, WA, USA

Department of Neurology, University of Washington, Seattle, WA, USA

Mike R. Schoenberg, PhD, ABPP, ABPN Department of Neurosurgery and Brain Repair, University of South Florida Morsani College of Medicine, Tampa, FL, USA

Dennis Shaw, MD Department of Radiology, Seattle Children's Hospital, Seattle, WA, USA

Department of Radiology, University of Washington, Seattle, WA, USA

Hillary Shurtleff, PhD, ABPP, ABPN Department of Psychiatry, Seattle Children's Hospital, Seattle, WA, USA

Department of Neurology, University of Washington, Seattle, WA, USA

Glenn Smith, PhD, ABPP Department of Clinical and Health Psychology, University of Florida, Gainesville, FL, USA

Mayo Clinic College of Medicine, Rochester, MN, USA

Jason R. Soble, PhD, ABPP Department of Psychiatry, Department of Neurology, University of Illinois College of Medicine, Chicago, IL, USA

Jeffrey A. Sordahl, PsyD, ABPP Boise VA Medical Center—V-IMPACT TeleHub, Boise, ID, USA

David Strand, PhD, CRC Neurological Vocational Services Unit, Department of Rehabilitation Medicine, Harborview Medical Center, University of Washington, Seattle, WA, USA

Emily H. Trittschuh, PhD Department of Psychiatry and Behavioral Sciences, University of Washington School of Medicine, VA Puget Sound Health Care System, Geriatric Research Education and Clinical Center, Seattle, Washington, USA

Doug Tynan, PhD, ABPP Center for Psychology and Health, APA, Washington, DC, USA

David G. Vossler, MD, FAAN, FACNS, FAES UW Medicine—Valley Medical Center Neuroscience Institute, Renton, WA, USA

Lucy Wang, MD Department of Psychiatry and Behavioral Sciences, University of Washington School of Medicine, VA Puget Sound Health Care System, Geriatric Research Education and Clinical Center, Seattle, Washington, USA

Molly Warner, PhD, ABPP, ABPN Department of Psychiatry, Seattle Children's Hospital, Seattle, WA, USA

Department of Neurology, University of Washington, Seattle, WA, USA

Michael B. Warren, PhD Independent Practice, Bellingham, WA, USA

Jordana Waxman, MA Psychology Department, York University, Toronto, ON, Canada

Michael Welner, MD The Forensic Panel, New York, NY, USA

Icahn School of Medicine at Mt. Sinai, New York, NY, USA

Robyn Westmacott, PhD, CPsych, ABPP Children's Stroke Program, Division of Neurology, Department of Paediatrics, The Hospital for Sick Children, University of Toronto, Toronto, ON, Canada

Department of Psychology, The Hospital for Sick Children, Toronto, ON, Canada

Tricia S. Williams, PhD, CPsych, ABPP Division of Neurology, Department of Psychology, The Hospital for Sick Children, Toronto, ON, Canada

Emily K. Wilner, PsyD Harvard Medical School Cambridge Health Alliance, Cambridge, MA, USA

Susan C. Woolley, PhD, ABPP Sutter Pacific Medical Foundation, Forbes Norris ALS Center, San Francisco, CA, USA

Annette Wundes, MD Department of Neurology, University of Washington School of Medicine, UW Medicine Multiple Sclerosis Center, Seattle, WA, USA

Department of Rehabilitation Medicine, University of Washington School of Medicine, UW Medicine Multiple Sclerosis Center, Seattle, WA, USA

Gaurav Yadava, MD Amita Health—Women and Children's Hospital, Center for Pediatric Brain, Hoffman Estates, IL, USA

Yadava Pediatric Neurology, Elmhurst, IL, USA

University of Chicago, Chicago, IL, USA

Part I
The Distinct Worlds of Neuropsychology and Medicine

Chapter 1
The Value of Neuropsychological Evaluation in Medical Practice

Michelle M. Braun

Physicians and other healthcare providers are often expected to provide guidance and treatment to patients who are concerned about memory, attention, language, and other aspects of cognitive functioning. Cognitive concerns may present as subjective complaints from the patient and/or family; through difficulty managing the cognitive demands of a previous level of functioning at work or school; as a change evident to a healthcare provider that has followed a patient over time; in the context of known neurological compromise (e.g., stroke, traumatic brain injury, Parkinson's disease, epilepsy, etc.), known medical compromise (e.g., liver failure, human immunodeficiency virus, cardiovascular issues, sleep apnea, etc.), or known psychiatric compromise (e.g., bipolar disorder, schizophrenia, posttraumatic stress disorder, etc.); and in the context of a number of other situations that may impact cognition (e.g., changes in medication, increased stress, alcohol or drug use, post-surgical compromise, toxic exposures, etc.). Because cognitive dysfunction may be symptomatic of multiple coexisting issues, cognitive assessment is a complex process that often requires the use of multiple diagnostic tools.

Common tools in the assessment of cognitive functioning include the neurological exam, structural neuroimaging (computed tomography/CT, magnetic resonance imaging/MRI), neurodiagnostic tests (electroencephalogram/EEG), laboratory measures, and neuropsychological evaluation. Each diagnostic tool has unique ability to inform diagnosis and to direct treatment (see Table 1.1). For example, the neurological examination helps determine whether abnormalities in sensory and motoric functioning contribute to cognitive symptoms. Common neuroimaging

M. M. Braun (✉)
Department of Neurology and Neurosurgery, Ascension|Wheaton Franciscan Healthcare, Racine, WI, USA
e-mail: Michelle.Braun@ascension.org

K. M. Sanders (ed.), *Physician's Field Guide to Neuropsychology*,
https://doi.org/10.1007/978-1-4939-8722-1_1

Key Point
Although non-neuropsychological measures provide important information about factors that may contribute to cognitive problems, neuropsychological evaluation provides a direct measure of cognitive functioning. Neuropsychological evaluation is a diagnostic procedure that synthesizes standardized comprehensive measures of cognitive functioning, variables that may impact the accuracy of test data (e.g., engagement in the testing process, emotional status), neurobehavioral information, and medical history.

techniques such as MRI and CT provide a measure of brain structure and help to identify whether obvious structural compromise such as stroke, tumor, or atrophy contributes to cognitive changes. However, given the significant structural variability in the normal brain [1], determination of subtle pathological changes with neuroimaging can also be challenging. Furthermore, cognitive functioning may be normal in spite of structural changes or abnormal in spite of normal brain structure. Neurodiagnostic tests such as EEG help to determine whether cortical electrical abnormalities due to seizures, metabolic disturbances, or other causes are contributing to cognitive symptoms. Similarly, laboratory measures help determine whether abnormalities in vitamin levels, metabolic functioning, hematologic functioning, or endocrinologic variables may impact cognitive functioning. Tests of cerebrospinal fluid and urine may also provide information about conditions that may impact cognitive functioning.

Cognitive screening tools are discussed in greater detail in Chap. 4. Computerized testing is another method that has been used to gather cognitive data in some settings, though several considerations should be addressed before using such programs in clinical settings, as discussed in Chaps. 2 and 3.

Key Point
Compared to neuropsychological testing, cognitive screening tools are limited in diagnosing neurocognitive syndromes because:

(a) They often do not sufficiently take into account variables that impact test interpretation, including the patient's level of education, ethnicity, level of engagement in the evaluation, and sensory abilities.
(b) Even if data are accurately interpreted, cognitive screening tools, given their brief nature, often do not provide adequate sensitivity or specificity and thus are limited in determining neurocognitive diagnosis.

When conceptualized in aggregate, data from multiple valid diagnostic tools provide a comprehensive understanding of the etiology and prognosis associated with cognitive symptoms [2].

Table 1.1 Comparisons of neurocognitive measures

	NP testing	CT/MRI	Neuro exam	Computer and COG screens
Dx endpoint	Yes	Yes	Yes	Limited
False +/–	Less likely	Less likely	Less likely	Likely
Dx utility	High	High	High	Limited
Detects subtle neurocog function	Yes	No	Limited	Limited
Normed/standardized	Yes	Some	NA	Limited
Directs treatment	Yes	Yes	Yes	Limited

NP neuropsychological testing, *neuro exam* neurological examination, *COG* cognitive, *CT* computed tomography, *MRI* magnetic resonance imaging, *Dx* diagnosis, *false +/–* false positive and negative, *neurocog* neurocognitive (table developed by Karen Sanders, PhD, ABPP)

Indications for Neuropsychological Evaluation

A neuropsychological evaluation can be helpful in determining the etiology and treatment for a wide variety of cognitive symptoms. Although memory complaints are a common referral issue, patients may also complain of problems with word finding, attention, information processing, problem solving, or other cognitive difficulties (see Table 1.2). Neuropsychological evaluations are also helpful in documenting baseline cognitive functioning and/or detecting subtle cognitive changes in patients with chronic medical or neurological disorders that have a likelihood of compromising future cognitive or behavioral functioning (e.g., Parkinson's disease, multiple sclerosis, diabetes). In such cases, baseline neuropsychological evaluations are valuable for early detection of cognitive changes, tracking of cognitive functioning (via comparison of baseline and serial test data), evaluating potential cognitive effects of treatments (e.g., medication, chemotherapy), evaluating and making treatment recommendations for emotional adjustment to cognitive symptoms in the context of chronic disease, connecting patients with supportive resources, and providing strategies to maximize daily cognitive functioning.

As detailed elsewhere [3, 4], neuropsychological evaluations are often a standard part of care for treatment selection and treatment outcome evaluations (e.g., deep brain stimulation, epilepsy surgery) and are the tool of choice when objective documentation of subjective cognitive complaints is indicated. In children, adolescents, and adults, an inability to develop expected knowledge, skills, or abilities required to adapt to new or changing cognitive, social, emotional, or physical demands may trigger a neuropsychological evaluation.

Table 1.2 Common clinical symptoms prompting neuropsychological evaluation

Changes in memory
Frequently loses items
Gets lost easily
Forgetting conversations
Poor attention and concentration
Does not appear to listen
Gets confused in conversations
Changes in language functioning
Aphasia
Word-finding problems
Changes in visuospatial abilities
Difficulty drawing
Difficulty navigating (using a map or understanding directions)
Misperceiving the environment
Impaired executive functioning
Perseverative
Poor judgment
Rigidity in thought
Changes in emotional functioning
Increased anxiety
Increased depression
Psychosis
Fluctuations in mental status
Confusion
Disorientation

Adapted from Kulas and Naugle [3]

Anatomy of a Neuropsychological Evaluation

Key Point
As detailed in other sources [5, 6], the neuropsychological evaluation consists of the following components:

1. Record review
2. Neurobehavioral status examination
3. Test selection
4. Test administration
5. Integration of findings
6. Feedback session

1. *Record review*

   The neuropsychologist reviews the medical records and referral question and determines whether a neuropsychological evaluation is appropriate.
2. *Neurobehavioral status examination*

   The evaluation begins with a neurobehavioral status examination conducted by the neuropsychologist. The neurobehavioral status examination includes a detailed analysis of the onset, course, and nature of cognitive symptoms. Aspects of history that will be integrated into the case conceptualization are gathered, including medical, academic, occupational, social, substance use, and psychiatric history. The interview of an informant, such as a relative or someone well known to the patient, is often a key part of the neurobehavioral status examination, given that the nature of some cognitive issues (e.g., memory problems) may lead the patient to misperceive the occurrence of cognitive difficulties and/or may impair the patient's ability to provide accurate historical information. The patient and family members may express different aims for the evaluation that can be incorporated into the assessment and recommendations (e.g., connection to community resources, management of problem behaviors, questions about independent living ability, etc.). Clinical behavioral observations are gathered, including analysis of the patient's functional memory (e.g., ability to recall autobiographical history and current information, repetitiveness, etc.), speech production, language comprehension, communication style, emotional functioning, social interaction, and motoric functioning.
3. *Test selection*

   Information from medical records, the neurobehavioral interview, and behavioral observations is integrated to guide the selection of specific neuropsychological tests. The selection of tests is a strategic process that varies due to patient characteristics (level of education, premorbid level of functioning, sensory abilities, physical limitations, fatigue level, age, ethnicity) and the goals of the evaluation (establishing a diagnosis, measuring treatment effects, etc.).
4. *Test administration*

   Tests are either administered directly by the neuropsychologist or by a trained technician supervised by the neuropsychologist. Test administration is a fluid process, such that different tests may be utilized or omitted as the data from tests completed earlier in the evaluation help to clarify the patient's abilities and difficulties. For example, impairments on measures of naming may lead to a more in-depth assessment of other language-related abilities such as spelling or arithmetic, or a shorter memory measure may be substituted for a longer measure based on patient fatigue. Neuropsychological tests are often presented in question-and-answer format and often involve object manipulation and responses to pictures or patterns. Paper-and-pencil or multiple-choice measures may also be utilized.

   Core cognitive and behavioral domains are listed in Table 1.3. A small sampling of commonly utilized measures in each domain is included, given that an exhaustive list of tests in each domain would be lengthy. *Because most neuropsychological tests simultaneously measure the functions of multiple cognitive*

Table 1.3 Common neuropsychological measures of core cognitive and behavioral domains

• **General intellectual ability**
– Wechsler Adult Intelligence Scale—IV
– Wechsler Test of Adult Reading
• **Reasoning, sequencing, problem-solving, and executive function**
– Delis-Kaplan Executive Function System
– Wisconsin Card Sort
– Tower of London
• **Attention and concentration**
– Continuous Performance Test
– Digit Span
• **Learning and memory**
– Wechsler Memory Scales—IV
– California Verbal Learning Test
• **Language and communication**
– Boston Naming Test
– Multilingual Aphasia Examination
• **Visual-motor praxis**
– Trails A
– Coding
• **Motor and sensory function**
– Finger Tapping
– Grooved Pegboard
– Reitan-Klove Sensory-Perceptual Examination
• **Mood, conduct, personality, quality of life, psychopathology**
– Beck Depression Inventory—II
– Minnesota Multiphasic Personality Inventory
– Personality Assessment Inventory
• **Adaptive behavior (activities of daily living)**
– Independent Living Scales
– Clinical Dementia Rating Scale
– Adaptive Behavior Assessment—II
• **Motivation and effort (e.g., performance validity testing)**
– Various measures that are self-standing and embedded

and behavioral domains, meaningful integration of results requires intra- and inter-domain analysis. It is the disease-specific, multivariable integration of test data across cognitive domains, in the context of clinical information and data from other diagnostic measures, that is the heart of specialty training and practice in neuropsychology.

5. *Integration of findings*

   The neuropsychological evaluation includes an integration of findings from the neurobehavioral interview, record review, and neuropsychological testing and provides a variety of deliverables that are designed to guide clinical management, as noted below. This information is sent to the referring physician or other healthcare provider and is often given to the patient and/or patient's caregivers.

Key Point

Typical Deliverables from the Neuropsychological Evaluation

1. Objective, norm-referenced test results for each cognitive domain (see Chap. 2 for more information on norm-referenced measures)
2. Diagnostic and etiological impressions
3. Recommendations for neurodiagnostic studies or other workup to assist in clarifying etiology, if needed
4. Recommendations for repeat neuropsychological testing, if needed
5. Connections to support organizations to enhance clinical outcome and quality of life (e.g., Alzheimer's Association, Aging and Disability Resource Center)
6. Recommendations to address any psychiatric issues that may have been detected
7. Customized cognitive strategies to enhance future cognitive functioning (e.g., use of specific memory strategies based on cognitive profile)
8. Behavioral strategies to enhance future cognitive functioning under the direction of a healthcare provider (e.g., enhancements in sleep, exercise, diet)
9. Strategies to manage difficult behaviors, if needed
10. Information on functional abilities and optimal living environment, if needed
11. Determination of the capacity to make healthcare decisions, if needed

6. *Feedback session*

   A post-evaluation feedback session with the patient and family members is a customary part of the neuropsychological evaluation [7]. The feedback session includes the following components, as detailed by Dr. Karen Postal in Section III of this book:

   (a) Discussion of the relationship between neuropsychological test results, diagnosis, and prognosis.
   (b) Explanation of treatment recommendations. In addition to those recommendations that are directly managed by the physician (e.g., changes in medication), patients are often provided with tailored behavioral strategies to maximize daily cognitive functioning, recommendations for nonpharmacological interventions, and connections to community resources to enhance quality of life and daily functioning.
   (c) Communication of results to family members is often provided and can help enhance compliance with treatment and behavioral recommendations. Feedback with family members may also have a significant impact on clinical treatment. For example, individuals with dementia may be able to live in their home for an average of 18 months longer when caregivers are provided with education and connected to caregiver resources [8].

The Value of Neuropsychological Testing

In a survey of physicians who utilize neuropsychological services, physicians indicated that they most often referred patients for diagnostic purposes and that information from neuropsychological evaluations was incorporated into their discharge summaries a majority of the time [9]. It is also noted that neuropsychology feedback is highly valued by patients [10] and significantly improves clinical outcomes and treatment satisfaction in individuals with traumatic brain injury [11]. In addition, as reviewed elsewhere [4], neuropsychological assessments predict functional abilities across a variety of neurocognitive disorders. With changes in healthcare reform, there has been an increased interest in demonstrating the cost-effectiveness of neuropsychological evaluations. A recent study of veterans showed decreased incidence and length of hospitalization in the year following a neuropsychological evaluation, as compared to the year prior, and decreased utilization of emergency room visits [12]. Additional research into the cost-effectiveness of neuropsychological evaluations is ongoing through grants from the American Academy of Clinical Neuropsychology Foundation and other sources.

Describing Neuropsychological Testing to Patients

Patients often ask referring physicians to describe what the neuropsychological evaluation process is and why it is necessary, especially given that some patients are unfamiliar with the term "neuropsychology" and assume it means they are being asked to complete a "psychological" evaluation. If a cognitive screening measure has been performed, it can be helpful to inform the patient that a neuropsychological evaluation is similar to an in-depth version of a cognitive screen that provides greater precision in measuring and diagnosing potential cognitive problems. Some patients benefit from learning that a neuropsychological evaluation is a "detailed test of memory and other thinking skills" that will help inform their treatment. Patients may also benefit from understanding that neuroimaging such as a head CT or Brain MRI "measures brain structure but not brain function" and that neuropsychological assessment directly measures brain function (i.e., the "software" of the brain). Patients who are nervous about the process may benefit from knowing that most previous patients report during the feedback session that they found the process to be engaging, beneficial, and worth the investment of time (typical evaluation time ranges from 2 to 4 hours, though can be longer for younger or more complicated patients). Patients also appear to value receiving brief written information about the evaluation process. To this end, the American Psychological Association Division of Neuropsychology (Division 40) has developed a brochure that provides information about the neuropsychology evaluation and is freely available [13]. Sharing these brochures with patients prior to the assessment can help provide additional information about the process of neuropsychological evaluation.

Neuropsychology Training

Patients and physician colleagues often inquire about the training of the neuropsychologist. A neuropsychologist typically holds a master's degree and doctoral degree (PhD or PsyD) in clinical psychology or neuropsychology from a graduate program or professional school that is accredited by the American Psychological Association (APA) or the Canadian Psychological Association (CPA). Completion of a master's thesis and doctoral dissertation are typically required. On average, neuropsychology training involves 8 years of post-baccalaureate course work and clinical supervision. Graduate school typically lasts 4–5 years and includes extensive didactics and clinical training in neuropsychology and clinical psychology, supplemented with training in neuroscience, functional neuroanatomy, behavioral neurology, research methods, statistics, psychotherapy, ethics, and tailored areas of specialization. A 1-year neuropsychology internship is completed after graduate school and is often followed by a 2-year neuropsychology fellowship. Components of graduate training, internship training, and the postdoctoral fellowship ideally follow the Houston Conference guidelines, which were developed to provide quality and consistency in neuropsychology training [14]. Professional organizations in neuropsychology are involved in ongoing effort to develop entry level practice competencies in neuropsychology.

Similar to physician practice, board certification is increasingly required by hospitals and other clinical care organizations to verify that a neuropsychologist has met practice competencies and achieved professional credentialing. The American Board of Professional Psychology (ABPP) is the primary organization for specialty board certification in psychology, and it facilitates specialty boarding in neuropsychology and subspecialty boarding in pediatric neuropsychology through the American Board of Clinical Neuropsychology (ABCN). Board certification through ABCN is a four-step process. The first step involves a credential review to ensure adequate specialty training in neuropsychology at the graduate and postgraduate levels. The second step involves successful completion of a written examination on neuropsychology, basic and clinical neuroscience, psychometrics, behavioral neurology, and clinical psychology. The third step requires peer-reviewed acceptance of two work/case samples. The fourth step involves successful completion of a three-part oral examination that requires the examinee to provide a diagnosis and recommendations for a clinical case through a "fact-finding" exercise, defend the previously submitted work samples, and pass an ethics examination. Other organizations offering neuropsychology board certification include the American Board of Professional Neuropsychology (ABN) and the American Board of Pediatric Neuropsychology (ABPdN).

Neuropsychological Evaluation Myths

There are several clinical myths associated with the process of neurocognitive diagnosis and neuropsychological evaluation that are helpful to clarify:

Myth #1: *Patients and their family members are accurate in reporting cognitive symptoms.*

Clarification #1: The report of patients and family members is subjective and often does not coincide with objective data. For example, patients and family members may lack insight into the existence of cognitive impairment, falsely attributing it to "normal aging," stress, medication effects, or other variables. This may lead to late diagnosis, missed treatment opportunities, and delayed ability to plan for future needs. Alternatively, patients may unknowingly pathologize normal age-related changes and become convinced they have a neurocognitive syndrome even though test data are normal, resulting in unnecessary treatment in the absence of neuropsychological data. In other situations, a patient may be motivated by external incentives to falsely report cognitive symptoms. Without the use of neuropsychological testing with embedded measures of validity ("performance validity testing"/PVT, as detailed in Chap. 2), unnecessary diagnosis and utilization of services may occur.

Myth #2: *Cognitive screening tools are sufficient to diagnose neurocognitive syndromes.*

Clarification #2: Interpretation of scores on cognitive screening tools may not sufficiently take into account variables that impact interpretation, including the patient's age, level of education, ethnicity, and sensory abilities. Even if data are accurately interpreted, cognitive screening tools, given their brief nature, often do not provide adequate sensitivity or specificity and thus are limited in informing neurocognitive diagnosis. Cognitive screening tools are discussed in greater detail in Chap. 2.

Myth #3: *Neurocognitive syndromes can be adequately diagnosed with neuroimaging.*

Clarification #3: Most neuroimaging does not measure cognitive functioning, which is necessary for the diagnosis of many neurocognitive syndromes. In addition, some neurocognitive conditions may have no associated structural findings (e.g., attention deficit disorder, learning disability, concussion, mild cognitive impairment). In addition, structural findings are often not helpful in neurocognitive differential diagnosis (e.g., determination of Lewy body dementia vs. Parkinson's dementia), cognitive symptoms may precede structural abnormalities [15], and cognitive functioning may be normal in the context of abnormal structural findings.

Myth #4: *Neuropsychological evaluation involves a straightforward interpretation of test data.*

Clarification #4: Interpretation of neuropsychological evaluation data requires extensive knowledge of the psychometric properties of each measure and expert analysis of test data based on years of clinical training and experience with multiple neurological, medical, and psychiatric populations. Similar to how physicians may interpret lab data differently based upon clinical presentation and other existing data, neuropsychologists interpret neuropsychological test data differentially based on clinical presentation and various premorbid and testing-related variables.

For example, a memory score at the 10th percentile may reflect a pathological change in some individuals and not in others. Interpretation is also dependent on the integration of performance validity tests (PVTs), which validate the accuracy of test data and are covered in greater detail in Chap. 2.

Myth #5: Neuropsychological assessment is a soft science that is not as valid as medical methods.

Clarification #5: Neuropsychological assessment is highly reliable and valid [16, 17]. Validity measures are equal to or stronger than medical tests, including neuroimaging [17].

Summary

Patients frequently request assistance from physicians in understanding and treating cognitive symptoms. Given that subjective reports of cognitive symptoms from patient and family members may under- or over-estimate actual cognitive ability, and given that cognitive screening devices provide limited diagnostic assistance and are often not sensitive to subtle cognitive deficits, a comprehensive neuropsychological assessment is often needed. Common neuroimaging techniques measure brain structure but do not measure cognitive functioning, and an objective assessment of cognitive functioning is often required to arrive at a neurocognitive diagnosis.

The neuropsychological evaluation is a highly valid, reliable, comprehensive assessment process that provides referral sources with diagnostic impressions, prognostic information, and tailored treatment recommendations for patients with cognitive symptoms and helps to tease apart multiple interacting variables that can impact cognitive functioning (e.g., underlying neurocognitive or medical disorders, medication effects, mood and stress issues, insufficient sleep, etc.). The interpretation of neuropsychological test results is not a straightforward process and is tailored to unique patient variables including age, education level, gender, ethnicity, medical status, sensory abilities, and emotional functioning. Neuropsychological evaluations also assess whether the obtained data are valid, based on measures of patient engagement in the evaluation. The neuropsychological evaluation is a valuable component of a multifaceted examination of cognitive symptoms and directly impacts medical management.

Specialty training in neuropsychology involves obtaining a master's and doctoral degree in psychology and requires an average of 8 years of education following receipt of the undergraduate degree, including completion of a neuropsychology internship and 2-year neuropsychological postdoctoral fellowship. Board certification is an increasing requirement for practice in hospitals and other clinical organizations and signifies competency in the discipline. Research suggests that physicians value neuropsychological evaluations and incorporate neuropsychological findings into discharge summaries a majority of the time. The cost-effectiveness of neuropsychological evaluations has been demonstrated through data showing reduced frequency and length of rehospitalizations following neuropsychological evaluation. There is ongoing research to investigate other aspects of cost-effectiveness and value.

Chapter Review Questions

1. A 78-year-old female with a master's degree reports increasing memory problems. Laboratory workup was normal, a brain MRI showed mild small vessel ischemia, and her score on the Mini-Mental State Examination (MMSE) was 28/30. Which would be the best course of action to take in response to her complaints?
   A. Reassure her that her cognitive complaints are likely due to normal aging, given her normal MMSE and laboratory workup.
   B. Inform her that although there are no serious concerns with her MMSE performance, a neuropsychological evaluation would provide a more sensitive measure to assess her cognitive functioning and potentially detect any subtle changes.
   C. Recommend a repeat brain MRI in 1 year to reassess her cognitive functioning.
   D. Inform her that individuals with higher educational levels are often sensitive to normal age-related cognitive changes and report memory problems that do not bear out on testing, so no further testing is needed, and she should follow up in 1 year.
2. A neuropsychological evaluation involves the following components:
   A. Test administration, interpretation, and report writing.
   B. Neurobehavioral interview, testing, and report writing.
   C. Neurobehavioral interview, record review, testing, interpretation, report writing, and feedback.
   D. Neurobehavioral interview, testing, interpretation, report writing, and feedback.
3. Which is typically not assessed in the neuropsychological assessment?
   A. Memory, attention, and executive functioning.
   B. Mood.
   C. Motivation and effort (e.g., performance validity testing).
   D. Cranial nerve function.

References

1. Damasia H. Human brain anatomy in computerized images. 2nd ed. Oxford: Oxford University Press; 2005.
2. Tanner JJ, Mellott E, Dunne EM, Price CC. Integrating neuropsychology and brain imaging for a referral of possible pseudodementia: a case report. Clin Neuropsychol. 2015;29:272–92.
3. Pritchard AE, Koriakin T, Jacobson LA, Mahone EM. Incremental validity of neuropsychological assessment in the identification and treatment of youth with ADHD. Clin Neuropsychol. 2014;28:26–48.
4. Braun MM, et al. Neuropsychology model LCD. https://www.theaacn.org/userdocuments/neuropsychology_model_lcd-1.pdf. Accessed 9 July 2015.
5. Braun MM, et al. Neuropsychological assessment: a valuable tool in the diagnosis and management of neurological, neurodevelopmental, medical, and psychiatric disorders. Cogn Behav Neurol. 2011;24(3):107–14.
6. Kulas JF, Naugle RI. Indications for neuropsychological assessment. Cleve Clin J Med. 2003;70(9):785–92.
7. American Psychological Association. Ethical principles of psychologists and code of conduct. http://www.apa.org/ethics/code/index.aspx. Accessed 9 July 2011.
8. Mittelman MS, Haley WE, Clay OJ, Roth DL. Improving caregiver well-being delays nursing home placement of patients with Alzheimer disease. Neurology. 2006;67:1592–9.
9. Temple RO, Carvalho J, Tremont G. A national survey of physicians' use of and satisfaction with neuropsychological services. Arch Clin Neuropsychol. 2006;21(5):371–82.
10. Westervelt HJ, Brown LB, Tremont G, Javorsky DJ, Stern RA. Patient and family perceptions of the neuropsychological evaluation: how are we doing? Clin Neuropsychol. 2007;21:263–73.
11. Pegg PO, Auerbach SM, Seel RT, Buenaver LF, Kiesler DJ, Plybon LE. The impact of patient-centered information on patients' treatment and outcomes in traumatic brain injury rehabilitation. Rehabil Psychol. 2005;50(4):366–74.
12. VanKirk KK, Horner MD, Turner TH, Dismuke CE, Muzzy W. Hospital service utilization is reduced following NP evaluation in a sample of US veterans. Clin Neuropsychol. 2013;27:750–61.
13. Clinical Neuropsychology: A Guide for Patients and Their Families. American Psychological Association, Division of Clinical Neuropsychology. 2001. http://www.div40.org/pdf/NeuropscyhBroch2.pdf. Accessed 10 July 2015.
14. Hannay JH, Bieliauskas LA, Crosson BA, Hammeke TA, Hammsher K d S, Koffler SP. Proceedings of the Houston conference on specialty education and training in clinical neuropsychology. Arch Clin Neuropsychol. 1998;13:157–250.
15. Lezak MD, Howieson DB, Loring DW. Neuropsychological assessment. 4th ed. New York, NY: Oxford University Press; 2004.
16. Matarazzo J. Psychological assessment versus psychological testing: validation from Binet to the school, clinic, and courtroom. Am Psychol. 1990;45:999–1017.
17. Meyer G, Finn S, Eyde L, Kay G, Moreland K, Dies R, et al. Psychological testing and psychological assessment: a review of evidence and issues. Am Psychol. 2001;56:128–65.

Chapter 2
The Integration of Neuropsychology in Pediatric Care Teams

Jennifer Queally and Tanya Diver

The Integration of Neuropsychology in Pediatric Care Teams

In the pediatric medical setting, many complex medical disorders are managed by teams of clinicians, including a coordinated team of physicians and specialists, as well as surgeons and therapists. These core teams follow patients and identify risk factors that may require referrals outside of the team and help to prioritize necessary treatments/interventions. Their goal is to establish individualized and comprehensive treatment plans that are responsive to changes in disease presentation and level of severity. These teams will often follow patients from birth through early adulthood, depending upon the disease/condition and availability of local adult providers.

In this context, teams often refer out for specialty care; at times, this can include consultations with psychologists, psychiatrists, or neuropsychologists. These consultations can be sufficient, particularly for patients with medical conditions that are not typically associated with substantial changes in cognitive development (e.g., asthma, cystic fibrosis, diabetes). However, for patient populations with known changes in brain development (e.g., hydrocephalus, cerebral palsy) or when the diagnosis is predicated on changes in brain development or trauma (e.g., brain tumor, head injury, stroke), a shift from a consultative model to the inclusion of a neuropsychologist on the medical treatment team becomes essential. Although the neuropsychologist continues to play a consultative role to families, their interaction with the medical team can have a direct influence on patient care and treatment planning.

J. Queally (✉) · T. Diver
Boston Children's Hospital, Boston, MA, USA
e-mail: Jennifer.Queally@childrens.harvard.edu; Tanya.Diver@childrens.harvard.edu

K. M. Sanders (ed.), *Physician's Field Guide to Neuropsychology*,
https://doi.org/10.1007/978-1-4939-8722-1_2

How Pediatric Medical Conditions Affect the Young Brain

Whole Child Model

The difference between pediatric and adult patients is not just the physical size of the patient. Children are inherently different patients as they are in the midst of ongoing brain development. For adults, we often assume that brain development has followed a normal trajectory and that a recent injury or disease has affected a typically developed brain. The goal of the evaluation is to determine how that illness or injury has altered their cognitive status and the magnitude of discrepancy between normal expectations and their current functioning. However, for children, this process is different because, by nature, the interruption alters not only their current cognitive status but their future brain development.

- *Timing/developmental status*: The timing of the insult for children has greater ramifications, as the effects on the developing brain vary based upon the child's age at the time of the injury or disease onset. For example, some children have underlying structural changes in brain development that may be secondary to a genetic disorder or changes in neuronal migration; these neurodevelopmental disorders change the child's whole developmental trajectory. From the time that these children are born, their access to information and learning style has been changed. Although babies who are born prematurely or experience trauma during birth also begin their lives on a different developmental trajectory, their course will be different due to the underlying etiology of the changes in brain development. Other children have a typical developmental course that is altered by the injury or disease onset at a later age, shifting the developmental trajectory after a period of typical development. Skills that have already begun to develop can be affected differently than those that have yet to emerge. Many skills which are known to develop later in childhood, such as executive functioning skills or abstract reasoning, are therefore affected by more frequent childhood medical disorders [1].
- *Localization/disease process*: It is essential to evaluate whether the change in brain development is isolated, such as an infarct or tumor, or more global, such as an anoxic episode or hydrocephalus. The age at diagnosis affects the relative state of brain development; therefore, using the adult literature to make assumptions about which skills would be affected by disease or injury in a specific location can at times lead to inaccurate conclusions. For example, there is some flexibility in brain development during childhood, often referred to as neural plasticity [2–4], to allow for skills to develop in the context of early changes in brain development or damage to neural tissue.
- *Cascading effects*: For patients who experience a more global insult, changes in speed of processing and the rate of developmental progression are often affected; even if children remain within typical expectations for age shortly after treatment, we expect for the patient to begin a different developmental trajectory

moving forward. We can then see slowed achievement of skills over time, relative to same age peers, resulting in increased discrepancies from expectations in the absence of skill regression [5, 6]. Some medical disorders can also include a profile of regression. In addition, we can see atypical developmental patterns, resulting in a more scattered skill development profile, with some age-appropriate skills and some domains of significant difficulty.

- At times, medical disorders can also change children's access to information (e.g., changes in vision secondary to the location of a brain tumor, hearing loss secondary to chemotherapy treatment), communication abilities (e.g., the loss of verbal speech secondary to a tracheostomy), or loss of mobility due to infarct or spinal cord tethering. These can also shift the child's developmental trajectory.
- *Intervention/treatment-related effects*: The effects of some medical treatments can also change brain development in its scope, frequency, and magnitude. Patients may experience both localized and global treatments, such as neurosurgery, focal radiation, and global chemotherapy, to treat a brain tumor, for example. While medical management of the disease is the priority, the late effects of the treatment can have lasting ramifications on developmental outcomes [7]. Therefore, when conceptualizing changes in brain development, all of these factors need to be carefully considered.
- *Changing expectations*: It is essential to consider that the environment is full of changing (typically increasing) expectations for children, as their environment shifts along with the developmental progress expected for typically developing children as they age. School demands tend to increase gradually each year, with more substantial changes in the independent functioning demands noted as children shift from elementary, to middle, and eventually to high school. Demands around functional independence also increase at home. However, also of importance are the decreasing supports that are typically available to children as they age; this decrease in support can be as problematic as the increases in demands.

For example, a child diagnosed with a left temporal lobe tumor at age 4, who was treated with surgery, radiation therapy, and chemotherapy, will have a different developmental trajectory than a child with a similar diagnosis and treatment at age 12. In addition, while their specific profiles may have some similarities due to the risk profiles associated with a tumor in the left temporal lobe, their strength and weakness profile (neurobehavioral profile) will be inherently different from a child whose medical diagnosis and treatments are of a different etiology.

Neuropsychological assessment is designed to carefully examine the brain-behavior relationship in the context of the child's current age, the age of injury or insult, and with consideration of both expected treatment-related effects and individual differences, including family history. These results are then related to expectations given important individual characteristics, the expected neurobehavioral profile given the patient's medical history, and age-related expectations.

Methods for Delivery of Neuropsychological Care

Historically, pediatric neuropsychologists have provided comprehensive assessments to evaluate changes in behavior that are linked to changes in brain development secondary to neurological diseases/disorders or brain-directed treatments (e.g., neurosurgery, chemotherapy, etc.). These evaluations were at times comprehensive, evaluating the whole child, including the assessment of intellectual abilities, language development, visual spatial reasoning skills, memory, attention, executive functioning skills, emotional functioning, and adaptive skill development. Given how integral school functioning is for children, particularly for those with (suspected) changes in brain development, full neuropsychological assessments have typically also included some screening of academic skills. These assessments are often repeated every couple of years given the significant changes in brain development as well as increasing environmental expectations as children age. For certain medical populations, more targeted assessments are warranted. This can occur with a sudden change in symptoms or cognitive functioning, evaluating changes in treatments, and prior to neurosurgery.

Referral Model

A comprehensive neuropsychological evaluation is warranted for most patients who have complex medical needs, particularly those with medical conditions that directly affect the central nervous system. In many institutions, this includes a referral to an outside clinician who can provide consultation to the family and medical team around a child's current functioning. Although most essential in early childhood (6–9 years) and as they are transitioning to adulthood (16–18 years), many neuropsychologists follow patients with evaluations every 3–4 years to monitor progress as environmental demands increase.

All pediatric neuropsychologists are trained in brain-behavioral relationships, child development, and behavioral health issues. However, like all providers, neuropsychologists tend to specialize. Many, for example, work with children who have developmental disabilities (e.g., autism), learning disabilities (e.g., dyslexia), or behavioral health issues (e.g., bipolar disorder). Although these specialists can certainly provide consultation to medical teams, they typically do not know the intricacies of specific medical conditions, the potential effects of treatments and procedures, the frequent presentations and comorbidities, and the typical developmental trajectory of these patients. Medical centers often have a group of trained providers who are familiar with a number of neurological and medical issues and can easily consult teams in medical systems; they are aware of the typical struggles of medically complex children and are well versed in brain-behavior relationships after changes in central nervous system development.

Integrated Team Care Models

The complexity of some pediatric conditions that involve multiple organ systems requires integrated care models that can flexibly adapt to the current needs of the patient; as more complex patients are surviving, clinics have evolved to include additional medical specialists, psychologists, and therapists. Ideally, pediatric neuropsychologists who specialize in medical and neurological conditions are embedded in specific pediatric treatment teams. This allows for the neuropsychologist who is specialized in a specific patient population to complete full evaluations and also provide more direct consultation to the medical team. For example, they can provide assessment of the patient's cognitive abilities, consult to the medical team on potential late effects or postsurgical changes, and facilitate targeted intervention planning for ongoing medical management. There are several different group treatment models that are currently used in practice; we have focused on multidisciplinary, interdisciplinary, and transdisciplinary.

- *Multidisciplinary*: Multidisciplinary team models are designed to include multiple different providers across disciplines that separately see the same patient and consult with other clinicians about the care of the patient. Many specialty clinics create multidisciplinary models; ideally, this provides access to multiple providers who tend to work together when providing care to specific populations. Families can come to one clinic visit in a "one-stop-shop" model and see several providers around individual aspects of need [8]. For example, a patient in spina bifida clinic would be able to meet with a neurosurgeon, urologist, orthopedic surgeon, and several other providers in an afternoon clinic to review imaging data and current concerns and create future plans.
- *Interdisciplinary*: "Interdisciplinary team approaches integrate separate discipline approaches into a single consultation" [9]. The integration of history and symptoms, assessment of current issue, and diagnostic formulation are completed as a team with the patient at one time, in conjunction with the creation of intervention plans and short- and long-term management goals [8, 9]. Psychological and neuropsychological assessments can be instrumental in evaluating the potential success or possible failure of some interventions; for example, cognitive and psychological evaluations are standard in the eligibility process for solid organ transplant and some surgical interventions, such as bariatric surgery for weight loss, in order to evaluate the patient's ability to follow complex instructions necessary for success following the procedures. In addition, information on future levels of independent functioning gathered through neuropsychological evaluations can be instrumental in the creation of recommended methods of surgical management for specific medical issues. For example, an oncologist, neurosurgeon, and radiologist work together to create a comprehensive treatment plan for a patient with a new diagnosis of a brain tumor. In interdisciplinary models, the care providers maintain their individual relationships with the patient but work together to create a comprehensive care plan.

- *Transdisciplinary*: Transdisciplinary team models also include multiple specialists but can be broader to include researchers and caregivers; the emphasis is on the creation of one comprehensive treatment plan that includes the collaboration of involved team members. The knowledge of the specialists and team providers is integrated into the treatment planning provided by all care providers. Given the sheer number of involved clinicians, the establishment of a transdisciplinary team can be extremely challenging. Epilepsy surgical teams often work in transdisciplinary models; when patients are evaluated for treatment options, neuroimaging, neuropsychological assessment, and Wada procedures are completed and reviewed by the team (e.g., neurologists, neurosurgeons, neuropsychologists, etc.) in the creation of a comprehensive treatment plan.

Contributions from Neuropsychologists to Group Models

Regardless of the design of the clinic, pediatric neuropsychologists can contribute to a variety of roles in patient care, in addition to conducting traditional comprehensive neuropsychological evaluations.

Consultation to the Medical Team

Neuropsychologists have the benefit of spending a great deal of time with patients over the course of an evaluation; this affords us the opportunity to informally gather information about family systems, compliance with medical regimens, engagement with the community, and trust in community systems and agencies that medical team members often do not get the opportunity to hear about. We interact with patients, their family systems, their school, and their provider networks and therefore can be privy to their personal belief systems and their methods of interacting with systems. For patients with complex medical needs, their medical appointments can often be brief and focused on physiological needs and problems despite the frequency of their visits with their physicians. In addition, in the pediatric medical model, neuropsychologists are also one of the few providers who meet with patients alone to complete assessments and often complete interviews and feedback sessions with parents/caregivers independently, allowing us to gather information that patients and their parents/caregivers may have been concerned about sharing in front of each other.

- *Cognitive problems*: In the context of multidisciplinary, interdisciplinary, and transdisciplinary clinic models, brief consultative appointments with patients (even 15–20 minutes) provide an opportunity to discuss the patient's current status, monitor their developmental progress for a new onset of problems or increasing difficulty, and evaluate the need for services. It is important to continue to evaluate for the onset of new medical/cognitive issues that result in problems with learning (in the academic, home, and community settings) given the developmental nature of pediatric patients. These visits can be billed through health and behavior codes designed to provide support to patients with medical diagnoses. However, many medical clinics subsidize the involvement of neuropsychologists as well, given their contributions to the team.

- Neuropsychologists also can speak to changes in child development secondary to complex neurocognitive profiles and/or behavioral health difficulties. Given medical complexity and changes in the rate of skill acquisition, we will often see differences in behavioral presentations. At times, these changes in presentation are consistent with their neurocognitive profiles, such as increased behavioral problems in children with language disorders. In contrast, it may be that a developmentally appropriate behavior is demonstrated at a later age than expected.
- Neuropsychologists often voice safety concerns that may influence treatments and procedures. For example, many patients are not capable of awareness of potential victimization, and the number of times per day they are disrobed for necessary medical cares (e.g., urinary catheterization) increases their risks; they may be safer with surgical intervention to create a stoma to reduce the need for catheterization through their urethra.
- *Noncompliance*: When noncompliance with medical regimens is broached as a concern, neuropsychologists are uniquely qualified to provide an understanding of the patient's ability to understand their medical treatment plans and recommendations, assess the patient's profile and potential cognitive factors related to their illness, evaluate the contribution of family history and environmental factors, and create a training model to evaluate compliance.
- Neuropsychologists can also help to differentiate between emotional, cognitive, and practical impediments to compliance. Once there is an understanding of their complex cognitive profile, behavioral health issues such as anxiety or depression can significantly affect compliance with medical regimens and confuse physical symptom profiles. For example, a patient with a brain tumor treated with chemotherapy and radiation therapy is expected to have slower information processing speed; this can be further slowed by symptoms of depression, which can be confused for a potential late effect of treatment.
- Medical teams often need to provide written instructions for those with memory impairments, to adjust recommendations for those with more limited vocabulary, and to be concrete and concise about potential side effects, complications, or other treatment information.
- Physicians can often be challenged by young adults who are noncompliant despite the best efforts of the teams and their families. In pediatric care facilities, teams are used to working with families, and at times community-based supports, to ensure that children have access to appropriate levels of care. However, these discussions can become more complex when young adults make choices about compliance with medical recommendations, particularly when the choices are in contrast to medical team recommendations and/or family wishes. In these instances, it is essential that the neurobehavioral profile of the young adult be

considered in the contract for medical care. When the medical team or provider feels it is necessary to terminate care due to noncompliance, significant cognitive or behavioral health impairments can complicate the picture. It is essential to have clear and up-to-date information on patients to ensure comprehension on the patient's behalf, as well as adequate and appropriate documentation for the medical team. It would be inappropriate, for example, to send a certified letter terminating care to a young adult with first-grade reading abilities, as they clearly do not have the requisite skills to ensure adequate comprehension.

- For example, one young adult patient with a moderate intellectual disability continued to gain weight despite concerns and repeated recommendations from her medical team, so much so that her airway was compromised. Discussions with the patient and her mother indicated she had stopped drinking soda and eating candy as had been recommended. However, it took further interview and a lengthy series of yes/no questions (rather than open-ended questions) to determine that she had replaced the soda with juice and did not understand recommended serving sizes. With concrete recommendations, such as "only drink water," "eat no portion larger than your hand," and "you must have five vegetables each day," she was able to lose weight without surgical intervention. In order to shift the manner of intervention by the medical team, careful consideration of the young adult's cognitive and emotional needs was necessary.

Consultation with Families

A significant role in any multidisciplinary clinic involves working with individuals to assume responsibility for their medical care, with a necessary understanding of typical physiological development, their medical condition(s), possible symptomology, and necessary treatment regimens. For any adolescent and young adult, management of medical emergencies and the logistics of insurance coverage can be a challenge. Children and young adults with chronic medical conditions have to develop an understanding of the symptoms and complexity of their medical disorder, acquire knowledge to understand the disorder and its management, and understand their own personal medical history (e.g., reactions, prior treatments). Given that many medical conditions can affect neurocognitive development, the ability to effectively acquire this information and the cognitive capacity needed to complete day-to-day care and effectively manage medical emergencies are even more of a challenge. In addition, parents of these children with chronic conditions have been managing their medical care for years; therefore, shifting the day-to-day management can be complicated by parent's understanding of their children's capacity, trust in their children's skills, the level of conflict in their relationship, and a history of noncompliance or poor engagement by teenagers. For many young adults, having a signed release on file for their parents allows for the young adult to continue to receive some level of support throughout this transition.

There are many pediatric medical disorders that up until the past few decades have not resulted in long-term survival. One of the starkest examples is the inclusion of central nervous-directed therapy in the treatment of pediatric leukemia. Up until the 1970s, when CNS-directed treatment was included in therapy, acute lymphoblastic leukemia's cure rates were extremely low; now, survival rates are estimated at 90% [10]. For patients with spina bifida, the use of intermittent catheterization to drain the bladder and protect the kidneys resulted in reduced mortality. There have been significant improvements in cystic fibrosis survival since the 1930s, when 70% of sufferers died in infancy, to a median predicted survival in 2015 of 45 years [11].

With the advent of more complex and successful medical care models, we have more patients surviving into young adulthood. Although they often transition to adult medical care models in their late 20s to early 30s, pediatric care must now also prepare young adults to assume responsibility for their own care. Independent functioning becomes an essential long-term goal despite significant medical needs and potential cognitive complications from their own medical disease and care.

The first step in helping parents share some responsibility with their adolescents is to accurately assess the cognitive capacity of the patient to understand and manage their own medical care. It is essential for parents to understand their child's ability to comprehend complex information, manage medical terminology, hold information in memory, and process information effectively and efficiently enough to ask questions and anticipate potential consequences (of treatments or noncompliance). For patients who have been closely followed over time, data is available on both cognitive capacity and the rate of development of adaptive skills and functional independence. Although serial assessments through middle childhood are helpful to understanding a child's general level of functioning, an updated assessment is essential as these adolescents are reaching adulthood (16–17 years of age). In young adulthood, the evaluation measures change to begin to evaluate more comprehensive and complex reasoning skills that are expected in adult development and are more consistent with the skills necessary for carefully evaluating medical procedures and treatment options. It also allows for an in-depth assessment of their current adaptive skills, including not only independence in activities of daily living but also their ability to manage money, manage a household, earn and maintain a job, and safely interact with the community. Although some of these domains are outside of the direct needs of the medical team, the information helps to create a more comprehensive picture of the young adult's capabilities and can directly affect their ability to engage in care.

For those young adults who are not able to successfully function independently, consideration of a legal guardian is critical. For some young adults, adolescence can be a time of experimentation and adherence issues; however, their ability to understand the potential ramifications of their actions is generally intact. For those with more intensive needs, particularly those who will have long-standing requirements for support, guardianship is often essential. While guardianship can be limited to medical decision making in most states, neuropsychological consultation can help to delineate specific domains of need. It is essential to understand that guardianship is not a panacea for noncompliance in young adults but is based upon careful examination of a young adult's capacity for decision making. Guardianship often includes decision making supports for medical care treatment (including behavioral health), financial decision making, and social decision making (e.g., job training, living placements, peer group access, etc.). For individuals with more transient needs—such as those with cognitive ramifications of their medical disorder, including those who are post-surgery or under treatment, or those patients who have behavioral health issues—the degree of support and length of guardianship can be modified by the legal system. In some states, such as Massachusetts where we practice, it is essential to clarify whether these skill deficits are global or more specific, as there are multiple vehicles for obtaining guardianship through the probate courts. It is important to be aware that many of these systems were put in place for aging adults who are losing skills over time, whereas our young adult patients have not yet developed these skills/abilities; therefore, the process can be overwhelming and challenging for families to navigate, particularly without a comprehensive understanding of their child's needs.

The management of symptoms is one of the most challenging aspects of assuming responsibility for their own care. For example, when patients with hydrocephalus have a headache, it could potentially be due to a shunt malfunction indicating an urgent need for neurosurgical intervention. However, it could also be due to stress, dehydration, high blood pressure, or sinus infection (or any other variety of reasons). The patient's ability to evaluate the severity and length of symptoms, to properly attend to other co-occurring symptoms, and to rule out potential issues due to a lack of symptoms is essential. Parents often complete this medical care decision tree modeling mentally, acquiring information through a series of what may seem like random questions to rule out other potential issues (e.g., Are you vomiting? Sniffling? Drinking water?). Adolescents learn this skill best through modeling and repeat exposure, which requires a lot of time; this is not a quick process that can occur in the few months before an adolescent turns 18 years of age. In order to develop these skills in their children, parents have to repeatedly provide explicit step-by-step explanations of their thought process, help children understand the implications of certain decisions, and repeatedly review emergency management strategies. Finally, it is also important to consider that many of our young patients have had traumatic experiences that may also be affecting their ability to actively participate in their medical care. Neuropsychologists are able to parse apart cognitive challenges that continue to be longstanding from more transient behavioral health issues that can also affect the patient's ability to engage in their own medical care.

For patients who are capable of assuming at least some level of independent functioning, neuropsychological assessment can help families understand ability levels and help to prioritize which skills should be acquired first. All skill acquisition is developmental in nature and typically requires that basic skills are taught and rehearsed first, prior to the development of more complex skills. Therefore, skills often need to be broken down and taught in an incremental fashion; however, many life skills are typically taught through observation and exposure, rather than via highly structured teaching models. Neuropsychological assessments can provide families with an understanding of their child's strengths and weaknesses, as well as the domains where they require assistance; therefore, they can better advocate for their young adult in the medical system. These are some of the necessary domains that neuropsychologists often work with families in order to facilitate skill development.

- *Awareness and significance of symptoms and medical conditions*: Patients need to be able to identify their medical conditions, affected parts of the body, current symptoms, and severity and to have a sense of who their medical team includes. For example, a young adult with spina bifida and shunted hydrocephalus who is on dialysis due to end-stage renal disease may tell an emergency room doctor that they are unable to walk but fail to mention their shunt, a history of seizures, and neurosurgical intervention or that they have medication allergies. Following a situation like this, neuropsychological evaluations can help to differentiate between issues with memory, problems with verbal comprehension, and management of emotions and pain in a stressful context.
- *Communication with medical providers*: Patients need to be able to greet medical team members, respond to basic questions, ask questions (even if rehearsed prior), and summarize information from medical visits. Patients need experiences participating in decision making in order to begin to assume the responsibility; many patients can use group meetings in the educational setting (for Individualized Education Programs) and/or medical visits to rehearse listening to complex material, identifying questions, and weighing different options. For complete functional independence in the medical setting, patients need to be able to advocate for themselves, even if in disagreement with medical team members, and the ability to effectively ask questions about their care. The ultimate goal is to be able to speak to medical teams freely and to request what they need (e.g., repetition of information, written step-by-step instructions, teaching/modeling, a private visit). Neuropsychological assessment and consultation become critical to understand the level of reasoning and complex problem-solving that the patient is able to manage independently. Social interaction skills, verbal communication, and memory functioning can also limit functional independence in this domain.
- *Management of daily regimen*: Patients must be able to know the names of their equipment (e.g., braces, hearing aids, catheters), cooperate with daily routines, assume more independent completion of these routines, and manage supplies of medications by alerting parents and eventually medical providers. Patients often require written reminders or electronic alarms in order to keep track of timing and task completion; working with families to identify the patient's ability to use reminders is important. Parent's methods of tracking task completion may be different from those of the children; for example, there are now smartphone applications that can be set to show images of the medication to take at that certain time (and allow for a check off if it was completed) rather than using a plastic pill sorter. In addition to the ability to evaluate the child's capacity for skill development in this domain, neuropsychologists also often help to mediate challenging conversations between adolescents or young adults with their parents; the transition of power and responsibility for many of these patients can

be extremely slow and fraught with emotion, as parents are concerned about their child's safety and well-being.

- *Managing access to records and payment information*: Patients need to understand that there is a medical record that they are able to access, use the information to prepare for future visits and extract recommendations, and manage payment/insurance issues. It is also essential that parents recognize that, with different skills, their children may need to complete tasks in a slightly different manner. For example, many of our parents would prefer to call and speak to an appointment coordinator, whereas their children may prefer to schedule through our online computer system (at 3 a.m.). Access to online medical record systems has diminished the need for the multiple three-ring medical binders that many parents used to bring with them to visits.
- *Management of lifestyle choices*: Adolescence and young adulthood are times that developmentally include separation from parents, engagement in social networks, and exposure to new experiences and potential risky behaviors. Although independence and the development of identity are essential tasks during this age range, engagement in risk-taking behaviors can have more dire consequences for those with medical conditions (e.g., seizure threshold is affected by alcohol consumption), and many of our patients are at elevated risk for victimization given their neurocognitive profiles. For example, patients with chronic medical conditions require treatments at school/day programs that involve physical touch (e.g., physical therapy, assistance with changing or walking) or nudity (e.g., catheterization, help dressing). At times, cognitive limitations can affect our patient's ability to discern appropriate from inappropriate touch; their typical high compliance with adult/care provider requests can further increase their risks in these contexts. In addition, the desire to be socially connected with others can increase the likelihood of victimization (both online and in person) and requires close monitoring and frequent supervision.

Closing Remarks

Overall, the roles of a neuropsychologist in a pediatric care model can vary significantly depending upon the nature of the disease, the complexity of the medical treatment regimen, and the cognitive status of the patients. Their active engagement can vary between consulting to other team members directly, patients, and families and working with others in the community to help bridge the gap between medical teams and educational and vocational programs. The transition into school, and out of childhood, is a significant transition where neuropsychological supports are most essential.

Chapter Review Questions

1. Why is the frequency of follow-up with neuropsychology different for children and adults?
2. Name three different roles that the neuropsychologist can offer to support patients as a member of the medical treatment teams.

References

1. Bernstein JH. Developmental neuropsychological assessment. In: Yeates KO, Ris MD, Taylor HG, editors. Pediatric neuropsychology: research, theory, and practice. New York, NY: Guilford Press; 2000. p. 405–38.
2. Ballantyne AO, Spilkin AM, Hesselink J, Trauner DA. Plasticity in the developing brain: intellectual, language and academic functions in c hildren. Brain. 2008;131:2975–85.
3. Dennis M, Spiegler BJ, Simic N, Sinopoli KJ, Wilkinson A, Yeates KO, Terry HG, Bigler ED, Fletcher JM. Functional plasticity in childhood brain disorders: when, what, how, and whom to assess. Neuropsychol Rev. 2014;24(4):389–408.
4. Pascual-Leone A, Amedi A, Fregni F, Merabet LB. The plastic human brain cortex. Annu Rev Neurosci. 2005;28:377–401.
5. Palmer SL, Gajjar A, Reddick WE, Glass JO, Kun LE, Wu S, Xiong X, Mulhern RK. Predicting intellectual outcome among children treated with 35–40 Gy craniospinal irradiation for medulloblastoma. Neuropsychology. 2003;17(4):548–55.
6. Reeves CB, Palmer S, Gross AM, Simonian SJ, Taylor L, Willingham E, Mulhern RK. Brief report: sluggish cognitive tempo among pediatric survivors of acute lymphoblastic leukemia. J Pediatr Psychol. 2007;32(9):1050–4.
7. Waber DP, Queally JT, Catania L, Robaey P, Romero I, Adams H, Alyman C, Jandet-Brunet C, Sallan SE, Silverman LB. Neuropsychological outcomes of standard risk and high risk patients treated for acute lymphoblastic leukemia on Dana-Farber ALL consortium protocol 95-01 at 5 years post-diagnosis. Pediatr Blood Cancer. 2012;58(5):758–65.
8. Choi BC, Pak AW. Multidisciplinarity, interdisciplinarity and transdisciplinarity in health research, services, education and policy: 1. Definitions, objectives, and evidence of effectiveness. Clin Invest Med. 2006;29(6):351–64.
9. Jessup RL. Interdisciplinary versus multidisciplinary care teams: do we understand the difference? Aust Health Rev. 2007;31(3):330–1.
10. Kansagra A, Dahiva S, Litzow M. Continuing challenges and current issues in acute lymphoblastic leukemia. Leuk Lymphoma Rev. 2017;11:1–16. https://doi.org/10.1080/10428194.2017.1335397.
11. Dodge JA, Lewis PA, Stanton M, Wilsher J. Cystic fibrosis mortality and survival in the UK: 1947–2003. Eur Respir J. 2007;29:522–6. https://doi.org/10.1183/09031936.00099506.

Chapter 3
A Model of Collaboration between Primary Care and Neuropsychology

Margaret Lanca and Kirsten Meisinger

Role of Neuropsychology in Medicine

Assessing cognitive dysfunction in patients with medical problems is imperative since cognitive impairments can contribute to poor medical treatment outcomes, lower their level of functioning, and increase their distress. The breadth and scope of cognitive assessments in primary care has proliferated, particularly as the field of neuropsychology has begun to integrate in primary care. This was not always the case. Neuropsychologists are trained as clinical psychologists with a specialization in assessing cognition and mood and understanding the medical, neurological, and psychiatric conditions that affect cognition. The field can trace its lineage to many roots, particularly to the early twentieth century when education psychologists were commissioned by the US government to assess intelligence [1]. This prompted a flurry of test developments, which began to examine not only how to capture cognition in healthy people with normal intelligence but also in people who were unhealthy and/or did not have normal intelligence. In the medical field, early neuropsychologists worked alongside neurologists and psychiatrists in particular, providing more in-depth characterizations of patients' cognitive functioning [1]. Modern-day clinical neuropsychologists, however, have expanded their expertise to many medical specialties such as geriatrics, oncology, and rehabilitation, to name a few, as medical research has underscored the crucial relationship between cognition, health, and emotional well-being. Now, following the trend in the Western medical system to predominantly ambulatory experiences of care, neuropsychologists are working alongside primary care providers (PCPs). Neuropsychologists'

M. Lanca (✉)
Harvard Medical School, Cambridge Health Alliance, Cambridge, MA, USA
e-mail: margaret_lanca@hms.harvard.edu; kmeisinger@challiance.org

K. Meisinger
Department of Public Health, Harvard University/Cambridge Health Alliance, Cambridge, MA, USA

K. M. Sanders (ed.), *Physician's Field Guide to Neuropsychology*,
https://doi.org/10.1007/978-1-4939-8722-1_3

expertise makes them well-suited collaborators with PCPs, who both appreciate quantifiable data-driven assessments of patients' health status and embrace their patients' health holistically with the understanding that many illnesses can affect their patients' cognition and vice versa.

Neuropsychologists provide assessments (pen-and-paper tests, with some computerized tests), integrating test results with patients' biopsychosocial history to formulate conclusions and make diagnoses. Tests resemble an extended mental status exam (lasting 1–3 h typically), but the administration is standardized, tests are normed, and analysis is evidenced-based. Neuropsychologists evaluate intelligence, alongside other cognitive domains such as expressive and receptive language, visuospatial processing, reasoning, problem-solving, learning, and memory. Test results provide information about the normal or abnormal functioning of the brain, which can be used for a variety of clinical purposes.

Key Point
Neuropsychological assessments are extended mental status examinations comprised of normed tests that are standardized, evidence-based, and interpreted within biopsychosocial context.

Purpose of Neuropsychological Testing

Providers refer their patient's neuropsychological testing for a variety of reasons [1]:

1. *Diagnosis*. Identifying significant neurocognitive deficits (e.g., impaired memory) that can suggest/confirm brain lesions, neurocognitive dysfunction, and/or a neurocognitive disorder (e.g., dementia).
2. *Management*. Testing reveals a patient's cognitive profile of strengths and weakness and sometimes impairments. Findings enable a patient, his/her medical provider, and family members to understand how his/her medical, neurological, and/or psychiatric conditions have affected them cognitively and how to manage it.
3. *Treatment*. A neurocognitive profile can be used to make treatment recommendations to the patient and his/her family about how to compensate for cognitive weaknesses/deficits or other kinds of treatment recommendations related to medication prescription, safety, self-care, treatment complication, etc. Rehabilitation programs for cognitive impairments and behavioral disorders can be improved by neuropsychological knowledge.
4. *Forensic*. Neuropsychological assessment undertaken for legal proceedings is common in situations whether there is personal injury with loss of cognitive function [2]. Most forensic questions are targeted to answering whether the claimant has suffered brain damage that may or may not be apparent by other neuroimaging tests.
5. *Educational*. Ascertaining a learning disability or attention-deficit hyperactivity disorder (AD/HD) is a quite commonplace assessment for neuropsychologists.

Although education evaluations for learning disabilities, or psychiatric evaluations for AD/HD, are possible, a comprehensive neuropsychological evaluation is invaluable to providing students, parents, and educators with comprehensive and detailed treatment evaluations that are both medically and educationally driven. Also, learning disabilities and AD/HD are highly comorbid with other psychiatric disorders and can be missed without a comprehensive psychiatric evaluation of the patient.

Key Point
Neuropsychological testing is used for diagnosis, management, treatment, forensic, and educational purposes in patient care.

Referrals for neuropsychological testing by primary care teams are typically related to all but the forensic category described above. Diagnostic evaluation is often requested to differentiate between neurocognitive disorders (e.g., dementia vs. pseudodementia) or to assist in elucidating a patient's cognitive complaints (e.g., with attention, memory, etc.). Neuropsychological testing can also identify the source of a patient's cognitive complaints. For example, a patient might complain of ongoing memory symptoms, but neuropsychological testing may reveal the etiology of the symptoms to be more attention- rather than memory-based. Neuropsychological testing is particularly helpful in assessing what is "normal" and what is "abnormal" cognition (e.g., Are my patient's memory symptoms normal age-related symptoms?). This is done by administering normed cognitive tests in which a patient's test score can be compared to the performance of healthy controls of the same age, gender, and/or level of education. By having these comparison scores, results can be deemed within the normal range for a particular patient or abnormal.

Identifying the source of the cognitive symptoms can assist in targeting appropriate compensatory strategies or medications for the symptoms (e.g., stimulant medication vs. anticholinesterase inhibitors). Sometimes primary care teams may wish to assist/improve their patient's ability to live with a medical condition or live independently. In these cases, a patient's cognitive profile can be used to formalize a treatment plan to improve everyday functioning and to make important determinations about the level of family or system support. In other cases, a patient's cognitive profile can be used to improve vocational training, inform cognitive rehabilitation programs, or design individual educational plans for school settings.

Key Point
Neurocognitive evaluation can help refine diagnoses across a wide spectrum of mental health disorders.

What Causes Cognitive Problems?

Cognitive disturbance can arise from many types of medical, neurological, and/or psychiatric conditions. Any brain disorder or medical condition, which affects the central nervous system (CNS), can potentially affect cognition. Obviously, diseases with direct CNS involvement are typically the most commonly known to affect cognition. Dementia, stroke, epilepsy, Parkinson's disease, multiple sclerosis, brain tumors, and hydrocephalus are some of the CNS diseases that impair cognition. Neurodevelopmental conditions can impact cognition; these may range from conditions known to affect cerebral morphology such as spina bifida or other milder neurodevelopmental conditions (i.e., (AD/HD), learning disorders), which result in abnormal cognitive functioning, but by clinical standards whose brain may be deemed "normal" on clinical neuroradiological tests such as a standard head MRI. Psychiatric conditions are also known to affect cognition, particularly in severe mental illness such as schizophrenia and bipolar disorder, of which neurocognitive deficits are considered cardinal symptoms [3]. Robust research has documented the disruptive effects of cognition due to mood disorders in the mild to moderate range (e.g., depression, anxiety, trauma) (for reviews see [4–6]).

Medical diseases can also secondarily impact cognition [7]. Because the brain is almost totally dependent on other organs and systems for maintaining its functional integrity, it is highly susceptible to dysregulation. Brain metabolism depends on the vascular system to transport oxygen, glucose, and nutrients. When an organ system is inefficient or unable to provide the brain with sufficient quantities of substances that are essential for normal functioning, it can alter brain functioning; for example, asthma can reduce oxygen levels to the brain [8]. Nutritional deficiencies due to either reduced storage or absorption of vitamins can also impair cognition (e.g., anorexia). Overly active organ systems can disrupt cerebral functioning (e.g., thyroid, pituitary, or adrenal glands) and can cause cognitive and affective disturbances. The liver and kidneys are responsible for detoxification and excretion of toxins for the body as a whole. Acute and chronic liver diseases typically induce an encephalopathy resulting in mild to severe cognitive impairment. Therefore, intact metabolic functioning of other organs is necessary for optimal brain function. When the finely tuned relationship between the brain and its other systems is disrupted by medical diseases, even transient ones, potentially adverse consequences of neurological functioning can occur. Neurotransmitter dysregulation typically occurs secondary to metabolic, biochemical, or endocrine disease [9].

Key Point

CNS as well as many other medical diseases can affect cognition, but this is not yet widely recognized as part of the management of many chronic diseases in primary care.

Regular assessment of cognitive disruption in patients with medical disease is critical.

While commonly accepted in the medical community that biologic disease can affect cognitive function, the effects and consequences of impairment have been underestimated, if not overlooked, until recently. Cognitive impairment can go undiagnosed and wreak havoc on medical treatment. Assessing the level of cognitive disruption in those patients with medical disease is therefore imperative since it can contribute to poor treatment outcomes for the primary medical condition and secondarily lower patients' overall health and functioning.

Interface between Primary Care and Neuropsychology

Modern Western medical practice is based on an interview format between physician and patient with supplementary testing to reach a "diagnosis" or hypothesis of what ails the patient. This format has been surprisingly long-lived, potentially dating back into prehistoric times [10]. The intellectual underpinning of medical interviews and tests relies on Bayesian principles [11]. Bayesian logic uses a combination of pre-event likelihood and outcomes to arrive at the soundest conclusion for a particular question. "Events" in the medical context are typically test results or patient complaints, and "outcomes" are the test results themselves and/or a conditional hypothesis of what the cause of the complaint is. A commonly cited example for PCPs is the use of testing for a pulmonary embolism based on a presenting patient complaint of shortness of breath. Scoring systems have been developed using Bayesian principles to aid providers in determining the likelihood of the pretest probability of a pulmonary embolism and whether to continue potentially invasive tests on the patient in order to prove or disprove the hypothesis [12]. Similarly, Bayesian logic is inherent in neuropsychology and neuroscience. Bayesian approaches to brain function investigate the capacity of the nervous system to operate in situations of uncertainty in a fashion that is close to the optimal prescribed by Bayesian statistics. This term is used in behavioral sciences and neuroscience, and studies associated with this term often strive to explain the brain's cognitive abilities based on statistical principles. It is frequently assumed that the nervous system maintains internal probabilistic models that are updated by neural processing of sensory information using methods approximating those of Bayesian probability [13, 14].

Western medicine also uses this probability theory technique to springboard from complaint to treatment, such as with gastroesophageal reflux disease. When presented with a complex complaint such as chest pain, experienced medical providers quickly narrow the likelihood of the different causes of chest pain with the initial interview and physical exam to arrive at a reasonable conclusion with little or no testing. The pretest probability of this diagnosis is so high when the interview results in answers confirmatory to reflux, rather than heart disease, that in standard medical practice, confirmatory testing is often skipped or delayed in favor of starting treatment immediately [15]. This rapid sequence logic model is now the primary method used in primary care practice around the world, partly as a result of unremitting pressures to treat as many people as possible in as short a time as possible. This methodology becomes orders of magnitude more challenging with more complex presentation of diseases and for those in which the pretest probability is low because there is a great deal of overlap in presenting complaints and no real-time testing available to help differentiate between potential diagnoses [10].

Key Point
Western clinical medicine is based on Bayesian logic models in which clinical judgements are made using probability theory techniques. Neuropsychology and behavioral neuroscience share these intellectual underpinnings.

Complex presentations are the standard in diagnosing psychiatric and often neurologic disease more than many other areas of medicine. Interestingly, primary care, not psychiatry or neurology, is resoundingly the setting in which most psychiatric and neurological diagnoses are now made [16]. The rapid fire primary care setting environment within which these diagnoses are made, managed, and treated has underscored the need for faster yet reliable testing for many complex psychiatric and neurological disorders such as AD/HD and dementia. The pretest probability of complex psychiatric diseases is consequently much lower than diseases with simpler mechanisms and expressions, so either testing or extended interviews become essential to making a diagnosis with reasonable certainty. Neuropsychological assessments can assist in some of these diagnostic conditions.

Psychiatry has hung its professional hat on the extended interview methodology, with hour-long consults and little confirmatory testing performed in support of the conclusions reached. Generally, this thorough interview technique results in narrowing the presenting complaints of patients to one or a handful of likely diagnoses with reasonable accuracy. It is, however, quite subject to cultural and intellectual overlays, as evidenced by the multiple versions of the *Diagnostic and Statistical Manual of Mental Disorders* published since 1917 [17]. In addition to these challenges, access to psychiatric care is limited around the world, and patients will also frequently decline evaluation by psychiatrists because of social stigma [18].

There have been few alternatives available within psychiatry to the extended interview technique until recently, largely because testing of the brain's expression and functions has not provided the certainty needed to reach a diagnosis with equal or improved certainty. The methodological similarities between medical practitioners and neuropsychologists make their collaboration substantially easier than medical and traditional psychiatric colleagues. In both medicine and neuropsychology, observation, interviewing, and testing are used to arrive at a diagnosis. Both fields are comfortable with the culture of testing and Bayesian logic, with its concepts of range of normal, screening cutoffs, and pretest probability. Not only are neuropsychologists familiar with the Bayesian concepts of diagnostic sensitivity and specificity but antecedent probability from Bayes theorem is also fundamental to diagnostic interpretation of neuropsychological test scores [19]. Further, new developments in statistical analysis of tests have led to the implementation of multiple-level likelihood ratios, which can improve diagnostic certainty [20].

The array of neuropsychological assessments described in this chapter provides solutions to both the lack of access to care for patients with psychiatric diseases and to the failures of the rapid throughput primary care system. Collaboration in a single primary care setting or across an integrated system leads to more efficient, patient-centered, and holistic care. Additionally, since cognitive health becomes part of standard medical practice, the Descartian artificial divide between the mind and body is mitigated. Considerations of cognitive functioning allow teams to focus diagnoses and treatments for patients at an effective and individualized level, improving treatment adherence, medication compliance, and behavioral interventions.

Key Point
Integrating neuropsychological testing in primary care improves access for patients, and the neuropsychological testing format resembles other results primary care teams often receive and so are easily incorporated into their thinking and workflow.

Neuropsychological Assessments in Primary Care

Neuropsychological integration in primary care is being facilitated by healthcare payment reform in the United States. Medical treatment is moving from fee-for-service to new payment arrangements centered on value. The triple aim, as defined by organizations such as the Institute for Healthcare Improvement, is one way to express this new paradigm: improve the health of populations and the patient experience of care and control costs. Moving the focus to outcomes rather than processes opens avenues for multidisciplinary care, often delivered in teams, with each member contributing to improve the health of the patients according to their individual training and expertise. This new structure is often described in primary care using the term "patient-centered medical home" model of care. Neuropsychological assessments and the integration of behavioral health into primary care teams are increasing arrays of services brought to patients where they typically seek care most often [21]. This has increased both access for patients and awareness in the medical community of important tools and partnerships for improved care like the routine use of neuropsychological assessments.

Neuropsychological contributions to primary care can take various forms. Many neuropsychologists are beginning to work more directly with primary care teams, and some are embedded in primary care clinics across the country to provide cognitive assessment and treatment recommendations to improve patient's level of functioning and well-being [22].

As many primary care clinics are reorganizing to medical home models with increased emphasis on providing greater integration and efficiency of medical care, treatment decisions are increasingly made according to an approach called stepped care [23]. In stepped care, the selection of treatment is directed according to three fundamental principles [24]: (1) medical treatment should be individualized, not only with regard to the presenting problem but also taking into account patient's wishes and the treatment availabilities; (2) treatments selected should be consistent with the contemporary research outcomes; and (3) the recommended treatment should be the least restrictive one that is appropriate, as based in Bayesian logic. The result is that more extensive treatments are reserved for more extreme problems [25]. When the treatment is initiated, the patient's medical status is monitored. If the patient responds to the least invasive treatment, then treatment is maintained for as long as necessary, but if the patient's status remains the same or is declining, then a more intensive level of treatment is implemented. Hypertension, depression, and other chronic diseases are treated in primary care using this approach, with the addition of specialist consultation at the higher steps of care.

Key Point
Medical care is moving to value-based arrangements and seeking the "triple aim," which seeks to improve population health and patient experience and reduce costs. Stepped care is how neuropsychology and primary care interface.

Stepped care involves individualized and evidence-based treatments which involve moving from lower levels of intervention to higher levels based on systematic feedback. For many neuropsychologists, integrated primary care work takes place within the framework of stepped care. This neuropsychology stepped model of care has resulted in an increased menu of deliverables; that is, the creation of varied types of neuropsychological assessments ranging from consultation to more comprehensive assessments with intervention.

Step 0: As can be seen in Fig. 3.1, in the least invasive assessment (i.e., step 0 level of care), primary care teams provide cognitive/mood screenings. Cognitive screens are an important element in assessing cognition in a community. They are quick (5–10 minutes) and can be administered by multiple healthcare professionals and paraprofessionals (e.g., Mini-Cog). The purpose is to identify patients who have not yet sought medical attention for cognitive symptoms. There are many different kinds of cognitive screens (see [26], for a review), but ideal screens are brief, well tolerated, and easily scored. They should have sufficient psychometric properties to alert primary care physicians that cognitive problems might be afoot and that a referral to specialty care (e.g., neurology, neuropsychology, or psychiatry) might be necessary (e.g., [27]). Screening instruments such as the Montreal Cognitive Assessment (MoCA) have respectable sensitivity and specificity to be able to detect changes in cognition [28]. These screens, however, can produce high false-positive and false-negative error rates [26], so they are not diagnostic in and of themselves

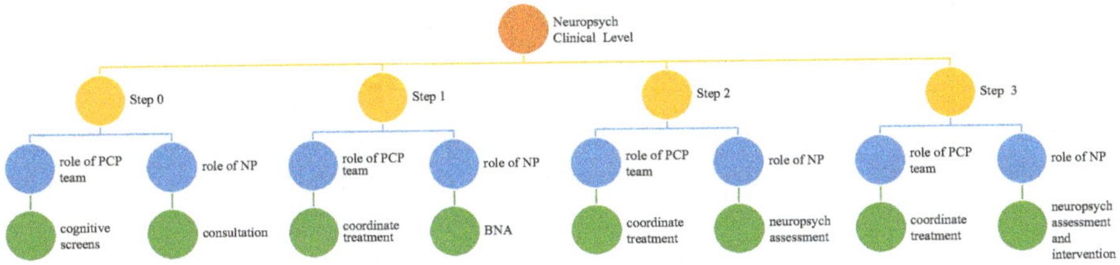

Fig. 3.1 Neuropsychological stepped model of care for neuropsychologists (NP) and primary care providers (PCP)

but rather serve as critical markers for potential further exploration [29, 30] define and delineate the scope of cognitive screening and how it is differentiated from cognitive testing and neuropsychological assessment. In Step 0 (as with the other steps), the primary responsibility for the patient is the PCP, and the role of the neuropsychologist (NP) is consultation, who can bring increased awareness of the cognitive deficits associated with chronic disease and better management when compensatory treatments and strategies are put into place for patients. Patient-administered symptom cognitive checklists, in conjunction with PCPs' own assessments of their patients, can raise concerns, and consultations can be sought in deriving next steps. If needed, increased neuropsychological intervention can then proceed from a consultation, to brief neuropsychological assessments, to more traditional neuropsychological assessments with or without intervention. The mere presence of neuropsychologists in primary care can raise awareness of the prevalence of cognitive dysfunction and often stimulates higher screening rates for vulnerable populations. An example of this step would be a patient who has just failed a Mini-Cog test but whose history and description of memory complaints seem relatively minor and appears discrepant with the screen outcome.

Step 1: The next level of cognitive evaluation is a brief neurocognitive assessment (BNA; [31]). Brief Neurocognitive Assessments can be especially suitable in primary care settings to offer a brief evaluation of cognitive abilities and emotional functioning. They are distinct from cognitive screens in that they require a longer appointment (typically 60–90 minutes) and tests are administered by a neuropsychological expert, trained to diagnose and make specific treatment recommendations. A BNA involves the use of fewer neuropsychological tests and targets specific referral questions (e.g., AD/HD, dementia) that can be addressed in a short period of time. The interview, testing, and feedback portions of the evaluation occur during the same appointment. BNAs are not meant to replace existing cognitive screens or neuropsychological evaluations; rather they target an intermediate stepped level of care (Step 1) between a comprehensive neuropsychological assessment and a cognitive screen. An example of Step 1 is a young adult patient who is having an increased trouble keeping up with coursework while in college. Symptoms may include distractibility, lack of focus, and memory problems. Routine drug and alcohol use have to be identified and stopped prior to evaluation, and the patient should screen negative and either be ruled out or optimally treated for depression and other additional confounders. The result of the BNA is frequently sufficient in this instance to rule in or out AD/HD and identify other kinds of cognitive dysfunction, such as executive dysfunction disorder. Appropriate strategies and/or psychopharmacologic treatment can then be put in place to improve functioning at home and/or in the school setting.

Step 2: The most comprehensive assessment typically requires a traditional neuropsychological evaluation (typically lasting 2–3 h), which integrates cognitive testing findings with an assessment of mood and biopsychosocial information gleaned from a detailed clinical interview. Conclusions are drawn from this biopsychosocial perspective, taking into account medical, psychiatric, and behavioral sources of information to inform diagnoses and provide treatment recommendations (e.g., medical, psychiatric, cognitive, adaptive functioning). Typically, the neuropsychologist provides feedback to patients and discusses treatment recommendations. Some patients referred for a comprehensive neuropsychological evaluation may have already completed a BNA; for example, a patient who screened positive for possible dementia in a BNA may be referred for a more comprehensive neuropsychological assessment to determine the scope and diagnostic specification of dementia subtype. Other CNS conditions such as multiple sclerosis, Parkinson's, seizures, and normal pressure hydrocephalus, to name a few, typically benefit from a comprehensive neuropsychological evaluation to identify the extent of cognitive deficits, especially if the CNS disease is complicated by other medical or psychiatric conditions and the patient has never before been cognitively evaluated.

Step 3: In some settings and for certain conditions, the neuropsychologist will also provide treatment interventions such as cognitive remediation. Cognitive remediation can be used to increase medication compliance, for example, or assist the patient to improve his/her level of functioning. For example, an AD/HD patient can be trained on executive function strategies to improve planning, efficiency, inattention, and distractibility. A schizophrenic patient can be trained on techniques to improve problem-solving, planning, and memory, which are typically affected by the illness. A patient with early dementia can be trained on strategies to improve and/or compensate for memory problems. This remediation problem is individually designed based on the patient's own cognitive profile.

Key Point

Steps 0–3 are the different levels of diagnosis and intervention in the stepped care model. Each step depends on systematic feedback about the state of the patient over time, and steps are taken sequentially when there is little or no improvement, although patients can start at any step based on their individualized needs.

Key Point
Cognitive assessments and interventions are an essential part of managing chronic disease in primary care, and the patient-centered medical home model welcomes these additional tools and expertise in the treatment of chronic disease.

Conclusions

The field of neuropsychology has developed its scope of practice in the last century and is currently making inroads in primary care as the importance of cognition in physical and mental health is increasingly acknowledged. The merging of neuropsychology and primary care has both theoretical and practice compatibility. The methodological similarities between primary care practitioners and neuropsychologists make their collaboration fluid. Primary care clinicians intuitively incorporate neuropsychological testing approaches into their diagnostic and treatment decisions because the Bayesian process used is identical to their own practice. Indeed, test results fit into the well-worn pattern of evaluation that primary care teams are adept at using in the ongoing care of their patients. Regardless of the level of care a patient receives from a neuropsychologist team member, the process of using neurocognitive evaluations in primary care involves combining the patient history, symptoms, and laboratory and testing results to reach a diagnostic conclusion. Once a satisfactory diagnosis has been established, treatment is initiated by the PCP and monitored and evaluated for efficacy in the primary care setting. Neuropsychologists become a team member in caring for patients, with their range of BNA and evaluations serving as both a baseline for cognitive health and stability and a "vital sign" that should be monitored regularly. With the integration of neuropsychologists into primary care, patients receive a range of cognitive assessments (e.g., screens, diagnostic tests, treatment recommendations, and direct interventions), all without having to navigate the specialty care medical system, making treatment more efficient and cost-effective.

Key Point
Cognition could be considered the sixth vital sign and has relevance across multiple chronic disease states.

Ultimately, cognition could be considered as the sixth vital sign in primary care (if pain is considered the fifth) where there is ongoing monitoring of cognitive health and, if needed, increased level of cognitive evaluations. Primary care clinics are no longer filled with acute illness amenable to a short course of antibiotics. Patients are living longer and healthier lives but are also living decades longer with chronic diseases. Chronic diseases impose a high burden on the patient to continually monitor, assess, and treat conditions outside of the medical arena. It is no surprise, therefore, that those with even mild cognitive deficits might be less successful in controlling the course of their illness, such that intact cognition is of critical import in maintaining health. As dictated by the triple aim, the integration of cognitive monitoring with biologic disease and psychiatric disorders can result in higher quality, patient-centered, lower cost care for patients with illnesses.

Chapter Review Questions

1. What are some of the reasons medical providers refer patients for neuropsychological testing?
   A. Diagnosis, treatment, and educational evaluations.
   B. Forensic, treatment, and bloodwork.
   C. Educational and treatment only.
2. True/False: Only diseases with direct CNS involvement affect cognition.
3. True/False: All neuropsychological referrals in primary care initially require a brief neuropsychological assessment before more comprehensive neuropsychological evaluation is undertaken undertaken.
4. True/False: Bayesian approaches to brain function investigate the capacity of the nervous system to operate in situations of uncertainty uncertainty.
5. In a Step 3 model of neuropsychological care:
   A. Patients are provided with a brief neuropsychological assessment.
   B. Patients are provided with a comprehensive neuropsychological assessment only.
   C. Patients are provided with cognitive intervention and treatment.
   D. All of the above.

References

1. Lezak MD, Howiesen DB, Loring DW. Neuropsychological assessment. 4th ed. Oxford: Oxford University Press; 2004.
2. Heilbronner RL, Pliskin NH. Clinical neuropsychology in the forensic arena. In: Prigatano GP, Pliskin NH, editors. Clinical neuropsychology and cost outcome research: a beginning. New York: Psychology Press; 2003.
3. Seidman LJ, Kremen WS, Koren D, Faraone SV, Goldstein JM, Tsuang MT. A comparative profile analysis of neuropsychological functioning in patients with schizophrenia and bipolar psychoses. Schizophrenia Res. 2002;53:31–44.

4. Elliott. The neuropsychological profile of unipolar depression. Trends Cogn Sci. 1998;2(11): 447–54.
5. Haman A, Ardal G. Cognitive functioning in major depression: a summary. Front Hum Neurosci. 2009;3(26):1–7.
6. Rogers MA, Kasai K, Koji M, Fukuda R, Iwanami A, Nakagome K, Fukuda M, Nobumasa K. Executive and prefrontal dysfunction in unipolar depression: a review of neuropsychological and imaging evidence. Neurosci Res. 2004;50:1–11.
7. Tarter RE, Edwards KL, VanThiel DH. Perspective and rational for neuropsychological assessment of medical disease. In: Tarter RE, VanThiel DH, Edwards KL, editors. Medical neuropsychology: the impact of disease on behavior. New York: Plenum Press; 1988.
8. Dunleavy RA, Baade LE. Neuropsychological correlates of severe asthma in children 9 to 14 years old. J Consult Clin Psychol. 1980;48:214–9.
9. Tarter RE, Butters R, Beers SR, editors. Medical neuropsychology. New York: Kluwer Academic/Plenum Publishers; 2001.
10. Lazare A, Putnam SM, Lipkin M Jr. Three functions of the medical interview. In: Lipkin Jr M, Putnam SM, Lazare A, editors. The medical interview: clinical care, education, and research. New York, NY: Springer; 1995. p. 3–19.
11. Jaynes ET. Probability theory: the logic of science. Cambridge: Cambridge University Press; 2003.
12. Neff MJ. ACEP releases clinical policy on evaluation and management of pulmonary embolism. Am Fam Physician. 2003;68(4):759–60.
13. Doya K, Ishii S, Pouget A, Rao RPN. Bayesian brain: probabilistic approaches to neural coding. Cambridge, MA: The MIT Press; 2007.
14. Knill D, Pouget A. The Bayesian brain: the role of uncertainty in neural coding and computation. Trends Neurosci. 2004;27(12):712–9.
15. Scott M, Gelhot A. Gastroesophageal reflux disease: diagnosis and management. Am Fam Physician. 1999;59(5):1161–9.
16. American Psychiatric Association. Collaboration between psychiatrists, primary docs vital to ensuring more people get mental healthcare. Psychiatric News. 1998.
17. American Psychiatric Association. Diagnostic and statistical manual of mental disorders: DSM-V. Washington, DC: American Psychiatric Association; 2013.
18. WHO Mental Health Action Plan 2013–2020. World Health Organization. 2013. http://apps.who.int/iris/bitstream/10665/89966/1/9789241506021_eng.pdf
19. Frederick R, Bowden S. The test validation summary. Assessment. 2009;16(3):215–36.
20. Bowden SC, Loring DW. The diagnostic utility of multiple-level likelihood ratios. J Int Neuropsychol Soc. 2009;15(5):769–76.
21. Hunkeler W, Katon L, Tang JW, Williams K, Kroenke E, Lin HB, Harpole LH, Arean P, Levine S, Grypma LM, Hargreaves WA, Unützer J. Long term outcomes from the IMPACT randomised trial for depressed elderly patients in primary care. Br Med J. 2006;332:259.
22. Mercury MG, Kehoe BA, Tshan MA. Neuropsychology for the PCP. Disease-a-Month. 2007;53:138–41.
23. Abrams DB. Treatment issues in tobacco dependence: towards a stepped-care model. Tobacco Control. 1993;2(Suppl):S17–37.
24. Sobell MB, Sobell LC. Stepped care for alcohol problems: An efficient method for planning and delivering clinical services. In: Tucker JA, Donovan DA, Marlatt GA, editors. Changing addictive behavior. Bridging clinical and public health strategies. New York: Guilford Press; 1999. p. 331–43.
25. Sobell MB, Sobell LC. Stepped care as a heuristic approach to the treatment of alcohol problems. J Consult Clin Psychol. 2000;68:573–9.
26. Mitrushina MN. Cognitive screening methods. In: Grant I, Adams M, editors. Neuropsychological assessment of neuropsychiatric and neuromedical disorders. 3rd ed. New York: Oxford University Press; 2009.

27. Ebell MH. Brief screening instruments for dementia in primary care. Am Fam Physician. 2009;79(6):497–8, 500.
28. Nasreddine ZS, Phillips NA, Bédirian V, Charbonneau S, Whitehead V, Collin I, Cummings JL, Chertkow H. The montreal cognitive assessment, MoCA: a brief screening tool for mild cognitive impairment. J Am Geriatr Soc. 2005;53(4):695–9.
29. Roebuck-Spencer T, Glen T, Puente A, Denney RM, Ruff R, Hostetter GJ, Bianchini K. Cognitive screening tests versus comprehensive neuropsychological test batteries: a National Academy of Neuropsychology Education paper. Arch Clin Neuropsychol. 2017;32:1–8.
30. Block, CK, Johnson-Green, D, Pliskin N. Boake, C. Discriminating cognitive screening and cognitive testing from neuropsychological assessment: implications for professional practice. The clin Neuropsychol. 2017; 31(3): 487–500.
31. Lanca, M. Integration of neuropsychology in primary care. Clin Neuropsychologist. 2017 (in press).

Chapter 4
Psychometrics of Assessment: Understanding What Neuropsychology Adds to the Physician's Understanding of the Patient

Mike R. Schoenberg, Jason R. Soble, and Katie E. Osborn

What Is Neuropsychology and What Can the Physician Gain from a Neuropsychological Study?

To briefly review, neuropsychology is a scientific subspecialty of clinical psychology focused on the study of brain-behavior relationships. Neuropsychologists are subspecialists who hold a doctoral degree in psychology and have also undergone specialized training in the clinical neurosciences. They incorporate knowledge from functional neuroanatomy, neuropathology, behavioral neurology, psychometrics, psychology, and psychiatry to assess and treat the neurocognitive, behavioral, and affective correlates of known or suspected neurological dysfunction. Evaluations provide crucial information for guiding patient care, with the types of questions answerable by a neuropsychologist generally falling into one of six categories (see [1], for a more expansive review):

M. R. Schoenberg (✉)
Department of Neurosurgery and Brain Repair, University of South Florida Morsani College of Medicine, Tampa, FL, USA
e-mail: mschoenb@health.usf.edu

J. R. Soble
Department of Psychiatry, Department of Neurology, University of Illinois College of Medicine, Chicago, IL, USA
e-mail: soble@uic.edu

K. E. Osborn
Vanderbilt University Medical Center, Nashville, TN, USA

K. M. Sanders (ed.), *Physician's Field Guide to Neuropsychology*,
https://doi.org/10.1007/978-1-4939-8722-1_4

Referral domain	Example referral questions
Diagnostic clarification, including differentiating neurodegenerative disease processes from psychiatric or otherwise reversible etiologies (e.g., depression, medication-based neurotoxic effects, normal age-related memory declines, etc.)	"Are the patient's memory problems suggestive of Alzheimer's disease or more characteristic of some other underlying cognitive/psychiatric dysfunction?"
Detailed assessment of the extent to which a disease or lesion is affecting cognitive, behavioral, and/or affective functioning	"What are the severity and specific nature of the patient's cognitive deficits resulting from a recent traumatic brain injury?"
Prognostic assessment and provision of treatment recommendations	"From a neurocognitive standpoint, is the patient expected to have a good outcome from temporal lobectomy for intractable epilepsy?" "From what sort of rehabilitation program(s) is the patient most likely to benefit in the context of a recent stroke?"
Identification of treatment effects and measurement of changes in functional status	"Has the child's individualized education plan (IEP) effectively addressed the academic problems associated with his/her learning disability?"
Data to test hypotheses for scientific research concerning central nervous system functioning	"Does investigational medication X result in any unknown cognitive, affective, or behavioral side effects?"
Forensic evaluations involving potential central nervous system dysfunction	"From a neurocognitive standpoint, is the defendant competent to stand trial?" "From a neurocognitive standpoint, is the defendant capable of managing financial affairs independently?"

The Underlying Rationale and Mechanics of a Neuropsychological Study

The practice of neuropsychology is not limited to the work of a clinical neuropsychologist. Indeed, physicians frequently assess aspects of cognitive status as a routine component of patient care. For instance, the completion of a neurological exam with basic mental status exam involves screening several neuropsychological functions. However, neuropsychological evaluations performed by a clinical neuropsychologist involve an in-depth, psychometrically based assessment that measures cognitive domains in more depth and breadth than is done in a routine mental status or neurological exam. An important component of this formal assessment process involves establishment of comparative standards for nomothetic and idiographic deficit measurements. In other words, a patient's performances on various tasks must be compared against benchmarks to allow the neuropsychologist to interpret whether deficits or strengths exist in relation to normative comparison standards (i.e., how the patient performs compared to others), as well as to individual comparison standards (i.e., how the patient's current performance compares to his/her own premorbid level of baseline functioning). The use of comparison standards is not unique to neuropsychology as species- and population-based comparison standards are used in a variety of laboratory and clinical tests throughout medicine. However, nuances in the application of these approaches to the measurement of neuropsychological deficits do carry some special considerations, which are discussed below.

Key Point

Neuropsychology is the science of brain-behavior relationships.

Neuropsychology measures brain function with behavior (e.g., learning/memory) using population-based normative (nomothetic) data.

Standardized Neuropsychological Assessment: How It Differs from Cognitive Screening

A neuropsychological evaluation differs from mental status exams and other cognitive testing in that it includes psychometrically derived data regarding the patient's neuropsychological functions, both in relation to performances of peers and to the individual's own premorbid level of functioning. Furthermore, the neuropsychologist draws from his/her specialized understanding of brain-behavior relationships to interpret findings in the context of neuropathological disease processes, functional neuroanatomy, and neuropsychological principals (see [1, 2] for reviews). In contrast, omnibus screening measures such as the Mini-Mental State Examination (MMSE) [3] and the Self-Administered Gerocognitive Examination (SAGE) [4], among others, have developed cutoff scores to identify when further evaluation is needed based on data to maximize sensitivity to identify the presence of neuropsychological deficits. Thus, falling below a cutoff score on a cognitive screener does not constitute evidence to warrant any particular diagnosis and does not typically provide data to identify the cause for a memory, attention, or language problem per se but instead indicates that further evaluation is needed to identify the likely cause(s) of cognitive dysfunction. Unlike cognitive screeners, neuropsychological evaluations provide specific and multifaceted findings across specific cognitive domains with regard to the exact nature and extent of the patient's neurocognitive dysfunction.

Normative Comparison Standards in Neuropsychology: Population-Based Norms

To illustrate the principle underlying deficit measurement in neuropsychological evaluations, consider how most laboratory tests in medicine are interpreted. In order to set laboratory ranges for what is considered normal versus abnormal, population studies are conducted to determine the normal distribution of values. Patients' laboratory values are then compared against these normally distributed comparison samples, and values are typically flagged as abnormal if they fall too far outside of the mean (typically two or more standard deviations). In some cases, value ranges are fairly consistent across all populations, so it is acceptable to incorporate all comparison sample values into a single distribution (i.e., species-specific comparison standards). An example of a species-specific standard in humans is development of language and bipedal gait. In other cases, it becomes necessary to develop population-specific comparison standards to account for relevant factors that may influence interpretation of findings (e.g., age, sex, etc.). For example, consider the maternal alpha-fetoprotein (AFP) test used to screen for potential fetal genetic abnormalities. Expected AFP levels vary based on several factors, including the mother's age and ethnicity, as well as the gestational age of the fetus. Accordingly, several specific population-based comparison standards must be developed in order for results to have any meaningful interpretive value in the context of each patient's unique demographic and gestational variables.

Neuropsychological tests follow similar normative procedures and assessment methods for comparisons, such that neuropsychological test scores typically follow a normal Gaussian distribution so neuropsychologists are able to compare each individual's performances to standardized comparison samples. Using the central limit theorem, it is possible to statistically calculate the exact position where each patient falls on the normal curve (i.e., the bell curve) for each score. As with the maternal AFP test example, a host of factors can influence expected performance ranges on neuropsychological measures [5]. For instance, premorbid cognitive abilities, age, education attainment, gender, ethnicity, and socioeconomic status are variables known to influence expected performance ranges for neuropsychological functioning.

Key Point

Neuropsychological tests vs. cognitive screen?

Neuropsychological tests are developed and normed to measure neurocognitive domains and can thus emphasize specificity for diagnosis.

Cognitive screens summarize cognitive function and emphasize sensitivity to identify a cognitive symptom.

Accordingly, careful considerations must be taken into account when developing and employing population-based comparison standards in order to produce the most accurate and clinically meaningful interpretations of scores.

Population-based normative samples are typically created from healthy peers who ideally approximate the patient in terms of relevant demographic factors. Thus, if a patient's score falls within two standard deviations of the sample mean, it suggests that the patient's performance is "normal" or within the expected range for a healthy, demographically matched sample. Conversely, if the patient's score falls outside the expected range of scores, an abnormal finding is obtained. From a statistical standpoint, this abnormal finding suggests it is highly unlikely (i.e., less than a 5% chance in the case of $p < 0.05$) that the patient's score is part of a healthy population. The patient's exclusion from the healthy population might be reflective of brain dysfunction, especially when clinical history, behavioral observations, and the patient exhibit concurrent clusters of neuropsychological deficits that correspond to functional neuroanatomical regions and known neuropathological disease processes. However, like other medical tests, it is important to rule out other explanations for abnormal scores, such as incorrect test administration, substandard collection of the data, poor patient cooperation, and/or feigning of symptoms. Neuropsychologists have developed sophisticated methods for detecting such confounding variables in neuropsychological measures that is discussed later in this section.

Key Point

Cut-off for cognitive impairment can differ to maximize sensitivity or specificity.

MMSE < 26 = potential deficit

MOCA < 26 = potential deficit

Individual Comparison Standards in Neuropsychology: Premorbid Ability Estimates

Population-based normative comparisons provide benchmarks for comparing a patient's performance to that of other, usually healthy, people. However, knowing a person's visual memory is at the seventh percentile (i.e., −1.5 SD below the mean) compared to a healthy population is not sufficient to determine that this score reflects a decline in the patient's memory. The individual may have had a weakness in visual memory since childhood. Even more difficult to determine is if the score obtained in your office was a decline greater than what might occur due to measurement error. Consider a 73-year-old male with history of hypertension and obstructive sleep apnea who presents to your office with concerns about his memory. You refer him for neuropsychological evaluation to determine if his memory problems are suggestive of Alzheimer's disease or due to normal age-related changes in memory. Upon testing, the neuropsychologist determines the man's verbal memory is at the 20th percentile relative to other healthy adults his age. Does this score constitute cause for concern? More data are required to answer this question, since this could reflect a normal score for some older adults but may indicate a dementia process for another patient that had a superior verbal memory (verbal memory at the 95th percentile). Thus, the interpretation of a verbal memory score at the 20th percentile is dependent on the neuropsychologist's ability to compare it to the patient's unique premorbid level of functioning (the individual comparison standard).

Comparison between current obtained scores and premorbid levels of ability would be most precise if a comparison of the current score could be made prior to neuropsychological test scores. Unfortunately, this is rarely (if ever) possible, and an estimate of premorbid neuropsychological functions of the individual is developed. The most common method for estimating premorbid functioning involves prediction of premorbid intelligence as a proxy of neuropsychological function because certain aspects of intelligence tend to be resistant to the effects of brain injury and aging. For example, tasks involving word recognition (word reading) and/or vocabulary knowledge and/or fund of information can be used to predict premorbid intellectual function in patients with known or suspected brain injuries, even among individuals with moderate to severe traumatic brain injuries and dementia. These predictors of premorbid intellectual function can be combined with individual demographic variables (e.g., educational attainment, vocational attainment, age, etc.) to improve accuracy of premorbid estimates for both adults and children with known or suspected neurological dysfunction [1, 6–10].

Key Point
Interpretation of neuropsychological abnormal lab values may be altered by premorbid factors:

A memory score at the 14th percentile may be entirely normal for a 70-year-old with 9 years of education, whereas this same score may be abnormal and suggestive of a neurodegenerative process for a 70-year physician.

Detecting Suboptimal Task Engagement: Performance Validity Tests (PVTs)

Another key element that differentiates cognitive screeners from neuropsychological evaluations is the administration of formal performance validity tests (PVTs) as a component of the latter to determine the reliability and validity of the obtained data [11]. Colloquially termed "effort measures," PVTs are integral to the neuropsychological evaluation because of the multitude of external/volitional (i.e., malingering, symptom exaggeration) and other extra-test variables (e.g., defensive or hostile test-taking approach, fatigue) that can influence a patient's approach to cognitive tests and potentially result in inadequate or inconsistent test engagement [12]. While a discussion of all available PVTs is beyond the scope of this chapter (see [13]), for a review), PVTs have been developed to be administered as a separate test or developed from other scores obtained from other tests. Although various algorithms have been proposed for detecting noncredible cognitive test performance, it has been recommended that noncredible test performance be determined on the basis of failures on at least two well-validated PVTs with strong psychometric properties (i.e., good specificity, minimal shared variance) in conjunction with behavioral evidence rather than relying on singular measures as a standard of practice [13, 14]. While assessment of performance validity may increase the time and cost of assessment, inclusion of PVTs in assessment has been found to be critical aspects of assessment [15]. Cognitive screening instruments do not include PVTs and thus limit the determination that an *impaired* score indicates actual neurocognitive deficits or is due to unreliable responding to the test.

Key Point

PVT = performance validity test. A test designed to measure validity on neurocognitive tests.

SVT = symptom validity test. A test designed to measure test validity on psychological tests.

Key Point

Effort/performance validity is important.

Effort accounts for more variance in neuropsychological test scores than severe traumatic brain injury or dementia.

Deconstructing and Understanding the Neuropsychological Study Report

A detailed discussion of all components of the neuropsychological report is beyond the scope of this chapter (see [16] and Chap. 3 in this text for greater detail); however, a few interpretive and psychometric issues are particularly salient.

1. Most reports will commonly assess the major domains of general cognitive functioning (intellectual function), processing speed, attention/executive, language, memory, and visuoconstructional functions along with mood/behavioral problems. Some studies will also assess sensory functions, particularly evaluating for hemi-inattention and hemi-neglect as well as psychomotor speed. Assessment of mood/behavioral problems will vary between adult and children but typically reflect assessment for depression, anxiety, and suicidal risk and evaluation of

psychosis. Within these domains, the interpretative process involves assigning a classification level to obtained test scores. Common classification descriptors include "Superior," "High Average," "Average," "Low Average," "Borderline," and "Impaired"(or "Extremely Low") that correspond to prescribed standard score and percentile ranges. Other qualitative descriptors of neuropsychological laboratory values include "within normal limits" (WNL), "above or below average" (i.e., above or below expectation), or "intact versus deficient." Regrettably, a universal reporting format does not exist [17]) with varying classification systems in use [18–21] and another recently proposed [22]. Thus, the criterion for determining impairment can vary among neuropsychologists.

2. Interpretation frequently involves examining profiles or patterns of scores to determine normality or abnormality as opposed to inferring this from single scores, which are subject to error variance and may not accurately represent the intended behavior [23]. Moreover, it is common for normal individuals to show a certain degree of scatter/variability that increases with the number of tests administered [24]. For instance, 67% of a cognitive healthy community-dwelling sample had discrepancies of three or more standard deviations between their highest and lowest neuropsychological scores on a battery of 21 tests [25]. Consequently, because relying on single scores can potentially over-pathologize a patient's performance and misinform conclusions, neuropsychological interpretation involves formulation of conclusions through careful analysis of overall score patterns, as well as relative score comparisons between domains.

Key Point

Low scores happen! One or two low scores should not be interpreted in isolation.

Variation in neuropsychological abilities is common in healthy people.

Beyond Localizing Lesions: What Neuropsychology Adds to Neuroradiology

Much has changed over the past 50 years in neuropsychology to expand the field beyond its initial focus of using behavioral data to lateralize and localize brain lesions. Once the cornerstone of their professional identity, neuropsychologists' roles in localizing neuropathology and seizure foci through pencil and paper measures have been substantially reduced in recent years due to technological advances in neuroimaging techniques. Even the Wada test, used to confirm language and memory lateralization prior to surgical treatment of epilepsy, is becoming phased out by less invasive clinical functional magnetic resonance imaging (fMRI) paradigms [26–28]. Despite these advances, neuroradiology has not reduced the need for neuropsychologists as members of healthcare teams. Quite to the contrary, neuropsychologists are serving more active roles to evaluate the extent, severity, course, and prognosis for known or suspected dysfunction of the brain due to direct injury to the CNS or secondarily due to systemic illness of other body organs/tissues or medications that affect the function of the brain.

Key Point
History + neuropathology = accuracy

Interpretation should be based on clinical history combined with known neuropathology and functional neuroanatomy and NOT based on neuropsychological test scores alone.

Neuropsychological examination contributes valuable diagnostic information for a variety of conditions involving cognitive and behavioral dysfunction, including but not limited to mild cognitive impairment (MCI) and dementia, mild traumatic brain injury (mTBI), toxic encephalopathies, and intellectual and learning disabilities. In other cases, the etiology for the brain dysfunction is known, but neuropsychological assessment establishes the extent and severity the known lesion(s) affect neuropsychological functions (e.g., moderate to severe traumatic brain injury, stroke, multiple sclerosis, epilepsy, etc.). Individual variability in functional neuroanatomy, neuroplasticity, and individual disease characteristics limit the value of other data about central nervous system abnormalities (e.g., neuroradiology) in inferring extent and nature of cognitive and behavioral dysfunction. For instance, symptom presentations can vary substantially from patient to patient following anatomically similar left hemisphere middle cerebral artery strokes (see [1, 2] for reviews). To this end, neuropsychological evaluation provides the only means for obtaining objective, quantified information about patients' capacities for engaging in self-care, following medical recommendations, or completing instrumental activities of daily living (IADLs). Neuropsychological evaluations are also able to predict disease progression, surgical outcome, and response to treatment or determine appropriate placement for cognitive, vocational, or occupational programs. The neuropsychological study provides unique predictive power beyond that obtained through neuroradiology and other clinical variables in multiple clinical contexts, such as TBI [29, 30], multiple sclerosis [31–33], Parkinson's disease [34], mild cognitive impairment [35], and surgical treatment for pharmacoresistant epilepsy [36–39].

Key Point
Neuroradiology is not sufficient to measure function.

Neuropsychology quantitatively measures cognition and behaviors, which is necessary to diagnose conditions in which change in functional status is needed.

Looking Ahead: Current Uses and Evidence Base for Computerized Neurocognitive Testing

Over the past two decades, computerized neurocognitive testing has become an increasingly popular tool, especially for the detection and management of sport-related concussion and detection of CNS effects of medications, as screening measures in pilot evaluations for the Federal Aviation Agency, and to evaluate neurocognitive status in settings in which formal in-person assessments are not possible [40, 41]. Individual computerized neurocognitive tests vary considerably both in terms of administration format (e.g., fully examiner-administered to self-administered) as well as scope (e.g., computerized version of a single traditional neuropsychological test vs. integrated batteries) [42, 43]. In general, increasing scientific evidence has been accumulating over recent years regarding the psychometric properties, accuracy, and clinical utility of specific computerized neurocognitive instruments with a multitude of clinical populations [42]. While a full review of computerized testing is beyond this chapter's scope, some common uses are outlined below to highlight the varied utility of computerized testing across settings, populations, and purposes. The reader is also referred to Wild et al. [43] for a systematic review of several available computerized batteries as well as the NIH Toolbox (www.nihtoolbox.org), which contains many royalty-free, computerized neurocognitive measures.

Computerized testing has a long history within the Department of Defense (DoD) and resulted in the development of the Automated Neuropsychological Assessment Metrics (ANAM) [44, 45], which allows for serial post-injury assessment and comparison to pre-deployment baseline testing for service members who sustained a concussion/TBI [46]. The ANAM Readiness Evaluation System (ARES) is an adaptation for handheld personal digital assistants (PDAs) that permits portable field assessment with minimal equipment needs [47]. ANAM tests also have been used in clinical trials to measure pharmacological treatment effects, such as subtle cognitive side effects or enhancement [48]. Computerized screening batteries also have demonstrated utility in differentiating controls from those with mild cognitive impairment (MCI) and dementia [49], as well as documenting cognitive outcomes following intervention [50]. Lastly, computerized testing has been widely used in sport-related concussion management to increase diagnostic accuracy and determine return to play [51, 52].

Many practical reasons exist for the use of computerized cognitive batteries, including conveniences associated with being able to administer baseline assessments to many individuals at once, minimizing error due to variations in administration procedures, ability to assess in dangerous environments, and capability to obtain scores to make a clinical decision quickly [53]. Nonetheless, while there are advantages to computerized cognitive batteries, these tests also have limitations both to their use and their interpretation. First, administration and score validity can be adversely affected by use of different computer operating systems, software required to run the programs, and hardware-to-software errors [54]. Second, the interpretation of rapid binary computer-based interpretation of scores using algorithms requires a knowledge of the tests' psychometric properties and limitations [55], as well as of brain-behavior relationships and the multitude of factors that can influence performance. A computerized version of an existing neuropsychological test also should be treated as a *new test* without assumption that the normative data derived from the examiner-administered test apply equally given the adaptation in administration. Rather, new normative data that consider key demographic and cultural factors should be developed [42]. Given these potential limitations, a thorough, systematic assessment of any computerized neurocognitive testing battery should occur prior to clinical implementation (see [56] for a quality assessment framework).

Key Point
When selecting a computerized neurocognitive testing battery, it is important to make sure that the computerized test battery and accompanying normative data are appropriate for the referral population being tested.

As the development and implementation of computerized cognitive tests become increasingly commonplace, federal regulatory guidelines will likely adapt to include tighter legal requirements for the marketing and use of these tools [42]. The Federal Food, Drug & Cosmetic Act Section 201(h) defines a medical device in the following manner: "an instrument, apparatus, implement, machine, contrivance, implant, in vitro reagent, or other similar or related article, including a component part, or accessory which is…intended for use in the diagnosis of disease or other conditions…" (FD&C; 21 U.S.C. 301). Given this definition, computerized cognitive tests theoretically fall under the FDA's regulatory purview. Accordingly, legal/regulatory issues will need to be increasingly considered along with issues related to the scientific evidence base and clinical appropriateness of these tools.

Summary

Neuropsychology is a scientific subspecialty of clinical psychology focused on the study of brain-behavior relationships. Neuropsychologists perform psychometrically based assessments that measure cognitive domains in more depth and breadth than is done in a mental status or neurological exam, and they interpret findings in the context of their training and expertise in the study of how neurological dysfunction influences cognitive abilities and behavior. Neuropsychological examination contributes valuable diagnostic information for a variety of clinical contexts and referral questions, such as potential mild cognitive impairment (MCI) and dementia, mild traumatic brain injury (mTBI), toxic encephalopathies, and intellectual and learning disabilities. Sometimes, the etiology for a brain dysfunction is known, but neuropsychological assessment helps elucidate the extent of functional decline from baseline in order to develop an accurate prognosis and appropriate treatment/rehabilitation recommendations.

This formal assessment process requires establishment of comparative standards for nomothetic and idiographic deficit measurements. Species-specific comparison standards are sometimes used, especially for more rudimentary aspects of a neurobehavioral status examination, but neuropsychologists more often employ population-specific normative standards in order to account for various factors known to influence neuropsychological performance (e.g., age, sex, education, etc.). Beyond these nomothetic comparisons, idiographic deficit measurements are also performed by comparing a patient's performance to his or her baseline level of functioning. Because actual baseline neuropsychological scores are rarely ever available, neuropsychologists have developed methods for estimating premorbid functioning, which typically involve some combination of evaluating "hold" measures known to be resistant to decline in brain injury/neurological insult, reviewing available academic and/or employment records, and accounting for demographic factors known to be associated with neuropsychological performance levels.

Another integral component of the neuropsychological evaluation process is the administration of formal performance validity tests (PVTs) to determine the reliability and validity of the obtained data. In this way, neuropsychologists are able to assess the degree to which a variety of external/volitional (i.e., malingering, symptom exaggeration) and other extra-test variables (e.g., defensive or hostile test-taking approach, fatigue) may have influenced a patient's observed test scores and performance patterns.

Over the past two decades, computerized neurocognitive testing has become an increasingly popular tool. Many practical reasons exist for the use of computerized cognitive batteries, but limitations are also present with regard to both their use and interpretation. Most importantly, results must be interpreted by an expert with knowledge of the tests' psychometric properties and limitations, as well as of the multitude of factors, neurocognitive-based and otherwise, that can influence performance.

Chapter Review Questions

1. A 69-year-old female is referred to her PCP for memory problems and increasing dysnomia. You complete a mental status examination and neurological examination on the patient and find an MMSE score of 24 and a nonfocal neurological exam. The patient medical history is positive for active problems of hypertension, hyperlipidemia, and Type II diabetes that is well controlled. A neuropsychological evaluation:
   A. Indicated in this case to better describe the extent and severity of cognitive deficits.
   B. Not indicated in this case since the MMSE score is below cutoff and indicates a "dementia."

   C. Indicated in this case to obtain a structural evaluation of the patient's brain.
   D. Not indicated in this case because the MMSE score was above cutoff and indicates no "dementia."

2. Neuropsychological assessments use tests that are normed against a reference sample. Comparison of test scores to this normative sample results in standardized scores that describe how rare or unusual a score is in relation to a demographically similar healthy population. This is called a:
   A. Species-specific comparison standard.
   B. Population-based comparison standard.
   C. Medical logic-based standard.
   D. Individual comparison standard.

3. A retired physician was referred by his neurologist for a neuropsychological evaluation following complaints of short-term memory problems, increasingly frequent incidents of getting lost in familiar settings, and evidence on MRI of hippocampal atrophy. Neuropsychological evaluation reveals the patient's verbal memory performance is in the eighth percentile relative to demographically similar peers. This performance level:
   A. Is definitely considered "abnormal," given the patient's high premorbid educational achievement level.
   B. Is definitely considered "normal," as it falls within 1.5 standard deviations of demographically similar peers.
   C. Depends; must be interpreted in the context of species-specific comparisons.
   D. Depends; must be interpreted in the context of the patient's estimated premorbid functioning level.

References

1. Lezak MD, Howieson DB, Loring DW. Neuropsychological assessment. 4th ed. New York: Oxford University Press; 2004.
2. Heilman KM, Valenstein E. Clinical Neuropsychology. New York: Oxford University Press; 2003.
3. Folstein MF, Folstein SE, Mchugh PR. "Mini-mental state". A practical method for grading the cognitive state of patients for the clinician. J Psychiatr Res. 1975;12(3):189–98.
4. Scharre DW, Chang SI, Murden RA, et al. Self-administered Gerocognitive Examination (SAGE): a brief cognitive assessment Instrument for mild cognitive impairment (MCI) and early dementia. Alzheimer Dis Assoc Disord. 2010;24(1):64–71.
5. Smith GE, Ivnik RJ, Lucas J. Assessment techniques: tests, test batteries, norms and methodological approaches. In: Morgan JE, Ricker JH, editors. Textbook of clinical neuropsychology. New York: Taylor & Francis; 2008. p. 38–57.
6. Axelrod BN, Vanderploeg RD, Schinka JA. Comparing methods for estimating premorbid intellectual functioning. Arch Clin Neuropsychol. 1999;14(4):341–6.
7. Schoenberg MR, Duff K, Scott JG, Adams RL. An evaluation of the clinical utility of the OPIE-3 as an estimate of premorbid WAIS-III FSIQ. Clin Neuropsychol. 2003;17(3):308–21.

8. Schoenberg MR, Duff K, Dorfman K, Adams RL. Differential estimation of verbal intelligence and performance intelligence scores from combined performance and demographic variables: the OPIE-3 verbal and performance algorithms. Clin Neuropsychol. 2004;18(2):266–76.
9. Schoenberg MR, Lange RT, Saklofske DH, Suarez M, Brickell TA. Validation of the child premorbid intelligence estimate method to predict premorbid Wechsler Intelligence Scale for Children-Fourth Edition Full Scale IQ among children with brain injury. Psychol Assess. 2008;20(4):377–84.
10. Strauss E, Sherman EM, Spreen O. A compendium of neuropsychological tests, administration, norms, and commentary. 3rd ed. New York: Oxford University Press; 2006.
11. Heilbronner RL, Sweet JJ, Morgan JE, Larrabee GJ, Millis SR. American Academy of Clinical Neuropsychology Consensus Conference Statement on the neuropsychological assessment of effort, response bias, and malingering. Clin Neuropsychol. 2009;23(7):1093–129.
12. Slick DJ, Sherman EM, Iverson GL. Diagnostic criteria for malingered neurocognitive dysfunction: proposed standards for clinical practice and research. Clin Neuropsychol. 1999;13(4):545–61.
13. Boone KB. Assessment of feigned cognitive impairment: a neuropsychological perspective. New York: Guilford; 2007.
14. Boone KB. A reconsideration of the Slick et al. (1999) criteria for malingered neurocognitive dysfunction. In: Boone KB, editor. Assessment of feigned cognitive impairment: a neuropsychological perspective. New York: Guilford; 2007. p. 29–49.
15. Meyers JE, Volbrecht M, Axelrod BN, Reinsch-boothby L. Embedded symptom validity tests and overall neuropsychological test performance. Arch Clin Neuropsychol. 2011;26(1):8–15.
16. Schoenberg MR, Scott JG. The Little Black book of neuropsychology: a syndrome-based approach. New York: Springer; 2011.
17. American Academy of Clinical Neuropsychology (AACN) practice guidelines for neuropsychological assessment and consultation. Clin Neuropsychol. 2007;21(2):209–31.
18. Groth-Marnat G. Handbook of psychological assessment. Hoboken, NJ: John Wiley & Sons; 2009.
19. Heaton RK, Grant I, Matthews CG. Comprehensive norms for an expanded Halstead-Reitan Battery: demographic corrections, research findings, and clinical applications. Odessa, FL: Psychological Assessment Resources; 1991.
20. Schretlen DJ, Testa SM, Pearlson GD. Hopkins neuropsychological normative system professional manual. Lutz, FL: Psychological Assessment Resources; 2010.
21. Wechsler D. Wechsler Adult Intelligence Scale-revised. New York: The Psychological Corporation; 1981.
22. Schoengerg MR. Towards reporting standards for neuropsychological study results: a proposal to minimize communication errors with standard qualitative score descriptors. Clin Neurol Neurosurg. 2017;162:72–9.
23. Hannay HJ, Lezak MD. The neuropsychological examination: Interpretation. In M. D. Lezak Howieson DB, Loring DW, eds. Neuropsychological assessment. 4th. New York: Oxford University Press; 2004:133–156.
24. Schretlen DJ, Testa SM, Winicki JM, Pearlson GD, Gordon B. Frequency and bases of abnormal performance by healthy adults on neuropsychological testing. J Int Neuropsychol Soc. 2008;14(3):436–45.
25. Donnell AJ, Belanger HG, Vanderploeg RD. Implications of psychometric measurement for neuropsychological interpretation. Clin Neuropsychol. 2011;25(7):1097–118.
26. Baxendale S, Thompson P. Beyond localization: the role of traditional neuropsychological tests in an age of imaging. Epilepsia. 2010;51(11):2225–30.
27. Baxendale S, Thompson PJ, Duncan JS. The role of the Wada test in the surgical treatment of temporal lobe epilepsy: an international survey. Epilepsia. 2008;49(4):715–20.
28. Duncan J. The current status of neuroimaging for epilepsy. Curr Opin Neurol. 2009; 22(2):179–84.

29. Sherer M, Novack TA, Sander AM, Struchen MA, Alderson A, Thompson RN. Neuropsychological assessment and employment outcome after traumatic brain injury: a review. Clin Neuropsychol. 2002;16(2):157–78.
30. Whyte J, Cifu D, Dikmen S, Temkin N. Prediction of functional outcomes after traumatic brain injury: a comparison of 2 measures of duration of unconsciousness. Arch Phys Med Rehabil. 2001;82(10):1355–9.
31. Achiron A, Polliack M, Rao SM, et al. Cognitive patterns and progression in multiple sclerosis: construction and validation of percentile curves. J Neurol Neurosurg Psychiatry. 2005;76(5):744–9.
32. Chelune GJ. Evidence-based research and practice in clinical neuropsychology. Clin Neuropsychol. 2010;24(3):454–67.
33. Chelune GJ, Stone L. Risk of processing speed deficits among patients with relapsing and remitting and secondary progressive multiple sclerosis. J Clin Exp Neuropsychol. 2005;11:52.
34. Dujardin K, Defebvre L, Duhamel A, et al. Cognitive and SPECT characteristics predict progression of Parkinson's disease in newly diagnosed patients. J Neurol. 2004; 251(11):1383–92.
35. Fleisher AS, Sun S, Taylor C, et al. Volumetric MRI vs. clinical predictors of Alzheimer disease in mild cognitive impairment. Neurology. 2008;70(3):191–9.
36. Chelune GJ. Hippocampal adequacy versus functional reserve: predicting memory functions following temporal lobectomy. Arch Clin Neuropsychol. 1995;10(5):413–32.
37. Chelune GJ, Najam I. Risk factors associated with postsurgical decrements in memory. In: Luders HO, Comair Y, editors. Epilepsy surgery. 2nd ed. New York, NY: Lippincott: Williams & Wilkins; 2001. p. 497–504.
38. Hermann B, Davies K, Foley K, Bell B. Visual confrontation naming outcome after standard left anterior temporal lobectomy with sparing versus resection of the superior temporal gyrus: a randomized prospective clinical trial. Epilepsia. 1999;40(8):1070–6.
39. Lineweaver TT, Morris HH, Naugle RI, Najm IM, Diehl B, Bingaman W. Evaluating the contributions of state-of-the-art assessment techniques to predicting memory outcome after unilateral anterior temporal lobectomy. Epilepsia. 2006;47(11):1895–903.
40. Meehan WP, D'hemecourt P, Collins CL, Taylor AM, Comstock RD. Computerized neurocognitive testing for the management of sport-related concussions. Pediatrics. 2012;129(1):38–44.
41. Randolph C. Baseline neuropsychological testing in managing sport-related concussion: does it modify risk? Curr Sports Med Rep. 2011;10(1):21–6.
42. Bauer RM, Iverson GL, Cernich AN, Binder LM, Ruff RM, Naugle RI. Computerized neuropsychological assessment devices: joint position paper of the American Academy of Clinical Neuropsychology and the National Academy of Neuropsychology. Clin Neuropsychol. 2012;26(2):177–96.
43. Wild K, Howieson D, Webbe F, Seelye A, Kaye J. Status of computerized cognitive testing in aging: a systematic review. Alzheimers Dement. 2008;4(6):428–37.
44. Reeves DL, Winter K, LaCour S, Raynsford K, Kay G, Elsmore T, Hegge FW. Automated neuropsychological assessment metrics documentation, Test administration guide, vol. I. Washington, DC: Office of Military Performance Assessment Technology; 1992.
45. Reeves DL, Winter KP, Bleiberg J, Kane RL. ANAM genogram: historical perspectives, description, and current endeavors. Arch Clin Neuropsychol. 2007;22(Suppl 1):S15–37.
46. Defense Centers of Excellence for Psychological Health and Traumatic Brain Injury. Indications and conditions for in-theater post-injury Neurocognitive Assessment Tool (NCAT) testing. Silver Spring, MD: Department of Defense; 2011.
47. Elsmore TF, Reeves DL, Reeves AN. The ARES test system for palm OS handheld computers. Arch Clin Neuropsychol. 2007;22(Suppl 1):S135–44.
48. Wilken JA, Sullivan CL, Lewandowski A, Kane RL. The use of ANAM to assess the side-effect profiles and efficacy of medication. Arch Clin Neuropsychol. 2007;22(Suppl 1):S127–33.
49. Gualtieri CT, Johnson LG. Neurocognitive testing supports a broader concept of mild cognitive impairment. Am J Alzheimers Dis Other Demen. 2005;20(6):359–66.

50. Masley S, Roetzheim R, Gualtieri T. Aerobic exercise enhances cognitive flexibility. J Clin Psychol Med Settings. 2009;16(2):186–93.
51. Lau BC, Collins MW, Lovell MR. Sensitivity and specificity of subacute computerized neurocognitive testing and symptom evaluation in predicting outcomes after sports-related concussion. Am J Sports Med. 2011;39(6):1209–16.
52. Van kampen DA, Lovell MR, Pardini JE, Collins MW, Fu FH. The "value added" of neurocognitive testing after sports-related concussion. Am J Sports Med. 2006;34(10):1630–5.
53. Resch JE, Mccrea MA, Cullum CM. Computerized neurocognitive testing in the management of sport-related concussion: an update. Neuropsychol Rev. 2013;23(4):335–49.
54. Cernich AN, Brennana DM, Barker LM, Bleiberg J. Sources of error in computerized neuropsychological assessment. Arch Clin Neuropsychol. 2007;22(Suppl 1):S39–48.
55. Harmon KG, Drezner JA, Gammons M, et al. American Medical Society for Sports Medicine position statement: concussion in sport. Br J Sports Med. 2013;47(1):15–26.
56. Schlegel RE, Gilliland K. Development and quality assurance of computer-based assessment batteries. Arch Clin Neuropsychol. 2007;22(Suppl 1):S49–61.

Part II
Case Examples

Chapter 5
Pediatric Case of Sickle Cell Disease

Melissa Gerstle, Katherine Baum, Charles T. Quinn, and Dean W. Beebe

Introduction

Children with sickle cell disease (SCD) often have cognitive, behavioral, and mood-related difficulties, in part due to the effect of their medical condition on the central nervous system. They are at high risk for neurological injury and insult, with as many as one-third having neurological complications [1]. This chapter details a pediatric case of SCD, assessed through repeated neuropsychological evaluations. It highlights the unique challenges of assessing a "moving target"—the interaction between a protean chronic illness and the developing brain.

Referral (Most Recent)

Patient: 16-year-old female
Education: attending 11th grade

Reason for referral: Jane Smith was diagnosed with SCD shortly after birth. She was first evaluated at age 10 years due to concerns with attention and learning and memory. That first evaluation offered diagnostic clarity that was then used to inform

M. Gerstle (✉) · K. Baum · D. W. Beebe (✉)
Division of Behavioral Medicine and Clinical Psychology, Cincinnati Children's Hospital Medical Center, Department of Pediatrics, University of Cincinnati College of Medicine, Cincinnati, OH, USA
e-mail: melissa.gerstle@cchmc.org; dean.beebe@cchmc.org

C. T. Quinn
Division of Hematology, Cincinnati Children's Hospital Medical Center, Department of Pediatrics, University of Cincinnati College of Medicine, Cincinnati, OH, USA
e-mail: Charles.Quinn@cchmc.org

K. M. Sanders (ed.), *Physician's Field Guide to Neuropsychology*,
https://doi.org/10.1007/978-1-4939-8722-1_5

medical and educational interventions. However, just as the medical effects of SCD can present new challenges with development, her neuropsychological concerns continued to pose challenges to her daily functioning. This follow-up evaluation was requested to re-assess her level of functioning, with an eye toward how to best help her transition to adulthood as she approached age 18 and the end of high school.

Case Presentation

Jane is a 16-year-old right-handed female with SCD (HbSC subtype), diagnosed by universal newborn screening for hemoglobinopathies. She was the product of full-term gestation without complications. Delivery was by Cesarean section due to maternal history of fibroid tumors. Birth weight was approximately 6 pounds. Early developmental motor and language milestones were met within age-appropriate timeframes. No concerns with development were present early on; however, her family became concerned about her attention and learning once she entered elementary school.

She has had multiple painful episodes and hospitalizations related to her illness (splenic sequestration, acute chest syndrome, pneumonia). Her last painful episode occurred about 1 month prior to the current evaluation, and she was able to manage the pain with over-the-counter analgesics. She was prescribed penicillin until age 5 years and has been receiving chronic erythrocytapheresis therapy monthly for several years. She has had two prior brain MRI/MRA studies, which have been normal. She has not had a transcranial Doppler study (TCD), as it is typically not performed for patients with HbSC.

Her mother earned a graduate degree, and her father completed high school. Immediate family history is notable for general learning difficulties. Extended family medical history is notable for dyslexia, suspected bipolar disorder, hypertension, stroke, diabetes (type 1 and 2), and obesity.

Prior to the current evaluation, she had been seen twice for neuropsychological evaluations, at ages 10 and 13 years. Problems at the initial evaluation included trouble with attention/focus, work completion, and excessing talking. She was also missing valuable academic instruction due to pain-related absences. She struggled in particular with math and reading comprehension. Test results indicated a fairly stable pattern of strengths and weakness. Her verbal skills were average and relatively stronger than visual skills, which were generally low average. She showed mild to moderate impairment in attention, executive skills, visual-spatial/visual-motor abilities, and speed and dexterity for her dominant (right) hand. Based on information from parents and teachers, which was consistent with behavioral observations and test results, she was diagnosed with attention-deficit/hyperactivity disorder (ADHD) at age 10 years. She briefly took stimulant medication for her ADHD symptoms but discontinued the medication due to unwanted side effects.

At the time of current evaluation, Jane was earning grades of C–F in her classes, with her lowest grades in math and science. Work completion remained an issue. Her mother described continued problems with distractibility, forgetfulness, disorganization, and poor time management. Jane had difficulty showing initiative and was struggling to manage daily routines on her own (e.g., getting up for school). Her mother expressed concern about Jane's ability to become more self-sufficient as she moves into young adulthood. She reported good peer relationships but noted Jane was also easily distracted by peers in the classroom. Problems with anxiety, depression, or risky adolescent behavior were denied.

Neurological Exams and Findings

MRI findings (most recent, age 13 years): The ventricles and extra-axial spaces were normal in size and shape. There was no mass lesion nor evidence of acute or past intracranial hemorrhage. Parenchymal signal and morphology were normal. There were no foci of abnormal enhancement or regions of restricted diffusion.
MRA findings (also at age 13 years): There was normal course and configuration of the intracranial arteries. No aneurysm, vascular malformation, or flow-limiting stenosis was demonstrated.
Neurological exam: cranial nerves, strength, sensation, and reflexes normal.

Preliminary Impressions

Jane's case illustrates one common scenario in patients with SCD. There is no evidence of overt neurological injury, and no history of overt stroke; however, she is functionally struggling to meet the demands of day-to-day life. There are a number of factors to consider in approaching such an evaluation, including medical factors, comorbid developmental and psychological disorders, and environmental and economic barriers.

SCD Overview

Sickle cell disease (SCD) is a broad term that refers to a group of autosomal recessive or codominant genetic disorders affecting the structure of hemoglobin, the molecule in red blood cells that delivers oxygen throughout the body. The abnormal hemoglobin is called sickle hemoglobin or hemoglobin S (Hb S). The most common form of SCD is the homozygous state for the Hb S mutation (HbSS), called sickle cell anemia (SCA). Other forms of SCD, such as Jane's subtype, result from coinheritance of the Hb S mutation with another interacting hemoglobin mutation, such as hemoglobin C or β-thalassemia. These compound heterozygous states result in different forms of SCD called sickle-hemoglobin C disease (HbSC), sickle-β^+-thalassemia (HbSβ^+), and sickle-β^0-thalassemia (HbSβ^0). The HbSS and HbSβ^0 genotypes are the most severe forms of SCD, and both may be referred to as SCA because they are clinically indistinguishable. On average, the HbSC and HbSβ^+ genotypes are less severe forms of SCD.

Hemoglobin should always remain soluble within red blood cells (RBCs), but Hb S polymerizes or gels upon deoxygenation. Cycles of oxygenation in the lungs and deoxygenation in the tissues (sickling and un-sickling) damage the RBC membrane, making RBCs in patients with SCD inflexible and prone to rupture. Consequently, the two main pathophysiologic features of SCD are chronic hemolysis and vaso-occlusion. The hallmark of SCD is the painful vaso-occlusive episode or "crisis." This acute debilitating complication is overt, in contrast to the many subtle or covert complications of SCD. While the lives of patients with SCD are punctuated with acute vaso-occlusive episodes that impair quality of life, such as pain, acute chest syndrome, and acute splenic sequestration, there is also a chronic, symptomatic anemia. Additionally, lifelong hemolysis and intermittent vaso-occlusion cause chronic organ damage that is often covert in young children but is progressive and increasingly problematic with age.

Key Point

Sickle cell disease (SCD) is a genetic condition in which red blood cells (RBC) contain abnormal hemoglobin that deforms (often producing the hallmark crescent or sickle shape) and destroys them prematurely. In addition to anemia, which decreases oxygen-carrying capacity, these RBCs are more likely to get trapped in small blood vessels and block the flow of blood. Vaso-occlusing leads to a host of problems, including debilitating painful episodes, acute chest syndrome, splenic sequestration, and stroke. The two most severe subtypes are HbSS (two Hb S mutations) and HbSβ^0 (one Hb S mutation and one β^0-thalassemia mutation).

There are both *direct* and *indirect* mechanisms that account for the effect of SCD on the developing brain. Direct effects on the central nervous system include cerebrovascular events (overt and silent cerebral infarction), acute and chronic anemia [2, 3], localized metabolic and perfusion deficits, and diffuse effects on neurons [4]. The increased risk for infections and use of opioid medications for pain crises can also affect brain functioning. Other factors indirectly affect brain development, including nutritional deficiencies, low-resource environments, parental educational attainment [5], and limited access to interventions and supports. The risk for neurological complications varies by subtype of the disease. Children with the HbSS subtype are at highest risk for cerebral ischemia and infarction, which are associated with significant morbidity and mortality [1].

In SCD broadly, the risk of overt stroke is 200 times higher than the general childhood population. In SCA specifically, the risk of stroke is even greater: 250–400 times higher than in children without SCD [6]. Without primary prevention, overt stroke occurs in 11% of children with HbSS by 18 years of age, with a peak yearly incidence of about 1% between 2 and 9 years of age. Stroke is much less common in HbSC and HbSβ^+. Most overt strokes in children are ischemic and are associated with occlusive cerebral arterial vasculopathy in large intracranial arteries.

Hemorrhagic strokes occur with increasing frequency beginning in young adulthood. Focal neurologic deficits that result from strokes can be detected by physical examination during scheduled (incidentally) or acute encounters. Brain MRI and MRA are the main imaging modalities to document past or current stroke. TCD ultrasonography can be used to identify children with HbSS at highest risk of overt stroke. Screening TCD examinations are now recommended at least yearly for children aged 2–16 years with SCA to direct the initiation of chronic transfusion therapy, which may need to be continued indefinitely for primary stroke prophylaxis. Chronic transfusion therapy is not only used as primary prevention of stroke but is standard care for children who have suffered an overt stroke (secondary prevention).

An even more common form of neurologic injury than overt stroke is a "silent stroke" or silent cerebral infarction (SCI), with a prevalence of about 40% in adolescents with SCA. Patients with other SCD subtypes are at lower risk, with lifetime SCI incidence in HbSC subtype estimated to be 5–31% [7]. SCI generally refers to small brain lesions visible on brain MRI without associated focal neurologic signs. The term SCI is actually a misnomer because these events are often not completely "silent." SCI is a morbid condition associated with increased risk for subsequent overt stroke and neurocognitive impairment, including difficulties with learning, attention, and behavior. These functional deficits may be due to accumulation of multiple small infarcts not seen on brain imaging [8]. Children with SCI may benefit from chronic transfusion therapy to prevent new or progressive cerebral infarction.

> **Key Point**
> The risk of cerebral infarction in SCD is highest in early childhood. Without primary prevention, 10–15% of children with sickle cell anemia (HbSS subtype, the most common subtype of SCD) will suffer overt stroke by age 15 years, and 20–25% will have SCI.

Role of Neuropsychology

Neuropsychologists are often consulted to determine mental or cognitive status or to assess for potential changes. Physicians may refer when a clear neurological event has occurred, such as a stroke (otherwise known as a cerebrovascular accident or CVA). In children with SCD, the lesions associated with CVAs tend to be localized to the deep white matter of the frontal, parietal, and temporal lobes [1]. These lesions can cause diffuse dysfunction, resulting in effects on attention, intelligence, learning, speed of processing, and mood. The effects can also be more focal, presenting as a language disorder such as aphasia or unilateral motor impairments.

Importantly, neuropsychological functioning can be disrupted even in the absence of an overt ischemic event. Therefore, physicians may refer for a neuropsychological evaluation when a patient is at high risk for stroke based on SCD subtype

(HbSS, HbSβ^0), a screening neuroimaging test is abnormal (e.g., TCD findings), there is suspected deficit or decline in cognitive functioning, or there is an adverse change in behavior of performance in school. MRI can detect SCI, but MRI is costly and many centers do not perform it regularly. Neuropsychological screening is a less invasive alternative that may help determine if a patient experienced one of these small strokes while simultaneously offering applied suggestions for how to improve medical, educational, and psychological care for the child. There is some evidence that performance on neuropsychological tests of memory and visual-spatial reasoning can accurately predict the presence of SCI [9].

Neuropsychologists play a unique role within the interdisciplinary sickle cell team. Their specialized training helps them to understand how disease processes affect neurological functioning in the context of a developing brain. They integrate knowledge about brain-behavior relationships with results of cognitive testing to determine the degree and severity of impairment for the individual patient. Physicians request neuropsychological evaluation to help identify these impairments and understand their effects on everyday functioning. Neuropsychologists can then guide diagnostic and treatment decisions, determine the effects of treatment, describe mental and cognitive status, and guide services and accommodations at school, work, or in the community [10].

Key Point

Neuropsychological evaluation is especially helpful for patients with significant neurological risk factors, abnormal neuroimaging findings, suspected cognitive deficit or decline, and/or significant change in behavior or academic performance. Neuropsychological evaluations can detect and clarify cognitive impairments and social-emotional factors and their bearing on treatment. Often even more importantly, neuropsychological evaluations consider the functional implications for the patient and family and offer concrete suggestions for the family, school, healthcare team, and other providers.

One common referral question for patients with SCD relates to comorbid diagnoses—*does this child have an intellectual disability or learning disorder? Does this adolescent need treatment for depression or attention-deficit/hyperactivity disorder (ADHD)?* In Jane's case, her family and medical team had concerns about her attention and learning. Her early neuropsychological evaluation results helped elucidate the nature of her difficulties, provide diagnostic clarity, and inform her medical-, academic-, and community-based care. Every case is different, but children and adolescents with SCD are at highest risk for learning disorders, ADHD, and internalizing disorders, such as anxiety and depression [8, 11]. A neuropsychologist can not only diagnose these conditions but can provide detailed recommendations to the family, school, and patient regarding how to support these challenges for each individual child. The neuropsychologist educates the family on the child's legal rights to educational services, as public schools are legally mandated to provide educational support and interventions for children who have medical conditions impacting their ability to benefit from academic instruction (see Individuals with Disabilities Education Act (IDEA) [12]). The multidisciplinary SCD team can then work with schools to ensure that these services are implemented.

Neuropsychologists can work with physicians to ensure that educational plans provide accommodations around medical needs for SCD, such as excused absences for medical appointments; permission for a school nurse to dispense medication; access to water, bathroom, and elevators; and increased monitoring during physical activity. Beyond this, the neuropsychologist uniquely addresses the patient's specific needs related to learning, behavior, and mood. Tailored instruction is often recommended as part of educational plans, but children with SCD may also need academic intervention; physical, occupational or speech/language therapy; or a structured behavioral plan. The earlier that children's difficulties are identified through an evaluation, the better their opportunity to benefit from targeted interventions.

Key Point

Neuropsychological evaluations are most helpful when there is a focused referral question. In SCD, examples include the following: What is this patient's cognitive capacity and how does that affect participation in medical, educational, and work settings? Does this patient have ADHD, learning disability, or an intellectual disability? Has this patient had a decline in their cognitive abilities? Should the parents of this young adult patient consider pursuing legal guardianship or power of attorney?

Serial Evaluation: Pediatric Considerations

Neuropsychologists use standardized measures that compare an individual's performance to normative data of age-matched, typically developing peers. In addition to these *between-person* comparisons, *within-person* comparisons can be conducted in cases like Jane's in which serial assessments have been completed. Ipsative comparisons allow neuropsychologists to document a patient's cognitive development and identify improvement or decline in a specific cognitive domain. Serial neuropsychological evaluations are important not only to assess disease progression and identify neurocognitive dysfunction as early as possible but also to assess how well a child is responding to targeted interventions (medical, psychological, and educational). Monitoring an individual's development over time is especially important given the risk for ischemic events. As noted, ischemic events are most likely to occur in the first decade of life, with the highest incidence occurring in children ages 2–5 years [13].

SCD-related neurological insults early in life can set children on a developmental trajectory similar to children with other early brain injuries. Children with SCD may not make age-appropriate gains in their skills or may fail to meet developmental expectations [11]. Therefore, regular follow-up evaluations allow neuropsychologists to more carefully assess this developmental path, guide services and accommodations, and consider alternative approaches. For Jane, follow-up evaluations were instrumental in helping to describe the trajectory of her cognitive development, monitor her ongoing psychological functioning, and guide the family, medical team, and school in how to accommodate her difficulties with the changing demands in her environment.

Neuropsychological testing and psychological and school intervention are key components of comprehensive SCD care. These services should certainly be provided to children experiencing overt problems (e.g., learning difficulties, behavioral problems, nonadherence to medical therapy), but ideally the need for these services and therapies should also be assessed by scheduled assessments throughout the life span.

Neuropsychological Testing

Clinical Findings and History

Historically, IQ has been used as the primary barometer of cognitive functioning in patients with SCD. However, the assessment of more specific cognitive skills is even more valuable and can show impairments even in the context of average IQ. Testing of specific cognitive domains is two to three times more sensitive to brain tissue injury than results of general intelligence tests [14]. Although a school psychologist or more general child clinical psychologist can give IQ tests, neuropsychological evaluations allow for better examination of attention, memory, executive skills, language, visual-spatial skills, and processing speed. Impairments in these cognitive areas are seen in children and adolescents with SCD and greatly affect a child's ability to be successful in daily life

Neuropsychological Domains

IQ. When compared to their siblings, children with SCD typically have lower scores on measures of intelligence [15, 16]. Even those with no evidence of cerebral infarction had a 4- to 5-point deficit in IQ compared to sibling and peer control groups [14]. Patients with low hematocrit (less than 27) tend to have lower full-scale IQ (influenced by lower scores on tests of verbal abilities and working memory) than those with higher hematocrit values [17]. When examined longitudinally, IQ declined over a 9-year period [18]. Jane's overall IQ score varied across evaluations largely due to her performance on working memory and processing speed subtests, but there was no clear pattern of overall decline.

Attention/Executive Functioning. The term "executive functioning" relates to the ability to approach problems with self-control and flexibility and in a sustained, organized manner. Conceptually and pragmatically, these abilities overlap with attention and impulse control. Domains of attention and executive functioning appear most consistently affected in children with SCD [14]. Compared to sibling controls, children with SCD had lower scores on tests of attention and executive functioning [8, 19]. Longitudinally, there is evidence of age-related declines on tests of psychomotor speed and focused attention [20]. Jane does not appear to have experienced a decline in these areas, and her deficits on testing were subtle; in fact, she showed improved performance on some aspects. However, attention and executive functioning deficits can be harder to detect on structured tests, so behavioral rating scales are often used to assess functioning in more complex real-world circumstances (e.g., at home, at school). Beyond the subtle deficits on objective testing, findings on rating scales completed by Jane, her mother, and her teachers clearly reflected persistent difficulties across environments. As she is asked to be more independent as she transitions into adulthood, the functional impact of these deficits becomes even more important.

Visual-Spatial/Visual-Motor. Less commonly studied than IQ and attention, children with SCD can show deficits in visual-spatial/visual-motor abilities [21]. As a result, math and science courses frequently prove more challenging for students with similar difficulties. Indeed, this domain represented stable areas of deficit for Jane, commensurate with her long-standing difficulties in math.

Effort/Validity. Although formal effort testing is less commonplace in pediatric evaluations, children may not put forth good effort for a multitude of reasons, including inattention, lack of interest or motivation, non-compliance/defiance, or feelings of inadequacy. Given Jane's history of ADHD, it was particularly important to assess her level of effort and ability to give a valid performance. Her performance on validity measures was within normal limits.

Additional Domains. Jane's other cognitive domains, such as language, learning and memory, and fine motor skills, were intact. In fact, when cued to pay close attention to new material being presented to her, her recall of it later was strong. At least for verbal information, problems with "memory" mostly reflected problems with attention and executive functioning. Academic achievement is typically also assessed during the course of neuropsychological evaluation. Although her reading and spelling skills were largely intact, her math skills remained weak. This pattern of academic skills is consistent with her cognitive strengths and weaknesses.

Data table			
	Age 10	Age 13	Age 16
1. Intelligence			
Wechsler Intelligence Scale for Children 4th Ed (WISC-IV)			
Verbal Comprehension Index (VCI)	102	102	98
Similarities	12	10	10
Vocabulary	10	10	9
Comprehension	10	12	–
Perceptual Reasoning Index (PRI)	88	90	82

(continued)

Data table			
	Age 10	Age 13	Age 16
Block Design	6	5	5
Picture Concepts	10	12	–
Matrix Reasoning	8	8	9
Working Memory Index (WMI)	77	77	80
Digit Span	8	4	9
Letter-Number Sequencing	4	8	5
Processing Speed Index (PSI)	85	88	97
Coding	7	8	9
Symbol Search	8	8	10
2. Academics			
Wechsler Individual Achievement Test 3rd Ed (WIAT-III)			
Word Reading	91	96	97
Reading Comprehension	100	99	–
Numerical Operations	97	85	75
Math Problem-Solving	–	–	79
Math Fluency	–	69	74
Spelling	94	92	–
3. Attention and Executive Function			
Delis-Kaplan Executive Function System (D-KEFS)			
Trail Making Test			
Visual Scanning	–	11	11
Number Sequencing	–	7	12
Letter Sequencing	–	10	11
Number/Letter Switching	–	9	9
Motor	–	11	12
Verbal Fluency			
Letter Fluency	–	9	14
Category Fluency	–	12	14
Category-Switching Correct	–	9	12
Category-Switching Accuracy	–	8	8
Color-Word Interference			
Color Naming	–	9	12
Word Reading	–	11	11
Inhibition	–	11	12
Inhibition-Switching	–	7	7
4. Memory			
Children's Memory Scale (CMS)			
Story Memory			
Immediate Recall	11	–	–
Delayed Recall	13	–	–
Recognition	12	–	–

Data table

	Age 10	Age 13	Age 16
Wide Range Assessment of Memory and Learning 2nd Ed (WRAML-2)			
Story Memory			
Immediate Recall	–	10	13
Delayed Recall	–	12	14
Recognition	–	11	13
Rey Complex Figure Test			
Immediate Recall	–	35	25
Delayed Recall	–	40	<20
Recognition	–	53	44
5. Visual-Spatial			
Beery-Buktenica Developmental Test of Visual-Motor Integration (VMI)			
VMI	65	73	76
Judgment of Line Orientation (JOLO)			
Total Correct—raw score (out of 30)	16/30	9/30	11/30
Rey Complex Figure Test			
Copy[a] (raw)	–	≤1 (24.0)	≤1 (27.5)
6. Motor			
Grooved Pegboard Test			
Right (raw)	−0.60 (83 s)	−1.38 (76 s)	−0.09 (67 s)
Left (raw)	−1.26 (99 s)	0.07 (71 s)	−0.77 (79 s)
7. Validity			
MSVT	–	–	WNL

[a]Expressed as percentile rank

Key Point
Patients with SCD are at risk for cognitive impairment and can show evidence of cognitive decline. Areas most affected include overall intelligence (IQ), attention, executive functioning, and visual-spatial skills. Learning difficulties are also common.

Conclusions

Collaborative Discussion

For patients with SCD, neuropsychological evaluations are often requested to determine if there is evidence of brain dysfunction, to describe the implications of impairment on everyday life, and to determine what can be done to minimize associated negative effects. Results of neuropsychological evaluations guide recommendations for healthcare, school, work, home, and community.

Although Jane had a generally less severe phenotype of SCD, even HbSC (sickle-hemoglobin C disease) can be associated with neuropsychological impairments. Findings from this latest follow-up evaluation indicate stable areas of cognitive weakness compared to results from 3 and 6 years earlier. Attention, executive skills, and visual-spatial/visual-motor skills remain significant weaknesses. She still struggles to stay focused and engaged and has trouble with efficiency and organization. Her untreated ADHD symptoms are continuing to interfere in daily life. For this reason, she and her mother were encouraged to revisit medication options for ADHD as well as to consider behavioral treatment. Organization and time management strategies were provided for the home environment. Specific strategies to support Jane in adopting greater responsibility for her medical care were also discussed. For purposes of school planning, an Individualized Education Program (IEP) was recommended to provide accommodations and academic intervention in math in high school and at the college level. Although Jane had not yet identified a particular college or possible major, the neuropsychologist and family discussed what type of college setting may be most appropriate and what kinds of careers or vocations fit with her cognitive strengths.

Screening vs. Comprehensive Evaluation

Despite the high risk of neuropsychological dysfunction in patients with SCD, comprehensive evaluations are not always feasible. For many children and families served in pediatric sickle cell clinics, lack of insurance and socioeconomic barriers to attending appointments (transportation issues, missed school, lost wages) present major issues. It is estimated that 70% of families of patients with SCD are insured through Medicaid [22], and insurance coverage often changes when adolescents transition to adult care, potentially jeopardizing care [23]. The socioeconomic challenges, in addition to the neuropsychological problems (cognitive, behavioral, psychological, and social problems), medical complications, and health-related disparities, make it difficult for patients to attend appointments, putting them at risk for being lost to follow-up. It is especially difficult for families to attend appointments beyond those required to manage their child's disease.

To minimize these barriers, for cases with no identified concerns (by the patient, family, or healthcare team), it can be very helpful to conduct neuropsychological screenings during patients' medical appointments. The goal of these screenings is to assess general level of functioning and triage more complex cases. However, for patients like Jane in whom there were concerns about her cognitive abilities and possible ramifications on her daily functioning, a comprehensive neuropsychological evaluation is warranted. Comprehensive evaluations are needed for complex cases requiring nuanced assessment of specific cognitive domains and individualized, detailed recommendations. In Jane's case, the need for more comprehensive evaluation was readily identified when she was young via astute queries by her healthcare team.

Educational and Vocational Planning

One of the main goals of neuropsychological evaluation is to assist patients and families with intervention planning in the school setting. Cognitive deficits associated with SCD place children at risk for poor school performance, but health-related and social/family factors also affect success at school [24]. Patients with SCD have poorer school attendance due to pain and frequent medical appointments as well as to socioeconomic factors, such as poverty, parental educational attainment, and limited resources [5]. Furthermore, their schools may have limited resources, making it less likely that their special learning needs will be identified and supported. All these factors contribute to the increased rates of grade retention and use of special education services in patients with SCD [24, 25]. Jane's initial evaluation helped identify areas of educational need and rally targeted resources to head off a further deterioration in educational functioning.

Planning in the primary or secondary school settings includes educational placement (i.e., special education/resource room, general education and advanced programming, vocational vs. traditional academic settings), appropriateness of curriculum, school-based therapies (i.e., speech/language, occupational, or physical therapy), testing accommodations, and teaching strategies—all within a developmental context.

Like Jane, older adolescents with SCD who are in high school or transitioning to adulthood may need resources about post-secondary educational opportunities, including college or employment guidance, information related to guardianship and powers of attorney, referrals to vocational rehabilitation, and identification of community supports. Patients with SCD may need adjustments to their class or work schedules to minimize fatigue or allowances for healthcare appointments and frequent breaks. Expectations within these settings may need to be altered if a patient has neuropsychological impairment, such as slowed processing speed, learning problems, or executive and memory difficulties. Extra time can be given to complete tasks, and multimodal presentation of information may maximize retention of information. Poor executive skills can be especially detrimental in high-demand adult settings, so ensuring the individual can identify and implement appropriate supports is critical.

Key Point

Results of neuropsychological evaluations translate into personalized recommendations that optimize a patient's success across multiple settings. Educational recommendations vary by age but often involve development of educational plans and determination of curriculum and therapeutic supports. In adolescents and young adults, neuropsychologists use test results to guide vocational decisions and supports, minimize barriers to functional independence, and provide targeted interventions and accommodations in "real-life" settings.

Supportive Healthcare Tools

Individualized care is important across all healthcare settings but is especially valuable for patients with SCD. Neuropsychological evaluation can guide the medical team's approach to care. Some patients may retain more information when both verbal and visual means of communication are employed. In addition to providing patients and families with verbal instructions, a written plan of care is a concrete tool and resource to which patients and families can refer. Jane has fairly marked executive dysfunction. For her, and other patients with similar challenges, creating external aides and tools to track and monitor their health status, medication, and hospital visits can be invaluable. Calendars, schedules, checklists, and electronic applications and alarms can all serve as external reminders when an individual's "internal" organization and structure are somewhat limited due to executive dysfunction.

Capacity/Competency

Neuropsychologists integrated into sickle cell teams are sometimes asked to make clinical judgments about a patient's decision-making capacity or competency. Although many young adult patients with SCD are capable of managing their own affairs, families and medical teams sometimes have questions about a patient's capacity to make medical, financial, and life-related decisions. In pediatric populations, these issues become especially prominent during adolescence, as the patient will soon obtain legal rights to make decisions, or in young adulthood if there has been a clear neurological event resulting in impaired functioning. While legal decisions must come from the courts, cognitive functioning is a critical factor that differentiates patients with impaired capacity from those who are unimpaired [26]. When addressing this referral question, neuropsychologists conduct cognitive assessments in addition to relying heavily on information gained through interviews with the patient, family, and/or medical team. Their role is to integrate all information about a patient's cognitive and developmental functioning, emotional regulation, and behavior to understand barriers to sound reasoning and judgment.

Patients with SCD are at risk for learning problems, inattention, and impulsive behavior, which may lead to poor decision-making. However, poor decision-making, in itself, does not indicate the patient is legally incompetent. There needs to be clear evidence that the patient does not understand, appreciate, or have the ability to reason through information related to a particular treatment decision [26]. If a patient is deemed unable to manage personal affairs in his/her own best interest, legal intervention is necessary to protect the person's welfare. Interventions can involve a family member obtaining legal guardianship or one of several types of powers of attorney, which may give limited (i.e., only related to medical or financial decisions) or general rights to act and make decisions on a patient's behalf. Importantly, the legal decision about capacity is ultimately at the determination of the judge. However, results of neuropsychological evaluations can shed light on cognitive and functional impairments and their implications for decision-making. With Jane, her family expressed particular concern about her ability to manage her complex medical care on her own once she moves away from home. After further exploration, their concern appeared grounded in her difficulties managing everyday demands at school and home related to her attention and executive deficits, more so than issues of competence. With discussion of evaluation findings with the family, use of a scaffolded approach to help her take greater responsibility of her medical care (while still under parental supervision) was determined to be a more appropriate solution.

Key Point
Neuropsychologists are well-positioned to understand the implications of a patient's cognitive, emotional, and behavioral challenges on their medical care. Armed with neuropsychological data and their clinical impressions, neuropsychologists can recommend specific strategies to the family, patient, and medical team to maximize the patient's understanding and communication in healthcare situations. They can broaden the team's understanding of the patient's limitations and guide the family toward necessary resources.

Transition to Adulthood

Transition to adulthood and to adult medical care is a major milestone for patients with SCD and can be challenging. Maximizing the structure and support during transition to adult healthcare is vital [27]. For example, many clinics have been successful by grouping medical appointments to minimize the burden on patients and families of repeated trips to the clinic. Joint appointments with a patient's pediatric and soon-to-be adult healthcare providers are also an effective approach [23]. Nearly all patients with SCD survive into adulthood (94–98%), but that transition time is associated with increased risk of mortality [28]. In a review of the transition literature in SCD [23], highlight the importance of a flexible patient-centered transition plan as well as education of adult health providers. Ideally, the transition plan includes an assessment of needs as a means of tailoring medical, educational, and developmental information to the patient. Neuropsychologists can be a valuable asset to the interdisciplinary transition team during this potentially vulnerable time. The primary role of the neuropsychologist during this time is to understand individual and systemic barriers to independence and provide appropriate recommendations to minimize barriers.

One approach is to provide neuropsychological assessment as a part of this routine transition care [22]. Although less studied in SCD, individuals with other neurological injury and insult that have clear neuropsychological impairment fare worse in young adulthood in terms of educational and vocational attainment [22]. Attention and executive functioning deficits can make it challenging for adolescents to independently manage their complex healthcare needs. Poor organization, planning, initiation, flexibility, and self-monitoring all contribute to difficulties remembering medication and appointments. The many demands on cognitive systems may be too much for the young adult to handle, resulting in internalizing disorders (anxiety, depression) and poor coping.

Neuropsychologists are well-positioned to identify these deficits and help the young adult and their family to identify effective strategies (i.e., use of planners, pill boxes with alarms) and interventions (i.e., cognitive-behavioral therapy, medication consultation). Armed with an understanding of the patient's strengths and weaknesses, the neuropsychologist can help the patient, their family, and the medical team make decisions about how to maximize independence while ensuring the patient has adequate support. In Jane's case, evaluation results helped guide her educational accommodations as she plans to enter college as well as channel career and vocational preparation. It also yielded patient-specific, concrete recommendations regarding strategies for medication adherence, the medical team's interactions, and pharmacological and therapeutic interventions. As part of an integrated care process, the neuropsychological evaluation facilitated Jane's transition to being a productive, well-adjusted member of adult society, successfully using support systems to navigate the challenges of her chronic illness.

Chapter Review Questions

1. Which subtype of sickle cell disease is the most common and most severe?
   A. HbSS.
   B. HbSC.
   C. HbSβ^{+}.
   D. HbSβ^{Ω}.

2. What is *not* an appropriate referral questions for a neuropsychologist treating a patient with sickle cell disease?
   A. Does this patient have an intellectual disability?
   B. Has the patient's cognitive abilities declined or stagnated compared to peers?
   C. What is the patient's cognitive capacity and implications for treatment?
   D. Can this patient get worker's compensation?

3. What mechanisms might account for neuropsychological deficits in SCD in the absence of abnormalities on neuroimaging or on neurologic exam?
   A. Obstruction of blood flow to organs and tissues.
   B. Low-resource environments.
   C. Disease complications (infections, splenic sequestration, acute chest syndrome).
   D. All of the above.

4. Which cognitive area is *least* likely to be affected in patients with sickle cell disease?
   A. IQ.
   B. Attention.
   C. Executive functioning.
   D. Language comprehension.
5. For Jane, her difficulties with math might be associated with deficits in what cognitive domain?
   A. Language comprehension.
   B. Language expression.
   C. Visual-spatial skills.
   D. Fine motor skills.
6. Neuropsychological evaluation typically makes recommendations in what areas?
   A. Healthcare.
   B. School/work.
   C. Home.
   D. All the above.
7. Which of the following might warrant a comprehensive neuropsychological evaluation (versus a shorter neuropsychological or psychosocial screening)?
   A. Suspected cognitive decline.
   B. Possible low mood related to parents' divorce.
   C. Concerns about test anxiety.
   D. Adjustment to chronic transfusion therapy.
8. Which of the following are examples of educational/vocational recommendations that may be found in a neuropsychological evaluation report?
   A. Consideration of a formal educational plan.
   B. Classroom placement decisions.
   C. Test or work setting accommodations.
   D. All the above.
9. Jane exhibited marked executive dysfunction. Which of the following is *least* likely to be helpful for her?
   A. E-mail reminders of upcoming medical appointments and medication refill dates.
   B. Alarms on her phone to alert her to take medication.
   C. Verbal checklist of treatment regimen and upcoming appointments.
   D. Written checklist of treatment regimen and upcoming appointments.

References

1. Kral MC, Brown RT, Hynd GW. Neuropsychological aspects of pediatric sickle cell disease. Neuropsychol Rev. 2001;11(4):179–96.
2. Dowling MM, Quinn CT, Plumb P, et al. Acute silent cerebral ischemia and infarction during acute anemia in children with and without sickle cell disease. Blood. 2012;120(19):3891–7.
3. Quinn CT, Dowling MM. Cerebral tissue hemoglobin saturation in children with sickle cell disease. Pediatr Blood Cancer. 2012;59(5):881–7.
4. Schatz J, Puffer ES. Neuropsychological aspects of sickle cell disease. In: Brown RT, editor. Comprehensive handbook of childhood cancer and sickle cell disease: a biopsychosocial approach. New York: Oxford University Press; 2006. p. 449–70.
5. King AA, Strouse JJ, Rodeghier MJ, et al. Parent education and biologic factors influence on cognition in sickle cell anemia. Am J Hematol. 2014;89(2):162–7.
6. Ohene-Frempong K. Stroke in sickle cell disease: demographic, clinical, and therapeutic considerations. Semin Hematol. 1991;28:213–9.
7. Solomou E, Kraniotis P, Kourakli A, Petsas T. Extent of silent cerebral infarcts in adult sickle-cell disease patients on magnetic resonance imaging: Is there a correlation with the clinical severity of disease? Hematol Rep. 2013;5(1):8–12.
8. Brown RT, Buchanan I, Doepke K, Eckman JR, Baldwin K, Goonan B. Cognitive and academic functioning in children with sickle-cell disease. J Clin Child Psychol. 1993;22:207–18.
9. White DA, Moinuddin A, McKinstry RC, Noetzel M, Armstrong M, DeBaun M. Cognitive screening for silent cerebral infarction in children with sickle cell disease. J Pediatr Hematol Oncol. 2006;28(3):166–9.
10. Schoenberg MR, Scott JG. The neuropsychology referral and answers to referral questions. In: Schoenberg MR, Scott JG, editors. The Little Black book of neuropsychology. New York: Springer Press; 2011. p. 1–37.
11. Schatz J, McClellan CB. Sickle cell disease as a neurodevelopmental disorder. Ment Retard Dev Disabil Res Rev. 2006;12:200–7.
12. Individuals With Disabilities Education Act (IDEA). Vol 20 U.S.C. § 1400. 2004.
13. Ohene-Frempong K, Weiner SJ, Sleeper LA, Miller ST, Embury S, Moohr JW. Cerebrovascular accidents in sickle cell disease: rates and risk factors. Blood. 1998;91(1):288–94.
14. Schatz J, Finke RL, Kellett JM, JH K. Cognitive functioning in children with sickle cell disease: a meta-analysis. J Pediatr Psychol. 2002;27(8):739–48.
15. Bernaudin F, Verlhac S, Fréard F, et al. Multicenter prospective study of children with sickle cell disease: Radiographic and psychometric correlation. J Child Neurol. 2000;15:333–43.
16. Wasserman AL, Wilimas JA, Fairclough DL, Mulhern RK. W W. Subtle neuropsychological deficits in children with sickle cell disease. Am J Pediatr Hematol Oncol. 1991;13:14–20.
17. Steen RG, Miles MA, Helton KJ, et al. Cognitive impairment in children with hemoglobin SS sickle cell disease: relationship to MR imaging findings and hematocrit. Am J Radiol. 2003;24:382–9.
18. Thompson RJ, Armstrong FD, Link CL, Pegelow CH, Moser F, Wang WC. A prospective study of the relationship over time of behavior problems, intellectual functioning, and family functioning in children with sickle cell disease: a report from the cooperative study of sickle cell disease. J Pediatr Psychol. 2003;28:59–65.
19. DeBaun MR, Schatz J, Siegel MJ, et al. Cognitive screening examinations for silent cerebral infarcts in sickle cell disease. Neurology. 1998;50:1678–82.
20. Wang W, Enos L, Gallagher D, et al. Neuropsychologic performance in school-aged children with sickle cell disease: a report from the Cooperative Study of Sickle Cell Disease. J Pediatr. 2001;139:391–7.
21. Berkelhammer LD, Williamson AL, Sanford SD, et al. Neurocognitive sequelae of pediatric sickle cell disease: a review of the literature. Child Neuropsychol. 2007;13:120–31.

22. Wills KE, Nelson SC, Hennessy J, et al. Transition planning for youth with sickle cell disease: embedding neuropsychological assessment into comprehensive care. Pediatrics. 2010;126:S151–9.
23. Jordan L, Swerdlow P, Coates TD. Systematic review of transition from adolescent to adult care in patients with sickle cell disease. J Pediatr Hematol Oncol. 2013;35:165–9.
24. Epping AS, Myrvik MP, Newby RF, Panepinto JA, Brandow AM, Scott JP. Academic attainment findings in children with sickle cell disease. J Sch Health. 2013;83(8):548–53.
25. King AA, Rodeghier MG, Panepinto JA, et al. Silent cerebral infarction, income, and grade retention among students with sickle cell anemia. Am J Hematol. 2014;89(10):E188–92.
26. Kolva E, Rosenfeld B, Brescia R, Comfort C. Assessing decision-making capacity at end of life. Pediatrics. 2014;36:392–7.
27. Crosby LE, Quinn CT, KA K. A biopsychosocial model for the management of patients with sickle-cell disease transitioning to adult medical care. Adv Ther. 2015;32(4):293–305.
28. Quinn CT, Roger ZR, McCavit TL, Buchanan GR. Improved survival of children and adolescents with sickle cell disease. Blood. 2010;115:3447–52.

Chapter 6
Pediatric Traumatic Brain Injury: Collaboration through Case Example

Paul C. Lebby and Jennifer V. Crocker

Introduction

Collaboration between the neuropsychologist and a variety of physicians involved in the care of a child with traumatic brain injury (TBI) is complex and critical to optimal patient outcomes. Management of TBI is best viewed as a dynamic process, beginning in the field with first responders, continuing through the emergency department (ED) and pediatric intensive care unit (PICU), and ultimately to the general medical floor and post-hospitalization. Primary neuropsychological and medical concerns change as the child progresses through these stages, with initial focus on life-sustaining measures and prevention or reversal of secondary brain injury. Primary brain injury from physical trauma to tissue is often irreversible, with recovery being related to neuroplasticity or compensatory mechanisms. However, secondary brain injury from the pathophysiological effects of the primary injury (edema, bleeding, hydrocephalus, increased intracranial pressure, vascular compromise, metabolic dysregulation, seizures, etc.) is often amenable to prevention or even reversal [1–3]. Initial management in the ED and PICU focuses primarily on minimizing the effects of secondary brain injury, in lieu of patient functioning. Once medically stable, focus moves to recovery of functioning, and maximizing independence via pharmacological and therapeutic interventions, and ultimately long-term treatments designed to optimize the child's future development, school success, and eventually transition to adulthood. Although there is considerable overlap between the initial treatment of concussions and TBI in children, the differing pathophysiologies for these two conditions result in disparate post-injury treatment planning and collaboration between the neuropsychologist and physician attending

P. C. Lebby (✉) · J. V. Crocker
Valley Children's Hospital, Madera, CA, USA
e-mail: plebby@valleychildrens.org

K. M. Sanders (ed.), *Physician's Field Guide to Neuropsychology*,
https://doi.org/10.1007/978-1-4939-8722-1_6

to the child. Similar to TBI, management of concussion is dynamic, although generally involves less intensive services, usually terminating after ED intervention and ongoing care from family, with outpatient follow-up as needed.

Pediatric Concussion

Concussion in children and adolescents continues to be a significant concern, especially given the drive for greater competitive edge in school sports, and with younger ages of participation in contact sports such as full-contact football. Further, the immaturity of a child's brain increases the potential for physiological disruption and risk of permanent damage when injuries are sustained at a younger age. Immature or incomplete myelination in children can result in greater metabolic disruption and risk of permanent pathology following concussion when compared to adults.

Differentiating concussion from mild traumatic brain injury (mTBI) is controversial, although more easily conceptualized if approached from a neuropathological perspective. Concussive injuries are considered functional conditions resulting in temporary acute neurophysiological changes at the cellular level, but without imaging evidence of permanent physical damage to brain tissues [4]. However, controversy arises as new advances in research and imaging technologies have demonstrated emerging evidence of microscopic damage such as tearing of axons or capillary level micro bleeds not previously identified with less sophisticated measures. This is true, even for concussive level injuries previously thought to cause no "physical damage" to the brain [5]. As such, although concussions can be considered primarily physiological in nature, there is clearly overlap between severe concussions and mild traumatic brain injuries, especially when considering the physiological effects at the microscopic level.

In general, concussions can be viewed as involving a rapid onset of acute neurophysiological disruption at the cellular level, resulting in temporary and theoretically reversible changes to brain functioning. Further, concussions place the brain in a state of susceptibility to more permanent damage during a vulnerability window that can last several weeks or even months. Concussion initiates a series of changes at the ionic, neurotransmitter, and vascular levels, resulting in a reversible period of cellular hypometabolism, along with cerebral blood flow uncoupling, all during a time when metabolic demands are elevated. Changes can begin within a minute and persist for weeks.

Any additional injury or overuse of vulnerable cells can result in irreversible energetic failure and cell death, a condition that mimics TBI. If the cells are allowed to regain metabolic homeostasis during the period of vulnerability, full return of functioning is expected. Common symptoms relate to the hypometabolic state of the brain and may include headache, difficulty concentrating or thinking clearly, memory problems, fatigue, sleep disturbance, irritability, dizziness, and loss of higher-level balance. Specialized assessment is often critical in differentiating the effects of transient metabolic disruption from more concerning longer-term difficulties associated with a TBI level injury. Brain imaging has a low yield and is not generally indicated for concussion. However, if there is suspicion of more severe injury, or acute deterioration, brain imaging should be considered. The most sensitive method to detect and monitor post-concussive symptoms is assessment by a specialist trained in brain injury such as a neuropsychologist, neurologist, or physical medicine and rehabilitation physician. The goal of management is to facilitate recovery by ensuring the child avoids activities and situations that may result in further injury or slowed recovery. With no additional injury and cognitive rest, symptoms should spontaneously resolve by a week or two. Symptoms resolve a week or two prior to full physiological homeostasis; the brain remains vulnerable for a short time following symptom resolution. Therefore, a gradual return to learning activities should be based on tolerance and cognitive recovery. Students should be performing at their cognitive "baseline" for a week or more prior to returning to sports, full physical activity, or other extracurricular activities to allow for complete resolution of the physiological vulnerability period. Protracted symptoms past 2 months are most strongly associated with noninjury factors, or the injury is better considered a TBI, and the child requires a higher level of care and more sophisticated assessments and treatment regimens.

Collaboration between the neuropsychologist and physician is especially important for children recovering from concussive type injuries, as risk of further damage is great, and potential for poor outcomes is disproportionate to the perceived severity of the initial injury. Monitoring of recovery can allow for return to activities more rapidly, something that is beneficial to the child's social and emotional functioning, while preventing premature return for those children that remain at risk or who require longer-term recovery periods, targeted therapeutic interventions, or accommodations and services within their school environments. For greater detail regarding concussive injuries, see the chapter in this book by Drs. Coppel and Herring.

Pediatric Traumatic Brain Injury

Approximately 500,000 children a year are seen in emergency departments due to TBI [6]. TBI in children is most common in two primary age ranges, young children from 0 to 4 years and adolescents from 15 to 19, and remains one of the leading causes of child mortality and morbidity [6–8]. The effects of TBI can be highly varied, making it difficult to describe a "common" or "standard" brain injury. However, even though no two brain injuries are alike, the symptom constellation, in addition to the cognitive and functional profiles following brain injury, share many similarities [9]. For example, one of the more common complaints following TBI includes disruption to higher-level cognitive processing involving speed and efficiency, mental flexibility, attention, and executive functioning. Additional common complaints involve poor arousal, compromised memory for new information, limited judgment and safety awareness, and ease of fatigue [10]. Dependent on the location of primary pathology, more specific deficits may be evident such as motor weakness/paralysis, aphasia, visual impairment, etc. Moderate to severe TBI may not permanently impair basic cognitive, motor, or sensory skills, although almost without exception, some degree of compromise will be evident for more complex cognitive processes involving memory and executive functioning, or subtle fine motor abilities [11]. Deficits generally persist for months to years following TBI with the most frequently expressed complaints a year or two following injury being related to speed and efficiency of cognitive information processing, higher-level reasoning skills, and memory for new information [12].

Traditionally, traumatic brain injuries have been divided into two categories, focal injuries affecting small areas of tissue or diffuse injuries affecting larger brain regions or systems [12, 13]. However, with severe TBI caused by physical trauma, the child will almost certainly experience both focal and diffuse damages to varying degrees. This results in some discrete functional deficits relating to focal areas of damage, in addition to more generalized or diffuse compromise to overall functioning. On neuroimaging, focal injuries such as hemorrhagic contusions are often more evident than diffuse injuries such as diffuse axonal shear injury due to the limitations of imaging technology. Brain imaging is not highly sensitive to microscopic axonal shear injury, although it is more sensitive to blood, edema, or inflammatory changes, often markers of underlying microscopic damage [14]. As such, it is easy to misinterpret neuroimaging, especially computer tomography (CT) as suggesting only minimal injury, when the child has actually experienced extensive diffuse axonal shear injury, especially to the white matter of the frontal lobes.

Focal injuries most often result from tearing of blood vessels (hemorrhages), bruising of tissue (contusions), or a combination of these pathologies. Although found in all regions of the brain, contusions are most common in areas where soft brain parenchyma is surrounded by the bony ridges of the eye orbits (orbital and inferior medial frontal) and the sphenoid ridge and temporal bones (anterior and medial temporal). As the sides of the cranium (frontal and parietal bones) are relatively flat and smooth, contusions are less common. This distribution of cranial features accounts for the most common symptoms of TBI. Orbital and inferior medial frontal contusions can disrupt emotional and behavioral regulation resulting in disinhibited behaviors, emotional lability, agitation, and irritability with low frustration tolerance. Contusions to the anterior and medial temporal lobes can result in disrupted ability to store new memories (post-traumatic amnesia, anterograde amnesia), and due to the amygdala and other limbic structures being located in this area, also can result in emotional dysregulation, especially that related to fear, anxiety, and aggression [14]. Of note, the structures of the anterior and medial temporal lobes are also highly prone to seizure activity, especially after injury, resulting in increased risk of acute post-traumatic seizures and a higher risk of lifelong seizures [15–17]. The clinical case described below had extensive hemorrhagic contusions within the frontal and anterior temporal lobe regions, as expected given the severity of physical injury sustained by the child.

Diffuse injuries are more often the result of shearing or twisting forces acting on delicate axons or capillaries. When soft brain tissue experiences rapid deceleration upon contacting the inner cranial surface, a compression wave can penetrate the brain, causing diffuse damage some distance from the point of impact. Twisting and shearing forces caused by distortion of the soft brain tissues and surrounding meninges can result in extensive tearing of bridging veins under the dura or arachnoid layers, resulting in subdural or subarachnoid bleeds. As a general rule, any force strong enough to result in a subdural bleed can also cause microscopic damage to the underlying brain parenchyma [18] and result in long-term functional deficits. The effects of forces traveling through soft brain parenchyma will differ depending on the density of brain tissue. Because gray matter and white matter have different densities, shear injuries are more common at the gray-white junctions, as these tissues tend to pull against each other severing delicate connections. Axonal shear injury at the gray-white borders is more common in infants and young children than in adolescents and adults, although shear damage of the corpus callosum is more common in adolescents and adults [9]. Petechial hemorrhages close to the gray-white junction on imaging suggest diffuse axonal shear injury, and the prognostic value of these tiny bleeds is greater than would be expected given the extent of bleeding [14]. Evidence of hemorrhagic contusions and diffuse axonal shear injury, especially to the corpus callosum, suggests a worse long-term prognosis. The clinical case study described below involved significant evidence of diffuse axonal shear injury and damage to the corpus callosum, making long-term prognosis poor, especially for higher-level integrated cognitive abilities. Diffuse injury to the brain can also be caused by secondary complications of TBI such as edema, vascular compromise, hypoxic ischemia, status epilepticus, etc.

Collaborative Care

Collaboration between the neuropsychologist and physician can assist in treatment planning based on realistic goals and expectations, a difficult topic for many with traumatic brain injuries. The cases with the clearest prognosis are often those with the most severe brain trauma or those with minimal brain trauma; prognosis is easiest at the extremes of severity. Prognosis in cases with injury to multiple areas of cortical and/or subcortical structures is more difficult to predict, especially early in recovery, while numerous physiological processes remain disrupted. Some predictive models for severe TBI have been developed and utilize a variety of baseline characteristics and pathological markers [19, 20], although as time progresses, prognosis generally becomes clearer. Because of this, predicting outcome for many cases of severe pediatric TBI should not be attempted within the first few weeks or until physiologic disruption such as edema or inflammatory changes have started to resolve. After a week or two, acute physiological disruption can resolve relatively rapidly, with functioning improving daily, a good prognostic indicator for the child.

The role of the neuropsychologist varies throughout the different phases of recovery and can range from providing general prognosis for functional recovery given the extent and severity of TBI to assessment of recovery and functional abilities and ultimately provision of therapeutic intervention or recommendations to maximize post-discharge functioning. Physician consultation is often more focused throughout the different phases of recovery, with attention primarily given to the patient's acute medical needs, medication management, coordination of care from a variety of specialists, and communication of complex medical issue to family members. The respective roles of the neuropsychologist and physician overlap at all stages of recovery, allowing for ongoing collaboration between these specialists. For example, both assess the patient's status and functional abilities, although neuropsychological evaluation provides more detailed information regarding cognitive, behavioral, or emotional strengths, weaknesses, or deficits, in addition to an overview of the individual's general functioning. The physician's assessment is more related to medical or physical concerns, especially those requiring pharmacological or structured therapeutic intervention; little time is spent on detailed assessment of cognitive, behavioral, or emotional functioning. In general, the information derived from neuropsychological assessment is often not available from other techniques, such as basic neurological or mental status examinations, neuroimaging, or electroencephalography (EEG). Although the physician evaluates the patient, additional information obtained from neuropsychological involvement can be critical in guiding the treatment direction for the physician.

Key Point

From an assessment standpoint, greater emphasis is placed on physician assessment during the critical care stages of recovery, with increasingly more reliance on neuropsychological assessment as the child recovers, and is able to participate in a more complex evaluation of higher-level cognitive or behavioral skills, or requires more sophisticated evaluation of emotional status. Follow-up neuropsychological assessment may last many hours and include a variety of age-appropriate tasks assessing cognitive integrity, behavioral functioning, and/or emotional status. Counseling is also provided and includes a discussion of the assessment findings, prognoses for each functional domain, and appropriate accommodations or intervention for ongoing recovery or use of compensatory strategies. During medical follow-up, the physician may only spend a few minutes evaluating medication or equipment needs, fill out prescriptions for services or referral to other specialists. Interactions between the neuropsychologist and physician are critical, as it is not helpful for a neuropsychologist to discover a condition requiring medical treatment, but not have the treatment initiated by the physician as soon as possible, or for the physician to discover a condition requiring neuropsychological assessment or intervention, but not communicate such to the specialist.

In the PICU, and during the critical care stage, the neuropsychologist acts as the expert on brain pathology and recovery from a functional perspective, while the physician provides expertise on the medical care of the patient. Emphasis is placed on minimizing or reversing complications responsible for secondary brain injury, such as edema, hemorrhages, seizures, increased intracranial pressure, reduced blood perfusion, etc. In the PICU, the role of the neuropsychologist can range from assessing changes to mental status that may suggest deterioration or recovery from pathological processes to reviewing the extent and severity of injury as it pertains to likelihood of recovery of cognitive, motor, sensory, and general adaptive functioning. The initial role of the physician in the PICU is to prevent further injury to the brain through secondary processes while also stabilizing the medical condition of the patient to facilitate recovery. As the patient becomes more stable, the neuropsychologist and physician can work together to formulate a pharmacological treatment plan that best matches the child's specific stage of recovery. For example, after initial stabilization, discussions may relate to appropriate rehabilitation therapies or medication options to maximize level of arousal, ability to interact with the environment or others, and ultimately communicate, process information, and regain functional mobility. Throughout the PICU stay, the neuropsychologist and physician often work together to communicate information to the child's family in a manner they are able to understand. The neuropsychologist may spend considerable time reviewing brain imaging, discussing the type and severity of damage, anatomical areas most involved along with general functioning, and recovery issues from a developmental perspective. The physician may spend time discussing the medical condition of the child, medication management of physical, cognitive, behavioral, or emotional symptoms, in addition to medical procedures such as external ventricular drains, intracranial pressure monitors, catheters, tracheostomies, gastronomy tubes, etc.

Once medically stable, the child is transferred to the general medical floor or the rehabilitation unit as appropriate given the severity of TBI, level of functioning, or therapeutic needs. Involvement of the neuropsychologist can increase at this stage of recovery, when the patient's abilities may change daily and affect how care is provided. Communicating changing cognitive abilities to the treatment team can optimize care and provision of therapeutic intervention. Ongoing assessment of functioning can assist in formulation of long-term prognosis, expectations for ongoing therapeutic needs or accommodations, school reintegration, and appropriateness of different recreational activities given safety concerns post TBI. During this stage of recovery, the physician works with the neuropsychologist and members of the treatment team to order appropriate interventions (speech therapy, occupational therapy, physical therapy, recreational therapy, etc.) and to assess for appropriateness of utilizing medications to optimize functioning and participation in the treatment regimen. Medication issues may relate to low arousal, apathy or abulia, and inability to sustain attention, in addition to behavioral and emotional difficulties such as agitation, emotional lability, anxiety, or depression. Pharmacological treatment of motor or sensory symptoms is also a focus of physician treatment at this stage of recovery. For example, the physician may treat increased tone or spasticity with baclofen or neuropathic pain with Neurontin. Systemic disruption relating to the bowel and bladder, gastrointestinal functioning, blood pressure, sleep-wake cycles, kidney functioning, hormone/endocrine functioning, etc., is also a focus of physician treatment of inpatient pediatric TBI. This is especially true for those cases with deep brain injuries involving diencephalic structures (thalamus, hypothalamus, etc.), pituitary system, in addition to frontal modulatory and limbic structures.

Following discharge from the hospital, appointments for neuropsychological or medical follow-up can be arranged at appropriate intervals depending on the specific needs of the child. Neuropsychological follow-up appointments may be necessary after only a month or two in order to coordinate changing needs for school services or accommodations, especially as this is the time when recovery is most rapid, and substantive functional changes may be apparent after only a few weeks. After the first year or two, when most acute recovery is complete, follow-up appointments may still be necessary to monitor the child's development relative to age- or grade-matched peers. For complex TBI cases, school psychologist evaluations focused on academics, and achievement or intelligence may not be sensitive to many of the child's difficulties, especially those related to complex attention, executive functioning, and memory. As such, even with ongoing assessment by the school, follow-up evaluation by a neuropsychologist trained and knowledgeable about brain injury in children is recommended. For babies and infants with TBI, follow-up appointments may be arranged 1 or 2 years following discharge and then every year or two as needed to monitor neurodevelopment and attainment of expected functional milestones. For the physician, outpatient follow-up appointments are frequently necessary for monitoring of, or discontinuation of, medications utilized during the acute stages of recovery, or if durable medical equipment is required (wheelchairs, orthotics, etc.), and to order new equipment as appropriate to the growing child's needs. Referral to other specialists is also a critical function of the physician in follow-up, in order to ensure appropriate care for a variety of medical or physical conditions related to TBI or the bodily injuries that often accompany TBI.

Key Point: Neuropsychologist and Physician Collaboration

There are numerous advantages to physicians who utilize neuropsychological services when working with pediatric traumatic brain injury patients. General prognosis for functional recovery is aided by accurate and timely cognitive and behavioral observation and standardized assessment to allow for comparison with age-based peer expectancies. Therapeutic interventions are guided by clear profiles of cognitive and behavioral strengths, weaknesses, and deficits. Recommendations from the neuropsychologist are critical in facilitating school reintegration and post-discharge functioning within a variety of personal and social domains. The roles of the neuropsychologist and physician overlap during all phases of treatment for pediatric TBI and allow for integration of similar but disparate bodies of expertise; the neuropsychologist provides expertise in neuropathology and patient cognitive and behavioral functioning, while the physician provides expertise in the medical management of the neurological, physical, and systemic effects of the TBI. With cognitive, behavioral, and emotional disruption negatively impacting patient care and ultimately transition back to more age-appropriate expectations, detailed clinical impressions involving these domains of functioning are critical in allowing the physician to most appropriately manage care, especially as it relates to medications and referral to a variety of healthcare specialists for ongoing intervention. Much of the information gained from neuropsychological evaluation is not available from basic neurological or mental status examinations or advanced diagnostic techniques such as neuroimaging or electroencephalography. Although clinic notes and assessment reports are available, the information obtained through review of reports does not come close to the information obtained during direct encounters between specialists. As such, integrating the findings and clinical impressions from neuropsychological assessment and observation is best done during direct collaboration between the neuropsychologist and the physician. Only when the context of the medical state and specific functioning of the patient, including subtle findings at that particular recovery stage, are considered together, can the accurate clinical picture of the patient be obtained and fully conceptualized.

Medication Management Post-PICU

Once a child is stable enough to be discharged from the PICU, the focus of medication management often transitions from critical care needs and secondary complications to management of motor/sensory disruption, in addition to cognitive, behavioral, or emotional difficulties. Below are some guidelines regarding medication use for a variety of common conditions exhibited by children following TBI, once they have been discharged from critical care.

Arousal: beyond therapeutic and environmental techniques, there are some pharmacological management tools to help stimulate arousal and maintain a state of readiness for sensory input. Prior to beginning a stimulant, it is prudent to carefully review the current medication list for potential drug-induced sedation. Sedative side effects of anticonvulsants, antihypertensive agents, and some gastrointestinal medications are magnified in brain-injured patients and generally underappreciated. Due to a neurotransmitter decrease following TBI, it is now suggested that some medications altering dopamine, norepinephrine, and serotonin may be beneficial in arousal disorders. One example in this case is the use of amantadine chloride, which has been shown to enhance neurotransmission in the dopamine-dependent nigrostriatal, mesolimbic, and frontostriatal circuits responsible for mediating drive, arousal, and attention [21, 22].

Attention: psychostimulants such as methylphenidate are commonly used to treat attention deficit hyperactivity disorder, a condition related to frontal-executive functioning and often caused or exacerbated by TBI. The agent is proposed to bind to the dopamine transporters, blocking reuptake and increasing extracellular dopamine levels, noted substantially in the frontal cortex. In the acute phase after TBI, it is thought that methylphenidate also increases norepinephrine and serotonin levels. Some patients treated with Ritalin have demonstrated better performance in attention, concentration, and motor memory testing at 1 month, but the benefits did not persist at 3 months. Long-term studies suggest that while psychostimulants may shorten recovery time, they do not change morbidity, and more studies are warranted [23].

Agitation: agitation has been shown to negatively affect the rate of recovery in pediatric acute inpatient rehabilitation. Symptoms can range from physical and verbal aggression, irritability, maladaptive behavior, and mood lability to explosive anger, akathisia, and disorientation. After non-pharmacological management has been utilized for environmental control of noise, visitors, and a behavioral plan is in place, some patients benefit further from pharmacological medical interventions. Research supports the use of beta-blockers such as propranolol for agitation reduction. The proposed mechanism of action is to reduce hyperadrenergic activity. Benzodiazepines work on the GABA receptor molecule to create anxiolytic, sedative, antispasticity, and amnestic effects. Effects are based on the duration of action. Short half-life medications include alprazolam and midazolam; intermediate effects for lorazepam, and longer duration medications, include diazepam and clonazepam. Side effects can include amnesia, fatigue, decreased alertness, and decreased concentration; and repeated or extended use of benzodiazepines may slow neuronal recovery. An alpha-adrenergic receptor agonist, clonidine, decreases sympathetic tone. Some studies show this may be useful for akathisia-induced agitation or for inattention. Anticonvulsants provide mood stabilization using various mechanisms (decrease excitatory neurotransmitter activity, increase inhibitor neurotransmitter activity, or reduce subclinical epileptic activity). Research on anticonvulsants in children is limited to epilepsy trials. Occasionally, agitation after a severe traumatic brain injury can progress to aggression, extreme emotional lability and dysregulation, motor and cognitive restlessness, and ultimately noncompliance and refusal to participate. In these cases, it may be prudent to consider an atypical neuroleptic or antipsychotic medication. Risperidone has a dual mechanism of antagonistic action affecting the serotonin-dopamine system, and has been reported to have fewer extrapyramidal side effects than typical antipsychotic medications, such as Haldol. Risperidone is known to block D2 and 5HT2A receptors. If other medication combinations have failed to curb agitation and aggression, short courses of low-dose risperidone have been shown to be helpful in patients with traumatic brain injury. Dosages of 0.25–1 mg are effective. There are some common adverse effects from risperidone, requiring monitoring of any patient receiving these medication. Anxiety, dizziness, vision changes, drowsiness, dystonia, nausea, constipation, tachycardia, and weight gain are the most common side effects. Thus, limited use is recommended, and there are very few complete studies on the effects of antipsychotic medications in pediatric brain injury.

For summaries of medication use after TBI, also consider Pangilinan et al. [24] and Suskauer and Trovato [25].

Unique Aspects of Working with Pediatric TBI

Neuropsychologists and physicians working with children face a variety of challenges not seen in most adult cases. TBI at a young age or during critical periods of brain maturation can disrupt the rate and extent of future brain development. Although a child may appear to experience a "good recovery" while still young, the child may fall behind peers in many areas of cognitive functioning over time due to disrupted neurodevelopment or manifestation of effects from early injury. For babies and infants, the full effects of TBI may not be apparent at the time of injury. The child may not have reached the developmental stage when abilities related to the injury are expected to emerge. For example, TBI in a 4-month-old involving the primary language cortices will not result in apparent changes to functioning as language has not yet developed in the child. However, early damage to dominant hemisphere peri-Sylvian language cortices will almost certainly disrupt future development of language in that child, a condition that will not become evident for several months to years. The same is true for TBI in children of elementary or middle school ages. Recovery of basic cognitive abilities reliant on old learning may be rapid and appear mostly complete. However, damage may result in disrupted development of higher-level cognitive processes expected later in adolescence, such as efficient complex or divided attention, executive functioning, mental flexibility, abstraction, and processing of complex concepts. As such, assessment of children with TBI must take into account the developmental age of the child, in addition to the acute effects of recovery or plasticity versus disruption to neurodevelopment of specific processes or functional systems. Additionally, the effects of damage to the brain differ depending on the specific stage of neurodevelopment.

As a general rule, TBI to an immature brain, especially prior to cell differentiation, can result in more diffuse cognitive and functional difficulties later in life, while the same TBI in a mature brain may affect only a specific cognitive process or system. Damage during critical neural growth spurts can be more disruptive to those systems undergoing rapid development than a similar injury at other times during the child's life [10]. Because of this, the stage of neurodevelopment becomes critical in formulating accurate prognoses following TBI, and general prognostic rules appropriate to adult TBI may not apply.

Key Point

The nature and extent of an insult to the brain may be silent at its onset and on evaluation of a young child. Problems may only appear once the child has developed to a point where the functioning would normally be expected to emerge. The child may appear to have experienced good recovery and be functioning normally for several years, but then may "grow into his or her pathology," experiencing increasing difficulty as expectations for more complex cognitive processes increase with advancing age or grade level.

An additional challenge involves the assessment and treatment of prelingual children, with their inability to verbally communicate symptoms. Symptoms must be derived from clinical examination and behavior, as you cannot just ask them about their difficulties. In addition, young children, especially those recovering from TBI, may not realize something is wrong with them due to a lack of reference or inability to self-assess their functioning. As an example, a child discovered to have subtle diplopia did not complain of double vision. However, during an assessment session, the child asked why there were two suns. Just prior to his assessment, the child had been outside with his parents during a break from physical therapy. He thought it was interesting that there were two suns out that day. This was not expressed as a symptom or as something wrong, just an interesting feature of the day. Further assessment confirmed diplopia due to mild dysconjugate gaze relating to a palsy in cranial nerve VI.

A final challenge to working with children with TBI relates to the family dynamics for each case. Every child with a TBI comes with a family or social environment that cannot be separated from the child. In reality, the neuropsychologist and physician treat the child and the family, with the family becoming integral members of the treatment team, "family-centered care." This can provide both benefits and complications and add many levels of complexity for the neuropsychologist and physician. See Seligman and Darling [26] for additional information and a multisystem perspective on childhood disability and its effects on family life.

Clinical Case: Cameron

Cameron sustained a severe traumatic brain injury with both focal brain stem and more diffuse bifrontal and bitemporal hemorrhagic contusions and diffuse axonal injuries requiring a variety of approaches to care throughout the various stages of recovery. This case highlights the wide range of clinical issues that can present in pediatric TBI, but also how one's approach to treatment changes with time due to the dynamic nature of brain injury. It also demonstrates the close interaction and collaboration between the neuropsychologist and physician caring for the child with TBI.

Patient: Cameron, 6-year-old male, status post motor vehicle accident, unrestrained passenger

Reason for hospital admit: multi-trauma including severe traumatic brain injury

Case Presentation

Cameron was a previously healthy 6-year-old male who was involved in a multiple vehicle collision as an unrestrained backseat passenger approximately 30 minutes prior to arrival in our emergency department. He was sitting in the back seat of his family vehicle with two other siblings when the vehicle was rear-ended at high speed. Emergency medical service reports indicate he was thrown forward and suffered extensive injuries to his head with positive loss of consciousness. Cameron was described as unresponsive at the scene with a Glasgow Coma Scale (GCS) of 3. The Glasgow Coma Scale is a basic measure of a patient's level of consciousness following TBI, with measures of eye opening, verbal response, and motor response [27]. He was emergently intubated due to bradycardia and facial trauma in order to protect his airway. Upon arrival to our emergency department, he was evaluated by the trauma service as well as neurosurgery. There was no motor movement and he was nonresponsive. His right pupil was 6 mm and unreactive, his left pupil was 3 mm and unreactive, and there were no corneal reflexes. He lacked a gag reflex; however, he did cough and was breathing occasionally over the ventilator. He was emergently scanned with CT identifying multiple subdural hematomas with minimal mass effect and some slight left to right midline shift. There was evidence of bifrontal and bitemporal contusions with significant bifrontal skull fractures comminuted through the frontal sinus. Basal cisterns were compressed although not completely obscured due to diffuse edema (brain swelling). The CT angiogram showed all the intracranial vasculature to be patent. He was placed on intracranial pressure (ICP) monitoring, and after he received multiple doses of 3% saline and mannitol, his ICPs dropped to the low 20s. He remained at a GCS of 3, but with some occasional spontaneous movement of his extremities. He had significant periorbital and frontal edema. Admit impressions to the PICU included but were not restricted to the following: severe TBI, diffuse axonal injury, multiple subdural and subarachnoid hemorrhages, bifrontal and bitemporal intraparenchymal hemorrhagic contusions, corpus callosum tearing, intracranial hypertension, acute respiratory failure requiring mechanical ventilation, extensive craniofacial injuries, and multiple physical/orthopedic injuries.

Past medical history was unremarkable, with the exception of some parental concerns regarding possible attention deficit hyperactivity disorder (ADHD), although without a formal diagnosis.

Pediatric Intensive Care: Physician Impressions

Overnight, Cameron's ICPs were trending up to the mid-20s, and they were expected to increase with ongoing evolution of edema, even with 3% saline and mannitol. At this point in the evolution of his brain injury, and with imminent increase in intracranial pressure, he was at risk of herniation and decrease in cerebral perfusion pressure (CPP). Accordingly, neurosurgery performed a bifrontal craniectomy to control his ICP and protect against herniation or hypoxic ischemia due to low CPPs. Decompressive craniectomy and hemicraniectomy are well-accepted surgical interventions for intracranial hypertension secondary to increased intracranial pressure when medical management has failed to control the pressure [2]. CT findings were discussed with the family who were at bedside. The rationale for proceeding with the hemicraniectomy given concerns regarding secondary damage to brain tissue and risk of herniation was also discussed. Norepinephrine (NE) was started and titrated for CPP of 60–70. He was placed on seizure prophylaxis as frontal and temporal contusions are very epileptogenic. Sodium was targeted to be between 145 and 155, his hemoglobin was maintained greater than 10, carbon dioxide levels were normalized, and his cerebral perfusion pressure was stabilized above 60. His cervical spine was cleared with MRI, and head MRI/MRA was obtained to provide more information regarding his brain injury. MRI revealed multifocal areas of hemorrhagic contusion and suggestion of extensive diffuse axonal injury throughout the bilateral frontal parenchyma and marked corpus callosum tearing. MRA of the cervical and intracranial arterial vasculature was unremarkable. Post craniectomy, ICPs were stabilized around 10–12 and his CPPs between 70 and 80; accordingly, his NE was weaned. Cameron's pupils remained nonreactive and he would occasionally bite on the endotracheal tube (ETT). No gag or cough was detected, and he presented without spontaneous movements. Intermittently, he exhibited reflexive movements of his upper and lower extremities.

Over the first few weeks of intensive care, Cameron was maintained on mechanical ventilation with sedation and Keppra for seizure prophylaxis. Serum sodiums were kept between 145 and 155. He was kept normothermic and normocapnic. He was started on meningitis dosing of ceftriaxone empirically. Aggressive therapies were continued. ETT cultures were found to be positive for MRSA for which he was started on clindamycin. Inotropic support was able to be weaned off. Sedation was minimized, and Cameron began to breathe above the vent, and eventually respirator support was able to be weaned. His nasogastric feeds were advancing to our goal. He regained a cough and gag reflex although failed extubation. Cameron was taken to surgery for tracheostomy and 1 week following the procedure was transferred out of the PICU to the medical rehabilitation unit.

Pediatric Intensive Care: Neuropsychology Impressions

Neuropsychology consultation was requested by the attending physician and medical team to assist in treatment planning and to meet with the family to discuss the type, extent, and severity of Cameron's brain injury, general prognosis, and expectations for recovery. Evaluation of functional abilities was also requested, in addition to the provision of counseling and support to the family during this difficult and confusing time for them.

Cameron had been extubated and was breathing through a tracheostomy with high flow oxygen. His sedation had been weaned, and he was stable without evidence of diencephalic storming, a concern given the severity of his brain injury that included midbrain structures. Cameron remained unresponsive to verbal or visual stimuli, and exhibited only generalized responses to tactile stimulation such as increased tone and posturing, in addition to sympathetic hyperarousal. Considerable time was utilized in consulting with family members, including parents, aunt and uncle, sister, and friends regarding my initial clinical impressions, general pathophysiology, severity and extent of his injury, and reasonable expectations from worst-case to best-case scenarios. It was clear that the provision of information was welcomed by Cameron's family and friends, and their questions were appropriate to this stage of recovery, with realistic expectations as they related to possible future outcomes.

Primary Clinical Considerations in the PICU for Neuropsychology and Physician

Prognosis is extremely difficult during the first few weeks following severe TBI. Inflammatory changes, swelling, electrolyte imbalance, disrupted vascular autoregulation, hypometabolic disruption at the mitochondrial level, and other acute physiological changes can temporarily disrupt functioning in excess of that expected given the extent of permanent physical trauma. As such, functioning during the initial week or two following injury may appear more impaired than physical damage would suggest due to temporary physiological or metabolic compromise to brain functioning. With respect to Cameron, for the first few weeks he remained mostly unresponsive and at a Rancho Los Amigos level I (no response to stimulation) with short periods of level II (generalized responses to stimulation). The Rancho Los Amigos Levels of Cognitive Functioning is a qualitative measurement of an individual's level of cognitive functioning following brain injury [28]. Due to the recency of his TBI, it was difficult to determine whether his initial low level of functioning was related to the effects of sedation, temporary neurophysiological compromise, or more permanent damage to his brain. As time progressed, and without rapid recovery after the first few weeks and weaning of sedation, it became clear his low level of arousal was related to damaged midbrain mesencephalic structures and pathways, with hemorrhage and contusion evident on MRI.

It is important to assess TBI not only on severity of injury but also the specific structures most damaged by the injury. Although most literature suggests recovery from severe TBI is likely to be incomplete and should progress in a roughly exponential fashion, with the most rapid recovery over the first few weeks to month and then recovery slowing after 6–9 months, and continuing for years, this is not always the case. As discussed above, recovery during the first week or two may have little relationship to long-term recovery and may be more related to neurochemical processes than healing of tissue per se. Further, recovery from mostly diffuse cortical injuries tends to follow the expected exponential recovery course described in the literature, while recovery from deeper injuries to the subcortical structures may be more protracted or even show changes over hours or days. Cameron is an interesting case because he sustained both focal subcortical injuries, in addition to more diffuse cortical and white matter damage. As such, predicting the extent and rate of recovery was more complex and the neuropsychological and medical counsel provided to his family reflected such. Specifically, it was likely his low arousal and inability to interact with the environment related to his mesencephalic (midbrain) injury (Figs. 6.1, 6.2, and 6.3, respectively). Note on Fig. 6.1, the bright region identified by the red arrow on the left represents hemorrhage, and the darker region identified by the red arrow on the right represents contusion to brain parenchyma.

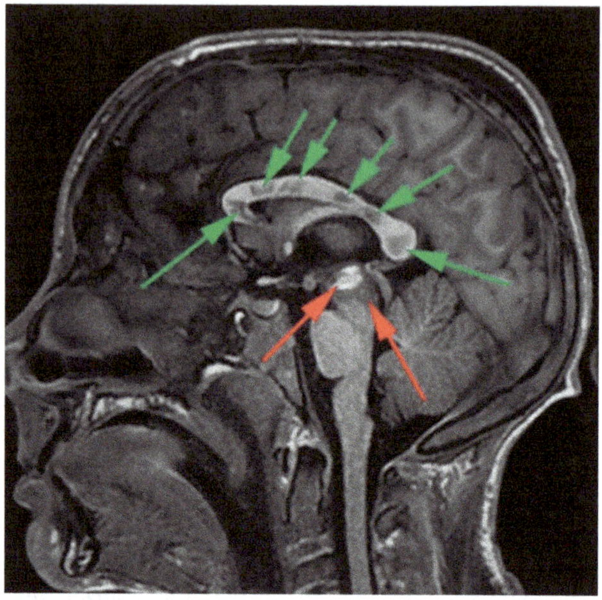

Fig. 6.1 Sagittal T1 (midbrain mesencephalic injury, red arrow; corpus callosum injuries, green arrows)

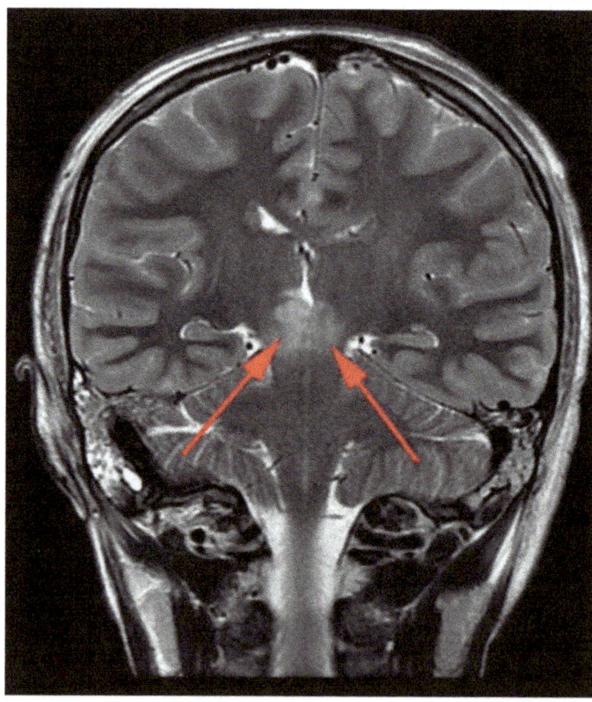

Fig. 6.2 Coronal T2 FSE (midbrain mesencephalic injury, red arrow)

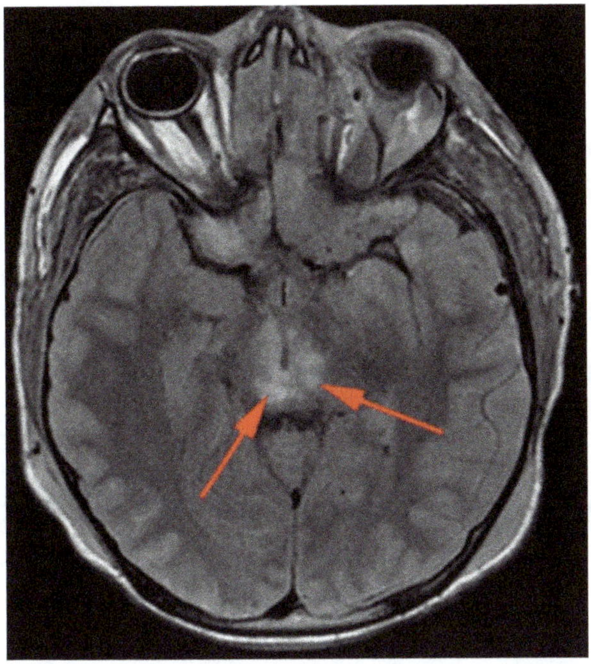

Fig. 6.3 Axial T2 FLAIR (midbrain mesencephalic injury, red arrow)

Recovery from midbrain injuries can be rapid and even complete, if there is minimal damage to supratentorial cortex. These conditions are sometimes referred to as "light-switch injuries," as the patient can remain unresponsive due to impaired mesencephalic functioning, but then with resolution of edema or ongoing recovery of midbrain structures, suddenly wakes up and exhibits rapid return of functioning. When counseling Cameron's parents, the analogy of a car was used to assist in understanding. The engine was used to represent the cortex, and the electrical system that activates the starter motor was used to represent the midbrain arousal systems. Put simply, until the midbrain injury heals, Cameron may not wake up, in the same way a car will not run if there is no power going to the starter motor. Once he wakes up, only then can the effects of his cortical injuries be assessed. Or using the car analogy, until one can start a car, it cannot be taken for a test drive to see how it runs. Cameron had two distinct neuropathological processes to be considered when providing prognosis and time course for recovery. First, the treatment team had to consider options to assist in providing activation to the arousal mechanisms of his midbrain. Then, if he exhibited improved arousal, his functioning could be assessed and a more accurate prognosis and long-term treatment plan could be provided to the family. At this point in his care, it remained possible he would never wake up from his midbrain injury, and this was communicated to his family.

After 3 weeks of hospitalization, Cameron remained unresponsive, although was medically stable and on room air through his trach. Sensory stimulation was ordered to facilitate improved arousal. Sensory stimulation, sometimes called "coma stimulation," is often used to improve arousal and awareness after severe brain injury.

In Cameron's case, the goal of coma stimulation was to activate reticular activating networks in an attempt to increase arousal and attention to the environment or incoming stimuli. Nurses and therapists employed techniques of tactile stimulation with varying degrees of pressure applied to arms, legs, torso, and gums. Mild temperature changes to skin areas, such as a cold wet cloth to the face, and vibratory sensation to fingertips and wrists were utilized. Auditory stimulation with music, soft bells, and verbal cadence change was utilized. Although olfactory stimulation can sometimes be helpful, many patients sustain cranial nerve injury to the olfactory bulbs, rendering this sensation limited or absent. Given Cameron's extensive orbital medial frontal lobe trauma in the region of his olfactory bulbs, this modality was not employed as part of his coma stimulation program. Given Cameron's vital signs were stable, a trial of amantadine, 100 mg twice a day, was considered to facilitate arousal. Following 4 days of amantadine, at almost 4 weeks post injury, assessment of functioning suggested subtle but continual improvements in general arousal. Over the next several days, Cameron exhibited increasing levels of arousal to the point where he was beginning to follow simple one-part commands (such as close your eyes, open your hand) and was able to visually orient and track objects and persons in the room. Given his stable medical state, increased arousal, and increasing ability to follow simple directions, he was transitioned to the medical rehabilitation unit for a higher level of therapeutic intervention.

Admit to Full Acute Inpatient Rehabilitation: Neuropsychology Impressions

Cameron was exhibiting improved reactivity to his environment and could sustain some limited interactions with family and staff. Arousal continued to improve; he appeared to be progressing to a stage of recovery consistent with Rancho Los Amigo's level IV (confused, agitated, restless). When his behavior was restricted, he would bite or try to strike the person interacting with him, with clear escalation of agitation and restlessness. He exhibited inconsistent and fleeting periods of awareness and would attempt to get out of bed. He had some communicative intent, although was still not verbalizing. Communication was achieved through changes in behavior and affect, or he would grab at items or reach for his groin to indicate a desire to urinate. He lacked appropriate self-directed behaviors and was almost completely reactive to his environment and the interventions of others. It was recommended he be transitioned from a standard hospital bed to a floor bed (mattress with soft siding on the floor) to allow him to move more freely and minimize any risk of him falling out of bed given his increased mobility, with lack of judgment or behavioral control. He was placed on full-time "one-on-one" supervision, as he would pull at tubes and his trach. Parents remained at bedside and were an excellent resource for him.

With his changing status, it was clear his symptoms were becoming less consistent with his previous midbrain mesencephalic injury and more representative of his bifrontal diffuse axonal injury with frontal-temporal contusions (Figs. 6.4 and 6.5),

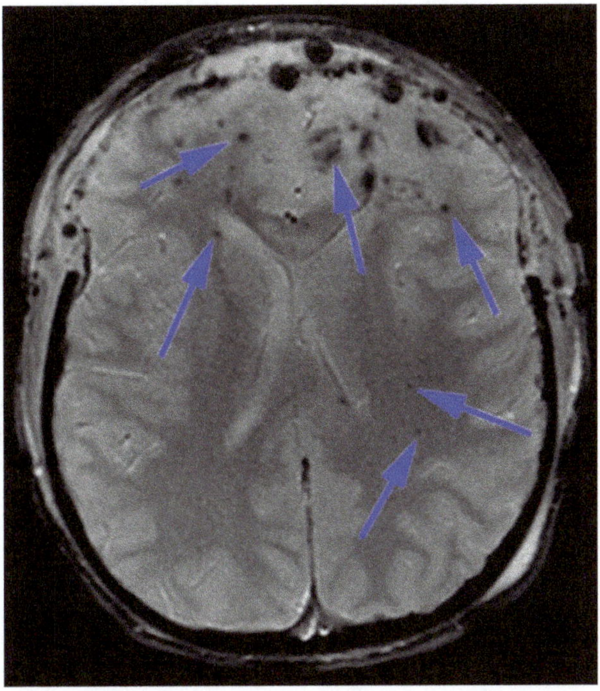

Fig. 6.4 Axial GRE (T2*) (hemorrhages shown as black patches—samples identified by blue arrows)

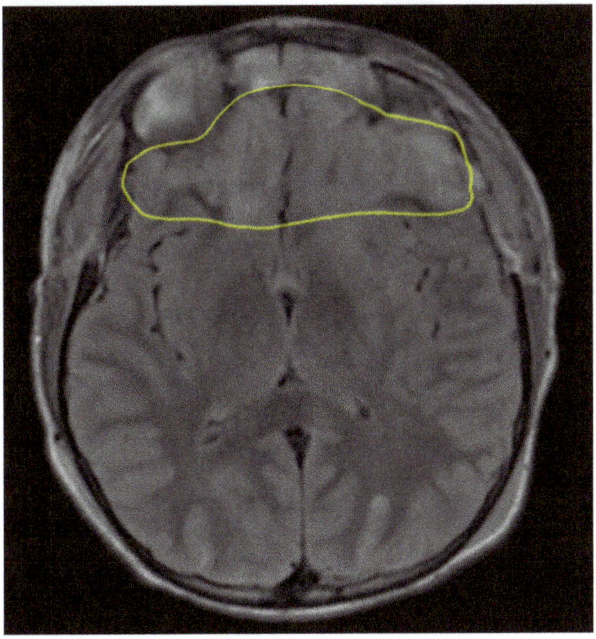

Fig. 6.5 Axial T2 FLAIR (frontal and temporal cortex contusions shown within yellow boundary)

in addition to tearing of the corpus callosum (Fig. 6.1—green arrows). Although diffuse axonal shear injury is not readily visible on MRI, the petechial hemorrhages evident on Fig. 6.4, especially those at the gray-white junction, are highly suggestive of such. Cameron's parents were counseled regarding his evolving condition and the reasons for his changing behavior and functional presentation. Current MRI imaging was reviewed with his parents to highlight the frontal, temporal, and white matter damage, something that was not emphasized while he was in the PICU. They were reminded of the car analogy provided in the PICU, paraphrased as, "we need to get his motor started first, and only then will we know the actual extent of his brain damage as it relates to his functioning." Given he was now awake and alert, discussion transitioned from one of "waking him up" to one focused on the effects of his cortical and white matter damage. They were counseled his behavioral difficulties were actually a sign of brain recovery, not deterioration. The fact that he had these new behavioral difficulties indicated improvement in his arousal mechanisms and neurological status, thus revealing problems not evident when he was in a coma. Discussion with his parents also covered issues relating to ways the brain heals, mechanisms for recovery, in addition to issues pertaining to the interaction between the benefits of neural plasticity and the detrimental effects of early injury on disrupted neural development.

Admit to Full Acute Inpatient Rehabilitation: MD Impressions

Cameron was now consistently alert and presented with inconsistent ability to follow directions and participate in intervention. Our neuropsychologist expressed concern regarding increasing agitation and restlessness, and some aggressive behaviors, likely related to improving but suboptimal awareness, physical limitations, and ongoing confusion, anxiety, and likely fear. Rancho Los Amigos level appears to be progressing from II (generalized responses to stimulation) to IV (agitation with restlessness and confusion). Pain was controlled with both ibuprofen and low-dose hydrocodone-acetaminophen (Norco) and environmental modifications such as a floor bed to allow more movement and minimize the need for restraints. Cameron remained nonverbal and our speech therapist was working with him to facilitate communication and attempted a Passy-Muir speaking valve upon clearance by pulmonology. Physical, occupational, and speech therapies were each provided 1 h per day, half hour in the morning and half hour in the afternoon. Pulmonology services followed for respiratory issues and worked toward preparing Cameron to have his trach removed prior to discharge from our service. Custom ankle-foot orthotics (AFOs) were utilized for standing and ambulation, and baclofen, 10 mg three times a day, had been added for spasticity and tone control. Botox was considered following a trial of baclofen, as his tone continued to increase and interfere with his ability to participate in therapies and with his general mobility.

Primary Clinical Consideration during Rehabilitation for Neuropsychology and Physician

Discussion between neuropsychology and the physician was focused on the following considerations for Cameron. First, he was more consistently awake, alert, and becoming aware of his surroundings but was also exhibiting agitation and restlessness. He continued to be confused and unable to act in a self-directed or functional manner and lacked safety awareness or control. When restless, he tried to pull at tubes and get out of bed, and exhibited irritability and some aggressive behaviors, requiring one-on-one supervision and a floor bed setup. With his changing status, discussion focused on discontinuing his amantadine, as he was consistently awake and alert. In addition, it was decided to begin lorazepam (Ativan) 0.5–1 mg as needed for excessive anxiety, agitation, and aggression, in addition to scheduled risperidone 0.25 mg daily for extreme emotional dysregulation, irritability, and aggression. Due to increased motor tone, baclofen was added as a way to control spasticity and allow for improved mobility during his rehabilitation regimen.

Discharge from Full Acute Inpatient Rehabilitation: Neuropsychological Impressions

Agitation, restlessness, and aggressive behaviors had resolved, and the Ativan and risperidone had been discontinued. Cameron was exhibiting improved awareness and insight into his condition, and he was exhibiting improved behavioral and emotional control. Cognitive abilities had continued to recovery, and Cameron had progressed to a Rancho Los Amigos level VI (ongoing confusion and memory impairment but with self-directed behaviors and appropriate object use). Cameron was more consistently communicative with basic receptive and expressive language abilities being mostly functional for communication of primary needs and wants. He was exhibiting self-initiated behaviors, although was exhibiting marked apathy and abulia, and an inability to sustain attention for more than a few seconds at a time. Attentional vigilance and task persistence were severely disrupted and limited his ability to participate in self-directed or structured activities, even with constant encouragement and reinforcement from others. He was unable to participate in comprehensive neuropsychological assessment, although was able to respond for short periods of time on individual tasks and on the Lebby-Asbell Neurocognitive Screening Examination for Children (LANSE-C) [10]. The LANSE-C measures a variety of cognitive domains for children from 6 to 11 years, 11 months, and the Lebby-Asbell Neurocognitive Screening Examination for Adolescents (LANSE-A) measures cognitive functioning in adolescents from 12 years to 17 years, 11 months, or older. These measures are useful in acute care or clinic setting when a child or adolescent is unable to tolerate lengthy assessment of neurocognitive functioning. The screening examinations can be administered in under 30 minutes, and each of the 14 subtests can be administered individually for children such as Cameron who struggled to sustain attention and task persistence for more than a few minutes at a time. Portions of standardized assessment batteries were also administered, as tolerated, and included such measures as the Wechsler Intelligence Scale for Children, Wechsler Preschool and Primary Scale of Intelligence, and the Children's Memory Scale.

Performance on examination of basic intellectual functioning suggested mildly impaired to low average abilities for his age. However, these levels did not fully represent his abilities in less structured settings and were more a function of old learning and premorbid skill acquisition than recovered higher-level cognitive processes per se. For example, when completing simple verbal and visual-perceptual problems, Cameron tended to process the surface structure or basic features, although lacked the ability to integrate information at a higher level of analysis expected for his age. In addition, he exhibited a high degree of frontal rigidity and perseverative interference, with Cameron often repeating responses from previous questions or using the same strategy to solve problems even when a new strategy was called for. In addition, his performance was optimized by a high degree of external structure to minimize the negative effects of his disrupted attentional vigilance and task persistence. Although formal measures of executive functioning were inappropriate given his young age, it was clear he struggled with internal mental organization and structure, and self-control, especially when in less structured settings. Memory for new information was improving each week, and Cameron could recognize members of his treatment team and was able to recall some salient activities of the day. However, on structured examination of new learning (anterograde memory), few details were retained after a short delay with distraction. Memory for information presented during therapy sessions was also compromised, with Cameron consistently failing to recall activities he had just completed with the therapist. Cameron's severe attentional limitation was considered a contributing factor for his memory disruption, as was his general apathy, abulia, and lack of task persistence or concern for his difficulties.

Mood was variable, although he generally presented as either indiscriminately happy or affectively flat, suggesting disruption to emotional regulatory systems. He exhibited little to no anxiety when around strangers, interacting with them in a manner not unlike that exhibited with family or known members of our staff. Social functioning remained immature and impulsive for his age, and his mood was often incongruent with the specific situation or environmental context. For example, at times he presented as happy when one would expect frustration due to significant difficulty completing tasks he found simple prior to his TBI. At other times, he remained emotionally blunted and affectively flat when one would expect excitement during visits from family and friends or when playing with the hospital's therapy dogs. Such capricious emotional responses suggested limited insight or awareness of his severe ongoing disabilities, in addition to disruption to frontal-limbic modulatory systems responsible for mood and affect regulation. Given his relatively unusual presentation, with Cameron frequently acting in a manner incongruous with the social or environmental context, a parental meeting was arranged with his neuropsychologist and physician to explain how the partial recovery from his TBI, and the specific structures impacted by his injury were influencing emotional and behavioral functioning. They were counseled about the dynamic nature of such injuries, and how this was likely a stage of recovery, and not his "new normal," as with further recovery, insight, and control of his emotional and behavioral functioning, significant improvements were expected. The time course for recovery was also discussed, with emphasis on this particular stage, with assurances provided such as "Remember, his recovery is only just beginning, and recovery from a brain injury is a marathon, not a sprint, we have barely left the starting gate." A school reintegration meeting was also arranged with his parents, the attending physician, rehabilitation therapists, and his educational team members to discuss his specific cognitive, behavioral, emotional, and physical strengths, weaknesses, and deficits.

Discharge from Full Acute Inpatient Rehabilitation: Physician Impressions

By discharge from the rehabilitation program, Cameron was no longer exhibiting marked behavioral dysregulation, agitation, restlessness, or aggressive tendencies. However, based on the ongoing neuropsychological assessments, it was clear Cameron was having difficulty with sustained and focused attention, self-initiation, and drive (abulia) and was densely apathetic. With his changing behavioral presentation, the Ativan and risperidone were discontinued, and a trial of methylphenidate (Ritalin) 5 mg morning and midday was administered, with subtle but noticeable improvements in functioning being evident. Ritalin was a good option during the final weeks of rehabilitation given his premorbid symptoms of mild ADHD, with exacerbation of these difficulties by his TBI. Ritalin was appropriate given his symptoms transitioning from low arousal, through a stage of agitation, and ultimately to consistently disrupted sustained and complex attention, limited cognitive vigilance and task persistence, and with some ongoing frontal apathy and abulia negatively impacting his ability to participate in many age-appropriate activities. Cameron's baclofen was discontinued as his muscle tone had improved, and the mild sedative effects of the medication may have been a contributing factor with his attentional difficulties, apathy, and abulia. Upon discharge, prescriptions were written for continuation of the Ritalin until he was seen for follow-up in the multidisciplinary rehabilitation follow-up clinic. Prescriptions were provided for IEP evaluation and services, in addition to adaptive physical education. A list of restrictions to recreational activities was provided to his parents and faxed to his school. Prescriptions were provided for ongoing physical, occupational, and speech therapy. Referrals were made for neurosurgery, neurology, and neuropsychology follow-up appointments.

Outpatient Follow-Up Examinations: The Next 10 Years—Neuropsychology and Physician

Cameron was seen for a 3-month post-discharge follow-up examination with his neuropsychologist and physician. Findings from his morning neuropsychological assessment were as expected, with clear evidence of ongoing recovery across all functional domains but with a pattern of strengths relating to basic processes and weaknesses and deficits for higher-level reasoning and problem solving. There had been significant resolution of his apathy and abulia, and he had improved ability to maintain focus on tasks presented to him without the need for constant redirection or prompting. Attentional functioning remained below age expectancies throughout his examination, and on specific measures of complex attention, performance remained mildly impaired for his age. Concerns were expressed regarding Cameron's behavior, with his parents describing situations where Cameron would become emotionally labile and distraught and have temper tantrums for even minor issues. During his afternoon clinic appointment with his physician, Cameron's parents described improved attentional functioning when taking his Ritalin, and so his prescription was renewed and a follow-up visit was scheduled to monitor medications.

Both his neuropsychologist and physician met with Cameron's parents following their respective assessments, to discuss findings and coordinate ongoing care. One of the primary topics of discussion was how Cameron's family and social dynamics changed following his injury and how this may be a factor in his behavioral and emotional difficulties. For example, since his injury, he had received disproportionate parental attention compared to his siblings, something that was necessary during his hospitalization, although can be disruptive following discharge home, and when transition to a more normal family dynamic is recommended. Put simply, although Cameron's brain injury had made him more prone to emotional dysregulation, the attention he was receiving each time he became upset was reinforcing his maladaptive behaviors, and he was becoming spoiled. The excessive attention from his parents was partly due to a lack of providing consequences as they believed his behavior was not his fault and was solely caused by his brain injury. In addition, his parents felt sorry for him given his ongoing difficulties functioning, as well as the recreational restrictions placed on him by his physician. Further, they were experiencing some self-guilt for failing to restrain him in the vehicle and causing his injuries and were trying to compensate for this by giving him everything he wanted. Cameron's parents were given explicit permission to begin normalizing his home environment, provide appropriate consequences both positive and negative for his behaviors, and place reasonable expectations given his abilities and age for family chores and duties. In addition, they were counseled regarding the effects of disproportionate attention to Cameron on their other children and ways to normalize this component of their lives. For a summary of contemporary theories of family dynamics with childhood disability, see Seligman and Darling [26].

Over the next several years, Cameron was seen for neuropsychological evaluation yearly at first and then every other year as needed. He was also followed by his neuropsychologist and physician in a joint clinic, every 6 months at first and then yearly to monitor his development and to make recommendations regarding his medications, therapeutic interventions, and educational program. Cameron's pattern of recovery followed the expected course for diffuse frontal and temporal injuries, with more rapid gains over the first few months to approximately a year, with slowing improvements after 1–2 years. After approximately 2 years of relatively rapid recovery, and quite marked gains, new difficulties began to emerge as expectations for higher-level reasoning and executive functioning increased. This suggested his brain injury had disrupted development of these higher-level integrated systems, with the effects of the pathology not being apparent when he was younger, or until such skills were expected to emerge.

Cameron's general pattern of cognitive strengths, weaknesses, and deficits was not unlike that identified during inpatient assessment. He continued to have little difficulty with basic cognitive processes, although he experienced disproportionate deficits with more complex tasks requiring mental manipulation, divided attention, and rapid efficient integration of information. He also struggled with higher-level reasoning requiring processing of abstract concepts or mental organization and strategy. When tasks could be completed without a high cognitive demand, his performance fell mostly within normal limits, although low normal to mildly diminished in some cases. Because of his specific profile of cognitive strengths and weaknesses, he was able to perform adequately on school-based academic assessment of basic skills, although consistently failed to meet expectations for classroom work or more advanced cognitive abilities. In the classroom, Cameron experienced the most difficulty with multitasking and dividing his attention, such as when required to listen to his teacher, review information in his textbooks, and write notes or when tracking the rapid flow of information during lectures. The discrepancy between his tested abilities and his classroom or homework performance was interpreted by his teachers as a function of his behavior. Specifically, they communicated to his parents their concerns such as, "he is not trying," and "he lacks effort," as a way to explain his failure in the classroom but adequate testing performance on measures of basic reading, spelling, and arithmetic.

Due to his declining classroom performance, Cameron's parents scheduled a joint clinic appointment with his neuropsychologist and physician. They expressed concerns regarding possible deterioration of neurological functioning as a way to explain declining school grades. Although his teachers had described poor effort, Cameron's parents noted he always seems to try his best and exert a good effort to his homework. His mother added, "He has been doing so well, and now is failing, I'm worried something is going bad with his brain." Physician evaluation included his neurological status, motor and sensory functioning, and reflexes, all unremarkable and without evidence of acute neurological decline since his previous clinic visit. On neuropsychological assessment, basic intellectual and academic functioning was mostly unremarkable and fell variably from the borderline impaired to average ranges, with the central tendency low average for his age. Qualitative assessment of his performance revealed disrupted ability to conceptualize abstractly or efficiently integrate information, with most responses being relatively concrete for his age. A neurodegenerative condition was ruled out as he continued to improve in all areas of functioning when comparing raw scores, even though his age-corrected (standardized) scores were declining over time. This pattern is indicative of Cameron gaining abilities but not at the rate expected given the passage of time, with his relative performance compared to age-matched peers declining. The gap between his abilities and that expected for his age was widening, especially for tasks involving complex attention and executive functioning, and to a lesser extent for higher-level reasoning. Over the next several years, even with assistance from his educational team and parents, Cameron fell further behind his peers as expectations increased for higher-level cognitive processing involving complex and divided attention, executive functioning, and ability to conceptualize abstractly. In addition, he experienced increasing difficulty functioning in a regular education classroom setting as presented material became more conceptual and complex, and required more active attention and integration, with his classroom grades suffering accordingly. Cameron didn't have a neurodegenerative condition or new brain pathologies; in contrast, he was experiencing the late effects of his diffuse TBI with extensive bifrontal white matter and corpus callosum injuries, along with the effects of disrupted neurodevelopment on neural systems that had not yet developed at the time of his early life brain trauma.

When comparing performance on primary cognitive processes over the decade following his TBI (Figs. 6.6 and 6.7), it is clear Cameron experienced the expected rapid recovery over the first 6 months to a year, with slowing gains over the next year or more. In Fig. 6.6, it is apparent Cameron's complex attention and executive functioning skills were more affected by his injury than basic verbal-linguistic and visual-spatial reasoning skills. Initially, and until approximately 9 years of age,

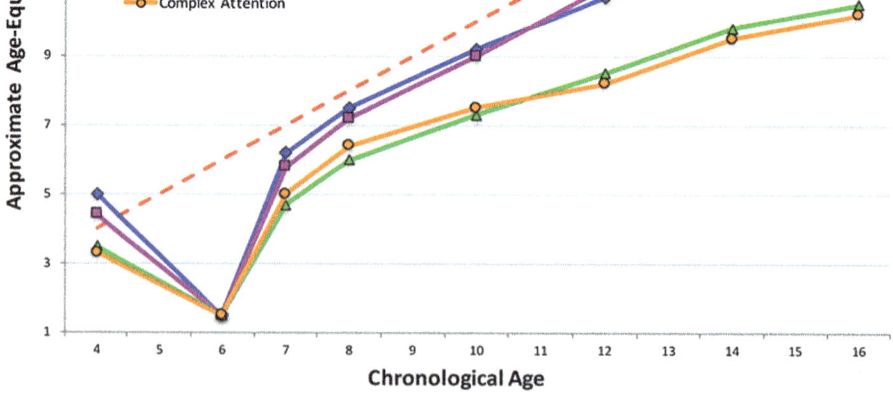

Fig. 6.6 Recovery and development for primary cognitive processes over 10 years post TBI

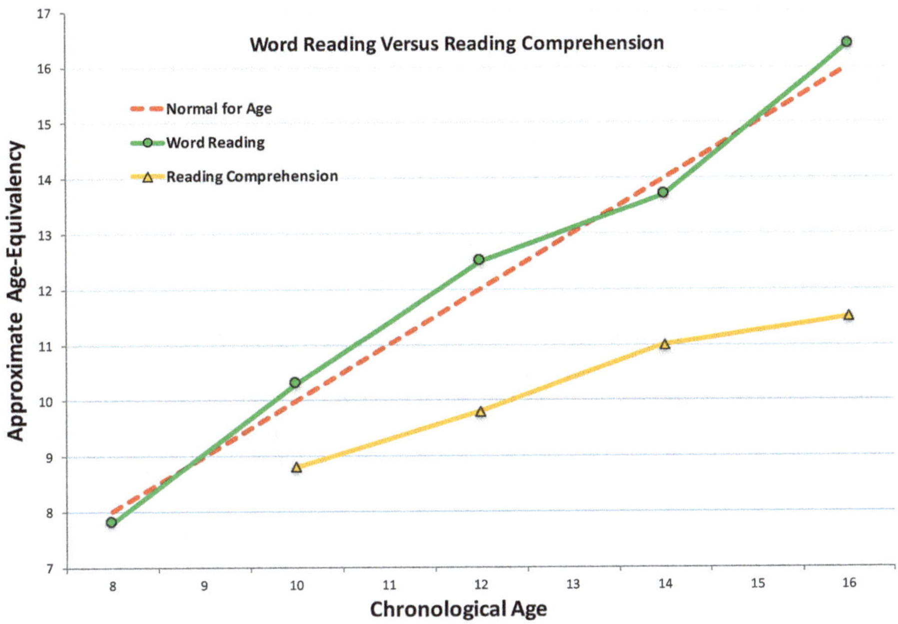

Fig. 6.7 Development of reading and reading comprehension skills

Cameron maintained improvements close to that expected for the passage of time. However, by 10 years of age, as expectations increased for higher-level cognitive processing, he began to experience disproportionate compromise to complex attention and executive functioning and to a lesser degree with higher-level reasoning requiring mental flexibility, abstract conceptualization, and complex integration of information. Assessment of basic word reading beginning at 8 years of age was unremarkable. More complex reading comprehension tests were added to his assessment beginning at 10 years of age due to parental concerns regarding declining school performance. The discrepancy between single word reading and reading comprehension was quite informative, as was the disproportionate relative decline in performance for reading comprehension tasks over the next 6 years. It was clear Cameron was having marked difficulty integrating and conceptualizing information on more advanced reading comprehension tests, with greater difficulty over time as expected given increasing grade-level requirements and expectations (Fig. 6.7). Such difficulties are not unexpected given his extensive diffuse white matter damage to the frontal lobes and corpus callosum, pathways critical for complex and efficient information processing, in addition to his ability to sustain attention to multiple details simultaneously and conceptualize and integrate across passages for reading comprehension tasks. A similar pattern was noted for basic arithmetic skills versus math reasoning skills or verbal math problems. Although basic arithmetic skills are necessary for these tasks, Cameron's difficulties related more to higher-level cognitive processes mediated by his frontal-executive system and white matter networks of his frontal lobes than basic arithmetic skills per se.

What had been interpreted as poor effort or a behavioral problem by his teachers was actually the expected presentation in a child with mostly preserved basic cognitive skills, but disproportionate deficits involving more complex higher-level processes. School-based assessment of basic academic skills was inadequate and not comprehensive enough to fully illuminate Cameron's profile of strengths, weaknesses, and deficits, all expected given the type, extent, and severity of TBI and his developmental age at the time of injury. Communication with his educational team, regarding his neuropsychological profile, with recommendations for specific accommodations and interventions assisted in formulating a more appropriate educational plan for Cameron.

Over time, and with continuing declines in classroom grades, and increasing difficulty in school, Cameron began to experience deterioration of his mood, ultimately struggling with frustration, low self-esteem, anxiety, and depression. All of these emotional difficulties can be caused by TBI involving the frontal and temporal lobes, and because of this, Cameron was at greater risk than other children his age. However, his struggles in school, and also with the expected adolescent social difficulties related to how he was perceived by peers, began to manifest as rapidly declining mood and confidence. Assessment of emotional status during neuropsychological assessment precipitated referral initially to school counseling services. Eventually, however, Cameron was referred to a private child psychologist at our hospital, with a trial of an SSRI antidepressant medication (Zoloft, 50 mg, daily), to be monitored by the neuropsychologist and physician on a regular basis and in consultation with his clinical psychologist.

Closing Remarks

While the symptoms of brain injury in children are similar to the symptoms experienced by adults, the functional impact is often markedly different. The cognitive and behavioral impairment of children may not be immediately obvious, and the nature of deficits transforms over time, maturation, and both academic and social expectations. It is essential to utilize a multidisciplinary team with expertise in child and adolescent functioning and the effects of TBI on neurodevelopment, on emotional maturation, and on the child's family or social system.

Chapter Review Questions

1. Secondary brain injury is:
   A. Brain injury caused by sedation and use of paralytic medications.
   B. Brain injury caused by the vascular, metabolic, epileptogenic, or other physiological processes caused by the initial trauma.
   C. Brain injury caused by the bouncing of the brain inside the cranium opposite the site of impact.
   D. Brain injury resulting from post-TBI disruption of neurodevelopment.

2. Recovery from TBI follows the following course:
   A. Slow while in intensive care, becoming more rapid in rehabilitation, and greatest after 6 months to 2 years.
   B. Linear beginning at the time of injury and following a consistent rate until recovery.
   C. Variable depending on the intensity of intervention provided following discharge from the hospital.
   D. Variable depending on the stage of recovery (acute versus post-acute) and the pathological processes being considered.

3. Pediatric TBI is different from adult TBI due to all of the following except:
   A. The child's developmental stage may mask deficits relating to the brain injury.
   B. An infant or young child with TBI may not recognize when his or her functioning is disrupted.
   C. Disruption to ongoing neurodevelopment may result in deficits later in life not evident during the acute stage.
   D. Family dynamics for children with TBI can be more complicated due to the child's dependency on care providers.
   E. Damage to an immature brain generally causes more focal injury than the same injury to an adult brain.

4. Most severe TBI injuries in children result in:
   A. Primarily focal injuries to the deeper subcortical structures of the brain.
   B. Primarily focal injuries to the cortical structures of the frontal, parietal lobes, and occipital lobes.
   C. Primarily diffuse injuries to the frontal lobes, parietal lobes, and occipital lobes.
   D. A combination of focal contusions to the frontal and temporal lobes with more diffuse white matter injuries at the gray-white junctions of the frontal and parietal lobes.
   E. Less severe damage to frontal and temporal lobes than the parietal and occipital lobes.

5. Methylphenidate is a stimulant that works to help increase alertness and some aspects of cognitive function in patients with brain injury by:
   A. Blocking calcium channels to prevent vasospasm.
   B. Blocking the reuptake of norepinephrine and dopamine into presynaptic neurons.
   C. Producing CNS depression and reducing intracranial pressure.
   D. Binding to the glycoprotein SV2A to inhibit presynaptic neurotransmitter release.

References

1. Chesnut RM. Secondary brain insults after head injury: clinical perspectives. New Horiz. 1995;3:366–75.
2. Haddad SH, Arabi YM. Critical care management of severe traumatic brain injury in adults. Scand J Trauma Resusc Emerg Med. 2012;20:12.
3. Unterberg AW, Stover JF, Kress B, Kiening KL. Edema and brain trauma. Neuroscience. 2004;129:1021–9.
4. McCrory P, Meeuwisse W, Dvořák J, et al. Consensus statement on concussion in sport—the 5th international conference on concussion in sport held in Berlin, October 2016. Br J Sports Med. 2017;51:838–47.
5. Helmer KG, Pasternak O, Fredman E, Preciado RI, Koerte IK, Sasaki T, Mayinger M, Johnson AM, Holmes JD, Forwell LA, Skopelja EN, Shenton ME, Echlin PS. Hockey Concussion Education Project, Part 1. Susceptibility-weighted imaging study in male and female ice hockey players over a single season. J Neurosurg. 2014;120(4):864–72.
6. Centers for Disease Control and Prevention, National Center for Injury Prevention and Control. Injury prevention & control: traumatic brain injury. Centers for Disease Control and Prevention. 18 March 2013.
7. Ganesalingam K, Yeates KO, Taylor HG, Walz NC, Stancin T, Wade S. Executive functions and social competence in young children 6 months following traumatic brain injury. Neuropsychology. 2011;25(4):466–76.
8. Lajiness-O'Neill R, Erdodi L, Bigler ED. Memory and learning in pediatric traumatic brain injury: a review and examination of moderators of outcome. Appl Neuropsychol. 2010;17(2):83–92.
9. Hutchison T, Lebby PC. Traumatic encephalopathies. In: David RB, editor. Clinical pediatric neurology. 3rd ed. New York: Demos Medical Publishing; 2009.
10. Lebby PC, Asbell SJ. The source for traumatic brain injury children and adolescents. East Moline, IL: LinguiSystems, Inc; 2007.
11. Ewing-Cobbs L, Prasad M, Landry S, Kramer L, DeLeon R. Executive functions following traumatic brain injury in young children: a preliminary analysis. Dev Neuropsychol. 2004;26(1):487–512.
12. Lebby PC, Pollock M, Mouanoutoua A, Lewey JH. Performance of children and adolescents with brain injury on the Lebby-Asbell neurocognitive screening examination for children and adolescents. J Child Neurol. 2015;30(10):1255–62.
13. Mayo Clinic. Traumatic brain injury. *Mayo Clinic.* 2012. http://www.mayoclinic.com/health/traumatic-brain-injury/DS00552.
14. Lebby PC. Brain imaging: a guide for clinicians. New York, NY: Oxford University Press; 2013.
15. Annegers JF, Hauser WA, Coan SP, Rocca WA. A population-based study of seizures after traumatic brain injuries. N Engl J Med. 1998;338(1):20–4.
16. Garga N, Lowenstein DH. Posttraumatic epilepsy: a major problem in desperate need of major advances. Epilepsy Curr. 2006;6(1):1–5.
17. Hahn YS, Fuchs S, Flannery AM, Barthel MJ, McLone DG. Factors influencing posttraumatic seizures in children. Neurosurgery. 1988;22(5):864–7.
18. Hoskote A, Richards P, Anslow P, McShane T. Subdural haematoma and non-accidental head injury in children. Childs Nerv Syst. 2002;18:311–7.
19. Hukkelhoven CW, Steyerberg EW, Habbema JD, Farace E, Marmarou A, Murry GD, Marshall LF, Maas AI. Predicting outcome after traumatic brain injury: development and validation of a prognostic score based on admission characteristics. J Neurotrauma. 2005;22(10):1025–39.
20. Tasaki O, Shiozaki T, Hamasaki T, Kajino K, Nakae H, Tanaka H, Shimazu T, Sugimoto H. Prognostic indicators and outcome prediction model for severe traumatic brain injury. J Trauma. 2009;66(2):304–8.

21. Giacino JT, Whyte J, Bagiella E, Kalmar K, Childs N, Khademi A, Eifert B, Long D, Katz D, Cho S, Yablon S, Luther M, Hammond FM, Nordenbo A, Novak P, Mercer W, Maurer-Karattup P, Sherer M. Placebo controlled trial of amantadine for severe traumatic brain injury. N Engl J Med. 2012;366(9):819–26.
22. Greb E. Amantadine may hasten functional recovery in patients with severe TBI. Neurol Rev. 2012;20(4):5.
23. Whyte J, Hart T, Vaccaro M, Grieb-Neff P, Risser A, Polansky M, Coslett HB. Effects of methylphenidate on attention deficits after traumatic brain injury: a multidimensional, randomized, controlled trial. Am J Phys Med Rehabil. 2004;83(6):401–20.
24. Pangilinan P, Giacoletti A, Shellhaas R, Hurvitz E, Hornyak E. Neuropharmacology in pediatric brain injury: a review. PMR J. 2010;2(12):1127–40
25. Suskauer S, Trovato M. Update on pharmaceutical intervention for disorders of consciousness and agitation after traumatic brain injury in children. PMR J. 2013;5(2):142–7.
26. Seligman M, Darling RB. Ordinary families, special children: a system approach to childhood disability. 3rd ed. New York, NY: Guilford Press; 2009.
27. Teasdale G, Jennett B. Assessment of coma and impaired consciousness. A practical scale. Lancet. 1974;2(7872):81–4.
28. Hagen C, Malkmus D, Durham P. Levels of cognitive functioning. Downey, CA: Rancho Los Amigos Hospital; 1972.

Chapter 7
Autism Spectrum Disorder with Seizures: Collaboration through Case Example

Amy V. Davis, Emma Cole, and Gaurav Yadava

Introduction

Anyone who evaluates children with an autism spectrum disorder (ASD) knows that they can be the most complex but rewarding patients. From a medical perspective, there are higher rates of seizure disorders [1], genetic disorders [2], in utero complications [3], and other abnormal neurological findings [4–6]. Parents of children with ASD are the fiercest advocates for their children. These parents seek out traditional but also nontraditional treatments and evaluations in pursuit of answers regarding their child, in hopes of a cure. The case selected here highlights the complexities associated with ASD but, more importantly, demonstrates the collaborative role that neurology and neuropsychology play in providing optimal care for an ASD child.

Referral

Patient: 7-year, 4-month-old male
Education: attending first grade

A. V. Davis (✉) · G. Yadava
Amita Health—Women and Children's Hospital, Center for Pediatric Brain—Hoffman Estates, Hoffman Estates, IL, USA
e-mail: Amy.Davis@amitahealth.org

E. Cole
Amita Health—Women and Children's Hospital, Center for Pediatric Brain—Hoffman Estates, Hoffman Estates, IL, USA

Department of Neuropsychology, Kennedy Krieger Schools, Kennedy Krieger Institute, Baltimore, MD, USA

K. M. Sanders (ed.), *Physician's Field Guide to Neuropsychology*,
https://doi.org/10.1007/978-1-4939-8722-1_7

Reason for Referral: Matt was referred for a neuropsychological evaluation in the context of previous diagnoses of Attention-Deficit/Hyperactivity Disorder (ADHD), Oppositional Defiant Disorder (ODD), Sensory Processing Disorder, and Anxiety Disorder, Not Otherwise Specified (NOS), as well as a medical diagnosis of absence seizures. There were also questionable diagnoses of gestational Lyme disease and hypothyroidism per parent report. Presenting concerns revolved around emotional and behavioral dysregulation, academic and memory difficulties, and inattention and impulsivity. In addition, there were concerns for fine motor deficits, sleeping and eating issues, poor social skills, sensory sensitivities, and specific concerns that he may be on the autism spectrum. Matt's parents sought diagnostic clarity and wished to obtain recommendations for supportive therapies and services.

Case Presentation

Matt was the product of a complicated early-term pregnancy and delivery. His mother had hyperemesis gravidarum for which she took medication. She had elevated alpha-fetoprotein levels on her quad screen, which required biweekly stress tests during the last 3 months of her pregnancy. Matt was born at 37 weeks gestation and spent 3 days in the NICU due to meconium aspiration. He was placed on a nasal capula and required stomach pumping. Matt's mother reportedly contracted Lyme disease 8 years prior to Matt's birth but was not diagnosed until Matt was 8 months old. Matt was evaluated by a Lyme specialist when he was 12 months of age and was treated with antibiotics for 3 months. He was diagnosed at age 5 with gestational Lyme disease by a DAN (Defeat Autism Now) doctor who prescribed Matt antibiotics and various supplements. Other medical history is positive for multiple ear infections requiring three sets of PE tubes, and adenoidectomy. Genetic testing at age four including microarray and Fragile X testing was normal. Dr. Yadava diagnosed Matt with abnormal gait, ADHD, combined type, sensory integration dysfunction with anxiety, and ODD when Matt was 5 years old. He was diagnosed with nonconvulsive, primary generalized epilepsy (i.e., absence seizures) by Dr. Yadava later that year. Matt has had multiple EEGs and MRIs. A 24 h EEG conducted when Matt was 5 years old was abnormal and suspicious of generalized seizure disorder with atypical features of an absence seizure disorder. An EEG completed when Matt was 7 years old was normal. Matt's last 48 h EEG was abnormal and indicated a lower threshold for primary generalized seizures. A brain MRI completed when Matt was 5 years old showed white matter hyperintensities bilaterally in the parietal lobes, but this was considered a normal myelination pattern for his age. A spine MRI completed when Matt was 5 years old was normal. Matt takes Focalin (10 mg bid) and Depakote (125 mg bid) managed by Dr. Yadava, and hydrocortisone (10 mg qid, 5 mg qid), levothyroxine (50 μg qid), liothyronine (15 μg qid), metoprolol (50 mg bid), and terazosin (3 mg tid) managed by his Lyme specialist. Immediate family history is significant for fibromyalgia, spina bifida occulta, and ADHD. Extended family history is positive for ADHD, dyslexia, and learning disabilities.

At the time of the evaluation, Matt had a limited diet. He preferred bland foods, was reluctant to try new foods, insisted that food was cut a certain way, and that he used the same dishware at each meal. Matt had good sleep initiation, but was a light sleeper, and occasionally grinded his teeth and snored. Motor milestones were on the later side of normal as Matt crawled at 10 months and walked at 14 months. His language and toileting milestones were met on time, although there was still nighttime enuresis. Matt had sensory sensitivity to auditory, olfactory, tactile, oral, and vestibular stimulation; he also overheated easily.

Matt received early intervention (EI) services including occupational therapy (OT), physical therapy (PT), and speech therapy (ST) from age 2 to 3. He attended 3 years of early childhood special education services from age three to five, where physical aggression, defiant behavior, and inattentive and impulsive behaviors were reported. Matt attended a half-day self-contained kindergarten program where he received social work (SW), OT, PT, and ST qualifying under the Developmental Delay category. He began first grade year in a self-contained classroom, but was moved to a general education setting with math and writing resource support after he began mimicking the poor behaviors of other students in his class. At the time of the evaluation, Matt was receiving OT, ST, SW, math, and writing supports under the category of Other Health Impairment (OHI). His parents reported that Matt had good reading skills but difficulty writing secondary to his fine motor deficits. They also reported that he was having difficulty retaining information. Matt had participated in multiple private therapies. He began private ST, OT, and PT at age three and was discharged from ST at age four, discharged from PT at age six, and was continuing with OT at the time of the neuropsychological evaluation. Matt also saw a social worker when he was 3 years old, and had recently restarted with both individual and group therapies.

Matt was usually a happy child whose mood could change quickly. He could be verbally and physically aggressive, defiant, argumentative, and noncompliant. Tight holds and brushing therapy helped regulate him. Behavior difficulties were not seen at school except during group instruction. Although Matt cried easily, there were no concerns for depression or low self-esteem. Matt worried about transitions, bad storms, and the dark. He had friends, but none were described as close or best friends. Matt was invited to birthday parties, but play dates were difficult to arrange because of Matt's poor behavior. Matt also had difficulty waiting his turn and was a "rule enforcer," which also impacted his social relationships. Matt got along better with girls and younger children. Matt's parents reported deficits in his social communication and interaction as he exhibited challenges with back-and-forth conversation and reciprocal play, and had difficulty with social approach. There were deficits in nonverbal communicative behaviors for social interaction including poor eye contact and difficulties reading social cues. His parents also reported that Matt had restricted interests for iPad, TV, and dinosaur books. Finally, his parents reported that Matt struggled with transitions and exhibited repetitive behaviors such as toe walking, spinning, lining up toys, echoing, scripting, and mixing up of pronouns.

Neurological Exams and Findings

Matt was awake, alert, and quite hyperactive in the exam room. He engaged in decent eye contact. He displayed difficulty with reciprocal and pragmatic interactions. He had mild diffuse hypotonia without weakness and deep tendon reflexes were 2+/symmetric. He had a tendency toward toe walking on casual gait examination. He was unable to copy basic shapes (i.e., circle, square). He was unable to hop on each foot independently.

EEG was ordered due to episodic staring noted by child's family. Routine EEG was abnormal showing generalized spike-and-wave activity at a frequency of 2.5–3.5 Hz. Due to his abnormal EEG and developmental issues, MRI brain was performed (in order to evaluate for structural abnormalities), which was normal for his age.

Preliminary Impressions

EEG is consistent with primary generalized epilepsy, in particular childhood absence epilepsy.

The MD Perspective

Children with developmental disorders are at higher risk for epilepsy. These children are also at increased risk for other social, cognitive, and behavioral issues. For example, patients with childhood absence epilepsy experience higher rates of comorbid ADHD. Therefore, inattention and learning difficulties in this population are often multifactorial [7]. Though clinical signs of cerebral dysfunction are evident in children with developmental disorders with and without epilepsy, many of these children have structurally normal neuroimaging.

> **Key Point**
> "Staring" episodes are commonly seen in children with developmental delays, in particular autistic disorders. In the majority of these children, staring is behavioral in nature (i.e., related to internal or external distractibility). However, EEG should be considered given higher rates of seizure disorders in this population.

Referring to Neuropsychology

Despite appropriate treatment of this child's ADHD and epilepsy, he continued to display behavioral dysregulation, atypical social skills, and learning difficulties. Neuropsychological assessment was advised in order to evaluate for the presence of coexisting neurodevelopmental disorders.

Role of Neuropsychology

Questions to be addressed via neuropsychological assessment: Does this child meet criteria for an autism spectrum disorder? What are his cognitive abilities? Are his attention and focus adequate on current medication?

Key Point
ADHD and hyperactive behaviors are common comorbid conditions in children with ASD. Recent data suggests that the diagnosis of ADHD can delay an appropriate diagnosis of autism [8]. Neuropsychological assessment is imperative for diagnostic clarity and in order to ensure appropriate management and interventions in children who often present with multiple possible diagnoses.

Evaluations: Pediatric Considerations

The MD Perspective

Research has shown differences in brain anatomy in children with ASD and that age and gender can play a moderating role [4, 6]. This is particularly evident in brain volumes that are found to be larger in ASD children during toddlerhood, normalizing by early school age and then declining into adolescence/adulthood. There are also structural brain abnormalities that have been linked to specific cognitive processes in ASD individuals including frontotemporal and amygdala regions associated with poor social-emotional processing, Broca's and Wernicke's areas to social and communicative language deficits, and orbitofrontal cortex and caudate nucleus playing a role in the repetitive and stereotyped behaviors associated with ASD [4]. Nonetheless, findings from neuroimaging studies are heterogeneous with few consistencies. Other neurological issues are often common in children with ASD, with epilepsy being the most common comorbid neurological condition. Children on the autism spectrum have a lifetime risk of seizures around 25–30% [1], and this risk is higher in those children with associated language impairments (up to 50%).

In children with developmental delays, neuropsychological evaluation, neurological assessments, and directed neurological studies (i.e., brain MRI, EEG, etc.) are indicated in order to clarify underlying diagnoses as well as common comorbidities. Results of comprehensive assessments can help guide educational accommodations, developmental therapies, and medication decisions (when appropriate) in order to maximize each child's functional potential.

Neuropsychological Testing

Neuropsychological Perspective of the ASD Child

Autism spectrum disorder (ASD) occurs in 1 in 68 children and is reported in all racial, ethnic, and social-economic groups [9]. The average prevalence of ASD is approximately 1–2% and is 4.5 times more common in boys than girls [9].

Research has definitively determined that there is a genetic contribution to autism disorders with at least half of the risk for being diagnosed with ASD originating from genetic factors [2]. Approximately 49% of ASD cases are the result of commonly inherited variants, 3% of cases result from de novo mutations, 3% of cases occur from rare inherited genetic variants, and 41% of cases have no apparent genetic component [10]. While larger chromosomal abnormalities are less common and found in only approximately 2% of cases [11], mild to severe deficits in intellectual abilities, language, seizures, motor skill deficits, and hypotonia are associated with such abnormalities [5]. More specifically, genetic syndromes such as Fragile X (25% of males), Prader-Willi (20–25%), tuberous sclerosis (20%), and Down's syndrome (6–15%) have high rates of autism symptomology [5].

Diagnosing ASD is challenging and many children are not identified as being on the spectrum because of the variability of symptom expression in ASD. Diversity in the presentation of ASD means that not one diagnostic test or instrument is sufficient to comprehensively assess for ASD. However, there are specific domains that the National Research Council Committee on Educational Interventions for Children with Autism have recommended be evaluated when diagnosing autism [12]. Among the most important domains are assessment of intellectual, developmental, and language testing. Evaluation of these areas is required to differentiate ASD from other developmental difficulties. The evaluation must also consist of, at a minimum, a parent interview and an observational assessment of the child by an experienced clinician. Observation of the child must occur in environments that allow for assessment of social-communicative skills, play, and/or peer interactions [13]. Specific instruments have been developed to help examiners interview parents and observe children's social skills. Two of the most validated instruments for autism diagnosis includes the *Autism Diagnostic Observational Schedule*, which is now in its second edition (ADOS-2; [14, 15]) and the *Autism Diagnostic Interview*, which is in its first revision (ADI-R; [16]). The ADOS-2 is a semi-structured play-based assessment that allows a clinician to assess various aspects of a child's social skills [14, 15]. The ADI-R is a 2 h semi-structured parent interview conducted by the clinician [16]). The ADI-R's significant administration time and training requirements may be prohibitive to many clinicians, and similar information can be completed utilizing the *Social Communication Questionnaire* (SCQ; [17]) in conjunction with the ADOS-2 [13].

There was a significant change to the conceptualization of diagnostic subtyping of ASD with the introduction of the DSM-5 [18]. Given that there was little empirical evidence to support diagnostic differences among the various subtypes of pervasive developmental disorders as outlined in the DSM-IV-TR [14, 15], the DSM-5 workgroup removed the subtypes of Asperger's disorder and pervasive developmental disorder not otherwise specified and subsumed it under the broader umbrella of autism spectrum disorder. Supported by empirical research, the three factor model was reduced to two: social communication deficits and restricted, repetitive behaviors [19]. There was removal of the strict requirement for onset prior to age three to allow for a later age of onset, with the notion that symptoms must be present in early childhood but may not become fully manifested until the social demands exceed the limited capacities of the child. Other changes included adding sensory abnormalities as a symptom, and specifiers to include intellectual and/or language impairments as well as catatonia. Coding also includes any associated known medical or genetic condition or environmental factors, or any comorbid neurodevelopmental, mental, or behavioral disorder, including ADHD. Finally, a symptom severity level scale was added to better communicate treatment needs.

While autism is a heterogeneous disorder, there are still general patterns of performance that have been described in many domains of neuropsychological functioning. Approximately 38% of children with autism present with an Intellectual Disability (ID; [20]). Children with autism differ from peers with primary ID in that ASD children typically exhibit a scattered pattern of test performances as opposed to evenly depressed skills that are characteristic of children with primary ID diagnoses [21]. Children with ASD exhibit a discrepancy between their verbal and nonverbal intellectual abilities 26–32% more frequently than typically functioning peers [22]. Younger children typically present with nonverbal skills that are higher than their verbal skills; however, as children age, discrepancies appear equally in favor of higher verbal or nonverbal abilities [22]. Skill discrepancy is important to examine as older children with discrepantly higher nonverbal than verbal abilities exhibit increased social impairments than their counterparts [22].

Communication and language deficits are the most commonly observed impairment in children with autism [23]. While a small number of autistic children do not exhibit delayed language milestones, most individuals begin to speak late and develop speech much more slowly than their typically developing peers [24]. A subset of children on the spectrum (25%) meet their early language milestones on time but then exhibit a regression of language skills, an event which is only observed in children on the spectrum [24]. Two language phenotypes have been proposed that are thought to describe verbal children with autism: children with normal language skills (i.e., typical phonological, vocabulary, syntax, and morphology) and children with language deficits similar to those identified in children with Specific Language Impairments [24]. However, even children without basic language deficits often exhibit unusual prosody, delayed grammar skills, and difficulty with language pragmatics [5].

Associated with language deficits are poor performances in areas of social cognition. Deficits in social reciprocity are one of the main diagnostic characteristics of autism [5, 25]. Social deficits are impaired in children with ASD regardless of their intellectual or language level [25]. Typical social impairments include poor social pragmatics, hyperfocusing on restricted topics of interest, difficulty understanding and expressing emotions, and difficulty interpreting nonliteral language such as sarcasm [25]. Furthermore, those on the spectrum have difficulty with appropriate perception of social stimuli, especially faces, and inappropriate use of nonverbal social skills (e.g., eye contact; [5]).

Memory is a neuropsychological domain where children with autism differ from their typical peers. Visual memory is usually stronger for children with autism, while verbal memory is often considered to be a characteristic area of deficit [26]. Children on the spectrum remember information best if it is less complex and consequently does not require significant organization to aid in retrieval [26]. It makes sense then that ASD children benefit when provided with supportive cuing to aid in memory organization and subsequent recall [26]. Overall, children on the spectrum generally have poor immediate and delayed memory for complex verbal and visual information, as well as for spatial information. Working memory for both verbal and visual information, however, remains intact [5].

Autistic children exhibit both attention and executive functioning deficits with approximately 23% of those with ASD also meeting criteria for ADHD [27]. Attention deficits impact children's ability to automatically attend to important stimuli, although sustained attention appears generally intact [5]. Children with autism also show deficits on select tasks of executive functioning including planning, organization, and flexibility, while their performance on tasks of response inhibition is unclear [28]. When compared to children with ADHD, children with ASD have better shifting and inhibition skills, but poorer flexibility, monitoring, and planning skills [28].

Children with ASD exhibit a variety of gross and fine motor impairments regardless of symptom severity level [5]. Research has shown that children with ASD often have poorer fine motor skills than age- and IQ-matched peers [29]. Gross motor deficits include poor upper limb coordination, gait balance, agility, speed, as well as postural impairments [5, 29]. Fine motor deficits often revolve around deficient handwriting, poor imitation, and impaired pantomiming skills [5, 29]. Another aspect of motor abnormalities includes frequent motor stereotypies (e.g., flapping, rocking, or finger flicking) and sensory modulation deficits [29].

Students with high-functioning autism exhibit select academic strengths and deficits. In the reading domain, strengths are often observed for basic reading and decoding skills [30]. As children age and reading instruction becomes more comprehension based, children with ASD begin to exhibit deficits especially for text requiring critical thinking such as inferential and abstract reasoning [30]. Such tests are especially difficult for children on the spectrum who have associated language impairments and/or poor verbal intelligence skills [30]. Research indicates that anywhere from 6% to 37% of students with ASD are eventually diagnosed with a learning disability in reading [30, 31]. The combination of graphomotor deficits and poor organization skills contributes to poorer performances on tasks of written expression. Approximately 60% of children with ASD also have a Learning Disorder with impairments in written expression [30]. Generally, children with ASD exhibit age-appropriate math calculation and fluency for simple rote math skills [30]. However, attention, reading comprehension, and organizational deficits often contribute to poor applied math skills, especially for complex word problems [30].

Approximately 17–23% of students with ASD meet criteria for a Learning Disorder with impairments in mathematics [30].

Finally, emotional or psychiatric comorbidities are common in children with ASD. Significant concerns with anxiety are among the most common complaints with approximately 41% of children with ASD meeting criteria for some sort of anxiety disorder [27]. The next most common co-diagnosis is conduct, and oppositional behavior disorders applying to 30% of children with ASD [27]. Significant depression, while rarer in children with autism, is still observed in approximately 1% of children [27].

Key Point

Only 10% of children on the spectrum are diagnosed during their initial evaluation for ASD [32]. A diagnosis of autism is often not made until a child is 2–3 years old, with the average age of diagnosis occurring at 6 years of age [32]. Delay in diagnosis is most often due to concerns by clinicians for inappropriately labeling or diagnosing the child with autism. To avoid delays in diagnosis, the American Academy of Pediatrics recommends that physicians screen for developmental delays at each well-child visit and if a child is found to have delays, administer a screener for autism [32]. These children should also be referred for more extensive assessments by clinicians with experience in diagnosing autism. The most accurate diagnoses of autism are made by autism experts who conduct observations of the child in conjunction with parent interview, while psychological evaluation alone produces the poorest diagnostic reliability [33]. Overall, the "gold standard" in the diagnosis of autism spectrum disorders occurs from a diagnostic consensus of at least two or more autism experts [34].

Neuropsychological Domains

IQ. Matt obtained an overall IQ score in the Average range. With respect to index composites, he showed significant variability, suggesting that his overall IQ was not the most reliable estimate of his intellectual ability. For specific index scores, he earned Average scores for Fluid Reasoning Index and Verbal Comprehension Index or verbal intelligence, Low Average scores for Visual Spatial Index and Processing Speed, and a Very Low score for Working Memory Index. Matt's overall FSIQ was the same as during prior school-based intellectual testing. Matt's pattern of intellectual performances is consistent with research of children with ASD in that he shows significant scatter among indices. However, he is not exhibiting significant discrepancies between his verbal and visual intelligence skills as is common in children within the spectrum. Positively, he is also not presenting with intellectual deficits that are also frequently associated with ASD.

Language and Social Cognition. Matt's expressive language skills fell within the average range, similar to his verbal intelligence; however, his receptive language skills were impaired. On various measures of social-pragmatic language, he performed within the low average to impaired range. He also performed poorly on tests involving identifying emotions in others. Matt's poor receptive language and social pragmatic skills are expected in children with an autism diagnosis. Additionally, his poor perspective taking and social problem-solving deficits, as well as impaired affect recognition, are consistent with expected deficits outlined in the ASD literature.

Attention and Executive Functioning. Matt's performances on various measures of visual and auditory sustained attention indicated difficulties with inattentiveness and sustained attention. He also performed poorly on measures of auditory divided attention and attention span. Parent and teacher rating forms indicated concerns for both Attention and Hyperactivity. Matt's performances on various executive functioning measures indicated impulsivity and impaired novel problem-solving skills. Parent and teacher report of executive functioning skills indicated significant concerns. Matt is exhibiting inattentiveness and problem-solving skills that the literature has shown are often associated with an ASD diagnosis. However, he exhibits additional weaknesses in his sustained attention and impulse control that is less consistent with what is expected given his ASD diagnosis. Overall, he is exhibiting symptoms of ADHD, which research has shown is a common co-diagnosis for children on the spectrum.

Memory and Learning. Verbal memory for stories was generally within the average range, with provision of cuing aiding retrieval. On a rote-list learning task, Matt exhibited difficulties with learning and retention. This would suggest that Matt does better at learning verbal information that is already organized for him within a meaningful format (i.e., story memory). Matt's face memory was low average (immediate) to mildly impaired (delay). He also was disorganized and imprecise in his copy of an abstract visual figure, resulting in poor immediate copy and subsequently impaired delayed recall. Research has shown that children with social challenges, particularly those on the autism spectrum, are poor at remembering names and faces and overall his performance suggests challenges with nonverbal memory. Matt's strength in his story memory is unexpected given the more complex nature of the information; however, he benefits from supportive curing which is consistent. Furthermore, Matt's difficulty for remembering faces, which is both socially mediated and visually complex, is expected. Poor planning and organization skills, which is common in children on the spectrum, likely impacted his copy and later recall of an abstract figure.

Visual Motor Functioning. Matt's performance was impaired for a copying task and low average for a visual-perceptual matching task. On a test of manual dexterity of fine motor coordination, he performed in the low average range for his dominant hand and in the average range for his nondominant hand. Matt was administered one test of sensorimotor processing and performed in the impaired range, sacrificing accuracy for speed. Matt's poor performances on tasks of fine motor skills are expected in children with autism, as is his strength on the visual matching task that had no motor component.

Academic Achievement. Matt performed in the average range on tests that assessed his fluency or automaticity of digit and number recognition. This is one of the earliest skills in reading development. He performed in the below average range on a measure of sentence reading fluency in the context of comprehending. On tasks measuring his awareness of basic phonemes, his ability to recognize individual subunits of sounds within words, and his ability to blend sounds into words was below average. Matt's phonemic decoding skills were further measured using tests of pseudoword and real word decoding, and were both average. A test measuring Matt's ability to read passages aloud accurately was also average. These findings would suggest that despite having weak phonological awareness skills, he had adequate decoding skills and might be relying on rote memory skills to decode. Matt's appropriate sight word and decoding skills are consistent with what is expected given his ASD diagnosis. Matt demonstrated average reading comprehension skills, which is an unexpected strength and an area where he would be expected to exhibit emerging difficulties as he ages and demands increase. Matt's writing skills were overall in the average range, with a relative weakness in spelling (below average), which is again unexpected given his ASD diagnosis and is likely related to lower demands in first grade. Matt's mathematical skills were below average overall for him and constituted a mild learning disability. Specifically, he earned below average scores for math calculation skills and for applied math skills (that involve more reasoning, problem-solving and application of learned concepts) and for his ability to quickly calculate simple math problems. Learning disorders in math are common in children with ASD, but his weaker math calculation skills are less consistent, especially for rote calculations that typically comprise a first grade curriculum.

Social-Emotional Ratings. Matt's parents and teachers rated concerns with conduct problems, anger control, and aggression on broad-based rating scales. Although Matt's behavioral difficulties are not severe enough to represent a behavioral disorder, conduct and oppositional behavior is frequently observed in children on the spectrum. Positively, Matt is not rated as exhibiting anxiety, which is the most comorbid psychiatric diagnosis in children with ASD.

Autistic Spectrum Behavior. On a semi-structured, standardized assessment instrument designed to obtain information in the areas of communication and reciprocal social interactions for diagnosing children who may have ASD, Matt's scores were consistent with a classification of autism (high probability). The examiner also rated symptoms related to autism and the total composite based on examiner rating fell within the "Mild to Moderate Symptoms" of autism spectrum disorder categorization, similar to parent report on a measure of social communication skills. Matt's parents also rated clinically significant concerns with Matt's social communication skills; with additional parent and teacher concerns for Matt's engagement in odd and unusual behaviors, his social withdrawal, his social skills, and his ability to recover from setbacks. Matt's social deficits are expected as this is one of the core impairments observed in children on the spectrum.

Key Point

A diagnosis of autism presents with a variety of neuropsychological implications. Intellectually, 38% present with Intellectual Disability with 56–62% of children exhibiting significant discrepancies between their verbal and nonverbal intelligence. Visual memory is typically stronger than verbal memory. Attention and executive functioning deficits are common in children with ASD, with approximately 23% also meeting criteria for ADHD. Furthermore, children with ASD exhibit a variety of gross and fine motor impairments regardless of symptom severity level. Academically, difficulty with reading comprehension, applied math word problems, and written expression skills are common.

Collaborative Discussion

Parents of children with ASD often pursue alternative, non-research-based treatments that can potentially be hazardous to the child. In the case of Matt, there was contradicting evidence as to whether or not he contracted Lyme disease. His parents had sought out treatment from a DAN doctor who had no formal training in immunology, and was boarded in internal medicine and emergency medicine. Some of the treatment protocols he utilized included chelation, hyperbaric medicine, biomedical therapy, and Lyme disease therapy. This same doctor was recommending to the parents that he be removed from his seizure medication, a dangerous proposition. When approaching such families, it is important to validate their concerns in a nonjudgmental manner. However, it is then imperative to reinforce validated medical treatments in regard to their children's conditions and to dissuade families from potentially dangerous interventions.

Key Point

Research has demonstrated that in utero exposure to maternal infectious disease (viral and bacterial) increases the risk for ASD [35]. In utero exposure to Lyme disease is controversial in and of itself, and no research to date has shown an association with ASD.

Recommendations

- *Medical Referrals*: Matt was referred back to Dr. Yadava, to reevaluate his medication regimen in order to further improve his inattention and impulsivity. He was also referred to a pediatric immunologist who specialized in Lyme disease given the questionable diagnosis and treatment regimen he was receiving for this.

- *Private Therapies*: It was recommended that Matt reinstate private ST, participate in feeding therapy, and receive in home Applied Behavior Analysis (ABA) therapy. Illinois-based insurance will pay upward of $38,000 per year for therapies for a child with a medical diagnosis of ASD.
- *School-Based Recommendations*: It was recommended that Matt's educational classification be primarily under Autism with secondary classifications under Specific Learning Disability and Other Health Impairment. Changing the classification to Autism expanded the level of school-based services made available to him, including autism itinerant services. It was recommended that Matt remain in the general education setting with continued pullout services in ST, OT, SW, and resource support. Additional academic goals were suggested to address spelling, mathematical fluency, calculation, applied math, phonemic awareness, and reading fluency skills. An OT goal to address attention regulation and executive functioning skills was offered. A SW goal specific to increased flexibility in play including sharing and engaging in others' interests was recommended. Further, ST goals were suggested related to pragmatic (maintaining reciprocal conversations around another's interest) and receptive language skills (following increasingly complex instructions). Finally, it was recommended that a Behavior Intervention Plan (BIP) be developed based on a Functional Behavioral Analysis (FBA), given concerns about poor work compliance and behavioral issues in the classroom (Table 7.1).

Table 7.1 Neuropsychological test results

	Standard/scaled score	Percentile
Wechsler Intelligence Scale for Children—Fifth Edition		
Full Scale IQ	91	27
Verbal Comprehension Index	98	45
Visual Spatial Index	84	14
Clinical Evaluation of Language Fundamentals—Fifth Edition		
Receptive Language	69	2
Expressive Language	100	50
Diagnostic Assessment of Nonverbal Accuracy		
Child Faces	66	1
Adult Faces	96	39
Child Paralanguage	85	16
Adult Paralanguage	91	27
NEPSY—Second Edition		
Affect Recognition	2	<1
Theory of Mind		<2

(continued)

Table 7.1 (continued)

	Standard/scaled score	Percentile
Test of Problem Solving—Third Edition, Elementary		
Total	80	9
Comprehensive Assessment of Spoken Language		
Pragmatic Judgment	<55	<1
Conners' Continuous Performance Test—Kiddie's Edition		
Omissions	90	>99
Test of Everyday Attention—Children's Version		
Score	5	5
Score DT	5	5
Code Transmission	3	1
Tower of London—Child Form		
Total Correct Score	78	7
Total Rule Violation Score	<60	<1
Children's Memory Scales		
Stories—Immediate Free Recall	8	25
Stories—Delayed Free Recall	7	16
Stories—Delayed Recog. (Cued)	9	37
Faces—Immediate Memory	6	9
Faces—Delayed Memory	4	2
Rey-Osterrieth Complex Figure Test		
Copy	<55	<1
Delayed Recall	<55	<1
California Verbal Learning Test—Children's Version		
List A Total (Trials 1-5)	62	1
List A Short-Delay Free Recall	85	16
List A Short-Delay Cued Recall	70	2
List A Long-Delay Free Recall	78	7
List A Long-Delay Cued Recall	55	<1
Wide Range Assessment of Visual Motor Ability		
Drawing	66	1
Matching	84	14
Pegboard—Dominant Hand	88	21
Woodcock-Johnson Tests of Achievement—Fourth Edition		
Letter-Word Identification	94	34
Word Attack	98	45
Passage Comprehension	95	37
Calculation	88	21
Applied Problems	86	18
Math Fluency	81	10
Writing Samples	98	45

(continued)

Table 7.1 (continued)

	Standard/scaled score	Percentile
Comprehensive Test of Phonological Processing—Second Edition		
Phonological Awareness	84	14
Childhood Autism Rating Scale 2nd Ed., High-Functioning Version		
Total Raw Score	33.5	50
ADOS-2 Module 3	**Raw Score**	
Social Affect	11	
Restricted and Repetitive Behavior	2	
Overall Total	13	
Comparison Score	8	
Behavior Rating Inventory of Executive Function		
	Parents	**Teacher**
Inhibit	67	60
Shift	73	61
Emotional Control	66	55
Initiate	65	62
Working Memory	75	58
Plan/Organize	65	55
Organization of Materials	66	52
Monitor	63	65

	T-Score		
BASC-2 Parent Rating Scale	Father	Mother	Teacher
Hyperactivity	73	79	68
Attention Problems	67	73	56
Aggression	66	68	65
Conduct Problems	62	65	85
Anger Control	72	75	64
Bullying	68	71	67
Depression	53	51	50
Anxiety	59	50	54
Atypicality	65	55	65
Withdrawal	73	71	50
Adaptability	42	35	43
Social Skills	41	37	34
Functional Communication	35	32	38

Chapter Review Questions

1. True/False: The average prevalence of ASD is approximately 1–2% and is 4.5 times more common in boys than girls.
2. True/False: A neurological evaluation and genetic testing are recommended for children with ASD given higher risk for seizures and genetic disorders.
3. True/False: The American Academy of Pediatrics recommends that physicians screen for developmental delays at each well-child visit, and if a child is found to have delays, an administration of a screener for autism is sufficient in making the diagnosis.
4. What is the prototypical neuropsychological profile in children with ASD?
5. The average prevalence of ASD is:
   A. Approximately 1–2% and is 4.5 times more common in boys than girls.
   B. Approximately 1–2% and is 4.5 times more common in girls than boys.
   C. Approximately 3–5% and is 4.5 times more common in boys than girls.
   D. Approximately 3–5% and is 4.5 times more common in girls than boys.
6. The following evaluations are recommended for children with ASD:
   A. A neurological evaluation.
   B. Genetic testing.
   C. Both.
   D. Neither.
7. The American Academy of Pediatrics recommends that physicians screen for developmental delays ___________. If a child is found to have delays the clinician should___________.
   A. At each sick and well-child visit; refer the child for more extensive assessments by clinicians with experience in diagnosing autism.
   B. At each well-child visit; refer the child for more extensive assessments by clinicians with experience in diagnosing autism.
   C. At each well-child visit; administer a screener for autism to determine whether to make an ASD diagnosis.
   D. At each sick and well-child visit; administer a screener for autism to determine whether to make an ASD diagnosis.
8. What is the prototypical neuropsychological profile in children with ASD?
   A. Language and intellectual impairments.
   B. Language impairments with variable intellectual functioning.
   C. Typical language and intellectual functioning.
   D. Variable language and intellectual functioning.

References

1. Canitano R. Epilepsy in autism spectrum disorders. Eur Child Adolesc Psychiatry. 2007;16(1):61–6.
2. De Rubeis S, Buxbaum J. Recent advances in the genetics of autism spectrum disorder. Curr Neurol Neurosci Rep. 2015;15(6):1–9.
3. Deykin E, MacMahon B. Pregnancy, delivery, and neonatal complications among autistic children. Am J Dis Child. 1980;134(9):860–4.
4. Ecker C, Bookheimer S, Murphy D. Neuroimaging in autism spectrum disorder: brain structure and function across the life span. Lancet Neurol. 2015;14:1121–34.
5. Fein D. The neuropsychology of autism. New York: Oxford University Press; 2011.
6. Lange N, Travers B, Bigler E, Prigge M, Froehlich A, Nielsen J, et al. Longitudinal volumetric brain changes in autism spectrum disorder ages 6–35 years. Autism Res. 2014;8(1):82–93.
7. Caplan R, Siddarth P, Stahl L, Lanphier E, Vona P, Gurbani S, Koh S, Sankar R, Shields WD. Childhood absence epilepsy: behavioral, cognitive, and linguistic comorbidities. Epilepsia. 2008;49(11):1838–46.
8. Miodovnik A, Harstad E, Sideridis G, Huntington N. Timing of the diagnosis of attention-deficit/hyperactivity disorder and autism spectrum disorder. Pediatrics. 2015;136(4):e830–7. https://doi.org/10.1542/peds.2015-1502.
9. Christensen D, Baio J, Van Naarden Braun K, Bilder D, Charles J, Constantino J, et al. Prevalence and characteristics of autism spectrum disorder among children aged 8 years—autism and developmental disabilities monitoring network, 11 sites, United States, 2012. Surveil Summ. 2016;65(3):1–23.
10. Yoo H. Genetics of autism spectrum disorder: current status and possible clinical applications. Exp Neurobiol. 2015;24(4):257–72.
11. Huguet G, Benabou M, Bourgeron T. The genetics of autism spectrum disorders. In: Sassone-Corsi P, Christen Y, editors. A time for metabolism and hormones. Cham: Springer International Publishing; 2015. p. 101–29.
12. Lord C, McGee P. Educating children with autism. Washington, DC: National Academy Press; 2001.
13. Huerta M, Lord C. Diagnostic evaluation of autism spectrum disorders. Pediatr Clin North Am. 2012;59(1):103–11.
14. Lord C, Petkova E, Hus V, Gan W, Lu F, Martin DM, et al. A multisite study of the clinical diagnosis of different autism spectrum disorders. Arch Gen Psychiatry. 2012;69:306–13.
15. Lord C, Rutter M, DiLavore P, Risi S, Gotham K, Bishop S. Autism diagnostic observation schedule. 2nd ed. Torrance, CA: Western Psychological Services; 2012.
16. Rutter M, LeCuteur A, Lord C. Autism diagnostic instrument, revised. Torrance, CA: Western Psychological Services; 2003.
17. Rutter M, Bailey A, Lord C. Social communication questionnaire. Torrance, CA: Western Psychological Services; 2003.
18. American Psychiatric Association. Diagnostic and statistical manual of mental disorders. 5th ed. Washington, DC: Author; 2013.
19. Frazier TW, Youngstrom EA, Kubu CS, Sinclair L, Rezai A. Exploratory and confirmatory factor analysis of the Autism Diagnostic Interview-Revised. J Autism Dev Disord. 2008;38:474–80.
20. Baio J. Prevalence of autism spectrum disorders—autism and developmental disabilities monitoring network, 14 sites, United States, 2008. Surveill Summ. 2012;61(SS03):1–19.
21. Klin A, Volkman F. Autism and other pervasive developmental disorders. In: Goldstein S, Renyolds C, editors. Handbook of neurodevelopmental and genetic disorders in children. New York, NY: Guilford Press; 1999. p. 247–74.
22. Joseph R, Tager-Flusberg H, Lord C. Cognitive profiles and social-communicative functioning in children with autism spectrum disorder. J Child Psychol Psychiatry. 2002;43(6):807–21.

23. Whitehouse A, Barry J, Bishop D. Further defining the language impairment of autism: is there a specific language impairment subtype. J Commun Disord. 2008;41:319–36.
24. Tager-Flusberg H, Paul R, Lord C. Language and communication in autism. In: Volkmar FR, Paul R, Klin A, Cohen D, editors. Handbook of autism and pervasive developmental disorders, vol. 1. 3rd ed. Hoboken, NJ: John Wiley & Sons, Inc.; 2005.
25. White S, Keonig K, Scahill L. Social skills development in children with autism spectrum disorders: a review of the intervention research. J Autism Dev Disord. 2007;37:1858–68.
26. Williams D, Goldstein G, Minshew N. The profile of memory function in children with autism. Neuropsychology. 2006;20(1):21–9.
27. Simonoff E, Pickles A, Charman T, Chandler S, Loucas T, Baird G. Psychiatric disorders in children with autism spectrum disorders: prevalence, comorbidity, and associated factors in a population-derived sample. J Am Acad Child Adolesc Psychiatry. 2008;47(8):921–9.
28. Happe F, Booth R, Charlton R, Hughes C. Executive function deficits in autism spectrum disorders and attention-deficit/hyperactivity disorder: examining profiles across domains and ages. Brain Cogn. 2006;61:25–39.
29. Bhat A, Landa R, Galloway J. Current perspectives on motor functioning in infants, children, and adults with autism spectrum disorders. Phys Ther. 2011;91(7):1116–29.
30. Whitby P, Mancil G. Academic achievement profiles of children with high functioning autism and Asperger syndrome: a review of the literature. Educ Train Dev Disabil. 2009;44(4):551–60.
31. Brown H, Oram-Cardy J, Johnson A. A meta-analysis of the reading comprehension skills of individuals on the autism spectrum. J Autism Dev Disord. 2013;43(4):932–55.
32. Filipek P, Accardo P, Ashwal S, Baranek G, Cook E, Dawson G, et al. Practice parameter: screening and diagnosis of autism: report of the Quality Standards Subcommittee of the American Academy of Neurology and the Child Neurology Society. Neurology. 2000;55:468–79.
33. Andersson G, Miniscalco C, Gillberg C. Autism in preschoolers: does individual clinician's first visit diagnosis agree with final comprehensive diagnosis? Sci World J. 2013;2013:1–10.
34. Mahoney W, Szatmari P, MacLean J, Bryson S, Bartolucci G, Walter S, et al. J Am Acad Child Adolesc Psychiatry. 1998;37(3):278–85.
35. Atladottir H, Thorsen P, Ostergaard L, Schendel D, Lemcke S, Abdallah M, et al. Maternal infection requiring hospitalization during pregnancy and autism spectrum disorders. J Autism Dev Disord. 2010;40(12):1423–30.

Chapter 8
Paediatric Neuro-Oncology: Medulloblastoma

Laura Janzen and Ute Bartels

Introduction

Children with brain tumours are at high risk for neuropsychological impairment. Tumour type and location, complications (e.g. posterior fossa mutism, seizures, hydrocephalus and hearing loss), age at diagnosis and whole brain radiation are among the many factors that are associated with long-term neuropsychological outcomes in this group [1–3]. This chapter details the medical and neuropsychological care of a child (DA) who was diagnosed at 5 years of age with standard-risk medulloblastoma. He experienced significant posterior fossa syndrome (PFS) following neurosurgical resection of the tumour, a complication which is known to negatively affect long-term cognitive functioning. Brain radiation, which is typically included in medulloblastoma treatment regimens for school-aged children, was avoided in this case due to concern about its additional neurocognitive impact. Instead, a chemotherapy-only regimen was utilized. DA was 7 years old and in the second grade at the time of his neuropsychological assessment. The case exemplifies collaborative patient care aimed at optimizing DA's functioning and quality of life.

L. Janzen (✉)
Division of Haematology/Oncology and Department of Psychology, The Hospital for Sick Children, Toronto, ON, Canada
e-mail: Laura.Janzen@sickkids.ca

U. Bartels
Division of Haematology/Oncology, The Hospital for Sick Children, Toronto, ON, Canada

Department of Pediatrics, University of Toronto, Toronto, ON, Canada
e-mail: Ute.Bartels@sickkids.ca

K. M. Sanders (ed.), *Physician's Field Guide to Neuropsychology*,
https://doi.org/10.1007/978-1-4939-8722-1_8

Physician Perspective

Medulloblastoma

Medulloblastoma is the most common malignant brain tumour in childhood. Since its first description in 1925, the prognosis of children affected by medulloblastoma has continuously improved. A deadly disease despite complete surgical removal at that time, it is now a potentially curable disease when adjuvant craniospinal radiation and chemotherapy are used after surgical resection. Over the last decade, molecular insights have led to the distinction of at least four subgroups of medulloblastoma [4, 5], and current clinical efforts are directed towards tailoring treatment strategies accordingly, with de-escalating radiation therapy and implementation of intensified chemotherapy or new targeted therapies where appropriate.

Medulloblastoma affects children of all ages. There is a gender predisposition with boys being two to three times more often affected than girls. This rapidly growing tumour is located within the posterior fossa and most often causes blockage of the cerebrospinal fluid (CSF) circulation, resulting in hydrocephalus. As a consequence, children typically present to medical attention with symptoms of headache, nausea and vomiting due to the increased intracranial pressure, as well as ataxia and cranial nerve deficits. The diagnostic workup includes clinical assessment, MRI of the brain and spine and surgical resection for pathological verification of the tumour. In the absence of metastatic disease on imaging and via CSF investigation, the degree of surgical resection influences prognosis and treatment. Previous trials showed that a residual tumour less than 1.5 cm^2 after surgery was favourable and doses of craniospinal radiation were therefore lower [6, 7]. So far, this still holds true in the molecular era [8]. There are ongoing trials evaluating the possibility of avoiding or reducing the dose of craniospinal radiation for children with favourable pathology and molecular profiles (such as desmoplastic/nodular and WNT-subtypes). Unfortunately, all previous trials which aimed at radiation avoidance or dose reduction in very young children were associated with a higher risk of relapse [9–11]. Nonetheless, craniospinal radiation is typically avoided for children under 3–5 years due to its especially negative impact on the developing brain, and intensive chemotherapy regimens are used instead.

Posterior Fossa Syndrome

Posterior fossa syndrome (PFS), also known as cerebellar mutism syndrome, refers to a severe post-operative complication of yet unclear aetiology which occurs in 20–25% of paediatric patients after resection of a cerebellar tumour. It includes symptoms of severely diminished or absent speech output, emotional instability and significant ataxia [12–14]. The onset of mutism is typically delayed and usually appears 24 h post-operatively, which has led to speculation that ischemic injury underlies this syndrome; however, other theories exist, and until now no definitive cause has been verified [12]. In children who develop PFS, speech function usually returns within days to months, but higher-order language deficits often persist. Patients with medulloblastoma who develop PFS have increased long-term neurocognitive, academic and psychosocial deficits relative to those who do not develop PFS [15, 16]. No established treatment exists for PFS, but case reports have suggested improvement with bromocriptine, aripiprazole and zolpidem, along with intensive physical, occupational and speech-language therapies [17–19].

The Patient

DA presented medically at 5 years of age. He was an appropriately developing, healthy boy with an unremarkable social and family history. He had started complaining about headaches 8 months preceding his diagnosis. At that time, it was found that he needed glasses. When his headaches worsened 6 months later and were associated with vomiting and balance difficulties, he was referred to a neurologist in the community who ordered an outpatient MRI. While awaiting diagnostic imaging, DA's balance worsened to the point of using his hands and knees to climb/descend stairs, and his headaches became severe. Subsequently, his parents brought him to the emergency room of a tertiary paediatric hospital, and the diagnosis of a posterior fossa tumour was made.

Diagnostic workup with CT and subsequently MRI of the brain and spine documented a single, large midline lesion centred in the fourth ventricle measuring about 5 cm in all dimensions that was causing severe obstructive hydrocephalus. The imaging characteristics were very consistent with the diagnosis of a medulloblastoma: the lesion was hyperdense on CT and on MRI, and it was hypointense on T1- and hyperintense on T2-weighted images. There was heterogeneous enhancement post-gadolinium contrast and evidence of diffusion restriction.

DA underwent emergent craniotomy, and a gross total resection of his tumour was achieved and documented on post-operative MRI. No intraoperative complications occurred. Pathology confirmed a classical medulloblastoma (subgroup 4). A lumbar puncture 14 days after surgical resection ruled out malignant cells in the cerebrospinal fluid, and hence DA was staged with average-risk medulloblastoma.

DA suffered from severe PFS following his surgery, with mutism, irritability and mood lability, ataxia and swallowing difficulties. For about 3 months after surgery, he had no expressive speech at all and initially did not follow verbal commands or respond consistently in a nonverbal manner. He was irritable, with regular emotional outbursts and crying. Intensive speech-language therapy was provided, along with a trial of bromocriptine, which resulted in gradual improvement. At the same time, DA was receiving a 6-month regimen of high-dose chemotherapy and autologous stem cell transplant. Following treatment and once he was medically stable, he received 3 months of extensive physiotherapy, occupational therapy and speech-language therapy at a paediatric rehabilitation facility to address his ataxia, balance difficulties, right-sided dysmetria (which led him to switch handedness) and speech difficulties.

Adjuvant treatment with the best chance of successful outcome for school-aged children with average-risk medulloblastoma consists of craniospinal radiation (23.4 Gy) plus a boost to the tumour bed/posterior fossa (to a total dose of 54 Gy) followed by a chemotherapy regimen [20, 21]. While the majority of neuro-oncologists would accept this radiation dose for a 5-year-old boy and not deviate from this therapy plan, the medical team and DA's parents were very concerned about DA's future independence and functioning if radiation therapy were to add to the already existing neurocognitive damage associated with the tumour itself and severe PFS, and thus, treatment was modified.

Key Point
Subsequent neuropsychological assessments would aid in measuring this patient's cognitive functioning and psychosocial status and provide his parents and the medical team with recommendations to optimize his functioning.

Neuropsychologist Perspective

Neuropsychological Impact

Neuropsychological assessment is the standard of care for children with brain tumours, and it is recommended that an initial assessment occur near the end of treatment, once the child is medically stable and returning to normal activities [22]. This initial assessment helps to gauge the impact of the tumour itself, related complications and their secondary effects (e.g. hydrocephalus, seizures, hearing loss) and neurosurgical interventions on cognitive functioning; the full implications of the adjuvant radiation and chemotherapy are not immediately evident. Reassessment is recommended every 2–3 years thereafter to provide updated recommendations in line with a child's functioning and development and in anticipation of major transitions (e.g. completing high school). Repeat assessments provide an indication of the cumulative radiation and chemotherapy effects on cognitive development and behaviour. Prospective, longitudinal assessment of neuropsychological outcomes is increasingly included in medulloblastoma clinical trials, leading to better understanding of the late effects of continuously evolving treatment regimens.

Children treated for medulloblastoma, as a group, show progressive intellectual and academic deficits and specific difficulties in attention, memory, processing speed and executive functioning [23]. Radiation therapy is particularly damaging to the developing brain, although neurosurgical resection and chemotherapy may also contribute to neuropsychological impairment [24]. For survivors, the impacts of medulloblastoma and its treatments are lifelong, affecting multiple neuropsychological domains. The vast majority of patients require accommodations in school for learning difficulties [25]. Reduced social functioning and quality of life are also reported in adult survivors [23]. There is typically a failure to make age-appropriate cognitive gains, resulting in a widening gap between patients and their peers, rather than a sudden loss of previously acquired information and skills [26]. Thus far, educational and pharmacological interventions have shown the most promise in remediating acquired deficits in childhood cancer survivors [27].

Assessment Process and Objectives

Establishing a positive, collaborative relationship with patients and their families early on is essential to provide psychoeducation about the late effects of treatment and to guide them through the coming years as neurocognitive effects become more evident. It is also an opportunity to gauge how the child is adapting to any experienced physical, cognitive, emotional or social difficulties and offer psychosocial supports when needed. Family functioning is a significant predictor of long-term cognitive and behavioural outcomes in brain tumour survivors [28]. In particular, it is important to support parents' adaptation to the changes that have occurred in the child since diagnosis, as parents often grieve the loss of their child's future potential [29].

While brief assessments, such as the DIVERGT battery [30], may be useful for screening and research purposes, most paediatric neuro-oncology patients require comprehensive neuropsychological assessment for diagnostic purposes, treatment and educational planning and eligibility determinations. Comprehensive assessment is essential when there are sensory, motor, cultural or language issues that might require adaptations to standardized assessment measures or use of alternative procedures. A comprehensive neuropsychological assessment involves solicitation of information from the child, parents, teachers and rehabilitation professionals familiar with the child's daily functioning and review of recent school records. A clinical interview with the child and parents is conducted to elicit information about current functioning and concerns. Use of standardized, norm-based measures allows for objective measurement of the child's cognitive, academic and emotional/behavioural status and to measure change over time. Test measures are chosen based on the child's age, estimated functional level, the referral question and knowledge of the domains most likely affected by the tumour and treatment. Fatigue, motor output difficulties and slowed processing speed are common in this population and may make it necessary to conduct the assessment over more than 1 day. Assessment results are interpreted in the context of the child's medical and personal history, and individually tailored recommendations are provided.

Clinically, this information may be used to determine the need for and access to interventions, special education or rehabilitation supports or other community-based services. Neuropsychologists communicate with school personnel regarding required accommodations and/or modifications and the child's Individual Education Plan (IEP). When emotional or behavioural difficulties are identified, appropriate referrals to psychological, psychiatric or behavioural therapists are provided. Recommendations may also be made for social skills groups or to enhance the child's social inclusion at school or in the community. Throughout the assessment process, parents, school professionals and others are educated about specific strategies that can help to improve the child's cognitive, academic and psychosocial functioning.

Key Point
Understanding a child's neuropsychological functioning allows the medical team to elicit information from the child and provide him/her with necessary information at an appropriate level. Cognitive, emotional and behavioural factors may impact the child's compliance with investigations and treatments and his/her capacity to consent to procedures or research.

The Patient

Prior to his diagnosis, DA had acquired school-readiness skills appropriately, and there were no learning or behavioural difficulties. At the time of his neuropsychological assessment (20 months following diagnosis), DA was medically stable. His intensive rehabilitation therapies had ended, and he had resumed normal activities. DA was not taking any medication. There were no concerns about fatigue, pain, sleep, appetite or vision (corrected with glasses). As a result of his chemotherapy treatment, he had sensorineural hearing loss bilaterally and wore hearing aids. DA had difficulty articulating some speech sounds. He was monitored by an occupational therapist every few months. He had nystagmus in both eyes and cranial nerve exam II to XII was normal. He continued to have balance difficulties although he was ambulating independently at the time of the assessment. Although improved, finger-to-nose testing continued to elicit mild right-sided dysmetria. Neuroimaging showed stable postsurgical changes in the posterior fossa (enlargement and distortion of fourth ventricle), stable cerebellar volume loss and mild to moderate dilatation of the lateral and third ventricles.

DA was living with his parents and two brothers. English was primarily spoken in the home, and both of his parents had completed college-level education. Within the immediate family, there was no history of attention, learning, neurological or psychiatric conditions.

He was in Grade 2 at the time of the assessment and was attending consistently. His educational instruction had been inconsistent the two prior years (kindergarten and Grade 1). He was supported by a full-time educational assistant and had an Individual Education Plan with accommodations mainly addressing his physical challenges (e.g. a scribe for writing due to his problems with fine motor and pencil control). DA was starting to identify letters and letter-sound associations and was able to recognize his name in print. His mother felt that DA was stronger in math than in reading.

DA reported having some friends and there were no social concerns. His parents noted that he struggled to recall names and was slow in processing information.

He tended to be a perfectionist and wanted to finish what he had started. He continued to display significant emotional dysregulation and had frequent temper tantrums. While the frequency had decreased since the initial post-surgical period, DA continued to have emotional 'meltdowns' once or twice a week.

Assessment Results

DA had generally low average to average cognitive abilities (see Table 8.1). This suggests a slight decline in his overall cognitive abilities, given that his premorbid functioning, based on parental education level, was estimated to be average. Reasoning skills were a relative strength for DA, and his verbal/language skills and verbal memory were intact, which was particularly encouraging in light of his hearing loss. His lowest cognitive performance was on tests of working memory and sustained attention (very low to extremely low range), indicating that DA struggled to actively hold information in mind as he was using it and stay on task. It is notable that these challenges were not reported by his mother or teacher in their ratings of his everyday functioning, which may indicate that these difficulties have recently

Table 8.1 Neuropsychological assessment data

	Age 7 years 5 months				
	Standard scores	Scaled score	*t*-score	*z*-score	
	100 ± 15	10 ± 3	50 ± 10	0 ± 1	Percentile
1. Intelligence					
Wechsler Intelligence Scale for Children 5th Ed (WISC-V)					
Full Scale IQ	83				13
Verbal Comprehension Index (VCI)	90				25
Similarities		11			63
Vocabulary		6			9
Visual Spatial Index (VSI)	86				18
Block Design		8			25
Visual Puzzles		8			25
Fluid Reasoning Index (FRI)	94				34
Matrix Reasoning		8			25
Figure Weights		10			50
Working Memory Index (WMI)	77				6
Digit Span		6			9
Picture Span		7			16
Processing Speed Index (PSI)	80				9
Coding		6			9
Symbol Search		7			16

(continued)

Table 8.1 (continued)

	Age 7 years 5 months				
	Standard scores	Scaled score	t-score	z-score	
	100 ± 15	10 ± 3	50 ± 10	0 ± 1	Percentile
2. Academics					
Wechsler Individual Achievement Test 3rd Ed (WIAT-III)					
Early Reading Skills	67				1
Word Reading	70				2
Pseudoword Decoding	69				2
Numerical Operations	85				16
Math Problem-Solving	92				30
Spelling	80				9
3. Language					
NEPSY-II					
Comprehension of Instructions		6			9
4. Attention and Processing Speed					
Conners K-CPT-2					
Omissions			90		99
Commissions			55		70
Hit Reaction Time			59		82
Hit Reaction Time Standard Deviation			61		86
Woodcock-Johnson III Tests of Cognitive Abilities					
Rapid Picture Naming	89				23
5. Memory					
Children's Memory Scale (CMS)					
Visual Immediate Index	88				21
Visual Delayed Index	94				34
Dot Locations—Learning		11			63
Dot Locations—Total Score		11			63
Dot Locations—Long Delay		11			63
Stories—Immediate		10			50
Stories—Delayed		8			25
Stories—Delayed Recognition		9			37
Faces—Immediate		5			5
Faces—Delayed		7			16
California Verbal Learning Test—Children's Version					
List A Total Trials 1-5			45		30
List A Trial 1 Free Recall				1.5	93
List A Trial 5 Free Recall				−1	16
List B Free Recall				−0.5	30
List A Short-Delay Free Recall				0.5	70
List A Short-Delay Cued Recall				−0.5	30
List A Long-Delay Free Recall				−0.5	30
List A Long-Delay Cued Recall				−1	16

(continued)

Table 8.1 (continued)

	Age 7 years 5 months				
	Standard scores	Scaled score	*t*-score	*z*-score	
	100 ± 15	10 ± 3	50 ± 10	0 ± 1	Percentile
6. Visual-Spatial					
Beery-Buktenica Developmental Test of Visual-Motor Integration (VMI)					
VMI	83				13
7. Motor					
Grooved Pegboard Test					
Left (now dominant)	48 seconds				4
Right	89 seconds				<1
8. Emotional and Behavioral Ratings					
Behavior Assessment System for Children—Second Edition (Parent)					
Hyperactivity			35		1
Aggression			46		40
Conduct Problems			40		12
Externalizing Problems			39		9
Anxiety			37		8
Depression			57		79
Somatization			63		91
Internalizing Problems			53		67
Atypicality			41		9
Withdrawal			37		5
Attention Problems			40		19
Behavioral Symptoms Index			40		14
Behavior Assessment System for Children—Second Edition (Teacher)					
Hyperactivity			40		15
Aggression			42		21
Conduct Problems			40		13
Externalizing Problems			40		13
Anxiety			54		70
Depression			47		50
Somatization			72		95
Internalizing Problems			60		86
Attention Problems			39		19
Learning Problems			58		79
School Problems			48		46
Atypicality			45		43
Withdrawal			56		76
Behavioral Symptoms Index			44		28

(continued)

Table 8.1 (continued)

	Age 7 years 5 months				
	Standard scores	Scaled score	*t*-score	*z*-score	
	100 ± 15	10 ± 3	50 ± 10	0 ± 1	Percentile
Behavior Rating Inventory of Executive Function (Parent Form)					
Inhibit			42		28
Shift			40		24
Emotional Control			68		95
Initiate			49		57
Working Memory			48		52
Plan/Organize			50		58
Organization of Materials			46		36
Monitor			47		43
Behavioral Regulation Index			51		58
Metacognition Index			48		47
Global Executive Composite			49		48
Behavior Rating Inventory of Executive Function (Teacher Form)					
Inhibit			43		45
Shift			57		77
Emotional Control			45		50
Initiate			49		53
Working Memory			51		55
Plan/Organize			55		67
Organization of Materials			44		50
Monitor			49		54
Behavioral Regulation Index			47		55
Metacognition Index			50		56
Global Executive Composite			48		54

emerged and although they are measurable, may not yet be obvious to others. Consistent with his known dysmetria, DA's fine motor function was found to be very limited with his right hand and below average when using his left (now dominant) hand. This impacted his writing speed and legibility.

Academically, DA's reading development was found to be limited, at least partly related to his inconsistent educational instruction, while his math abilities were stronger and low average to average for his age. Ratings of his emotional and behavioural functioning were age-appropriate, and he was coping quite well but had continued emotional regulation difficulties and outbursts. DA showed strengths in his social functioning and adaptability (e.g. adjusts well to change or new situations). Ongoing monitoring was recommended, with planned reassessment in 2–3 years.

Recommendations

Specific recommendations were provided to accommodate for DA's emerging difficulties with working memory and sustained attention. In light of his young age, most of the suggestions involved changing the environment (e.g. minimizing distractions, offering frequent, short breaks when working on focused activities) and means of interacting with him (e.g. prompts to return his attention to the task when he is distracted, providing instructions and explanations in a clear, orderly manner, in manageable chunks rather than expecting him to hold multiple steps in mind). Greater insight into his attention difficulties and self-management of attention strategies might be expected as he gets older. Given that attention difficulties tend to worsen over time in brain tumour survivors and may impair academic and social functioning, stimulant medication may be warranted for DA in the future, as it has been shown to be safe and efficacious in this population [31].

In light of his delayed reading development, a systematic, phonetically based reading intervention was recommended for DA. It was thought to be particularly important to offer this reading support in a small group or individual setting to optimize DA's variable attention and to ensure that his hearing was optimized. His parents were eager to work with him at home to improve his reading, and they were provided with strategies to build on his current skills while ensuring that reading remained a pleasurable activity for him. DA was also struggling with writing, and a scribe had already been provided for him at school. Additional accommodations were recommended such as consistent note-taking supports and the option to respond orally rather than in writing. Continued monitoring and assessment by an occupational therapist was also suggested. In addition, his parents and teachers were advised on assistive technology (e.g. voice to text software) that could help DA compensate for his writing challenges.

DA's parents were reassured that they were handling his emotional outbursts quite well and were encouraged to continue to remain calm and to guide him in using simple words to describe his emotions (e.g. 'my feelings are getting *hot* and I need to *cool* down'). The impact of DA's fatigue, stress and over-stimulation was also explored as contributing to his difficulties with emotional control and frustration. Regular physical exercise and use of relaxation and breathing exercises were promoted, and specific resources were provided. The plan for future neuropsychological assessments was discussed, with particular emphasis on the need to monitor DA's emerging cognitive difficulties and to reassess his reading progress after a reasonable period of intervention.

Collaboration Discussion

For paediatric neuro-oncology patients, clinical care is optimized by the collaborative efforts of oncologists, neuropsychologists and many other health professionals. Ensuring that medical treatment is effective and results in the highest possible chance of survival, while at the same time minimizing adverse treatment-related effects, is a delicate balance that must be carefully considered for each patient. Reducing treatment intensity for certain medulloblastoma patients (e.g. those with favourable molecular subtypes or those who are neurologically compromised) may be one way of preventing later, additional, neuropsychological deficits. Systematic assessment of a range of long-term outcomes, including neuropsychological, is of utmost importance to understanding the impact of these treatment decisions. Multidisciplinary teams are required to provide the ongoing support required by the increasing cohort of paediatric brain tumour survivors in dealing with the long-term impacts of their disease/treatments and to navigate complex medical, mental health, and educational systems to access interventions and support services.

Chapter Review Questions

1. Which of the following symptoms is *not* usually associated with posterior fossa syndrome (PFS)?
   A. Seizures.
   B. Emotional lability.
   C. Ataxia.
   D. Mutism.

2. Which of the following subgroups of children with medulloblastoma are *least likely* to be treated with craniospinal radiation?
   A. Cranial nerve deficits.
   B. Without metastatic disease.
   C. Incomplete surgical resection.
   D. Aged 0–3 years.

3. What are the most common presenting symptoms in children with a posterior fossa tumour?
   A. Chronically reduced appetite and growth failure.
   B. Acute headache, vomiting, ataxia.
   C. Status epilepticus.
   D. Delirium.

4. Which of the following statements is *true* regarding the neuropsychological performance of children who have been treated for medulloblastoma?
   A. Cognitive deficits typically improve within 1–2 years of diagnosis.
   B. Following surgery, radiation and chemotherapy, children often lose previously acquired skills, such as knowledge of the multiplication tables.
   C. Specific difficulties in attention, memory, processing speed and executive functioning are common.
   D. Cognitive deficits cannot be reliably assessed.

References

1. Lassaletta A, Bouffet E, Mabbott D, Kulkarni AV. Functional and neuropsychological late outcomes in posterior fossa tumors in children. Childs Nerv Syst. 2015;31(10):1877–90.
2. Robinson KE, Fraley CE, Pearson MM, Kuttesch JF Jr, Compas BE. Neurocognitive late effects of pediatric brain tumors of the posterior fossa: a quantitative review. J Int Neuropsychol Soc. 2013;19(1):44–53.
3. Schreiber JE, Gurney JG, Palmer SL, et al. Examination of risk factors for intellectual and academic outcomes following treatment for pediatric medulloblastoma. Neuro Oncol. 2014;16(8):1129–36.
4. Ramaswamy V, Remke M, Bouffet E, et al. Risk stratification of childhood medulloblastoma in the molecular era: the current consensus. Acta Neuropathol. 2016;131(6):821–31.
5. Taylor MD, Northcott PA, Korshunov A, et al. Molecular subgroups of medulloblastoma: the current consensus. Acta Neuropathol. 2012;123(4):465–72.
6. Lannering B, Rutkowski S, Doz F, et al. Hyperfractionated versus conventional radiotherapy followed by chemotherapy in standard-risk medulloblastoma: results from the randomized multicenter HIT-SIOP PNET 4 trial. J Clin Oncol. 2012;30(26):3187–93.
7. Zeltzer PM, Boyett JM, Finlay JL, et al. Metastasis stage, adjuvant treatment, and residual tumor are prognostic factors for medulloblastoma in children: conclusions from the Children's Cancer Group 921 randomized phase III study. J Clin Oncol. 1999;17(3):832–45.
8. Thompson EM, Hielscher T, Bouffet E, et al. Prognostic value of medulloblastoma extent of resection after accounting for molecular subgroup: a retrospective integrated clinical and molecular analysis. Lancet Oncol. 2016;17(4):484–95.
9. Ashley DM, Merchant TE, Strother D, et al. Induction chemotherapy and conformal radiation therapy for very young children with nonmetastatic medulloblastoma: Children's Oncology Group study P9934. J Clin Oncol. 2012;30(26):3181–6.
10. Duffner PK, Horowitz ME, Krischer JP, et al. The treatment of malignant brain tumors in infants and very young children: an update of the Pediatric Oncology Group experience. Neuro Oncol. 1999;1(2):152–61.
11. Rutkowski S, von Hoff K, Emser A, et al. Survival and prognostic factors of early childhood medulloblastoma: an international meta-analysis. J Clin Oncol. 2010;28(33):4961–8.
12. Bodranghien F, Bastian A, Casali C, et al. Consensus paper: revisiting the symptoms and signs of cerebellar syndrome. Cerebellum. 2016;15(3):369–91.
13. Robertson PL, Muraszko KM, Holmes EJ, et al. Incidence and severity of postoperative cerebellar mutism syndrome in children with medulloblastoma: a prospective study by the Children's Oncology Group. J Neurosurg. 2006;105(6 Suppl):444–51.
14. Wells EM, Walsh KS, Khademian ZP, Keating RF, Packer RJ. The cerebellar mutism syndrome and its relation to cerebellar cognitive function and the cerebellar cognitive affective disorder. Dev Disabil Res Rev. 2008;14(3):221–8.
15. Palmer SL, Hassall T, Evankovich K, et al. Neurocognitive outcome 12 months following cerebellar mutism syndrome in pediatric patients with medulloblastoma. Neuro Oncol. 2010;12(12):1311–7.
16. Wolfe-Christensen C, Mullins LL, Scott JG, McNall-Knapp RY. Persistent psychosocial problems in children who develop posterior fossa syndrome after medulloblastoma resection. Pediatr Blood Cancer. 2007;49(5):723–6.
17. Adachi J, Nishikawa R, Hirose T, Matsutani M. Mixed neuronal-glial tumor of the fourth ventricle and successful treatment of postoperative mutism with bromocriptine: case report. Surg Neurol. 2005;63(4):375–9.
18. Shyu C, Burke K, Souweidane MM, et al. Novel use of zolpidem in cerebellar mutism syndrome. J Pediatr Hematol Oncol. 2011;33(2):148–9.
19. Yap JL, Wachtel LE, Ahn ES, Sanz JH, Slomine BS, Pidcock FS. Treatment of cerebellar cognitive affective syndrome with aripiprazole. Journal of Pediatric Rehabilitation Medicine. 2012;5(3):233–8.

20. Gajjar A, Chintagumpala M, Ashley D, et al. Risk-adapted craniospinal radiotherapy followed by high-dose chemotherapy and stem-cell rescue in children with newly diagnosed medulloblastoma (St Jude Medulloblastoma-96): long-term results from a prospective, multicentre trial. Lancet Oncol. 2006;7(10):813–20.
21. Packer RJ, Gajjar A, Vezina G, et al. Phase III study of craniospinal radiation therapy followed by adjuvant chemotherapy for newly diagnosed average-risk medulloblastoma. J Clin Oncol. 2006;24(25):4202–8.
22. Annett RD, Patel SK, Phipps S. Monitoring and assessment of neuropsychological outcomes as a standard of care in pediatric oncology. Pediatr Blood Cancer. 2015;62(Suppl 5):S460–513.
23. Ribi K, Relly C, Landolt MA, Alber FD, Boltshauser E, Grotzer MA. Outcome of medulloblastoma in children: long-term complications and quality of life. Neuropediatrics. 2005;36(6):357–65.
24. Hanzlik E, Woodrome SE, Abdel-Baki M, Geller TJ, Elbabaa SK. A systematic review of neuropsychological outcomes following posterior fossa tumor surgery in children. Childs Nerv Syst. 2015;31(10):1869–75.
25. Edelstein K, Spiegler BJ, Fung S, et al. Early aging in adult survivors of childhood medulloblastoma: long-term neurocognitive, functional, and physical outcomes. Neuro Oncol. 2011;13(5):536–45.
26. Palmer SL, Goloubeva O, Reddick WE, et al. Patterns of intellectual development among survivors of pediatric medulloblastoma: a longitudinal analysis. J Clin Oncol. 2001;19(8):2302–8.
27. Castellino SM, Ullrich NJ, Whelen MJ, Lange BJ. Developing interventions for cancer-related cognitive dysfunction in childhood cancer survivors. JNCI J Natl Cancer Inst (2014) 106(8): dju186. https://doi.org/10.1093/jnci/dju186
28. Carlson-Green B, Morris RD, Krawiecki N. Family and illness predictors of outcome in pediatric brain tumors. J Pediatr Psychol. 1995;20(6):769–84.
29. Woodgate RL, Tailor K, Yanofsky R, Vanan MI. Childhood brain cancer and its psychosocial impact on survivors and their parents: a qualitative thematic synthesis. Eur J Oncol Nurs. 2016;20:140–9.
30. Krull KR, Okcu MF, Potter B, et al. Screening for neurocognitive impairment in pediatric cancer long-term survivors. J Clin Oncol. 2008;26(25):4138–43.
31. Smithson EF, Phillips R, Harvey DW, Morrall MC. The use of stimulant medication to improve neurocognitive and learning outcomes in children diagnosed with brain tumours: a systematic review. Eur J Cancer. 2013;49(14):3029–40.

Chapter 9
Pediatric Stroke

Robyn Westmacott, Jordana Waxman, and Nomazulu Dlamini

Introduction

Arterial ischemic stroke (AIS) occurs when there is a disruption of arterial blood supply to the brain, causing focal injury in a vascular territory. It is one of the leading causes of acquired brain injury in the pediatric population. Acute neonatal stroke (onset from birth to 28 days of life) occurs in approximately 1 in every 4000 live births [1]. Childhood stroke (onset between 1 month and 18 years of age) is less common, with reports of annual incidence ranging from 2.3 to 13 cases per 100,000 children [2]. It is important to differentiate between neonatal and childhood stroke, as they are markedly different in terms of etiology, risk factors, and clinical presentation. For both of these groups, however, the increased plasticity of the young brain has traditionally been thought to protect against significant neurological and neuropsychological deficits [3]. In fact, a significant amount of research highlights the vulnerability of the young brain and the widespread, long-term neuropsychological

R. Westmacott (✉)
Children's Stroke Program, Division of Neurology, Department of Paediatrics, The Hospital for Sick Children, University of Toronto, Toronto, ON, Canada

Psychology Department, The Hospital for Sick Children, Toronto, ON, Canada
e-mail: robyn.westmacott@sickkids.ca

J. Waxman
Psychology Department, York University, Toronto, ON, Canada

N. Dlamini
Children's Stroke Program, Division of Neurology, Department of Pediatrics, The Hospital for Sick Children, Toronto, ON, CA

K. M. Sanders (ed.), *Physician's Field Guide to Neuropsychology*,
https://doi.org/10.1007/978-1-4939-8722-1_9

deficits that often result from early disruption of brain function and subsequent brain development [4, 5]. An increasing body of work indicates that children with a history of neonatal and childhood stroke are at increased risk for difficulties in a number of neurological, cognitive, academic, and psychosocial domains that emerge over the course of development (see [6] for review). Heterogeneity in outcomes within the pediatric stroke population has been linked to a range of clinical and demographic factors, including those related to the brain (e.g., lesion location, size, and volume), the child (e.g., age at stroke, age at assessment, co-occurring neurological conditions, stroke etiology, genetic predispositions), and the environment (family stress/functioning, parent mental health, sibling interactions, educational support, rehabilitation therapy) [6]. Our understanding of how these factors interact to impact neuropsychological outcome and resiliency is far from complete, but evidence to date suggests that these relationships are very complex.

This chapter details a case of childhood stroke, assessed through multiple neuropsychological assessments across development. The case highlights the unique cognitive and psychosocial difficulties that emerge across development following early childhood stroke and the importance of long-term follow-up and team collaboration in this population.

Case Presentation

Reason for Referral: Sarah is a nearly 14-year-old girl in Grade 8 who experienced a left hemisphere stroke involving the basal ganglia and temporoparietal cortex at 2 years of age in the context of myocarditis. As a result of the stroke, Sarah has moderate right spastic hemiparesis and right hemidystonia. Her first neuropsychological assessment was carried out at 4 years of age, revealing difficulties with articulation, expressive language, attention, and visual-motor integration. Subsequent assessments at ages 6, 8, and 10 documented emerging deficits in working memory, literacy, and numeracy, as well as ongoing challenges with attention and complex expressive language. She was referred for a follow-up assessment to track her development and assist with high school transition planning.

Family and Medical History: Sarah lives with her parents and 17-year-old brother. Both parents have college diplomas and are currently employed full time. No family history of any learning, attention, or intellectual deficits was reported, though several members of the family were described as having mild symptoms of anxiety.

Sarah was born at full term weighing 8 lbs. 11 oz. after a typical pregnancy and delivery. She met early motor and language milestones without difficulty, and, by 2 years of age, Sarah was speaking in phrases, running, and interacting well with other toddlers at daycare. There were no developmental or medical concerns until Sarah was diagnosed with pneumonia at the age of 2 years and 5 months. Five days into her illness, Sarah's parents noticed some subtle right facial droop and weakness of her right arm and leg. By the time of her admission to hospital, Sarah exhibited a dense right hemiparesis, global aphasia, and lowered level of consciousness. Brain imaging revealed an acute infarct involving the left basal ganglia, left internal capsule, and left temporoparietal cortex. Further investigations, including echocardiography, cardiac MRI, coronary angiogram, and myocardial biopsy, indicated a diagnosis of acute myocarditis as well as intracardiac left atrial clot. Thus, the etiology of Sarah's stroke was cardioembolic. An infection of the heart led to the formation of a blood clot, which traveled to her brain and occluded the middle cerebral artery, causing an ischemic stroke. Sarah was treated for approximately 2 months with steroids and enoxaparin and then switched to aspirin, which she continues to take for secondary stroke prevention. Cardiac function returned to baseline quickly following treatment, and she was discharged from cardiology after her first follow-up visit. However, Sarah's recovery and development have been followed closely in neurology, and her story illustrates many of the common challenges faced by individuals with a stroke in early childhood.

Post-stroke Recovery and Development: Forty-eight hours after the onset of her stroke, Sarah began to show some return of motor function on her right side by wiggling her right foot and leg. At 6 days post-stroke, she began to use some single words again. Sarah was discharged from the hospital at 8 days post-stroke and transferred to an inpatient rehabilitation program where she received intensive occupational, physical and speech-language therapies. She made significant gains in motor function, but continued to exhibit a significant right hemiparesis, with her arm and hand impacted to a greater extent than her leg. Sarah had been showing clear signs of right-handedness prior to the stroke, but she was forced to switch hand dominance to the left. Language recovery occurred gradually, but, by 4–5 months post-stroke, Sarah was judged to be back to her baseline of using short phrases to communicate. However, subsequent language development was challenging, as significant difficulties with articulation, grammar, and word finding emerged over the course of her preschool years. Approximately 4 months following her stroke, Sarah also began to develop right hemidystonia—a movement disorder characterized by involuntary muscle contractions and limb posturing. Due to worsening dystonia symptoms over the following year, Artane was prescribed, but Sarah experienced some negative side effects (i.e., imbalance, mood changes) and was subsequently switched to baclofen. Sarah continues to take baclofen, with slight reported improvement in her dystonia symptoms.

In addition to traditional rehabilitation therapy, Sarah has received regular Botox injections in her right ankle and arm to facilitate movement, and she participated in two sessions of constraint-induced therapy in which her left arm was constrained in a cast for 2 weeks to promote motor recovery of her right arm function. Some additional improvement was noted following constraint therapy, but Sarah continues to have limited use of her right hand. Sarah is also described as a clumsy and poorly coordinated girl who frequently trips, falls, and bumps into things.

The Neurology Perspective: Overview of Pediatric Stroke

Definitions and Epidemiology of Pediatric Stroke: Stroke is defined as an acute neurological deficit, accompanied by CT or MRI evidence of ischemic injury in a vascular territory consistent with the neurological presentation. It remains one of the top ten causes of death in childhood and causes lifelong disability with socioeconomic implications for the children, their families, and society [7–9]. Ischemic perinatal stroke (IPS) is defined as "a group of heterogeneous conditions in which there is focal disruption of cerebral blood flow secondary to arterial or cerebral venous thrombosis or embolization, between 20 weeks of fetal life through the 28th postnatal day, confirmed by neuroimaging or neuropathologic studies" [10]. Neonatal arterial ischemic stroke (NAIS) and neonatal cerebral sinovenous ischemic stroke (NCSVT) are subcategories of IPS diagnosed following acute symptomatic presentation with a corresponding ischemic infarct in the arterial (NAIS) or venous (NCSVT) vascular territory. In neonates the most common clinical presentation is acute encephalopathy with altered mental status and focal seizures typically with onset beyond 12 h after delivery. Children with a delayed presentation of a focal neurological deficit, for example, presenting with early hand preference and imaging findings of a chronic infarct on neuroimaging, are subcategorized as having a presumed perinatal ischemic stroke (PPIS). This too can be arterial (PPAIS) or venous (PPVIS).

Management of Pediatric Stroke: Timely neuroimaging is essential for diagnosis and selection of hyperacute and acute treatments. Magnetic resonance imaging (MRI) of the brain with diffusion-weighted sequences and MR angiography are the imaging modalities of choice for the diagnosis of pediatric stroke. Management is based on early institution of neuroprotective measures and antithrombotic therapy (antiplatelet or anticoagulant). Neuroprotective measures aim to minimize the extent of ischemic injury to the brain. The aim of antithrombotic therapy is to reduce the risk of recurrent thrombosis in childhood arterial stroke, neonatal cardioembolic arterial ischemic stroke, or thrombus propagation in CSVT.

Key Point
Importance of Neuropsychological Assessment: Neuropsychological assessment is considered to be part of the standard of care for patients and families impacted by pediatric stroke. Concerns about cognitive, academic, social, and emotional functioning are consistently among the top priorities of parents and other family members, and these are best addressed by a neuropsychologist. Unlike motor function, neuropsychological issues tend to change dynamically over the course of childhood and adolescence, making longitudinal follow-up evaluation and consultation an essential part of care for these families.

Pediatric Stroke Outcome: Outcomes following pediatric stroke include death in up to 10%, recurrent stroke in 10–50% depending on the cause, neurological deficits in 60–70%, and seizures in up to 30%. The spectrum of neurological outcome following stroke includes loss of focal sensorimotor function causing hemiparesis, spasticity, and/or a movement disorder such as dystonia, dysphasia, and dysphagia, as well as cognitive and behavioral difficulties. Sensorimotor and cognitive outcomes in pediatric stroke vary widely, and although lesion volumes of greater than 10% are shown to be associated with poor outcomes, no independent and specific effect of lesion size or lesion has been demonstrated in childhood stroke [11]. Acute Wallerian degeneration remote from the area of infarction (also termed pre-Wallerian degeneration) and appearing as restricted diffusion MRI signal within descending corticospinal tracts has been correlated with motor outcome in neonatal ischemic stroke [12–14]. However, imaging predictors of outcome in pediatric CSVT cannot simply be extrapolated from the findings in AIS given the difference in underlying pathology [15]. The Pediatric Stroke Outcome Measure (PSOM) is a validated tool used for the standardized assessment of sensorimotor, language, and behavioral and cognitive outcomes following stroke in childhood [16]. Functional status at 1 year post-stroke is strongly predictive of long-term outcome, and mental health issues are emerging as a significant area of need [17].

Sarah's Neurological Outcome and Dystonia: Sarah's post-stroke hemiparesis and dysphasia represent a typical recovery trajectory following stroke in childhood. In addition to hemiparesis, many children with basal ganglia stroke, like Sarah, develop dystonia—a movement disorder characterized by excessive, involuntary muscle contractions resulting in repetitive movements, twisting movements, and/or abnormal posturing [18, 19]. The underlying mechanisms of post-stroke dystonia are not well understood but thought to result more from disruption in functional networks and connectivity, rather than a single lesion [20]. Preliminary estimates suggest that 21% of children with unilateral basal ganglia stroke develop hemidystonia, with slightly higher incidence following left compared to right hemisphere lesions [21]. The onset of dystonia is typically 6–12 months following the stroke, leading some to suggest that maladaptive neuroplasticity and reorganization may contribute to its manifestation [20, 22]. Interestingly, there is some evidence to suggest that children who develop post-stroke dystonia exhibit more pronounced difficulties with cognitive inhibition and poorer overall intellectual and academic outcomes when compared to children with similar basal ganglia strokes but no dystonia [23]. Sarah's case is consistent with this, as her overall intellectual abilities were moderately weak, and she exhibited significant challenges with attention, cognitive inhibition, literacy, and math. Maladaptive reorganization following basal ganglia stroke may help explain the emergence of dystonia and associated neurocognitive deficits.

Rehabilitation Strategies: Current understanding of how the brain responds and modifies its structure and function after injury—referred to as neuroplasticity—has evolved into the concept of a recovery continuum between plasticity and vulnerability in pediatric acute ischemic stroke [24]. Multimodal rehabilitation strategies targeting motor deficits, language and intellectual impairments, behavioral and social disabilities, and epilepsy are often required to enhance neuroplasticity and support recovery, so as to improve outcome. However, as in Sarah's case, the intervention required may change over time as the neurological deficits evolve.

The Neuropsychology Perspective: Predicting and Tracking Development

Neuropsychological assessment is a routine part of standard clinical care for children with perinatal, neonatal, or childhood stroke. As with other pediatric populations, the goals of assessment include tracking development across a broad range of domains, helping parents and educators understand the child's neuropsychological profile in the context of the stroke and subsequent response to that brain injury, providing recommendations based on individual strengths and challenges, advocating for access to services, and predicting long-term outcome and anticipating needs that may arise in the future. Serial assessments and long-term follow-up throughout childhood and adolescence are critical due to the gradually emerging nature of neuropsychological deficits in this population.

Key Point

Cognitive Screening vs. Comprehensive Neuropsychological Assessment: When children are school age or older at the time of stroke, some cognitive screening may be warranted in the first few months post stroke. Helpful tools for early post-stroke cognitive screening include brief intellectual batteries such as the Reynolds Intelligence Assessment Scales—2nd Edition (RIAS-2)—or the Kaufman Brief Intelligence Scale, 2nd Edition (KBIT-2). Screening of basic vocabulary and core academic skills is also helpful in some cases. Obtaining a detailed description of premorbid functioning through parent interview and standardized questionnaires is extremely valuable and important for evaluating post stroke changes. A comprehensive neuropsychological assessment is generally not recommended until at least 5–6 months post stroke, at which point recovery has typically slowed, and the child's new baseline level of function can be accurately determined.

Tracking Sarah's Development: As is typical within our program, Sarah was first seen for neuropsychological assessment at 4 years 3 months of age in order to prepare for her entry into junior kindergarten. In addition to the impact of her right-side weakness and dystonia on day-to-day functioning and independence, her parents were concerned about Sarah's speech and language development at that time. Her articulation was poor, she struggled to find words, and she often became frustrated when trying to communicate her ideas. Oral-motor control, specifically drooling, was also an issue. Standardized testing revealed age-appropriate single-word vocabulary, verbal and visual reasoning, factual knowledge, and concept formation. However, Sarah struggled on tasks that required verbal expression beyond single-word answers, and her sentence structure and grammatical expression were poor. Visual-motor integration and visual-spatial construction were also very weak, in part due to her reliance on one hand to complete these tasks. Finally, impulsive response tendencies were noted, and Sarah required a significant amount of redirection during testing. Recommendations included ongoing speech-language and occupational therapy, opportunities for small-group learning in kindergarten, support from a Special Needs Assistant, and accommodations for her physical disability. Sarah's elevated risk for academic difficulties in the future was highlighted, and the importance of follow-up assessment was emphasized.

A follow-up assessment at 6 years of age indicated ongoing challenges with verbal expression, grammar, and organization of ideas, though single-word vocabulary and nonverbal reasoning abilities continued to be largely age-appropriate. Early academic difficulties in reading, printing, and math were starting to emerge, as were challenges with sustained attention and working memory. Sarah had become more adept at using her left hand for pencil tasks, but she still struggled with letter formation and drawing, and broader deficits in visual-spatial organization and visual-motor integration were apparent. Moreover, Sarah's parents reported some emerging tendencies toward anxiety and low mood. Sarah was becoming increasingly aware of being different from her peers and made negative self-comments (e.g., "I can't run like the other kids," "I'm not very smart"), though she was still successful in friendships. Sarah had also started expressing significant fears about death, illness, aging, and separation from loved ones. Her parents reported that she had multiple episodes of intense crying each week and that she was starting to show reluctance to go to school. A diagnosis of language disorder was given at that time, and specific strategies to facilitate attention, language, and academic development were provided. Resources and strategies to help Sarah manage feelings of anxiety and sadness were also discussed with her parents.

By the time of her next neuropsychological at 8 1/2 years of age, Sarah was struggling in Grade 3, and symptoms of anxiety had worsened to the point of interfering with daily functioning at home, at school, and with peers. Sarah was having particular difficulty in math and oral language expression, and her teacher suggested that Sarah move into a small class for students with academic and language difficulties. Cognitive testing revealed emerging difficulties with both verbal and nonverbal reasoning, lowering estimates of overall intellectual function, and there were ongoing challenges with verbal expression, word finding, organization of ideas, visual-spatial organization, and visual-motor integration. Core reading skills were developing adequately, but weaknesses in reading comprehension, math calculation, and math problem solving were becoming apparent. Challenges with attention, working memory, cognitive inhibition, processing speed, and executive function were also clearly evident in standardized testing and on parent and teacher reports of daily functioning. A diagnosis of attention deficit hyperactivity disorder (ADHD)-inattentive presentation was given, and Sarah was referred to a clinical psychologist for a combination of individual and family therapy targeting anxiety and mood.

Summary of Current Neuropsychological Assessment: Sarah was seen for a follow-up assessment halfway through Grade 8, at 13 years 11 months, in order to reassess her educational needs prior to beginning high school. Following her previous assessment, she was enrolled in the aforementioned specialized classroom for students with learning challenges. However, in Grade 7, she was transferred into a classroom for students with mild intellectual disability. Sarah's mother reported that she had made great gains since her previous assessment but continues to struggle academically in both literacy and math. Related to this, Sarah continued to have difficulties with complex language skills, such as word finding and expression of complex ideas. Additionally, ongoing challenges with attention and organizational skills were reported by her mother and teacher. For example, Sarah continues to be easily distractible, loses track of what she is doing or saying, and has difficulty with multitasking. Though significant improvements in Sarah's anxiety were noted, her parents endorsed several broad symptoms of anxiety (i.e., nervousness and worry) on standardized questionnaires. Additionally, Sarah was noted to have difficulties with social maturity, which may be related to her difficulties with complex language.

Cognitive testing revealed that Sarah's intellectual abilities were continuing to develop somewhat more slowly than her peers, though significant gains had been made in her ability to reason with verbal information (see Table 9.1). Despite these improvements in more basic language skills (including grammar and sentence structure), most of Sarah's reasoning abilities were still falling in the low average range. Indeed, she continued to have significant difficulty with fluent word retrieval and word generation. Moreover, visual-spatial processing with an additional motor component continued to be most difficult for Sarah. This added difficulty above and beyond her visual-spatial processing highlighted her significant gross and fine motor deficits. Additionally, despite her largely low average intellectual profile, her core and applied academic skills were still significantly lower than expected. Moreover, continued challenges were noted with sustained attention, filtering out distractions, mental manipulation of information, initiation, organization, and novel problem solving. As such, she continued to meet criteria for ADHD-inattentive presentation. A new diagnosis of learning disorder (as opposed to language disorder) was given as well, with an emphasis on teaching Sarah applied- or basic-level courses. The importance of a structured environment and meaningful context when learning was highlighted for Sarah, and her parents were given specific recommendations in order to improve her higher-order language skills. A follow-up assessment was also recommended to facilitate the transition to postsecondary education as well as adult neuropsychological follow-up.

Table 9.1 Data from Sarah's most recent neuropsychological assessment

Test name	Description	Percentile
Cognition		
WISC-V Verbal Comprehension Index	**Index of verbal comprehension skills**	13
Similarities	Classifying objects and words into categories based on concrete & abstract similarities	16
Vocabulary	Describing the meaning of words	16
WISC-V Visual-Spatial Index	**Index of visual-spatial skills**	6
Block Design	Copying geometric patterns using colored blocks	16
Visual Puzzles	Mental rotation of puzzle pieces to make a whole	9
WISC-V Fluid Reasoning Index	**Ability to reason with unfamiliar information in novel ways**	2
Matrix Reasoning	Visual pattern completion, nonverbal reasoning and problem solving	9
Figure Weights	Solving nonverbal problems, quantitative reasoning	2
WISC-V Working Memory Index	**Index of attention and mental manipulation skills**	1
Digit Span	Repetition of digit strings read aloud	1
Picture Span	Keeping track of pictures and the order in which they were shown	9
WISC-V Processing Speed Index	**Index of visuomotor processing speed**	1
Coding	Speeded transcription of numbers into symbols	<1
Symbol Search	Speeded visual search	9
WISC-V Optional subtests		
Comprehension	Answering open-ended questions, social and practical reasoning	9
WISC-V Full Scale IQ	Overall intellectual abilities	Not reported due to variability
Academics		
WIAT-III	**Academic achievement**	
Reading Comprehension	Measures untimed reading comprehension of text	2
Math Problem Solving	Untimed math problem solving skills	4
Word Reading	Single-word reading skills	2
Pseudoword Decoding	Ability to decode nonsense words	2
Numerical Operations	Measures untimed written math computational skills	<1
Oral Reading Fluency		1
(Oral Reading Accuracy)	Measures accuracy of contextualized oral reading	2
(Oral Reading Rate)	Measures speed of contextualized oral reading	2
Spelling	Spelling single words dictated by the examiner	3

(continued)

Table 9.1 (continued)

Test name	Description	Percentile
Executive functioning		
DKEFS Word Fluency	**Measures of Language Fluency**	
Letter	Rapidly generating words that start with a particular letter	5
Category	Rapidly generating words that belong to a particular category	16
Category Switching Accuracy	Rapidly generating words that belong to 2 alternating categories	9
DKEFS Color Word	**Test of processing speed, attention regulation, and inhibitory control**	
Color Naming	Rapid naming of colors	<1
Word Naming	Rapid reading of color words	<1
Inhibition	Inhibition of automatic responses, e.g., naming color of ink rather than reading word	<1
Inhibit/Switch	Measure of inhibition and cognitive flexibility	<1
DKEFS Tower Test	**Executive function, strategy formation, problem solving, ability to follow rules**	
Total Achievement Score	Index of problem-solving ability	50
Move Accuracy Ratio	Total moves relative to minimum moves required—measures problem-solving efficiency	25
DKEFS Trails	**Tests of visual scanning, number and letter sequencing, cognitive flexibility, and motor speed**	
Visual Scanning	Ability to rapidly cross-off target symbols using a pencil	1
Number Sequences	Ability to rapidly navigate visual "trails" by using a pencil to connect numbers in a sequence	16
Letter Sequences	Ability to rapidly navigate visual "trails" by using a pencil to connect letters in sequence	<1
Number-Letter Switching	Ability to rapidly navigate visual "trails" by using a pencil to alternate between numbers and letters in a sequence	2
Wisconsin Card Sorting Test	**Problem solving, cognitive flexibility, abstract thinking, hypothesis testing**	
Total errors	Index of overall problem solving ability	4
Perseverative Responses	Tendency to get "stuck" in one response pattern	70
Memory		
CVLT-C	**Rote memory and learning**	
List A Total Trials 1-5	Memory for a list of words over 5 trials	3
List A Trial 1 Free Recall	Memory after hearing a list of words one time	31
List A Trial 5 Free Recall	Memory after hearing a list of words five times	16
List B Free Recall	Memory for a second, competing list of words after one presentation	2

(continued)

Table 9.1 (continued)

Test name	Description	Percentile
List A Short Delay Free Recall	Recalling a list of words after a brief delay	16
List A Short Delay Cued Recall	Recalling words from the first list, by category	16
List A Long Delay Free Recall	Recalling a list of words after a long delay	2
List A Long Delay Cued Recall	Recalling words from the first list, after a long delay, by category	7
Delayed Recognition	Yes/No recognition of words after a delay	69
RCFT		
Immediate Recall	Ability to recall and recreate a complex visual figure from memory, 3 minutes after copying	<1
Delayed Recall	Ability to recall and recreate a complex visual figure from memory, 30 minutes after copying	<1
Delayed Recognition	Ability to recognize parts of the figure that were part of the design that was copied and drawn	<1
Attention		
TEACH	**Tests of Attention**	
Sky Search-Total Attention Score	Speeded visual search, focusing on relevant information and filtering out distracters	<1
Sky Search #Correct	Number of correctly circled targets	2
Sky Search-Time per target	Average time taken to circle each target	<1
Score-Total	Sustained auditory attention	<1
Sky Search DT	Divided attention to simultaneous visual search and sustained auditory tasks	<1
Motor and Visuomotor Integration		
Grooved Pegs	**Test of fine motor control**	
Grooved Pegs-Dominant Hand	Fine motor dexterity and speed with the left hand	<1
Grooved Pegs-Nondominant hand	Fine motor dexterity and speed with the right hand	Not administered due to hemiparesis
RCFT		
Copy	Ability to copy a complex visual figure	<1
Beery Visuomotor Integration	Copying designs of increasing complexity	3
Beery Perceptual	Matching designs of increasing complexity	5
Beery Motor Coordination	Pencil control, accurate tracing between lines	2
DKEFS Trails		
Motor Speed	Ability to rapidly navigate visual "trails" by using a pencil to connect circles	16

Abbreviations: *WISC-V* Wechsler Intelligence Scale for Children—version V, *Tea-Ch* Test of Everyday Attention for Children, *CVLT-C* California Verbal Learning Test for Children, *RCFT* Rey Complex Figure Task, *DKEFS* Delis-Kaplan Executive Function Systems, *WCST* Wisconsin Card Sorting Test, *WIAT-III* Wechsler Individual Achievement Test 3rd Edition, and *Beery VMI* Beery-Buktenica Developmental Test of Visual-Motor-Integration

Collaborative Discussion

Sarah's story highlights many themes in the neuropsychological research literature in this population. A substantial number of children with pediatric stroke experience neuropsychological sequelae that emerge over time, despite the static nature of their focal lesions. In this collaborative discussion, we will utilize Sarah's case to review relevant literature on intellectual outcomes, language development, attention, executive function, and psychosocial outcomes in the pediatric stroke population. In addition, we will discuss the impact of dystonia of neuropsychological functioning, factors within the family and environment that promote resilience, the role of the neuropsychologist within the pediatric stroke medical team, and the importance of supporting children and families as they transition to the adult medical system.

Intellectual Ability: Sarah's overall intellectual abilities continue to develop at a moderately slow rate compared to her peers. Sarah's development mirrors research to date, indicating that global intellectual outcomes of children with stroke are within the broad range of average, although compromised compared to normative samples [25–27]. Because children with stroke often present with multiple areas of cognitive dysfunction, psychometric estimates of overall intelligence may be misleading—scores may be depressed due to specific neurocognitive deficits, not due to a global impairment in all aspects of cognitive function. Certainly, many children with early stroke do go on to develop widespread intellectual disabilities, but many others (like Sarah) have a unique combination of strengths and deficits and are grossly misrepresented by a single test score. The fact that Sarah's stroke occurred at a very young age and that it involved both cortical and subcortical regions places her at increased risk for negative cognitive outcome. Combined cortical-subcortical lesions are more detrimental to cognitive outcomes compared to isolated cortical or subcortical lesions alone [26–30]. Moreover, there is some evidence to suggest that cortical lesions in the early childhood period (between 1 month and 5 years of age) are more likely to be associated with negative cognitive outcome than cortical lesions occurring before or after this period [27]. Further, there is significant evidence to suggest that younger age at brain insult is associated with increased risk of poor cognitive outcome [4, 25, 31, 32].

Language: Sarah's stroke affected the left basal ganglia and also the left temporoparietal cortex, which is considered to be part of the classic language network [33]. Consistent with the research literature, Sarah exhibits a combination of preserved core language abilities (e.g., vocabulary, comprehension of simple instructions) and impaired higher-level language skills (e.g., verbal fluency, organization of complex ideas, grammatical expression, written expression, and reading comprehension). Specifically, higher-level language and verbal deficits often emerge gradually as children with early left hemisphere brain injuries grow older, and younger age at injury is in fact associated with poorer long-term outcome [31, 34–38]. Although younger children often do recover more quickly from acute-stage aphasic deficits than older children or adults, many go on to develop significant challenges with more sophisticated aspects of language and verbal ability as they get older [36,

39, 40]. This clearly illustrates how enhanced plasticity is not necessarily associated with positive outcome. Compensatory mechanisms may be insufficient to support higher-level skills, and plasticity may be maladaptive and cause disruption of later-developing abilities [4]. The functional neuroimaging literature supports this view, with several studies showing an advantage for typical left hemisphere language organization patterns following early left hemisphere stroke [41–43]. Indeed, there is a wealth of evidence that language lateralization begins early in life [44] and increases throughout childhood [45]. With increased lateralization, the likelihood of successful reorganization of language within the right hemisphere appears to decrease [46].

Attention and Executive Functioning: Sarah's long-standing difficulties with attention, working memory, and executive functioning (e.g., inhibitory control, cognitive flexibility, goal setting, organization) represent some of the key deficits encountered by children with a history of stroke [30, 32, 47–51]. Although heterogeneity of type of stroke (ischemic, hemorrhagic, venous) and location (cortical, subcortical, combined) have been predictive of attention and executive functioning deficits in certain studies [28, 47, 48, 50], deficits in these domains are frequently documented regardless of many clinical factors that are known to affect other cognitive abilities in this population [25, 30, 51, 52]. Attention, working memory, and executive function are extremely complex skills that are represented by widespread diffuse but integrated functional areas of the brain [51], which may explain their vulnerability in pediatric stroke regardless of specific lesion location. Moreover, early injury is posited to disrupt the normative process of myelination, particularly in the frontal lobes, thereby rendering the developing brain less able to support higher-level cognitive skills needed for executive functioning [31]. Related to these difficulties, Sarah met criteria for the diagnosis of attention deficit hyperactivity disorder (ADHD). Max et al. [47, 48] reported that 46% of the children in their sample fulfilled diagnostic criteria for ADHD, suggesting that this is a common disorder diagnosed post-pediatric stroke. The basal ganglia has complex interconnections with prefrontal cortex (including dorsolateral prefrontal, cingulate gyrus, and medial prefrontal regions), and these fronto-striatal networks have been strongly implicated in the manifestation of ADHD and a variety of executive function disorders [53–55]. Thus, Sarah's lesion in the left basal ganglia can help to contextualize her difficulties in executive functioning and attention, as well as her diagnosis of ADHD. As neuropsychologists and neurologists, we need to be aware of the increased prevalence in this special population and help families and educators understand that the diagnosis of ADHD may be largely secondary to the stroke. Additionally it will be important for healthcare professionals to understand the complications with recommending medications in a neurological population such as pediatric stroke.

Academic Skills: Sarah's case provides an example of the academic difficulties that come in conjunction with deficits in higher-level language ability, executive functioning, and attention. Although much of the research on academic outcomes has been in neonatal strokes, findings suggest that in preschool and school-aged children, academic skills in math, reading, writing, and spelling are all significantly lower than controls [56–58]. As well, children who experience stroke earlier in development may be most vulnerable to academic challenges [59]. A slower acquisition of skill instead of arrested development has been posited, as time since stroke was not a predictive factor of academic achievement over a 3-year period of the longitudinal study [56]. In Sarah's case, she was not diagnosed with a learning disorder until adolescence, as her academic difficulties only appeared once deficits in higher-level language, attention, and executive functioning emerged. Preliminary results from our group corroborate this hypothesis and suggest that working memory and certain aspects of executive functioning may be predictive of poorer performance in math and spelling [60, 61]. It is important for the neuropsychologist to understand the unique learning profile that may emerge as a child with a history of pediatric stroke develops, in order to make adequate recommendations to implement in the school and at home. Additionally, it is important to understand the vulnerability of academic skills in a population that is prone to difficulties with executive functioning and attention [6].

Psychosocial Outcomes: Quality of life is poor among a significant minority of pediatric stroke survivors [62, 63]. These poorer outcomes may be related to social participation and adjustment being lower, and rates of mental health problems being higher, in comparison to controls and children with chronic illnesses [34, 47, 48, 63–65]. Recent work has elucidated clinical, neurological, as well as proximal and distal environmental factors that may predict worse outcomes. Specifically, poor neurological outcomes were predictive of lower quality of life and social participation, which seem to exacerbate other risk factors such as cognitive and behavioral deficits, stroke type, female gender, older age at stroke, as well as larger lesion size and subcortical location [29, 62]. Interestingly, proximal (family functioning, parent mental health) and distal (parent education) family factors were of utmost importance for social competence and reducing internalizing problems [63, 64]. Certainly Sarah's case was complicated by significant challenges with anxiety that emerged throughout middle childhood. According to her parents, there were early signs of fearfulness and separation anxiety following her stroke, but clear symptoms of anxiety began around 8 years of age. Although they had decreased in severity after participating in sessions of play therapy and cognitive-behavioral therapy with a clinical psychologist over several years, Sarah's most recent assessment in adolescence revealed that she was still endorsing symptoms of anxiety, and her parents reported concerns with her social maturity. Although Sarah has poorer neurological functioning and a host of clinical risk factors, her supportive family environment provides a protective factor for her quality of life, social participation, and mental health. Sarah's difficulties highlight the importance of assessing quality of life and psychosocial functioning in our neuropsychological test batteries, as these difficulties may impact the child or adolescent's ability to put their best effort forth during testing. Additionally, it underscores the importance of targeting support at the family level to promote more adaptive psychosocial outcomes.

The Role of the Neuropsychologist with the Stroke Team: The primary role of the pediatric neuropsychologist is to conduct a comprehensive neuropsychological assessment; interpret the results within the context of brain, child, and environmental factors; and communicate the findings and recommendations to the child (as appropriate) and those involved in his/her care. In addition to formal psychometric testing of intelligence, language, visual-spatial abilities, learning and memory, attention, executive function, academics, psychosocial functioning, and effort, the neuropsychologist gathers detailed information about the child's medical history, developmental history, and day-to-day functioning from a variety of sources including medical and school records, standardized parent and teacher questionnaires, and interviews with the child, caregiver, and educators [66]. The neuropsychological assessment provides a foundation for understanding the child's cognitive profile in the context of his/her medical history, making relevant diagnoses, monitoring recovery and development over time, and assisting with treatment planning and educational programming. As highlighted by Sarah's case, diagnoses and conclusions are not based on individual scores but rather on patterns of data at a single time point and over multiple time points to track that child's developmental trajectory and assist with prediction of long-term outcome [5]. Moreover, although neuropsychologists do not treat mental health disorders, it is imperative for them to carefully assess for anxiety, depression, and other psychosocial problems and to understand how these issues typically present in children of different ages.

When working with children who have a history of stroke, the neuropsychologist must keep in mind several unique considerations. First, it is critical to have a good understanding of the research literature to date on the complex interactions among brain, child, and environmental factors and their impact on long-term neuropsychological outcome. Brain-behavior relationships evolve over the course of development, and assessment data must be interpreted in the context of these changing dynamics. Second, it is important to recognize that the impact of an early focal lesion will unfold and evolve gradually over time and to help parents make the connection between their child's current struggles and the remote brain injury. However, with this understanding should also come the recognition that parents, educators, and other professionals have the capacity to alter the child's trajectory with various treatments, interventions, and styles of interaction. Longitudinal follow-up assessments are also critical in the pediatric stroke population, as illustrated in Sarah's case. An initial assessment can assist in documenting recovery of lost skills and providing a baseline for later follow-up, but the nuances of the child's cognitive profile often do not become clear until higher-level skills have started to come online [5]. Third, many children with stroke have focal motor deficits that must be accommodated during the assessment and taken into consideration when interpreting findings. A stroke impacting the dominant hand often results in switched hand dominance, the ramifications of which are poorly understood. Fourth, pediatric stroke remains under-recognized and poorly understood within the general population and even within some healthcare settings [67]. The neuropsychologist must assist in educating family members and educators about the impact of stroke on the developing brain and must advocate for access to services within the education system and the broader community. Sarah did meet the criteria for two well-known diagnoses (learning disorder and ADHD), but her needs cannot be understood solely in the context of these labels. Sarah experienced an early stroke involving systems in her brain that are critical for attention, executive function, language processing, academic skill development, and motor control. The implications of this early brain injury must be clearly communicated by the neuropsychologist to all relevant parties. Finally, the transition to adult care can be challenging and overwhelming for patients and families. In the case of those with pediatric stroke, it may be difficult to find an adult neurologist with experience working with young people impacted by stroke. Pediatric stroke and adult stroke differ tremendously in terms of etiology, associated medical issues, and outcome, and the young adult with a history of pediatric stroke may feel quite out of place in an adult neurology setting. In our clinic, we often extend neuropsychological services to young adults who require follow-up assessment for the purposes of educational support, job accommodations, or disability funding [68].

Key Point

Conclusions: This case example illustrates many of the themes that have emerged from research on pediatric stroke, as well as important considerations for clinicians working with this population.

- Neuropsychological assessments must be comprehensive in this population, covering a wide range of cognitive, academic, and psychosocial domains.
- The importance of longitudinal follow-up cannot be overstated, as many children grow into their deficits during the school-age and adolescent years.
- There is significant heterogeneity in neuropsychological outcome following pediatric stroke, depending on a host of factors related to the child, the brain, and the environment.

We are just starting to understand the complex interactions among these factors and how they impact neuropsychological development. Individual differences in the response to brain injury have not been well explored in research to date, but this promises to be an important avenue for future studies. Neuropsychological outcomes following pediatric stroke highlight the vulnerability of the developing brain, and the idea that neuroplasticity can be adaptive or maladaptive, depending on a variety of individual factors.

Chapter Review Questions

1. Which of the following statements is *not* supported by current research?
   A. Pediatric strokes rarely result in significant intellectual disability.
   B. Early left hemisphere stroke does not usually result in aphasia.
   C. Deficits in attention are common following pediatric stroke.
   D. Earlier age at stroke is associated with poorer intellectual outcome.

2. A unique consideration for neuropsychologists working in the area of pediatric stroke is that:
   A. Traditional psychological diagnoses cannot be given.
   B. Longitudinal follow-up is rarely necessary.
   C. Stroke later in childhood may necessitate a switch in hand dominance.
   D. Most children with stroke present with dystonia and cannot participate in traditional neuropsychological assessment.

3. Which of the following statements is *not* true?
   A. Neonatal stroke is more common than childhood stroke.
   B. Stroke is a leading cause of brain injury in the pediatric population.
   C. Neonatal stroke, childhood stroke, and adult stroke have similar etiologies.
   D. Antithrombotic therapy and neuroprotective measures are important parts of acute stroke management for children.

4. Long-term neurological deficits following pediatric stroke are more common when:
   A. Infarcts involve subcortical regions only.
   B. Acute Wallerian degeneration of the corticospinal tract is observed on the acute diffusion-weighted MRI.
   C. The infarct impacts the right hemisphere.
   D. When there are no seizures at the time of the stroke.

References

1. Härtel C, Schilling S, Sperner J, Thyen U. The clinical outcomes of neonatal and childhood stroke: review of the literature and implications for future research. Eur J Neurol. 2004;11(7):431–8. https://doi.org/10.1111/j.1468-1331.2004.00861.x.
2. Lynch JK, Hirtz DG, DeVeber G, Nelson KB. Report of the National Institute of Neurological Disorders and Stroke workshop on perinatal and childhood stroke. Pediatrics. 2002;109(1):116–23. https://doi.org/10.1542/peds.109.1.116.
3. Woods BT, Teuber HL. Early onset of complementary specialization of cerebral hemispheres in man. Trans Am Neurol Assoc. 1973;98:113–7. http://ovidsp.ovid.com/ovidweb.cgi?T=JS&PAGE=reference&D=med1&NEWS=N&AN=4784915
4. Dennis M, Spiegler BJ, Juranek JJ, Bigler ED, Snead OC, Fletcher JM. Age, plasticity, and homeostasis in childhood brain disorders. Neurosci Biobehav Rev. 2013;37(10):2760–73. https://doi.org/10.1016/j.neubiorev.2013.09.010.
5. Dennis M, Spiegler BJ, Simic N, et al. Functional plasticity in childhood brain disorders: when, what, how, and whom to assess. Neuropsychol Rev. 2014;24(4):389–408. https://doi.org/10.1007/s11065-014-9261-x.
6. Fuentes A, Deotto AA, Desrocher MM, DeVeber G, Westmacott RR. Determinants of cognitive outcomes of perinatal and childhood stroke: a review. Child Neuropsychol. 2014;22(November):37–41. https://doi.org/10.1080/09297049.2014.969694.
7. Fullerton HJ, Wu YW, Zhao S, Johnston SC. Risk of stroke in children: ethnic and gender disparities. Neurology. 2003;61(2):189–94. https://doi.org/10.1212/01.WNL.0000078894.79866.95.

8. Lo W, Gordon AL, Hajek C, et al. Pediatric stroke outcome measure: predictor of multiple impairments in childhood stroke. J Child Neurol. 2014a;29(11):1524–30. https://doi.org/10.1177/0883073813503186.
9. de Veber G, Canadian Paediatric Ischemic Stroke Study Group. Canadian paediatric ischemic stroke registry: analysis of children with arterial ischemic stroke. Ann Neurol. 2000;48:514.
10. Raju TNK, Nelson KB, Ferriero D, Lynch JK. Ischemic perinatal stroke: summary of a workshop sponsored by the National Institute of Child Health and Human Development and the National Institute of Neurological Disorders and Stroke. Pediatrics. 2007;120(3):609–16. https://doi.org/10.1542/peds.2007-0336.
11. Ganesan V, Ng V, Chong WK, Kirkham FJ, Connelly A. Lesion volume, lesion location, and outcome after middle cerebral artery territory stroke. Arch Dis Child. 1999;81(4):295–300. https://doi.org/10.1136/adc.81.4.295.
12. Kirton A, Shroff M, Visvanathan T, DeVeber G. Quantified corticospinal tract diffusion restriction predicts neonatal stroke outcome. Stroke. 2007;38(3):974–80. https://doi.org/10.1161/01.STR.0000258101.67119.72.
13. McKinstry RC, Miller JH, Snyder a Z, et al. A prospective, longitudinal diffusion tensor imaging study of brain injury in newborns. Neurology. 2002;59(6):824–33. https://doi.org/10.1212/WNL.59.6.824.
14. De Vries LS, Van der Grond J, Van Haastert IC, Groenendaal F. Prediction of outcome in new-born infants with arterial ischaemic stroke using diffusion-weighted magnetic resonance imaging. Neuropediatrics. 2005;36(1):12–20. https://doi.org/10.1055/s-2005-837544.
15. Kaseka ML, Moharir M, DeVeber G, MacGregor D, Askalan R, Dlamini N. Prognostication value of descending corticospinal tract DWI signal in neonatal cerebral sinovenous thrombosis. Pediatr Neurol. 2016;59:90–4. https://doi.org/10.1016/j.pediatrneurol.2016.02.004.
16. Kitchen L, Westmacott R, Friefeld S, et al. The pediatric stroke outcome measure: a validation and reliability study. Stroke. 2012;43(6):1602–8. https://doi.org/10.1161/STROKEAHA.111.639583.
17. Elbers J, deVeber G, Pontigon A-M, Moharir M. Long-term outcomes of pediatric ischemic stroke in adulthood. J Child Neurol. 2013;29(6):782–8. https://doi.org/10.1177/0883073813484358.
18. Mink JW. The basal ganglia: focused selection and inhibition of competing motor programs. Prog Neurobiol. 1996;50(4):381–425. https://doi.org/10.1016/S0301-0082(96)00042-1.
19. Sanger TD, Chen D, Fehlings DL, et al. Definition and classification of hyperkinetic movements in childhood. Mov Disord. 2010;25(11):1538–49. https://doi.org/10.1002/mds.23088.
20. Tibussek D, Mayatepek E, Klee D, Koy A. Post stroke hemi-dystonia in children: a neglected area of research. Mol Cell Pediatr. 2015;2(1):14. https://doi.org/10.1186/s40348-015-0026-2.
21. Soman T, Askalan R, Martin M, et al. Predictors of dystonia in childhood basal ganglia stroke. Neuropediatrics. 2006;37(S1):121.
22. Quartarone A, Hallett M. Emerging concepts in the physiological basis of dystonia. Mov Disord. 2013;28(7):958–67. https://doi.org/10.1002/mds.25532.
23. Westmacott R, McDonald K, Williams T, Deveber G. Maladaptive reorganization following pediatric basal ganglia stroke: motor, intellectual and academic outcomes. In: Abstract presented at the annual meeting of the American Academy of Clinical Neuropsychology; 2016.
24. Anderson V, Spencer-Smith M, Wood A. Do children really recover better? Neurobehavioural plasticity after early brain insult. Brain. 2011;134(8):2197–221. https://doi.org/10.1093/brain/awr103.
25. Allman C, Scott RB. Neuropsychological sequelae following pediatric stroke: a nonlinear model of age at lesion effects. Child Neuropsychol. 2013;19(1):97–107. https://doi.org/10.1080/09297049.2011.639756.
26. Studer M, Boltshauser E, Datta A, et al. Factors affecting cognitive outcome in early pediatric stroke. Neurology. 2014;82(9):784–92.
27. Westmacott R, Askalan R, Macgregor D, Anderson P, Deveber G. Cognitive outcome following unilateral arterial ischaemic stroke in childhood: effects of age at stroke and lesion location. Dev Med Child Neurol. 2010;52(4):386–93. https://doi.org/10.1111/j.1469-8749.2009.03403.x.

28. Hajek CA, Yeates KO, Anderson V, et al. Cognitive outcomes following arterial ischemic stroke in infants and children. J Child Neurol. 2013;29(7):887–94. https://doi.org/10.1177/0883073813491828.
29. Lo W, Gordon A, Hajek C, et al. Social competence following neonatal and childhood stroke. Int J Stroke. 2014b;9(8):1037–44. https://doi.org/10.1111/ijs.12222.
30. Long B, Spencer-Smith MM, Jacobs R, et al. Executive function following child stroke: the impact of lesion location. J Child Neurol. 2011;26(3):279–87. https://doi.org/10.1177/0883073810380049.
31. Dennis M. Developmental plasticity in children. J Commun Disord. 2000;33(4):321–32. https://doi.org/10.1016/S0021-9924(00)00028-9.
32. Everts R, Pavlovic J, Kaufmann F, et al. Cognitive functioning, behavior, and quality of life after stroke in childhood. Child Neuropsychol. 2008;14(4):323–38. https://doi.org/10.1080/09297040701792383.
33. Catani M, Jones DK, Ffytche DH. Perisylvian language networks of the human brain. Ann Neurol. 2005;57(1):8–16. https://doi.org/10.1002/ana.20319.
34. Bates EA. Explaining and interpreting deficits in language development across clinical groups: where do we go from here? Brain Lang. 2004;88(2):248–53. https://doi.org/10.1016/S0093-934X(03)00102-0.
35. Bates E, Reilly J, Wulfeck B, et al. Differential effects of unilateral lesions on language production in children and adults. Brain Lang. 2001;79(2):223–65. https://doi.org/10.1006/brln.2001.2482.
36. Dennis M. Discourse in children with neurodevelopmental disorder, early focal brain injury, or childhood acquired brain injury. Brain Lang. 1998;307(61):305–7. https://doi.org/10.1006/brln.1997.1881.
37. Reilly JS, Bates EA, Marchman VA. Narrative discourse in children with early focal brain injury. Brain Lang. 1998;61(3):335–75. https://doi.org/10.1006/brln.1997.1882.
38. Reilly JS, Wasserman S, Appelbaum M. Later language development narratives children with perinatal stroke. Dev Sci. 2013;16(1):67–83. https://doi.org/10.1111/j.1467-7687.2012.01192.x.
39. Eisele JA, Lust B, Aram DM. Presupposition and implication of truth: linguistic deficits following early brain lesions. Brain Lang. 1998;61(3):376–94. https://doi.org/10.1006/brln.1997.1883.
40. Woods BT, Carey S. Language deficits after apparent clinical recovery from childhood aphasia. Ann Neurol. 1979;6(5):405–9. https://doi.org/10.1002/ana.410060505.
41. Ilves P, Tomberg T, Kepler J, et al. Different plasticity patterns of language function in children with perinatal and childhood stroke. J Child Neurol. 2014;29(6):756–64.
42. Raja Beharelle A, Dick AS, Josse G, et al. Left hemisphere regions are critical for language in the face of early left focal brain injury. Brain. 2010;133(6):1707–16. https://doi.org/10.1093/brain/awq104.
43. Tillema J, Byars AW, Jacola LM, et al. Brain & language. Language (Baltim). 2008;106(2):184–94. https://doi.org/10.1016/j.bandl.2007.07.127.
44. Dehaene-Lambertz G, Dehaene S, Hertz-Pannier L. Functional neuroimaging of speech perception in infants. Science. 2002;298(5600):2013–5. https://doi.org/10.1126/science.1077066.
45. Schlaggar BL, Brown TT, Lugar HM, Visscher KM, Miezin FM, Petersen SE. Functional neuroanatomical differences between adults and school-age children in the processing of single words. Science. 2002;296(5572):1476–9.
46. Liégeois F, Connelly A, Cross JH, et al. Language reorganization in children with early-onset lesions of the left hemisphere: an fMRI study. Brain. 2004;127(6):1229–36. https://doi.org/10.1093/brain/awh159.
47. Max JE, Mathews K, Lansing AE, et al. Psychiatric disorders after childhood stroke. J Am Acad Child Adolesc Psychiatry. 2002;41(5):555–62. https://doi.org/10.1097/00004583-200205000-00013

48. Max JE, Fox PT, Lancaster JL, et al. Putamen lesions and the development of attention-deficit/hyperactivity symptomatology. J Am Acad Child Adolesc Psychiatry. 2002;41(5):563–71. https://doi.org/10.1097/00004583-200205000-00014.
49. Max JE, Mathews K, Manes FF, et al. Attention deficit hyperactivity disorder and neurocognitive correlates after childhood stroke. J Int Neuropsychol Soc. 2003;9(6):815–29. https://doi.org/10.1017/S1355617703960012.
50. Max JE, Manes FF, Robertson BAM, Mathews K, Fox PT, Lancaster J. Prefrontal and executive attention network lesions and the development of attention-deficit/hyperactivity symptomatology. J Am Acad Child Adolesc Psychiatry. 2005;44(5):443–50. https://doi.org/10.1097/01.chi.0000156661.38576.0f.
51. O'Keeffe F, Liegeois F, Eve M, Ganesan V, King J, Murphy T. Neuropsychological and neurobehavioral outcome following childhood arterial ischemic stroke: attention deficits, emotional dysregulation, and executive dysfunction. Child Neuropsychol. 2014;20(5):557–82. https://doi.org/10.1080/09297049.2013.832740.
52. Everts R, Lidzba K, Wilke M, et al. Lateralization of cognitive functions after stroke in childhood. Brain Inj. 2010;24(6):859–70. https://doi.org/10.3109/02699051003724978.
53. De La Fuente A, Xia S, Branch C, Li X. A review of attention-deficit/hyperactivity disorder from the perspective of brain networks. Front Hum Neurosci. 2013;7(May):192. https://doi.org/10.3389/fnhum.2013.00192.
54. Moreno-Alcázar A, Ramos-Quiroga JA, Radua J, et al. Brain abnormalities in adults with Attention Deficit Hyperactivity Disorder revealed by voxel-based morphometry. Psychiatry Res Neuroimaging. 2016;254:41–7. https://doi.org/10.1016/j.pscychresns.2016.06.002.
55. Teicher MH, Anderson CM, Polcari A, Glod CA, Maas LC, Renshaw PF. Functional deficits in basal ganglia of children with attention-deficit/hyperactivity disorder shown with functional magnetic resonance imaging relaxometry. Nat Med. 2000;6(4):470–3. https://doi.org/10.1038/74737.
56. Ballantyne AO, Spilkin AM, Hesselink J, Trauner DA. Plasticity in the developing brain: Intellectual, language and academic functions in children with ischaemic perinatal stroke. Brain. 2008;131(11):2975–85. https://doi.org/10.1093/brain/awn176.
57. Rodrigues SDD, Ciasca SM, Guimarães IE, da Freiria Elias KMI, Oliveira CC, de Moura-Ribeiro MVL. Does stroke impair learning in children? Stroke Res Treat. 2011;2011:369836. https://doi.org/10.4061/2011/369836.
58. Woolpert D, Reilly JS. Investigating the extent of neuroplasticity: writing in children with perinatal stroke. Neuropsychologia. 2016;89:105–18. https://doi.org/10.1016/j.neuropsychologia.2016.06.005.
59. Max JE, Bruce M, Keatley E, Delis D. Pediatric stroke : plasticity, vulnerability, and age of lesion onset. J Neuropsychiatry Clin Neurosci. 2010;22(1):30–9.
60. Deotto A, Fuentes A, Desrocher M, Westmacott R, deVeber G. Executive function and academic achievement outcomes in children with arterial ischemic stroke. In: Canadian Psychological Society; 2014.
61. Fuentes A, Westmacott R, Deotto A, DeVeber G, Desrocher M. Working memory outcomes following unilateral arterial ischemic stroke in childhood. Child Neuropsychol. 2016;18:1–19. https://doi.org/10.1080/09297049.2016.1205008.
62. Friefeld SJ, Westmacott R, Macgregor D, Deveber GA. Predictors of quality of life in pediatric survivors of arterial ischemic stroke and cerebral sinovenous thrombosis. J Child Neurol. 2011;26(9):1186–92. https://doi.org/10.1177/0883073811408609.
63. Greenham M, Hearps S, Gomes A, et al. Environmental contributions to social and mental health outcomes following pediatric stroke. Dev Neuropsychol. 2015;40(6):348–62. https://doi.org/10.1080/87565641.2015.1095191.
64. Anderson V, Gomes A, Greenham M, et al. Social competence following pediatric stroke: Contributions of brain insult and family environment. Soc Neurosci. 2014;9(5):471–83. https://doi.org/10.1080/17470919.2014.932308.

65. Neuner B, von Mackensen S, Holzhauer S, et al. Health-related quality of life in children and adolescents with hereditary bleeding disorders and in children and adolescents with stroke: cross-sectional comparison to siblings and peers. Biomed Res Int. 2016;2016(group 1):1–8, 8p. https://doi.org/10.1155/2016/1579428.
66. Baron IS. Neuropsychological evaluation of the child. New York, NY: Oxford University Press, Inc; 2004.
67. Rafay MF, Pontigon AM, Chiang J, et al. Delay to diagnosis in acute pediatric arterial ischemic stroke. Stroke. 2009;40(1):58–64. https://doi.org/10.1161/STROKEAHA.108.519066.
68. Dyer A, Yau I, Westmacott R. Moving from paediatric to adult health-care: the transitional needs of childhood survivors of stroke. In: Congress of the World Federation of Neuroscience Nurses; 2009.

Chapter 10
Neuropsychological Assessment of Extremely Preterm Children

Tricia Williams, Samantha Roberts, and Vann Chau

Introduction

In the United States, one out of every nine infants is born premature [1], and preterm birth (<37 weeks gestational age) is estimated at 11.1% worldwide [2]. There has been a steady improvement in obstetric and neonatal practice care that has resulted in increasing numbers of preterm deliveries and an increase in the proportion of extreme preterm infants who survive to childhood [3]. Although there is considerable diversity in neuropsychological outcomes among preterm children, results of several meta-analyses consistently show lower intellectual, academic, and behavioral outcomes among preterm cohorts compared to children born at term [4–8]. As such, children born preterm continue to represent a substantial number of children in need of follow-up care both medically and cognitively. This chapter describes the early learning years of a child born at 27 weeks with multiple medical risk factors of prematurity, assessed through two neuropsychological evaluations (at 4 and 6 years of age). It highlights the importance of assessing children born preterm at multiple stages in their early development, as well as the still common comorbid cognitive and behavioral issues observed in this population.

T. Williams (✉) · S. Roberts
Division of Neurology, Department of Psychology, The Hospital for Sick Children, Toronto, ON, Canada
e-mail: tricia.williams@sickkids.ca

V. Chau
Division of Neurology, Department of Pediatrics, The Hospital for Sick Children, Toronto, ON, Canada

K. M. Sanders (ed.), *Physician's Field Guide to Neuropsychology*,
https://doi.org/10.1007/978-1-4939-8722-1_10

Referral (Most Recent)

Patient: 6-year-old female
Education: completed senior kindergarten, to start grade 1

Reason for Referral: Helen was born at 27 weeks (Twin A) with several complications common among children born at this age as described in the case presentation. She was first evaluated at 4 years of age, which informed early developmental intervention. At the time of the current assessment, Helen was 6 years old, and reassessment was recommended by her neurologist to support her transition to grade 1.

Case Presentation: Helen was born at 27 weeks weighing 780 g and described as small for gestational age (her twin was 1140 g). She had many complications associated with prematurity including bilateral subependymal hemorrhage, patent ductus arteriosus (spontaneously closed after failure to respond to indomethacin), sepsis, chronic lung disease, retinopathy of prematurity, and poor growth. She also required prolonged ventilation, was extubated at day 62 of life, and was discharged from hospital on day 137 on low-flow oxygen. She was initially followed through her local hospital's neonatal clinic and a respiratory care clinic. She also participated in early intervention (physical, occupational, and speech therapy) at a local children's treatment center.

When she was 4 years old, Helen was referred to our hospital's neonatal neurology clinic given concerns regarding her gait. A neurological exam indicated ataxia as well as positive cerebellar signs (e.g., broad-based gait, intention tremor) with some hypotonia and spasticity. She was referred for her initial neuropsychological assessment at that time. This evaluation offered diagnostic clarity that was then used to inform interventions specific to her expressive language disorder as well as early signs of attention deficit hyperactivity disorder (ADHD).

A reevaluation was requested to update Helen's development when she was 6 years old and inform an individual education plan (IEP) for grade 1. At the time of this assessment, Helen was well without any new medical concerns. She had just completed senior kindergarten. She had an educational assistant who she shared with her twin sister and was described as working very well with 1:1 support. Her individual education plan from kindergarten highlighted her alternative curriculum in fine motor, focus/attention (e.g., small group, reduced distraction, multisensory, Raz-Kids), and language (e.g., modeling proper pronunciation of words, increasing vocabulary). Her report card noted variability in her reading and numeracy skills. Outside of school, Helen continued to participate in occupational therapy and had intermittent access to speech and language services that were mostly consultative.

Parents' main concern during this reassessment was the widening gap between Helen's abilities and those of other students, as well as her twin sister. Her mother and father both commented on the variability in her early cognitive and academic development. Specifically, they shared "*Helen will surprise you. One day she will know her letters and numbers, but the next day she will not.*" They also observed a regression in her writing skills, attributing this to the lack of structure in the play-based kindergarten curriculum. Helen's attention span and memory continued to be limited, with poor sense of time and recollection of past events. She remained very impulsive, without a sense of danger or fear of strangers. Overall, her parents wanted to use this assessment to update Helen's needs and how to support her early academic development.

Neurological Exams and Findings

Helen's most recent brain imaging (MRI) was when she was 4 years and 6 months of age (Fig. 10.1). Results indicated small head size (microcephaly), which was measured just below the second percentile for corrected age. There was some prominence of the lateral ventricles (fluid-filled spaces of the brain), which seemed to be worse in the posterior portion of the brain and more on the left side, but there was no thinning of her corpus callosum. Small foci of abnormal signals were also seen in the white matter bilaterally, around the ventricles. Together, these findings were suggestive of bilateral periventricular leukomalacia (PVL), a commonly seen type of brain injury in children born preterm.

Neurological Exam: At her last clinic visit, Helen's neurological exam showed normal cranial nerves, but there was bilateral convergent squint. The motor exam showed diffuse hypotonia (axial more than peripheral) and mild distal spasticity over both ankles. However, this spasticity was less obvious on later exams. Reflexes were normal throughout, except for an upgoing plantar reflex in her right foot. Helen had a broad-based gait and tended to tiptoe intermittently on either foot. There was mild intentional tremor and past pointing on cerebellar testing.

Preliminary Impressions

Helen's case illustrates common outcomes in children born preterm with the additional medical risk factors including abnormal brain imaging (i.e., severe grades of IVH, as well as persistent periventricular leukomalacia on follow-up imaging in childhood).

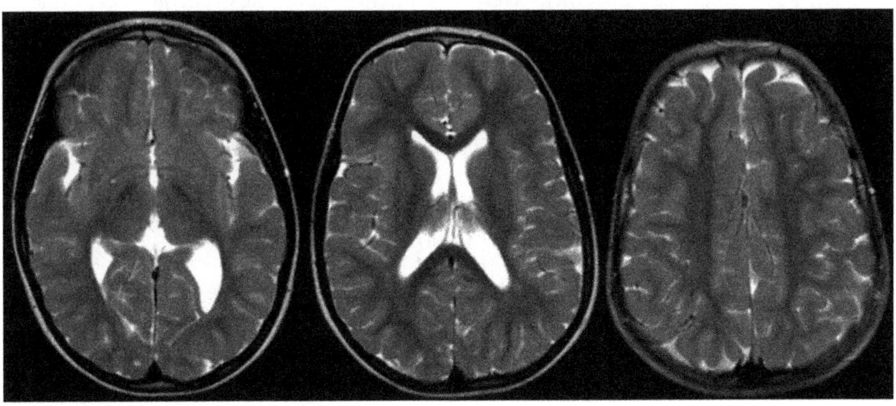

Fig. 10.1 MR image at 4 years of age

The MD Perspective

Key Point
- Neuropsychologists play an essential role in supporting families and children following preterm birth.
- Through assessment and follow-up, the child's current challenges and learning needs are identified which directs home, school, and community support.
- Neuropsychologists provide critical answers to what parents, clinicians, and educators really want to know:
  - *Does this child have an intellectual disability, learning disability, ADHD, or ASD?*
  - *What support and intervention will be needed at home and school to optimize this child's success?*
  - *How do these issues fit with the child's early medical risks associated with preterm birth?*

Preterm Overview

Definitions: Preterm infants are typically described by gestational age and birth weight. Using gestational age, delivery <37 weeks meets criteria for preterm birth. Birth at 34–36 weeks is designated as "late preterm," at 32–33 week birth as "moderate preterm," at <32 weeks as "very preterm," and at <28 weeks as "extremely preterm." Birth weight of <2500 g is considered low birth weight (LBW), <1500 g as very low birth weight (VLBW), and <1000 g as extremely low birth weight (ELBW). The term "small for gestational age" is also used if the newborn's birth weight falls below the 10th percentile for gestational age, and the term "intrauterine growth retardation" is used if there has been fetal growth restriction.

Both gestational age and birth weight influence outcomes, but neither alone is sufficiently predictive of later neuropsychological functioning. There is a wide and complex range of mediating and moderating medical, psychological, and socioenvironmental variables, and we highlight specific patterns of brain injury environmental factors below.

Brain Injury in the Premature Newborn

Periventricular leukomalacia (PVL), an important pattern of brain injury in the premature newborn, refers to injury of cerebral white matter that consists of periventricular focal necrosis in a characteristic distribution, with subsequent cystic formation or more diffuse cerebral white matter injury [9]. Over the last decade, the incidence of cystic PVL in premature newborns has decreased dramatically [10, 11].

In contrast, multifocal non-cystic white matter injury (WMI) is increasingly recognized as the most prevalent pattern of brain injury in this population [10].

The severity of WMI, best visualized with MRI, is associated with adverse neurodevelopmental outcome at 12–18 months of age [12–14]. The MR signal changes that characterize this form of WMI (i.e., multifocal WMI) are most easily recognized in the first weeks of life, becoming harder to detect near term-equivalent age [13].

Experimental studies attribute the exquisite vulnerability of the preterm brain to WMI as resulting from specific developmentally regulated cell populations that are vulnerable to oxidative stress [15], ischemia [16], and inflammation [17]. More specifically, perinatal infection [18, 19] and elevated inflammatory cytokines [20–22] are recognized risk factors for WMI. Myelination failure associated with WMI results primarily from arrested maturation of the oligodendrocyte lineage at the pre-oligodendrocyte stage [23]. The persistence of this "susceptible" cell population also maintains white matter vulnerability to recurrent insults [24]. Furthermore, there is now increasing recognition of gray matter involvement in preterm neonates, with abnormalities increasingly recognized in the cerebral cortex, thalamus, and cerebellum [9, 25, 26].

Intraventricular hemorrhage (IVH) occurs only in 4–5% in preterm infants born with a very low birth weight; however, the incidence seems to rise markedly in specific populations (i.e., 24–26 week gestation or birth weight <750 g) [27–29]. IVH typically occurs in a sick and premature infant who is receiving mechanical ventilation. The largest hemorrhages are usually seen in the more immature infants (<28 weeks gestation). The cause is related to the fragile germinal matrix, which persists in prematurity and can be injured and bleed in the intensive care setting [30]. Located ventrolateral to the lateral ventricles, the germinal matrix houses a network of complex capillaries, which matures throughout fetal development.

When severe, IVH can be associated with periventricular hemorrhagic infarction, which can injure the pre-oligodendrocytes and axons of the overlying white matter and lead to secondary maturational disturbances and tissue loss. Consequences include interruption of thalamocortical fibers and impairment of cortical development [9, 31, 32]. IVH may extend to the lateral ventricular system. Some estimates put the rate of hydrocephalus at more than 50% [33]. Ventriculomegaly may also occur related to posthemorrhagic hydrocephalus and may progress, causing either a transient or progressive ventriculomegaly.

Most studies suggest that ineffective autoregulation of blood flow and fluctuations in perfusion in the germinal matrix lead to rupture of vessels and IVH. These fluctuations can be linked to irregular breathing, hypercarbia, hypovolemia, restlessness, seizures, patent ductus arteriosus, and excessive handling [34]. As a premature brain is unable to accommodate increased systolic blood pressure, these risks are increased by elevation in blood flow caused by the pressure passive state of the cerebral circulation [35]. Exchange transfusions, rapid infusion of colloid, and rapid volume expansions are among the most common treatment-related causes [36]. Other risk factors include thrombocytopenia, acute umbilical inflammation or chorionic vasculitis, coagulation disorders, twin-twin transfusion, fetomaternal transfusion, and fetal distress.

Environmental Risk Factors

In addition to medical risk factors, neurocognitive development is also influenced by environmental factors. There is increasing attention to the influences of socioeconomic status (SES), neonatal pain, as well as the specific NICU environment and parenting experience. There is evidence that the prevalence of cognitive delay is higher in preterm populations that are socioeconomically disadvantaged [37]. Higher maternal educational level has also been found to be associated with cognitive improvement over time as well as protective against a lack of deterioration in cognitive scores over time [38]. Furthermore, many studies have linked spontaneous preterm birth with low maternal socioeconomic status [39]. As a result, the presence of biological risk factors combined with higher prevalence of preterm births in socioeconomically disadvantaged environments put preterm children at double risk of poor cognitive outcome [40].

Infant pain is increasingly recognized as contributing to long-term outcomes among preterm children. In a recent systematic review [41], studies were reported to find statistically significant associations between neonatal pain experience and early development of preterm infants, including postnatal growth, neurobehavioral, cortical activation, and brain development outcomes. More specifically, neonatal procedural pain was associated with delayed early postnatal body and head growth in preterm infants at 32 weeks post-conceptional age, independent of other medical confounding variables [42]. In addition, greater numbers of skin-breaking procedures (used as a proxy for early neonatal pain-related stress) during NICU hospitalization were significantly associated with reduced white matter and subcortical gray matter maturation at term age equivalent in very preterm infants [43]. The independent association between neonatal procedural pain and early brain development persisted even after controlling for multiple confounding clinical variables, such as infection, illness severity, and analgesic medication. Taken together, these findings suggest that preterm infants who undergo early repeated painful procedures during NICU hospitalization are at risk for altered brain activation and development.

The impact of the NICU environment and extent of parental involvement are also influential to the outcomes of preterm children. Single-family rooms (SFR) and allowing maternal presence and participation during the hospitalization of the preterm infant have been shown to have tremendous benefits to the infant health and the developing brain. Indeed, providing facilities for parents to stay in the neonatal unit from admission to discharge has been shown to reduce the total length of stay for infants born prematurely, lower rates of rehospitalization, and better feeding post discharge [44, 45]. Infants in single-family room have also been found to have fewer apneic events, reduced sepsis and mortality, as well as earlier transitions to enteral nutrition [46]. Infants in the single-family room tend to weigh more at discharge, require fewer medical procedures, and show better attention, less physiologic stress, hypertonicity, lethargy, and pain [47].

Early interventions targeting developmentally supportive care in the NICU environment and at home have also been found to promote optimal neuropsychological outcomes of children born preterm. Well-known examples include the Newborn

Individualized Developmental Care and Assessment Program, and kangaroo care, which involves skin-to-skin contact between mother and infant [48]. Across several randomized trials, these and similar programs have been shown to decrease parent distress and anxiety, as well as improve long-term intellectual and behavioral outcomes in children (e.g. [49–51]). Perhaps most compelling is the benefit to actual brain development observed in infants of parents exposed to such interventions, with improved white matter microstructure of the developing brain at term corrected age [52, 53].

Referring to Neuropsychology

Developmental Assessments: Children born preterm are routinely offered developmental assessments as part of their follow-up at many medical centers. Common follow-up ages, at our institution, are 12, 18, and 36 months. These assessments often include developmental cognitive screeners such as the Bayley-III. These screeners offer gross estimates of the child's abilities to identify those in need of early intervention support such as physical, speech, and occupational therapy.

Role of Neuropsychologists. Over the past 20 years, neuropsychologists have been increasingly utilized in follow-up of preterm [54]. Neuropsychological measures were introduced in preterm studies beginning around the 1990s to better understand more discrete behavioral effects of disruptions to the early brain development associated with preterm birth. Neuropsychological assessment helps provide clinicians and parents a more detailed understanding of their child's ability beyond general cognitive functioning to assist in supporting early learning and intervention [55–59].

Neuropsychological assessment can help identify emergent delay or dysfunction in functioning in the initial school years and offer earlier identification and advocacy for support. These years also offer an ideal time to intervene given the dramatic brain growth and cognitive development that occurs during this period [60].

Neuropsychologists play an important role in recognition of the child's current needs and projecting anticipated support to best maximize and scaffold early learning experiences and functional success. Information from neuropsychological assessments guides formal diagnoses and related treatment decisions, determine the effects of treatment, describe cognitive and socio-emotional status, and guide services and accommodations at school, at work, and in the community. The most common differential questions for children with preterm history relate to comorbid learning and behavioral diagnoses. Common questions parents, clinicians, and educators may have about the child are:

- *Does this child have an intellectual disability or learning disability?*
- *Do this child's symptoms warrant diagnosis and treatment for attention deficit hyperactivity disorder?*
- *Are the child's early history and symptoms concerning for social communication disorders such as autism spectrum disorder?*

Clinical Challenges in Early School-Age Assessments

Behavioral Engagement: One of the biggest challenges in testing young children is behavioral engagement—i.e., getting children to willingly go along with test instructions. These difficulties are heightened among children with less formal preschool exposure or discomfort separating from their parents. Although tests are designed to be engaging, fun, and motivating for young children, there is still variability due to behavior and attention. As such, test scores may be attributed to engagement and not cognitive ability, and the neuropsychologist must have a keen perception of these influences on testing and readily acknowledge how these issues affect the child's profile. There is also well-established normal variability in performance in typically developing school-age children to take into account in interpreting neuropsychological profiles [61–63].

Age Correction: There is ongoing debate on how long cognitive age-standardized test scores should be corrected for prematurity. The American Academy of Pediatrics recommends use of corrected scores for preterm children up to 3 years of age [64]. At later ages, correcting for prematurity may mask developmental differences and delay access to educational support. However, not correcting for prematurity may lead to an underestimate of the preterm child's abilities. Recent studies have shown significant and sizeable differences between corrected and uncorrected intellectual scores, particularly among children of average intellectual functioning and among children with lower gestational age [65, 66].

Neuropsychological Testing: Clinical Findings and History

Global versus Selective Vulnerability

Neuropsychological outcomes of children born preterm or with very low birth weight can have both global and selective neuropsychological deficits [67]. Global vulnerability/disability includes depressed scores across batteries assessing intellectual as well as distinct neuropsychological domains, profiles that are often associated with more severe brain injury, and/or presence of other disabilities such as cerebral palsy and/or visual impairment [68]. Specific or selective cognitive impairment has also been established among preterm children with average cognitive functioning, with common specific deficits of nonverbal/visual-spatial abilities, as well as attention and executive functioning [56, 69–71].

Helen's overall neuropsychological profile reflected a global vulnerability, highlighting the multiple medical risk factors associated with her preterm experience. Many of her scores across domains of language, visual-spatial, memory, academic, and adaptive functioning were well below age expectations. However, she also had heightened difficulties with attention and behavioral regulation, beyond that explained by her intellectual, comprehension, and learning challenges that warrant more specific treatment directions in addition to general learning support.

Intellectual Outcomes: The assessment of intelligence has long been the primary index or proxy of overall cognitive functioning in studies of children and youth born preterm. Intelligence scores are often inversely related to the child's birth weight and gestational age with mean IQ scores consistently below those of term controls [6, 8, 72]. These differences have been observed at different ages in follow-up and found to persist into early adulthood [73]. Consistency in intellectual differences between preterm and term cohorts has been observed across meta-analyses of different birth cohorts and publication date suggesting consistency in intellectual deficits in preterm cohorts over time, despite advancement in early medical interventions [6]. It is important to consider, however, that more recent cohorts will include children born at potentially lower birth weights and/or gestational ages than those in earlier studies given these advances in medical treatment [74].

Helen's overall intellectual full-scale score as measured by the Wechsler Intelligence Scale for Children, Fifth Edition, was substantially below age expectations and fell in the extremely low range according to test descriptors.

Attention and Executive Functioning: Attention and executive functioning difficulties are among the most common and challenging issues for preterm children throughout their lives [74, 75]. Children born preterm were found to be three times more likely to have an ADHD diagnosis than term control cohort [76]. This vulnerability is thought to occur given the abnormally protracted development of frontal subcortical cerebral regions as well as the preterm brain's increased susceptibility to white matter abnormalities [77–79].

Helen had tremendous difficulty paying attention during this 1:1 assessment. She was extremely busy, exploring the testing room, frequently sliding under the table, scribbling on test manuals, and going through the personal items of the psychometrist. She had a lot of difficulty sustaining her attention and regulating her behavior for brief time periods, even with 1:1 or 2:1 support. Her working memory span remained limited. She was able to remember two to three pieces of information at a time (i.e., numbers, pictures, or instructions). Both parent and teacher questionnaire ratings reflected Helen's substantial difficulties with inattention and behavioral regulation that significantly interfered with her learning. Formal assessment of her attention was discontinued, as she began responding randomly. This is consistent with research documenting differences between extremely low birth weight children and term controls, as well as the greater difficulties preterm children have in actually completing the tasks at all [80].

Language: Language outcomes of preterm cohorts have generally been considered less affected than other cognitive domains but still vulnerable to deficits compared to term controls [81, 82]. Although preterm children may fare worse than term controls in both simple and complex language (i.e., understanding of complex concepts, relational terms), there has been some evidence of catchup or improvement over time in receptive vocabulary among a cohort of preterm without neurosensory impairment and higher maternal education [83].

Consistent with this literature, across both assessments, Helen's vocabulary remained among the highest scores she achieved in the test battery. In her second assessment, Helen made the most improvement in her single-word vocabulary, with scores approaching age expectations. However, on tests of complex language, verbal reasoning, and comprehension tasks, Helen's scores were lower.

Visual Perceptual and Motor Skills: Visual and motor functioning are often compromised among preterm children [84]. Medical complications including retinopathy of prematurity, in addition to low birth weight and low gestational age, negatively influence visual and motor development [85, 86]. However, visual motor control issues have been identified in children without such medical risks [87]. There is also emerging MEG evidence of alterations in posterior parietal and inferior temporal regions associated with these selective difficulties in visual perceptual ability in very preterm children [88, 89].

Helen's visual perception was accurate, and she did well on a test of *visual matching by quantity and color*. However, her scores on tests of visual-spatial construction and problem solving were well below age expectation. Consistent with parent concern, Helen made few gains in her visual motor drawing skills over the 2 years since her last assessment, with a score now below age level.

Memory and Learning: Relative to term controls, preterm children have been reported to have deficits in all memory domains, including immediate memory, working memory, and long-term memory, across both visual and verbal modalities [90]. Memory deficits have been associated with slower information processing [91, 92] as well as receptive language skills [93]. For Helen, however, it was her limited attention span that most significantly affected her learning with no gains made despite repetition on formal memory measures.

Academic Skills: There is long-standing evidence of the academic difficulties among preterm children. Very preterm children are reported to be less school ready and display less early academic skill in the preschool years [94]. As such they are more likely to require additional special education services, with elevated need among children with history of neonatal brain injury [95]. In her second assessment, Helen's early academic skills were only emerging—with good understanding of color but inconsistent identification of letters and numbers, their related sounds and quantity, as well as concepts related to size and shape. Of note, this is with intensive daily support from her parents throughout the school year and summer.

Adaptive Functions: Given the plethora of potential neuropsychological difficulties that preterm children may experience, it is not surprising that their overall adaptive functioning and skills of independence are similarly affected [4]. Both parents and teacher voiced significant concerns about Helen's adaptive functioning and understanding in the world around her.

Psychosocial Health: Children born preterm are at increased risk for psychological disorders such as anxiety and depression [76]. There is also an increased rate of autism spectrum disorder diagnoses [96, 97]. A recent study also highlighted the restrictions in social and extracurricular experiences of children born preterm [98]. In interview and on psychosocial rating scales, parent and teacher ratings highlighted several concerns about Helen's social skills, e.g., not being able to appropriately approach or play with her peers. However, despite these issues, Helen was described as a positive and outgoing young girl who readily tries new activities and is not overly aware of her differences from others.

Diagnostic Summary: Overall, the extent of Helen's intellectual and adaptive difficulties observed during this assessment was consistent with the diagnosis of intellectual disability (mild). Given the persistence of her attention and behavioral regulation issues since her last assessment and the substantial interference in her life at home and school, the diagnosis of attention deficit hyperactivity disorder (combined presentation type) was also given.

Collaborative Discussion

Helen's issues remain highly consistent with her medical history of extreme prematurity with several complications, as well as the updated imaging showing periventricular leukomalacia. Her difficulties are common among kids with early neurodevelopmental injury and made worse by the associated difficulties regulating her attention and behavior.

Next Steps

Educational Planning and School Support: It is paramount that Helen participate in intense early academic intervention to optimize her chance at developing functional literacy and numeracy skills. An unquantifiable strength is her easygoing nature and flexibility, which will be an invaluable asset as she transitions to grade 1.

Specific recommendations for Helen emphasized increased opportunities for 1:1 and small-group learning environments to build her fundamental literacy and numeracy skills. Specialized assistive technology (dedicated laptop/tablet, related software such as print to speech in reading or word prediction software) was also recommended. Finally, errorless learning strategies were suggested to help build her ability to learn new things. The principle of errorless learning involves learning that takes place when virtually all errors are prevented during the training process. Errorless learning opportunities are often more effective for students who do not remember repeated learning experiences and the feedback that they receive.

Recommendations for Attention and Behavioral Regulation: Stimulant medication, behavioral interventions, and especially the combination of the two have become the most often recommended treatments for ADHD by leading associations and governmental entities (e.g., [99–102]). A stimulant trial was discussed with the family's physician with monitoring as needed with the neuropsychologist. Many environment and behavioral-based strategies were already in place in the home (e.g., predictable structure and routine). Setting realistic expectations for her learning (e.g., how much she can learn and how long she can focus at one time) was also discussed as well as the importance of increasing these expectations very gradually to build attention capacity and behavioral regulation.

Improving Social Skills: To foster cooperative learning activities, simple adult-directed turn-taking games and life skills opportunities are strategies that may promote social contact with peers. Emphasizing experientially based, "real-life," concrete experiences such as repeated practicing of skills in her daily environments will be most effective (and better than more verbally mediated/discussion-based approaches).

Additional speech and language support was also strongly recommended. Specific goals included building Helen's pronunciation, social communication skills, and use of instructive technology.

Family Support: There is increasing awareness of the emotional toll on parents of preterm children and the importance of supporting parents on this journey [103]. Although much of the attention has been to support offered in the early months to years following birth, it remains equally important as parents traverse educational and social development in school-age years. This family was directed to local Community Care Access Centre (CCAC) about potential services specific to children with intellectual disabilities as well support and advocacy for parents.

Reassessment: A third evaluation was recommended for Helen. Often these are most helpful to the student, family, and school around the time of a transition (i.e., to high school) or as curriculum demands increase (i.e., grades 4–6). In the interim, it is helpful when the neuropsychologist remains available to family for school meetings and consultations as needed.

Conclusion: Helen's neuropsychological assessment results highlight the many risks being born preterm still involves. Her profile of scores fits within that of global vulnerability but with specific needs to intervention for her attention and behavioral regulation to optimize her learning experience.

Helen's example highlights the need for additional emphasis on early intervention to monitor and promote preterm outcomes beyond typical follow-up periods in neonatal care. This may be through extended early rehabilitation directed specifically to maximizing early language and cognitive development, as well as parenting and individual support to address the effects of attention and behavioral regulation, potentially through traditional psychopharmacological as well as behavioral-based therapies.

Finally, Helen's story highlights preterm resilience through her positive and upbeat attitude and never letting her limitations get in her way. Additionally, it accentuates the importance of family support. Her parents have tirelessly promoted Helen's development from attending countless therapy sessions, providing daily learning support, and now the needed advocacy at school and in her community.

Key Points

- Clinical neuropsychological assessment offers an integral service in supporting long-term learning for children born preterm.
- Case examples such as Helen's serve as important reminders of the extent of cognitive disability that can be anticipated in a sizeable number of children born preterm.
- It is important that medical and psychosocial interventions that aim to reduce the frequency, magnitude, and impact of these neurodevelopmental impairments are developed, evaluated, and available to children and families.
- Clinicians need to be aware of the comorbidity between intellectual disability and attention deficit hyperactivity and not attribute these issues solely to low cognitive functioning (i.e., diagnostic overshadowing) [104, 105].

Chapter Review Questions

1. Identify key neurocognitive vulnerabilities following preterm birth:
   A. Global cognitive abilities.
   B. Visual-spatial skills.
   C. Language/communication skills.
   D. Attention and executive functioning.
   E. Academic progress.
   F. All of the above.
2. True/False: Children with intellectual disability cannot be simultaneously diagnosed with ADHD.
3. What is currently the most common pattern of brain injury following preterm birth (check all that apply)?
   A. Cerebellum.
   B. Periventricular leukomalacia (PVL).
   C. Multifocal non-cystic white matter injury (WMI).
   D. Basal ganglia.

References

1. Centers for Disease Control and Prevention. National prematurity awareness month; learn more about premature birth, risk factors, and what you can do. 2015. www.cdc.gov.
2. Blencowe H, Cousens S, Oestergaard MZ, Chou D, Moller A-B, Narwal R, et al. National, regional, and worldwide estimates of preterm birth rates in the year 2010 with time trends since 1990 for selected countries: a systematic analysis and implications. Lancet. 2012;379(379):2162–72.

3. Saigal S, Doyle LW. An overview of mortality and sequelae of preterm birth from infancy to adulthood. Lancet. 2008;371(9608):261–9.
4. Anderson PJ, Doyle LW. Neurobehavioral outcomes of school-age children born extremely low birth weight or very preterm in the 1990s. JAMA. 2003;289(24):3264–72. https://doi.org/10.1001/jama.289.24.3264.
5. Aylward GP. Neurodevelopmental outcomes of infants born prematurely. J Dev Behav Pediatr. 2005;26(6):427–40. https://doi.org/10.1097/00004703-200512000-00008.
6. Bhutta AT, Casey PH, Cradock MM, Anand K, Cleves AM. Cognitive and behavioral outcomes of school-aged children who were born preterm. JAMA. 2002;288(6):728–37.
7. Hack M, Taylor G, Drotar D, Schluchter M, Cartar L, Wilson-Costello D, et al. Poor predictive validity of the Bayley Scales of infant development for cognitive function and extremely low birth weight children at school age. Pediatrics. 2005;116(2):333–41.
8. Kerr-Wilson CO, MacKay DF, Smith GCS, Pell JP. Meta-analysis of the association between preterm delivery and intelligence. J Public Health (Oxf). 2011;34(2):209–16. https://doi.org/10.1093/pubmed/fdr024.
9. Volpe JJ. Brain injury in premature infants: a complex amalgam of destructive and developmental disturbances. Lancet Neurol. 2009;8(1):110–24. https://doi.org/10.1016/S1474-4422(08)70294-1.
10. Hamrick SEG, Miller SP, Leonard C, Glidden DV, Goldstein R, Ramaswamy V, et al. Trends in severe brain injury and neurodevelopmental outcome in premature newborn infants: the role of cystic periventricular leukomalacia. J Pediatr. 2004;145(5):593–9. https://doi.org/10.1016/j.jpeds.2004.05.042.
11. Van Haastert IC, Groenendaal F, Uiterwaal CSPM, Termote JUM, Van Der Heide-Jalving M, Eijsermans MJC, et al. Decreasing incidence and severity of cerebral palsy in prematurely born children. J Pediatr. 2011;159(1):86–91.e1. https://doi.org/10.1016/j.jpeds.2010.12.053.
12. Chau V, Synnes A, Grunau RE, Poskitt KJ, Brant R, Miller SP. Abnormal brain maturation in preterm neonates associated with adverse developmental outcomes. Neurology. 2013;81(24):2082–9. https://doi.org/10.1212/01.wnl.0000437298.43688.b9.
13. Miller SP, Ferriero DM, Leonard C, Piecuch R, Glidden DV, Partridge JC, et al. Early brain injury in premature newborns detected with magnetic resonance imaging is associated with adverse early neurodevelopmental outcome. J Pediatr. 2005;147(5):609–16. https://doi.org/10.1016/j.jpeds.2005.06.033.
14. Woodward LJ, Anderson PJ, Austin NC, Howard K, Inder TE. Neonatal MRI to predict neurodevelopmental outcomes in preterm infants. N Engl J Med. 2006;355:685–94.
15. Back SA. Perinatal white matter injury: the changing spectrum of pathology and emerging insights into pathogenetic mechanisms. Ment Retard Dev Disabil Res Rev. 2006;12(2):129–40. https://doi.org/10.1002/mrdd.20107.
16. Back SA, Han BH, Luo NL, Chricton CA, Xanthoudakis S, Tam J, et al. Selective vulnerability of late oligodendrocyte progenitors to hypoxia-ischemia. J Neurosci. 2002;22(2):455–63. http://doi.org/22/2/455
17. Degos V, Favrais G, Kaindl AM, Peineau S, Guerrot AM, Verney C, Gressens P. Inflammation processes in perinatal brain damage. J Neural Transm. 2010;117(8):1009–17. https://doi.org/10.1007/s00702-010-0411-x.
18. Chau V, Brant R, Poskitt KJ, Tam EWY, Synnes A, Miller SP. Postnatal infection is associated with widespread abnormalities of brain development in premature newborns. Pediatr Res. 2012;71(3):274–9. https://doi.org/10.1038/pr.2011.40.
19. Dammann O, Kuban KCK, Leviton A. Perinatal infection, fetal inflammatory response, white matter damage, and cognitive limitations in children born preterm. Ment Retard Dev Disabil Res Rev. 2002;8(1):46–50. https://doi.org/10.1002/mrdd.10005.
20. Dammann O, Leviton A. Maternal Intrauterine infection, cytokines, and brain damage in the preterm newborn. Pediatr Res. 1997;42(1):1–8.
21. Yoon BH, Jun JK, Romero R, Park KH, Gomez R, Choi J-H, Kim I-O. Amniotic fluid inflammatory cytokines (interleukin-6, interleukin-1β, and tumor necrosis factor-α), neonatal brain white matter lesions, and cerebral palsy. Am J Obstet Gynecol. 1997;177(1):19–26.

22. Yoon BH, Romero R, Kim CJ, Koo JN, Choe G, Syn HC, Chi JG. High expression of tumor necrosis factor-alpha and interleukin-6 in periventricular leukomalacia. Am J Obstet Gynecol. 1997;177:406–11. https://doi.org/10.1016/S0002-9378(97)70206-0.
23. Buser JR, Maire J, Riddle A, Gong X, Nguyen T, Nelson K, et al. Arrested preoligodendrocyte maturation contributes to myelination failure in premature infants. Ann Neurol. 2012;71(1):93–109. https://doi.org/10.1002/ana.22627.
24. Segovia KN, McClure M, Moravec M, Ning LL, Wan Y, Gong X, et al. Arrested oligodendrocyte lineage maturation in chronic perinatal white matter injury. Ann Neurol. 2008;63(4):520–30. https://doi.org/10.1002/ana.21359.
25. Tam EWY, Miller SP, Studholme C, Chau V, Glidden D, Poskitt KJ, et al. Differential effects of intraventricular hemorrhage and white matter injury on preterm cerebellar growth. J Pediatr. 2011;158(3):366–71. https://doi.org/10.1016/j.jpeds.2010.09.005.
26. Vinall J, Grunau RE, Brant R, Chau V, Poskitt KJ, Synnes AR, Miller SP. Slower postnatal growth is associated with delayed cerebral cortical maturation in preterm newborns. Sci Transl Med. 2013;5(168):168ra8.
27. Bassan H, Feldman HA, Limperopoulos C, Benson CB, Ringer SA, Veracruz E, et al. Periventricular hemorrhagic infarction: risk factors and neonatal outcome. Pediatr Neurol. 2006;35(2):85–92. https://doi.org/10.1016/j.pediatrneurol.2006.03.005.
28. Larroque B, Marret S, Ancel PY, Arnaud C, Marpeau L, Supernant K, et al. White matter damage and intraventricular hemorrhage in very preterm infants: the epipage study. J Pediatr. 2003;143(4):477–83. https://doi.org/10.1067/S0022-3476(03)00417-7.
29. Murphy BP, Inder TE, Rooks V, Taylor GA, Anderson NJ, Mogridge N, et al. Posthaemorrhagic ventricular dilatation in the premature infant: natural history and predictors of outcome. Arch Dis Child Fetal Neonatal Ed. 2002;87(September 1997):37–41. https://doi.org/10.1136/fn.87.1.F37.
30. Hambleton G, Wigglesworth JS. Origin of intraventricular haemorrhage in the preterm infant. Arch Dis Child. 1976;51(9):651–9. https://doi.org/10.1136/adc.51.9.651.
31. Counsell SJ, Dyet LE, Larkman DJ, Nunes RG, Boardman JP, Allsop JM, et al. Thalamo-cortical connectivity in children born preterm mapped using probabilistic magnetic resonance tractography. Neuroimage. 2007;34(3):896–904. https://doi.org/10.1016/j.neuroimage.2006.09.036.
32. Marin-Padilla M. Developmental neuropathology and impact of perinatal brain damage. II: White matter lesions of the neocortex. J Neuropathol Exp Neurol. 1997;56(3):219–35.
33. Whitelaw A. Intraventricular haemorrhage and posthaemorrhagic hydrocephalus: pathogenesis, prevention and future interventions. Semin Neonatol. 2001;6(2):135–46. https://doi.org/10.1053/siny.2001.0047.
34. Rennie JM. Cerebral blood flow velocity variability after cardiovascular support in premature babies. Arch Dis Child. 1989;64(7 Spec No):897–901. https://doi.org/10.1136/adc.64.7_Spec_No.897.
35. Perry EH, Bada HS, Ray JD, Korones SB, Arheart K, Magill HL. Blood pressure increases, birth weight-dependent stability boundary, and intraventricular hemorrhage. Pediatrics. 1990;85(5):727–32. http://pubmed.gov/2330232
36. Kadri H, Mawla AA, Kazah J. The incidence, timing, and predisposing factors of germinal matrix and intraventricular hemorrhage (GMH/IVH) in preterm neonates. Childs Nerv Syst. 2006;22(9):1086–90. https://doi.org/10.1007/s00381-006-0050-6.
37. Wong HS, Edwards P. Nature or nurture: a systematic review of the effect of socio-economic status on the developmental and cognitive outcomes of children born preterm. Matern Child Health J. 2013;17(9):1689–700. https://doi.org/10.1007/s10995-012-1183-8.
38. Wang LW, Wang ST, Huang CC. Preterm infants of educated mothers have better outcome. Acta Paediatr. 2008;97(5):568–73. https://doi.org/10.1111/j.1651-2227.2008.00738.x.
39. Blumenshine P, Egerter S, Barclay CJ, Cubbin C, Braveman PA. Socioeconomic disparities in adverse birth outcomes: a systematic review. Am J Prev Med. 2010;39(3):263–72. https://doi.org/10.1016/j.amepre.2010.05.012.

40. Parker S, Greer S, Zuckerman B. Double jeopardy: the impact of poverty on early child development. Pediatr Clin North Am. 1998;35(6):1227.
41. Valeri BO, Holsti L, Linhares MBM. Neonatal pain and developmental outcomes in children born preterm: a systematic review. Clin J Pain. 2014;31(4):1–31. https://doi.org/10.1097/AJP.0000000000000114.
42. Vinall J, Miller SP, Chau V, Brummelte S, Synnes AR, Grunau RE. Neonatal pain in relation to postnatal growth in infants born very preterm. Pain. 2012;153(7):1374–81. https://doi.org/10.1016/j.pain.2012.02.007.
43. Brummelte S, Grunau RE, Chau V, Poskitt KJ, Brant R, Vinall J, et al. Procedural pain and brain development in premature newborns. Ann Neurol. 2012;71(3):385–96.
44. Erdeve O, Arsan S, Yigit S, Armangil D, Atasay B, Korkmaz A. The impact of individual room on rehospitalization and health service utilization in preterms after discharge. Acta Paediatr. 2008;97(10):1351–7.
45. Ortenstrand A, Westrup B, Broström EB, Sarman I, Akerström S, Brune T, et al. The Stockholm Neonatal Family Centered Care Study: effects on length of stay and infant morbidity. Pediatrics. 2010;125(2):e278–85. https://doi.org/10.1542/peds.2009-1511.
46. Domanico R, Davis DK, Coleman F, Davis BO. Documenting the NICU design dilemma: comparative patient progress in open-ward and single family room units. J Perinatol. 2011;31(4):281–8. https://doi.org/10.1038/jp.2010.120.
47. Lester BM, Hawes K, Abar B, Sullivan M, Miller R, Bigsby R, et al. Single-family room care and neurobehavioral and medical outcomes in preterm infants. Pediatrics. 2014;134(4):754–60. https://doi.org/10.1542/peds.2013-4252.
48. Als H, McAnulty GB. The Newborn Individualized Developmental Care and Assessment Program (NIDCAP) with Kangaroo Mother Care (KMC): comprehensive care for preterm infants. Curr Womens Aust Health Rev. 2011;7(3):288–301. https://doi.org/10.2174/157340411796355216.
49. Kaaresen PI, Rønning J. a, Ulvund SE, Dahl LB. A randomized, controlled trial of the effectiveness of an early-intervention program in reducing parenting stress after preterm birth. Pediatrics. 2006;118(1):e9–e19. https://doi.org/10.1542/peds.2005-1491.
50. Koldewijn K, Wolf M-J, van Wassenaer A, Meijssen D, van Sonderen L, van Baar A, et al. The Infant Behavioral Assessment and Intervention Program for very low birth weight infants at 6 months corrected age. J Pediatr. 2009;154(1):33–38.e2. https://doi.org/10.1016/j.jpeds.2008.07.039.
51. Spittle AJ, Ferretti C, Anderson PJ, Orton J, Eeles A, Bates L, et al. Improving the outcome of infants born at <30 weeks' gestation—a randomized controlled trial of preventative care at home. BMC Pediatr. 2009;9:73. https://doi.org/10.1186/1471-2431-9-73.
52. Als H, Duffy FH, McAnulty G, Butler SC, Lightbody L, Kosta S, et al. NIDCAP improves brain function and structure in preterm infants with severe intrauterine growth restriction. J Perinatol. 2012;32(10):797–803. https://doi.org/10.1038/jp.2011.201.
53. Milgrom J, Newnham C, Anderson PJ, Doyle LW, Gemmill AW, Lee K, et al. Early sensitivity training for parents of preterm infants: impact on the developing brain. Pediatr Res. 2010;67(3):330–5. https://doi.org/10.1203/PDR.0b013e3181cb8e2f.
54. Baron IS, Rey-Casserly C. Preterm birth outcomes in adolescence and young adulthood. In: Pediatric neuropsychology: medical advances and lifespan outcomes. New York, NY: Oxford University Press; 2013. p. 237–56.
55. Aarnoudse-Moens CSH, Weisglas-Kuperus N, van Goudoever J, Oosterlaan J. Meta-analysis of neurobehavioral outcomes in very preterm and/or very low birth weight children. Pediatrics. 2009;124(2):717–28. https://doi.org/10.1542/peds.2008-2816.
56. Bohm B, Smedler AC, Forssberg H. Impulse control, working memory and other executive functions in preterm children when starting school. Acta Paediatr. 2004;93(10):1363–71. https://doi.org/10.1080/08035250410021379.
57. Marlow N, Hennessy EM, Bracewell MA, Wolke D. Motor and executive function at 6 years of age after extremely preterm birth. Pediatrics. 2007;120(4):793–804. https://doi.org/10.1542/peds.2007-0440.

58. Nosarti C, Giouroukou E, Micali N, Rifkin L, Morris RG, Murray RM. Impaired executive functioning in young adults born very preterm. J Int Neuropsychol Soc. 2007;13(4):571–81. https://doi.org/10.1017/S1355617707070725.
59. Pizzo R, Urben S, Van Der Linden M, Borradori-Tolsa C, Freschi M, Forcada-Guex M, et al. Attentional networks efficiency in preterm children. J Int Neuropsychol Soc. 2010;16(1): 130–7. https://doi.org/10.1017/S1355617709991032.
60. Baron IS, Anderson PJ. Neuropsychological assessment of preschoolers. Neuropsychol Rev. 2012;22(4):311–2. https://doi.org/10.1007/s11065-012-9221-2.
61. Brooks BL. A study of low scores in Canadian children and adolescents on the Wechsler Intelligence Scale For Children, Fourth Edition (WISC-IV). Child Neuropsychol. 2011;17(3):281–9. https://doi.org/10.1080/09297049.2010.537255.
62. Brooks BL, Iverson GL. Comparing actual to estimated base rates of "abnormal" scores on neuropsychological test batteries: implications for interpretation. Arch Clin Neuropsychol. 2010;25(1):14–21. https://doi.org/10.1093/arclin/acp100.
63. Brooks BL, Iverson GL, Feldman HH, Holdnack JA. Minimizing misdiagnosis: psychometric criteria for possible or probable memory impairment. Dement Geriatr Cogn Disord. 2009;27(5):439–50. https://doi.org/10.1159/000215390.
64. Engle WA. Age terminology during the perinatal period. Pediatrics. 2004;114(5):1362–4.
65. Van Veen S, Aarnoudse-Moens CSH, Van Kaam AH, Oosterlaan J, Van Wassenaer-Leemhuis AG. Consequences of correcting intelligence quotient for prematurity at age 5 years. J Pediatr. 2016;173:90–5. https://doi.org/10.1016/j.jpeds.2016.02.043.
66. Wilson-Ching M, Pascoe L, Doyle LW, Anderson PJ. Effects of correcting for prematurity on cognitive test scores in childhood. J Paediatr Child Health. 2014;50(3):182–8. https://doi.org/10.1111/jpc.12475.
67. Taylor HG, Klein N, Drotar D, Schluchter M, Hack M. Consequences and risks of <1000-g birth weight for neuropsychological skills, achievement, and adaptive functioning. J Dev Behav Pediatr. 2006;27(6):459–69. http://doi.org/00004703-200612000-00002
68. Hoff Esbjorn B, Hansen BM, Greisen G, Mortensen EL. Intellectual development in a Danish cohort of prematurely born preschool children: specific or general difficulties? J Dev Behav Pediatr. 2006;27(6):477–84. https://doi.org/10.1097/00004703-200612000-00004.
69. Bayless S, Stevenson J. Executive functions in school-age children born very prematurely. Early Hum Dev. 2007;83(4):247–54. https://doi.org/10.1016/j.earlhumdev.2006.05.021.
70. Joseph RM, O'Shea TM, Allred EN, Heeren T, Hirtz D, Jara H, et al. Neurocognitive and academic outcomes at age 10 years of extremely preterm newborns. Pediatrics. 2016;137(4). https://doi.org/10.1542/peds.2015-4343.
71. Lind A, Korkman M, Lehtonen L, Lapinleimu H, Parkkola R, Matomäki J, Haataja L. Cognitive and neuropsychological outcomes at 5 years of age in preterm children born in the 2000s. Dev Med Child Neurol. 2011;53(3):256–62. https://doi.org/10.1111/j.1469-8749.2010.03828.x.
72. Baron IS, Rey-Casserly C. Extremely preterm birth outcome: a review of four decades of cognitive research. Neuropsychol Rev. 2010;20(4):430–52. https://doi.org/10.1007/s11065-010-9132-z.
73. Stålnacke J, Lundequist A, Böhm B, Forssberg H, Smedler A-C. Individual cognitive patterns and developmental trajectories after preterm birth. Child Neuropsychol. 2015;7049(September):1–20. https://doi.org/10.1080/09297049.2014.958071.
74. Anderson PJ. Neuropsychological outcomes of children born very preterm. Semin Fetal Neonatal Med. 2014;19(2):90–6. https://doi.org/10.1016/j.siny.2013.11.012.
75. Howard K, Anderson P, Taylor HG. Executive functioning and attention in children born preterm. In: Executive functions and the frontal lobe: a lifespan perspective. Philadelphia: Taylor & Francis; 2008. p. 219–41.
76. Trevaud K, Ure A, Doyle LW, Lee KJ, Rogers CE, Kidokoro H, Inder TE, Anderson P. Psychiatric outcomes at age seven for very preterm children: Rates and predictors. J Child Psychol Psychiatry. 2013;54(7):772–9.
77. Edgin JO, Inder TE, Anderson PJ, Hood KM, Clark CA, Woodward LJ. Executive functioning in preschool children born very preterm: relationship with early white matter pathology. J Int Neuropsychol Soc. 2008;14(1):90–101. https://doi.org/10.1017/S1355617708080053.

78. Murray AL, Scratch SE, Thompson DK, Inder TE, Doyle LW, Anderson JFI, Anderson PJ. Neonatal brain pathology predicts adverse attention and processing speed outcomes in very preterm and/or very low birth weight children. Neuropsychology. 2014;28(4):552–62. https://doi.org/10.1037/neu0000071.
79. Murray AL, Thompson DK, Pascoe L, Leemans A, Inder TE, Doyle LW, et al. White matter abnormalities and impaired attention abilities in children born very preterm. Neuroimage. 2016;124:75–84. https://doi.org/10.1016/j.neuroimage.2015.08.044.
80. Baron IS, Kerns KA, Müller U, Ahronovich MD, Litman FR. Executive functions in extremely low birth weight and late-preterm preschoolers: effects on working memory and response inhibition. Child Neuropsychol. 2012;18(6):586–99. https://doi.org/10.1080/09297049.2011.631906.
81. Reidy N, Morgan A, Thompson DK, Inder TE, Doyle LW, Anderson PJ. Impaired language abilities and white matter abnormalities in children born very preterm and/or very low birth weight. J Pediatr. 2013;162(4):719–24. https://doi.org/10.1016/j.jpeds.2012.10.017.
82. van Noort-van der Spek IL, Franken CJ, Weisglas-Kuperus N. Language functions in preterm-born children : a systematic review and meta-analysis. Pediatrics. 2012;129(4): 745–54. https://doi.org/10.1542/peds.2011-1728.
83. Luu TM, Vohr BR, Allan W, Schneider KC, Ment LR. Evidence for catch-up in cognition and receptive vocabulary among adolescents born very preterm. Pediatrics. 2011;128(2):313–22. https://doi.org/10.1542/peds.2010-2655.
84. Böhm B, Lundequist A, Smedler AC. Visual-motor and executive functions in children born preterm: the bender visual motor gestalt test revisited. Scand J Psychol. 2010;51(5):376–84. https://doi.org/10.1111/j.1467-9450.2010.00818.x.
85. Grunau RE, Whitfield MF, Petrie-Thomas J, Synnes AR, Cepeda IL, Keidar A, et al. Neonatal pain, parenting stress and interaction, in relation to cognitive and motor development at 8 and 18 months in preterm infants. Pain. 2009;143(1–2):138–46. https://doi.org/10.1016/j.pain.2009.02.014.
86. Heineman KR, La Bastide-Van Gemert S, Fidler V, Middelburg KJ, Bos AF, Hadders-Algra M. Construct validity of the Infant Motor Profile: relation with prenatal, perinatal, and neonatal risk factors. Dev Med Child Neurol. 2010;52(9):209–15. https://doi.org/10.1111/j.1469-8749.2010.03667.x.
87. Gerner EM, Katz-Salamon M, Hesser U, Soderman E, Forssberg H. Psychomotor development at 10 months as related to neonatal health status: the Stockholm Neonatal Project. Acta Paediatr Suppl. 1997;419(i):37–43. https://doi.org/10.1111/j.1651-2227.1997.tb18307.x.
88. Doesburg SM, Chau CM, Cheung TPL, Moiseev A, Ribary U, Herdman AT, et al. Neonatal pain-related stress, functional cortical activity and visual-perceptual abilities in school-age children born at extremely low gestational age. Pain. 2013;154(10):1946–52. https://doi.org/10.1016/j.pain.2013.04.009.
89. Doesburg SM, Moiseev A, Herdman AT, Ribary U, Grunau RE. Region-specific slowing of alpha oscillations is associated with visual-perceptual abilities in children born very preterm. Front Hum Neurosci. 2013;7(November):791. https://doi.org/10.3389/fnhum.2013.00791.
90. Omizzolo C, Thompson DK, Scratch SE, Stargatt R, Lee KJ, Cheong J, et al. Hippocampal volume and memory and learning outcomes at 7 years in children born very preterm. J Int Neuropsychol Soc. 2013;19(10):1065–75. https://doi.org/10.1017/S1355617713000891.
91. Rose AS, Feldman JF. Memory and processing speed in preterm children at eleven years: a comparison with full-terms. Child Dev. 1996;67:2005–21.
92. Rose SA, Feldman JF, Jankowski JJ. Information processing in toddlers: continuity from infancy and persistence of preterm deficits. Dermatol Int. 2009;37(3):311–20. https://doi.org/10.1016/j.intell.2009.02.002.
93. Briscoe J, Gathercole SE, Marlow N. Everyday memory and cognitive ability in children born very prematurely. J Child Psychol Psychiatry Allied Discip 2001;42(6):749–754. http://ovidsp.ovid.com/ovidweb.cgi?T=JS&PAGE=reference&D=med4&NEWS=N&AN=11583247\nhttp://ovidsp.ovid.com/ovidweb.cgi?T=JS&PAGE=reference&D=emed5&NEWS=N&AN=2001324733. PMID: 11583247.

94. Roberts G, Lim J, Doyle LW, Anderson PJ. High rates of school readiness difficulties at 5 years of age in very preterm infants compared with term controls. J Dev Behav Pediatr. 2011;32(2):117–24. https://doi.org/10.1097/DBP.0b013e318206d5c9.
95. Luu TM, Vohr BR, Schneider KC, Katz KH, Tucker R, Allan WC, Ment LR. Trajectories of receptive language development from 3 to 12 years of age for very pretermchildren. Pediatrics. 2009;124(1):333–41. https://doi.org/10.1542/peds.2008-2587.
96. Johnson S, Hollis C, Kochhar P, Hennessy E, Wolke D, Marlow N. Autism spectrum disorders in extremely preterm children. J Pediatr. 2010;156(4):525–531.e2. https://doi.org/10.1016/j.jpeds.2009.10.041.
97. Karmel BZ, Gardner JM, Meade LS, Cohen IL, London E, Flory MJ, et al. Early medical and behavioral characteristics of NICU infants later classified with ASD. Pediatrics. 2010;126(3):457–67. https://doi.org/10.1542/peds.2009-2680.
98. Kodjebacheva GD, Sabo T. Influence of premature birth on the health conditions, receipt of special education and sport participation of children aged 6-17 years in the USA. J Public Health (Oxf). 2015;38(2):e47–54. https://doi.org/10.1093/pubmed/fdv098.
99. CADDRA. n.d. http://www.caddra.ca.
100. CHADD. n.d. http://www.chadd.org/.
101. .National Institute of Mental Health. n.d.
102. Subcommittee on Attention-Deficit/Hyperactivity Disorder, & Steering Committee on Quality Improvement and Management. ADHD: clinical practice guidelines for the diagnosis, evaluation, and treatment of attention-deficit/hyperactivity disorder in children and dolescents. Pediatrics. 2011;128(5):1007–22.
103. Spittle A, Orton J, Anderson PJ, Boyd R, Doyle LW. Early developmental intervention programmes provided post hospital discharge to prevent motor and cognitive impairment in preterm infants. Cochrane Database Syst Rev. 2015;11(12):CD005495. https://doi.org/10.1002/14651858.CD005495.pub4.
104. Neece CL, Baker BL, Crnic K, Blacher J. Examining the validity of ADHD as a diagnosis for adolescents with intellectual disabilities: clinical presentation. J Abnorm Child Psychol. 2013;41(4):597–612. https://doi.org/10.1007/s10802-012-9698-4.
105. Simonoff E, Pickles A, Wood N, Gringras P, Chadwick O. ADHD symptoms in children with mild intellectual disability. J Am Acad Child Adolesc Psychiatry. 2007;46(May):591–600. https://doi.org/10.1097/chi.0b013e3180323330.

Chapter 11
Neuropsychology's Contributions to a Pediatric Epilepsy Surgery Team

Molly Warner, Hillary Shurtleff, Catherine Amlie-Lefond, Russell Saneto, Edward Novotny, Jonathan Lopez, Sandra Poliachik, Andrew Poliakov, Dennis Shaw, and Jeffrey Ojemann

Neuropsychologists have played integral roles in comprehensive epilepsy centers for decades [1–3] (also see chapters by Queally and by Brandling-Bennett and Vossler in this book). In pediatric settings, neuropsychologists provide assessment of children's cognitive skills as needed for clinical purposes and document levels of functioning pre- and post-interventions such as neurosurgery for epilepsy [4]. Additional roles for neuropsychologists specific to the epilepsy surgery setting may

M. Warner (✉) · H. Shurtleff
Department of Psychiatry, Seattle Children's Hospital, Seattle, WA, USA

Department of Neurology, University of Washington, Seattle, WA, USA
e-mail: molly.warner@seattlechildrens.org

C. Amlie-Lefond
Department of Neurology, Seattle Children's Hospital, Department of Neurology, University of Washington School of Medicine, Seattle, WA, USA

R. Saneto · E. Novotny · J. Lopez
Department of Neurology, Seattle Children's Hospital, Seattle, WA, USA

Department of Neurology, University of Washington, Seattle, WA, USA

S. Poliachik
Department of Neurology, Seattle Children's Hospital, Seattle, WA, USA

Applied Physics Laboratory, University of Washington, Seattle, WA, USA

A. Poliakov
Department of Radiology, Seattle Children's Hospital, Seattle, WA, USA

D. Shaw
Department of Radiology, Seattle Children's Hospital, Seattle, WA, USA

Department of Radiology, University of Washington, Seattle, WA, USA

J. Ojemann
Department of Neurological Surgery, Seattle Children's Hospital, Seattle, WA, USA

Department of Neurological Surgery, University of Washington, Seattle, WA, USA

K. M. Sanders (ed.), *Physician's Field Guide to Neuropsychology*,
https://doi.org/10.1007/978-1-4939-8722-1_11

include managing the behavioral and cognitive aspects of medical procedures designed to identify localization and lateralization of eloquent brain cortex [4]. These procedures provide information for neurosurgeons and epileptologists who must plan for surgical interventions that minimize risk of causing additional neurologic deficits, with the goal of stopping seizures by eliminating the epileptogenic focus. Neurosurgery for epilepsy is almost always an elective procedure. The process of arriving at a decision to operate is multifaceted, in which a series of factors must all point toward a good probability of a successful outcome and all parties, including the family, agree to move forward.

In this setting, neuropsychologists help to provide some of the data on which to base those decisions. Their roles require nuanced understanding of the effects of perturbations on brain development, a firm grasp of the practice of pediatric psychology with children and their parents in a hospital setting, and the ability to communicate with others who interact with these children in their everyday environments. The two neuropsychologist authors above are employed at Seattle Children's Hospital (rather than being outside consultants) and are members of the epilepsy surgery team which includes physicians (neurology, neurosurgery, radiology, and genetics), imaging analysts, nurses, EEG technicians, neuropsychologists, psychometrists, social workers, and administrators involved in coordination and scheduling.

At our institution, in the traditional role of cognitive assessment, a team of neuropsychologists and psychometrists [4] together evaluate the patients referred by physicians. The neuropsychologist works with the accompanying parent to complete a clinical intake interview, covering multiple aspects of patient history and current functioning. At the same time, the psychometrist, who works under the supervision of the neuropsychologist, works with the patient to administer selected psychological and neuropsychological test measures that cover multiple domains. The psychometrist scores the tests and observes the patient's behavior during the test session. The neuropsychologist is responsible for integrating all information and giving feedback to the family members (and the patient, when appropriate) about the assessment results and their implications. The neuropsychologist then writes an integrative report incorporating behavioral and test data with information on family, medical, and educational variables. Recommendations may include suggestions for treatment, further information, and social support.

Additional roles for the neuropsychologist in the epilepsy surgery setting include coaching patients through functional MRI (fMRI), the intracarotid amobarbital injection procedure (Wada test, described with the second case below), and cortical stimulation mapping [4]. Cortical stimulation mapping for localization of a specific function may be accomplished either extra-operatively using the same intracranial electrode array used to record seizures or intraoperatively during a surgical resection procedure in which the patient is awakened after the brain is exposed. The neuropsychologists' roles in all of these procedures are to teach the patients the tasks, guide them through the procedures, comment on the patient's responses, and for the Wada test provide interpretation of the motor, language, and memory findings. All of these procedures require cooperation and practiced coordination between the neuropsychologist and other medical professionals: radiology imaging and image processing team for the fMRI; interventional radiology, nursing, and EEG teams for the Wada test; neurologist and neurodiagnostics team for grid mapping in patient rooms; and neurosurgeon, neurodiagnostics team, and operating room staff for awake mapping during brain surgery.

We present here the journeys through the epilepsy surgery program of three cases that illustrate the different aspects of the neuropsychologists' contributions to the epilepsy surgery team (NB: references are representative but not exhaustive).

Case 1

Case 1 was a 6-year-old, left-handed boy who presented with new-onset focal seizures that became refractory to medications within months of onset and was referred for epilepsy surgery evaluation. He performed well in kindergarten and was at the beginning of his first-grade year in a regular education class; however, he was struggling with learning to read. Prior to seizure onset, the child had been noted to walk on his toes with his right foot but walked normally with his left foot. A neurological evaluation identified very mild right hemiparesis; his EEG monitoring showed a left frontal seizure focus; his magnetic resonance imaging (MRI) of the brain identified an area of left frontotemporal encephalomalacia suggestive of a small perinatal stroke (Fig. 11.1); and his positron emission tomography (PET) showed hypometabolism in the same left posterior frontal area. He continued to have up to five short focal seizures per day while on three antiepileptic medications (levetiracetam, lamotrigine, and oxcarbazepine, with nasal midazolam available as a rescue medication in case of status epilepticus).

A neuropsychological evaluation included measures of intellect, attention, language, memory, executive functioning, motor and sensory functioning, and parent ratings of behavior. Results indicated decreased right upper extremity sensory and motor functioning as well as mild difficulties with measures of processing speed and motor control. Otherwise, his cognitive functioning was within the normal range for his age (see Table 11.1 for selected test scores). He presented as a sweet boy who was a pleasure to work with, who had friends at school, and who was generally well behaved at school and at home. Academically, this beginning first grader knew the basic building blocks of reading, spelling, and math, although was not yet combining sounds to read words.

At this point in his evaluation for possible surgery, it was imperative to discover the spatial relationship between his left posterior frontal lesion and the cortical location of his speech/language functions, as the lesion was in the normal region for expressive language in right handers [5]. To prepare the child for a functional MRI, the neuropsychologist (MW) trained the child on two simple tasks that he could easily master: (1) a motor task involving blocks of time of finger tapping with right versus left hand and (2) a verb generation task in which he thought of verbs (action words) associated with black-and-white line drawings of objects or animals. The verb generation task was presented in blocks of time contrasted with blocks of time of resting while fixating on a plus sign. The task was practiced first out loud and then silently [6]. With a child of this young age, holding still during the procedure was an important aspect to rehearse, and his parent was tasked with helping the child practice at home while lying on a couch, without wiggling.

The first fMRI session coached by the neuropsychologist identified right-hand activation immediately superior to the area of encephalomalacia in the left hemisphere. Language lateralization was unclear due to motor movements as the child had a persistent cough. The second fMRI session was successful as the child was able to hold still throughout the session while performing the desired tasks. The radiology image processing team analyzed the data and co-registered the functional and anatomical brain imaging. This analysis showed that the child's language functions appeared to be right hemisphere dominant with a lateralization index of right, 0.26, versus left, 0.09. Signal change in each hemisphere was defined as a percentage of average BOLD (blood oxygen level dependent) signal over a certain region of interest, in this case using Brodmann areas 44 and 45, combined and symmetrized [7]. Thus, for Case 1, eloquent language cortex appeared to be safely distant from the site of surgical interest in the contralateral hemisphere (Fig. 11.1).

To pinpoint the seizure focus within the left frontal lobe, the child was implanted with a subdural intracranial electrode grid over the left posterior frontal and parietal areas. Prior to the grid implantation and over two teaching sessions, the neuropsychologist prepared the child for further language mapping. Several days after the grid placement and over a period of 3 h, stimulation mapping of the cortex under the grid was performed. The neurologist handled the cortical stimulation, and the EEG technician recorded the cortical responses, while the neuropsychologist coached the child, presented the pictorial stimuli to be named, managed his behaviors, and interpreted his responses. This process identified motor and sensory cortical areas associated with the right shoulder, arm, hand, and fingers superior and posterior to the lesion, but as expected, no changes were elicited in language (naming or speaking abilities). Thus, fMRI and cortical mapping results were congruent in indicating that a left hemisphere surgery would be unlikely to disrupt language skills.

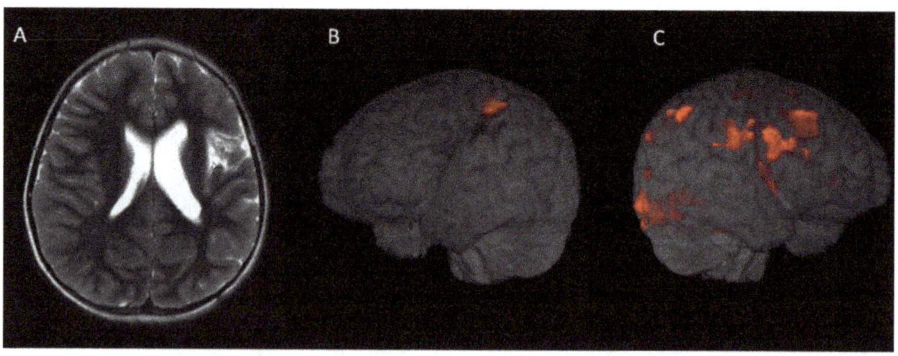

Fig. 11.1 Case 1. (**a**) Presurgical T2 axial MRI scan illustrating the left frontal lesion. (**b**) 3D volume rendering of presurgical functional MRI showing right-hand finger tapping activation (in red) superior to the adjacent lesion (the dark area). (**c**) 3D volume rendering of presurgical functional MRI showing right frontal lobe activation by language tasks. The occipital lobe activation reflects the patient's viewing of the line drawing stimuli

Table 11.1 Selected neuropsychological test scores pre- and post-surgery for Case 1

Wechsler Intelligence Scale for Children-IV	Age 6 years and 6 months (2.5 months pre-surgery)			Age 7 years and 3 months (6.5 months post-surgery)		
Intellectual summary scores	**Standard score**[a]			**Standard score**[a]		
Verbal comprehension	99			98		
Perceptual reasoning	88			90		
Working memory	91			88		
Processing speed	83			80		
Full Scale IQ	88			87		
Developmental Test of Visual-Motor Integration-VI:	**Copy**	**Visual**	**Motor**	**Copy**	**Visual**	**Motor**
Standard score[a]	93	86	74	91	84	61
Age equivalent (years:months)	5:11	4:8	3:9	6:3	5:1	3:7
Wide Range Assessment of Memory and Learning-II	**Standard score**[a]			**Standard score**[a]		
Memory Screener Index	92			101		
Verbal Memory Index	97			97		
Visual Memory Index	94			106		
Wide Range Achievement Test-IV	**Standard score**[a]	**Grade equivalent**		**Standard score**[a]	**Grade equivalent**	
Reading	78	K.0		101	2.0	
Spelling	90	K.6		89	1.2	
Arithmetic	99	1.1		96	1.7	
Motor functioning (mild right hemiparesis)	**Non-dominant right hand**	**Dominant left hand**		**Non-dominant right hand**	**Dominant left hand**	
Finger tapping	26 taps/10 s	34 taps/10 s		20 taps/10 s	37 taps/10 s	
Name writing speeds	0.40 letters/s	1.00 letters/s		0.36 letters/s	1.33 letters/s	
Strength of grip	3.5 kg	8.0 kg		4.5 kg	10 kg	

[a]Standard Scores have a mean of 100 and a standard deviation of 15 at any age

The lesion and EEG focus were close to motor areas, but the neurosurgeon had enough room to avoid further disruption of the weaker right-body side motor skills. At age 6 years and 9 months, the child underwent resection of the inferior frontal lobe area identified during EEG monitoring as the seizure focus, an area of the gliotic tissue.

Following his resection the child became seizure-free. Six and a half months after his surgery, he underwent another neuropsychological evaluation, in which his cognitive profile was very similar to before surgery (Table 11.1). However, by the end of his first grade year, he had learned to read at grade level; his grade-equivalent score on the reading subtest of the Wide Range Achievement Test-IV had improved from beginning kindergarten level before surgery to beginning second grade level at the end of his first grade year. At age 8 years and 2 months, he began tapering off the last of his three antiepileptic medications.

Physician Perspective

In Case 1, the neuropsychologist guided a relatively normal 6-year-old and his family through a series of stressful preoperative diagnostic procedures that required his total cooperation. Particularly important was ensuring the child's active role in cooperating with the functional MRI that identified eloquent cortex for language in the hemisphere contralateral to his seizure focus [8, 9]. Cortical stimulation mapping through the intracranial electrode grid was easier for him than the functional MRI because the pace was much slower and breaks in testing could be taken, but still his cooperation was crucial. He became scared and upset briefly the first time that an electrical stimulus to the brain caused his right arm to move, but once consoled and encouraged, he continued cooperating.

A recent publication [10] from our institution examined cognitive and seizure outcomes of 15 pediatric epilepsy surgery patients who were operated on between ages 2 and 6 for benign lesion-related, early-onset epilepsy; Case 1 was one of those subjects. The study concluded that surgical treatment of focal seizures in cognitively intact preschool children is likely to result in seizure remediation, discontinuation of antiepileptic medications, and no significant decrement in intelligence. This latter finding is particularly significant in light of the long-standing concern associated with performing resections in the language-dominant hemisphere (in this case the lesion was in the hemisphere contralateral to language). Importantly, shorter seizure duration prior to surgical resection resulted in improved cognitive outcome, suggesting that earlier surgery for certain populations is important to improve cognitive outcomes. In this case, the child underwent surgery within 8 months of his first seizure, with all indicators for the appropriateness of a surgical intervention well documented by that time.

Atypical language lateralization and localization such as illustrated by Case 1 has been associated with early brain lesions in areas of normally eloquent cortex, with language developing either in the hemisphere contralateral to the lesion [8] or elsewhere within the ipsilateral hemisphere [9]. The study of neuroplasticity in establishment of language has been furthered by the availability of functional MRI [5, 11, 12, 13]. A variety of fMRI language protocols can illustrate different integrated language networks [5, 13] but may not necessarily identify areas that are critical to support language. Of particular interest to neurosurgeons and epileptologists is the issue of defining more narrowly a brain area that should be resected so that the operation can be tailored to the patient. Cortical stimulation mapping is the appropriate tool once fMRI has identified a region of interest. Case 1 is an example where fMRI was helpful in alleviating the concern about resecting critical language

Key Point
An fMRI can be helpful in alleviating the concern about resecting critical language areas. Cortical mapping confirmed the absence of naming sites near the lesion under the grid in the left hemisphere, and concordance of results of both procedures facilitated earlier intervention.

areas. Cortical mapping confirmed the absence of naming sites near the lesion under the grid in the left hemisphere, and concordance of results of both procedures facilitated earlier intervention.

Case 2

Case 2 was a right-handed teenage girl with seizures associated with the left mesial temporal lobe. She had her first febrile seizure at 9 months of age, with medically refractory focal seizures of anterior temporal origin ongoing since 4 years of age. At age 6 she was worked up at another children's hospital for possible left temporal lobe epilepsy surgery, but her seizures ceased without surgery and eventually she was weaned off medications. Her seizures reappeared when she was 9 years old. Seizures were treated with topiramate (varying doses, see Table 11.2) and became more problematic with time. In addition to her seizures, she was followed for a rheumatological condition, pauci-immune glomerulonephritis, treated with Prednisone and other medications (see Table 11.2).

At age 13 the patient was referred by the rheumatology service for neuropsychological evaluation and was seen by a non-epilepsy service neuropsychologist at Seattle Children's Hospital. Her test scores were generally within the normal range, but she exhibited somewhat slow processing speed (Table 11.2).

Worsening seizures resulted in a referral from her local neurologist to the epilepsy surgery program at Seattle Children's Hospital. The patient lived out of state; her visit here was planned to include clinic appointments with the neurosurgeon and epileptologist, a neuropsychological re-evaluation with epilepsy service neuropsychologist HS, and a functional MRI under her direction. Compared to her previous test scores at age 13 and at age 14 years and 10 months, the patient performed more poorly on intellectual and memory measures (Table 11.2), raising the issue of possible cognitive decline due to increased seizures. Her scores were particularly low on verbal memory tasks involving list-learning of unusual word pairs (Children's Memory Scale), a pattern that has been documented in individuals with left temporal epilepsy and left hemisphere lateralization for both speech and verbal memory, whose seizures have contributed to loss of verbal memory skills [14, 15]. However, the neuropsychologist also noted that between the two neuropsychological evaluations, the patient had been prescribed a higher dose of her anticonvulsant medication topiramate, a drug with a known dose-dependent dampening effect on cognitive functioning [16, 17]. She was concerned that the more aberrant neuropsychological profile could be the result of a drug effect rather than an effect of increased seizures.

The patient was coached by the neuropsychologist for a functional MRI that used motor, language, and memory paradigms [18]. This procedure identified left hemisphere cortical activation for language measures (lateralization index [7]: Left 0.3, Right 0.08, Fig. 11.2a). With memory paradigms, activity was recorded in the right but not the left posterior hippocampus [19], with asymmetry (R > L, lateralization index: left, −0.002; right, 0.02) in activation of the parahippocampal region

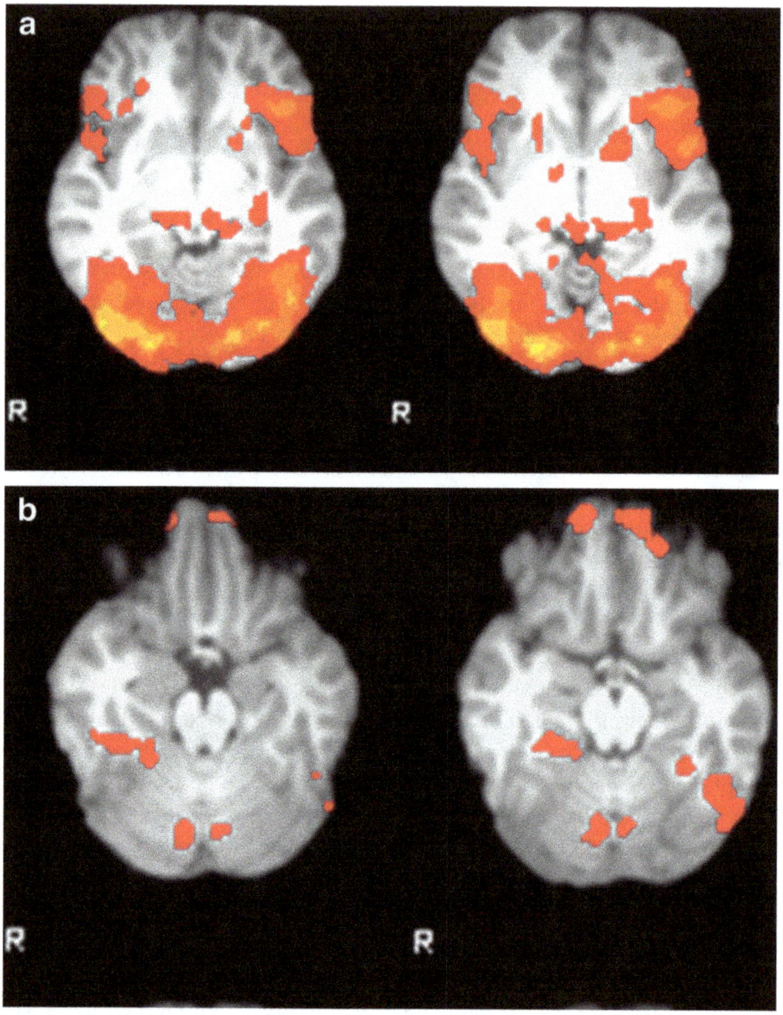

Fig. 11.2 Case 2: (**a**) The fMRI language paradigms resulted in predominantly left-sided language activation in sensorimotor and Broca's areas. Lateralization index: left, 0.3; right, 0.08. The occipital lobes were also activated due to visual presentation of the stimuli. Red, orange, and yellow areas indicate statistically greater increases in blood oxygen levels during the language tasks when compared to the contrast task. (**b**) The fMRI memory paradigms resulted in primarily right hemisphere activation in the mesial temporal lobes (posterior hippocampus and parahippocampal gyrus). Lateralization index: left, –0.002; right, 0.02

(Fig. 11.2b; the mask partially overlapped Brodmann areas 20, 30, and 37). This finding suggested the possibility of early brain reorganization with crossed speech and verbal memory functions (as opposed to the expected left hemisphere language and ipsilateral verbal memory localization found in most right handers) [15].

The epileptologist and the neurosurgeon both judged that the patient would be a likely candidate for a left temporal lobectomy but first ordered further evaluation by EEG monitoring to confirm the seizure focus, an updated MRI of the brain, and an intracarotid amobarbital procedure (IAP or Wada test) for confirmation or refutation of the fMRI results that had suggested crossed language and memory lateralization. The neuropsychologist recommended screening to confirm or rule out the effect of topiramate on test scores and thus help address lateralization of, and integrity of, function.

At age 15 years and 0 months, the patient returned for further evaluations prior to her surgery. Her MRI of the brain confirmed the left mesial temporal sclerosis (small left hippocampus) reported earlier from other institutions. During her inpatient EEG monitoring, topiramate was discontinued from her drug regimen in order to induce seizures. Two days after discontinuation of topiramate, a brief neuropsychological screening showed dramatically better results on verbal memory tests (Table 11.2), a finding that supported the hypothesis of a drug effect dampening previously better verbal memory scores.

The Wada test [4] is conducted in the interventional radiology suite and involves both a cerebral angiogram and brief suppression of cortical functioning by administration of sodium amytal separately to each internal carotid artery (catheter access via the femoral artery). Testing by the neuropsychologist of the patient's language and memory capabilities during drug presence continues until the effect of the drug has worn off and the patient's responses return to baseline. Test paradigms vary between institutions; here at Seattle Children's Hospital the particular stimuli used for object naming and reading distractors are adjusted to the ability of the child. Case 2 was able to cooperate well with the procedure. Results of the patient's Wada test indicated that her left hemisphere supported speech and that her right hemisphere supported memory functions.

Since memory results of the fMRI and the Wada test were congruent in indicating right hemisphere localization remote to the seizure focus, the epilepsy surgery team felt that left temporal lobe surgery would be unlikely to result in a decline in her verbal memory skills. A week later, she underwent a surgical resection (selective left amygdalohippocampectomy) for the purposes of seizure remediation.

The patient experienced no seizures after surgical resection. Neuropsychological re-evaluations at 6 and 18 months postoperatively resulted in successively better intellectual and memory scores (Table 11.2), up to or exceeding presurgical levels on some tasks. By 6 months after surgery, her topiramate had been reduced to the previously tolerated level, and by 18 months after surgery, topiramate had been discontinued entirely.

Table 11.2 Selected neuropsychological test scores for Case 2 pre- and post-surgery (left mesial temporal sclerosis)

Timing relative to surgery	Pre-surgery			Post-surgery	
Age (years-months)	**13-0**	**14-10**	**15-0**	**15-6**	**16-6**
Medications (including prednisone and mycophenolate mofetil)	Topiramate (150 BID)	Topiramate (200 BID)	Omeprazole	Topiramate (150 BID)	Omeprazole
Wechsler Intelligence Scale for Children IV (WISC-IV)	**Standard Score[a]**	**Standard Score[a]**	**Standard Score[a]**	**Standard Score[a]**	**Standard Score[a]**
Verbal Comprehension Index	100	95	–	99	99
Perceptual Reasoning Index	110	100	–	115	127
Working Memory Index	126	77	104	102	120
Processing Speed Index	83	91	–	94	109
Full Scale IQ	107	89	–	105	118
Wide Range Assessment of Memory and Learning	**Scaled Score[b]**	**S.S.[a]/s.s.[b]**	**S.S.[a]/s.s.[b]**	**S.S.[a]/s.s.[b]**	**S.S.[a]/s.s.[b]**
Memory Screener Index	–	89	–	100	103
Verbal Memory Index	–	91	–	105	111
Visual Memory Index	–	91	–	94	94
Story memory	10	7	–	10	12
Picture memory	–	9	–	8	12
Design memory	–	8	–	10	6
Verbal learning	11	10	–	12	12
Children's Memory Scale, Word Pairs Subtest		**Scaled Score[b]**	**Scaled Score[b]**	**Scaled Score[b]**	**Scaled Score[b]**
Learning	–	4	12	9	14
Total score	–	4	11	10	14
Long delay	–	6	11	9	12
Delayed recognition	–	11	11	11	11
Wide Range Achievement Test IV (WRAT-IV)		**Standard Score[a]/ Grade Equivalent**		**Standard Score[a]/ Grade Equivalent**	**Standard Score[a]/ Grade Equivalent**
Reading	–	98/7.5	–	100/8.9	103/11.2
Spelling	–	104/10.3	–	107/11.6	106/12.2
Arithmetic	–	112/>12.9	–	101/9.8	123/>12.9

[a]Standard Scores (S.S.) have a mean of 100 and a standard deviation of 15
[b]Scaled Scores (s.s.) have a mean of 10 and a standard deviation of 3

Physician Perspective

Case 2 had her surgery in 2011; she was one of our early fMRI cases in which we were able to elicit subcortical activation in individual patients using a memory paradigm adapted from an adult paradigm (by neuropsychologist HS) for a pediatric population [18]. These memory tasks require the patient to imagine him or herself moving through very familiar environments (home and school; these tasks are based on visualization and retrieval of well-learned information, as opposed to encoding and retrieval of novel information). With eyes closed, the patient relies on tactile cues from an accompanying parent to alternate between blocks of the memory tasks and blocks of the contrasting counting task. In general, adolescents can successfully manage these memory tasks more easily than younger children. When the patient is able to comply with this paradigm, the temporal mesial areas are activated (middle and posterior more than the anterior mesial structures) [19]. Our epilepsy surgery team is preparing a study summarizing our experiences to date with regard to the outcome of pediatric temporal lobe surgeries and the utility of the fMRI memory protocols in the workup of these cases.

The results of the fMRI for Case 2 correlated well with the results of the Wada test (the gold standard [20]), with both procedures identifying verbal memory lateralized to the right cerebral hemisphere. For this patient, whose verbal memory scores normalized once topiramate was removed, the left temporal surgery did not pose a threat to her memory skills. Case 2 is another example of neuroplasticity in a child with early focal seizures related to a benign brain lesion (in this case, mesial temporal sclerosis).

The epilepsy surgery team at our institution now relies heavily on the noninvasive fMRI to address questions of lateralization and localization of speech and memory functions. Wada tests may still be requested when fMRI language results are inconclusive or suggest bilateral speech and when fMRI memory results are inconclusive. Wada tests are more expensive, more time consuming, and involve more personnel than fMRIs. Additionally, the Wada tests are invasive and therefore more physically and emotionally challenging for the patients (especially for younger children). Thus, the efforts of neuropsychologist HS to develop a workable fMRI memory procedure and adapt other fMRI paradigms for our pediatric epilepsy population [18] have resulted in lowered costs, a more patient-friendly procedure for an important aspect of presurgical diagnostic workup, and an increased ability to identify eloquent cortex in younger patients.

Key Point

Neuropsychologists develop workable fMRI memory procedures and adapt other fMRI paradigms for the pediatric epilepsy population. This has resulted in lowered costs, a more patient-friendly procedure for an important aspect of presurgical diagnostic workup, and an increased ability to identify eloquent cortex in younger patients.

Case 3

Case 3 was a left-handed boy who was born prematurely at 30 weeks gestation, weighing 5 lbs. 9 oz., and who began having seizures at age 4 days secondary to perinatal brain injury associated with hypoglycemia. Seizures of occipital lobe origin were well controlled for a while but increased in frequency over time. Medical treatment for epilepsy (oxcarbazepine) was started at age 7.

By age 11 he was having focal seizures several times per month, sometimes in clusters, and sometimes seizures occurred at school. He also had prolonged generalized tonic-clonic seizures that required administration of rectal diazepam to abort the seizures. He was referred by his local neurologist for evaluation to undergo epilepsy surgery. EEG monitoring suggested predominantly left occipital seizure origin. Medications at this point included zonisamide, lamotrigine, and oxcarbazepine to treat seizures, as well as fluoxetine for depression and anxiety. His brain MRI was notable for T2 signal hyperintensity in the bilateral occipital cortex near the calcarine fissure, more so on the left; PET demonstrated decreased uptake of radiolabeled tracer in a similar distribution (Fig. 11.3).

As a result of the early injury to his occipital lobes, the boy had abnormal visual and secondary ocular motility deficits. At age 2, he underwent superior oblique tendon expansion for Brown syndrome (ocular motility abnormalities) of his right eye and began an extensive trial of occlusion therapy (patching) for amblyopia of his left eye. In a later evaluation at Seattle Children's Hospital, he was also noted to have dissociated vertical deviation and latent nystagmus. He failed two attempts at Humphrey visual field evaluation of the right eye due to unreliable performances with high rates of false-negative and false-positive results. He was suspected to have a right hemianopia; however, an untrained observer would not perceive any abnormality in his visual system.

At age 9, in third grade, the boy had been evaluated at school for special education services due to his epilepsy and difficulty with reading and especially writing. At that time his intellectual evaluation using the Kaufman Brief Intelligence Test (K-BIT) resulted in a Verbal Ability standard score of 106, a Performance Ability score of 93, and a Composite IQ of 100 (normal range, compared to average for age of 100). Discrepancies between parent and teacher ratings of behavior indicated significant dysfunction in the school setting with respect to behavioral self-control and ability to organize that was less severe in the home environment. The history of visual disorders was mentioned but not integrated into the clinical picture in the child's individual educational plan (IEP). His academic performance was noted to be far below same-aged peers, with difficulties in abstract reasoning and following multiple-step directions, but reading was a relative strength. Some teachers had misinterpreted his inefficiencies at school as willful idleness (rather than visual processing problems), adding to his discouragement and resulting lack of cooperation.

Neuropsychological evaluation at age 11 years and 6 months yielded a different picture, indicating mildly reduced verbal intellectual skills, poor visuospatial skills, and very slow visual processing speeds (Table 11.3). He was an unhappy child who had developed a habit of refusal at school, was suffering from frequent seizures, and was burdened by three antiepileptic medications. The neuropsychological evaluation was discontinued prematurely when he ceased cooperating. At his next visit 2 months later, he was in a better frame of mind and did marginally better but was still challenged by memory tasks and measures of processing speed (NB: his earlier intellectual evaluation at age 9 with the K-BIT did not include a measure of visual processing speed).

The boy was prepared for a functional MRI. We suspected incomplete cooperation for some of the fMRI trials; motion artifact was moderate to severe during the procedure and was mitigated by removing time points compromised by motion. Activation during language tasks was seen predominantly in the right cerebral hemisphere in Broca's and Wernicke's areas as well as the supplementary sensorimotor area, with cerebellar activation predominantly on the left. Language activation was strongly dominant in the right hemisphere with a lateralization index for Broca's areas of left, 0.26, and right, 0.49 [7]. Visual activation occurred over a smaller area than expected in the occipital lobes (possibly due to closing of the eyes during part of the task or to pre-existing injury). A confirming Wada test for language lateralization was not performed as it was felt that the child would not tolerate the demands of the procedure.

At age 11 years and 11 months, he underwent presurgical intracranial EEG grid monitoring during which his medications were temporarily weaned off to provoke seizures. He had several habitual seizures that originated near the left posterior hemisphere and one seizure that was not typical of his previous seizures that rapidly spread over the right occipital lobe. Because of his bilateral occipital damage, he and his family were counseled that he would be at risk for further seizures postsurgically without continuing protection by antiepileptic medications, although his chance for sustained seizure freedom on medications was good. He, his family, and his team decided to proceed with a surgery in which epileptogenic tissue in the left occipital lobe was removed (Fig. 11.3).

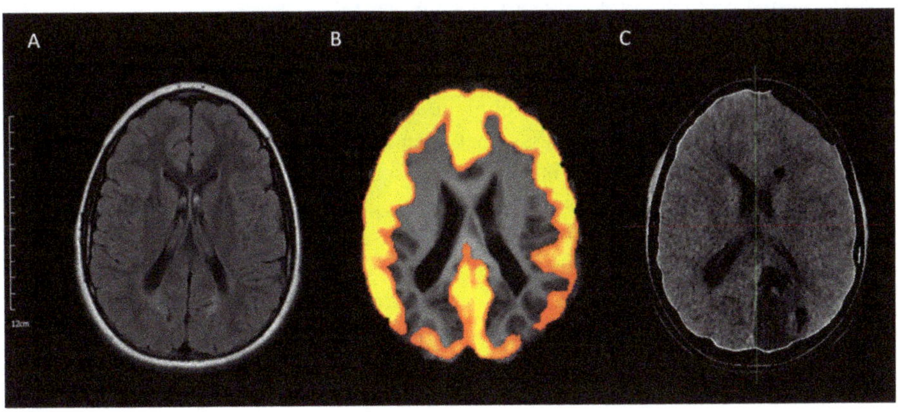

Fig. 11.3 Case 3. (**a**) Preoperative axial FLAIR MRI showing bilateral occipital lobe injury; (**b**) preoperative PET depicting hypometabolism in the occipital lobes, more pronounced on the left side (areas in yellow indicate normal cortical metabolism); and (**c**) postoperative CT showing the resection in the left occipital lobe

The boy returned for postsurgical re-evaluation at age 12 years and 7 months. The oxcarbazepine and fluoxetine had been discontinued. He now took only lamotrigine and zonisamide for seizure control, with rectal diazepam and nasal midazolam available as rescue medications. His mood had improved, and he had been seizure-free except for two brief episodes of seeing rainbows throughout his visual fields and one focal motor seizure that occurred several months postoperatively during a medication wean. The ophthalmologist determined that the boy definitely now had, as previously suspected, a right hemianopia related to his occipital lobe injury and subsequent surgery, in addition to his earlier documented oculomotor issues.

His neuropsychological evaluation 8 months after surgery (Table 11.3) was notable for better verbal skills including verbal memory scores and better spatial processing as long as speed was not a factor. He now had greater difficulty with visual processing speed and perception of some visual material due to the right-sided hemianopia. He did more poorly on language tasks where the stimuli were pictorial in nature. His behavioral measures were much improved. He appeared to be a happier, more confident, and more mature young man.

At the request of the boy's parent, the neuropsychologist (MW) met via remote telecommunication with his new teachers when he moved from elementary to middle school. The content of the meeting included teaching the basics of the anatomy of the visual system to school staff, with illustrations showing how breaks in different segments of the system result in different kinds of visual field deficits, as well as discussion of how the visual system of this boy was affected. After his occipital lobe surgery to remove epileptic tissue, he had a clear right hemianopia, so he was essentially "blind to objects on his right side," but he could adequately perceive objects to the left of the midline. The neuropsychologist explained that the blindness was not in his eyes but was due to the injury and removal of the portion of the brain that would normally process visual information coming in from his right visual field. This right-side blindness would not be apparent to the casual observer, and the concept of one-sided blindness is not intuitive to those without an understanding of the neuroanatomy. His history of abnormal control of eye movements was also explained in nontechnical terms (side-to-side and up-down, with differences in control and steadiness between the two eyes). School staff also had the support of a vision specialist from the educational district offices. The boy's individual education plan was adjusted to integrate information about his visual system with other cognitive and medical factors. His combined visual and oculomotor disabilities are permanent and will continue to hinder his ability to perform at the expected pace in school and later in life. With better understanding from teaching staff, the boy felt better supported in school and became more engaged in his education.

Table 11.3 Selected neuropsychological test scores for Case 3 pre- and post-left occipital lobe surgery

Timing relative to surgery	Pre-surgery		Post-surgery
Wechsler Intelligence Scale versions	Wechsler Intelligence Scale for Children IV	Wechsler Abbreviated Scale of Intelligence II	Wechsler Intelligence Scale for Children IV
Age	**11-6**	**11-8**	**12-7**
Intellectual summary scores	**Standard Score[a]**	**Standard Score[a]**	**Standard Score[a]**
Verbal Comprehension Index	89	92	93
Perceptual Reasoning Index	69	72	82
Working Memory Index	59	–	91
Processing Speed Index	62	–	50
Full Scale IQ	65	79	75
General Ability Index	78	–	87
Boston Naming Test			
Raw score	42	–	35
Z score (avg. = 0.0) boys/peers	−0.86/−0.98	–	−2.79/−3.56
NEPSY subtest	**Scaled Score[b]**	**Scaled Score[b]**	**Scaled Score[b]**
Comprehension of Instructions	5	7	8
Wide Range Assessment of Memory and Learning II	**Standard Score[a]**	**Standard Score[a]**	**Standard Score[a]**
Memory Screener Index	–	77	77
Verbal Memory Index	–	82	100
Visual Memory Index	–	79	60
Developmental Test of Visual-Motor Integration VI			
VMI (copy) standard score[a]	79	–	60
Age equivalent (years:months)	7:6	–	6:3
Achenbach Child Behavior Checklist	**Mother's ratings (T-score[c])**	**Mother's ratings (T-score[c])**	**Mother's ratings (T-score[c])**
Internalizing problems[a]	73	–	61
Externalizing problems[a]	71	–	60
Total problems[a]	73	–	61
Behavior Rating Inventory of Executive Function	**Mother's ratings (T-score[d])**	**Mother's ratings (T-score[d])**	**Mother's ratings (T-score[d])**
Behavior Regulation Index	74	–	60
Metacognition Index	68	–	62
General Executive Composite	72	–	63

[a]Standard Scores have a mean of 100 and a standard deviation of 15
[b]Scaled Scores have a mean of 10 and an SD of 3
[c]T-score: average = 50, normal range = 50–64, borderline range = 65–69, clinical range = 70 and above
[d]T-scores of >65 are in the clinical range

Physician Perspective

Case 3 was a child who presented initially as discouraged and unhappy due to his seizures and the burden of medications and being misunderstood by his school community who had incomplete understanding of his disabilities. With access to the complete medical and academic record, the neuropsychologist was able to integrate the behavioral and cognitive test results with the data from imaging, ophthalmological and neurological evaluations, and epilepsy surgery team conferences in order to paint a picture of the "invisible" challenges for this child within his environment of a normal school setting. In this case, the role of the neuropsychologist as educator and communicator to the child's community [4] was particularly useful, as prior to the intervention some of his school behaviors had been attributed merely to willful lack of effort.

This case also illustrates a situation sometimes encountered in the field of epilepsy surgery, in which a sacrifice of skills may be made in order to stop the debilitating seizures. The increase in a visual field defect that was felt to be present prior to surgery was considered an acceptable trade-off to having frequent seizures that were incompletely controlled by medications and contributed to his cognitive and behavioral disabilities. Indeed, the boy and his family are pleased with this outcome.

A similar situation may occur in cases where functional hemispherectomy [21] is the most effective way to stop seizures, where the sacrifice of motor and sensory abilities on one side of the body may sometimes be made. These children, whose seizures result from large brain lesions related most frequently to perinatal strokes or to widespread unilateral cortical malformations, usually have contralateral motor and sensory impairments prior to surgery, sometimes with contralateral visual field deficits. Language functions and hand dominance develop in the more normal hemisphere, with varying degrees of cognitive delay. Depending on the details, further losses of motor or sensory function due to surgery may be anticipated, particularly with vision. For the casual observer of children who have undergone hemispherectomy, a hemianopia is somewhat easier to understand once this is explained, as easily perceived motor impairments are on the same body side as the hemianopia. Neuroplasticity with regard to the development of motor functioning in these hemispherectomy patients has been addressed in a recent publication from our institution [21].

Due to the complex, very specific, and early-developing neural connections between the eyes and the occipital lobes ("hard-wiring"), the opportunity for neuroplasticity in the visual system is minimal in comparison to some other systems where neural connections develop later. As the young child's cortex grows, there is more flexibility for development of language, motor, and even memory systems in non-normal cortical areas following very early focal damage to the usual brain locations for these functions.

Key Point
When collaborating with neuropsychologists pediatric epilepsy teams are better able to discover these idiosyncratic, atypical patterns of brain organization that develop following focal damage in many pediatric epilepsy surgery patients.

Thanks to collaborative efforts with our neuropsychologists, we are better able to discover these idiosyncratic, atypical patterns of brain organization that develop following early focal damage in many of our pediatric epilepsy surgery patients.

In summary, neuropsychologists working within a pediatric epilepsy surgery team may serve in several different roles for a given patient and family over the course of their journey through the epilepsy surgery process, depending on the details of each case. Their job requires considerable flexibility within a structured environment and uses the full range of their clinical skills, including integrating information from multiple sources, addressing parental concerns, managing and guiding children of varying ages and abilities through complex procedures, and coordinating and communicating effectively with team members and with other involved persons outside the hospital.

Key Point

- Neuroplasticity (development of atypical lateralization/localization of cognitive or motor functions) occurs in some children with early focal brain abnormalities that lead to medically intractable focal seizures.
- Presurgical identification of critical functional brain areas, whether typically or atypically sited, assists physicians in planning neurosurgical procedures that minimize possible harm.
- Neuropsychologists in pediatric epilepsy surgery settings train and guide selected child and adolescent patients through complex multidisciplinary procedures that require their cooperation, designed to identify eloquent cortex unique to each child.
- Especially if antiepileptic medications can eventually be discontinued, successful control of seizures by safely removing the seizure focus can be life-changing for children with focal epilepsy and their families.
- Neuropsychologists integrate knowledge of cognitive development and behavior with medical issues pertinent to each patient and track their development pre- and post-surgery. They can help parents and school personnel understand and manage these children in their normal environments to optimize future development.

Presentation of these de-identified cases from Seattle Children's Hospital is covered by IRB #15721, "Seizure and functional outcomes after surgical treatment of epilepsy" (Jeffrey Ojemann, MD, Principal Investigator), and IRB #13690, "Functional MRI in pediatric populations, Part 2" (Andrew Poliakov, Ph.D., Principal Investigator).

Chapter Review Questions

1. These cases all involve some degree of neuroplasticity (the development of function in another cortical area following early focal brain lesion or insult to the normal location). These three cases illustrate neuroplasticity for:
   A. Language systems.
   B. Motor systems.
   C. Visual systems.
   D. Memory systems.
   E. All of the above.
   F. A, B, and D only.
   G. A and B only.
   H. B, C, and D only.

2. Perusal of the intellectual test scores from these cases will show that the Full Scale IQ scores are a combination (but not an average) of indices covering different domains. Why might these indices (and hence the Full Scale IQ) fluctuate over time in individual pediatric epilepsy patients?
   A. Degree of frequency and severity of seizures affecting attention and alertness.
   B. Types and doses of medications.
   C. Differences in amount of effort by the patient.
   D. Exposure to the test materials over time.
   E. All of the above.
   F. A and B only.

3. Neuropsychologists employed in a pediatric epilepsy surgery setting work together with the radiology team to provide patient data on:
   A. Brain structure using PET.
   B. Brain function using fMRI.
   C. Brain structure using the intracarotid amobarbital procedure (IAP or Wada test).
   D. Brain function using the intracarotid amobarbital procedure (IAP or Wada test).
   E. Brain structure using fMRI.
   F. B and D only.
   G. A and C only.

4. One of the neuropsychologist's roles is to be able to interpret the implications of the pattern of test scores, the medical condition and its treatments, and even the particular neuroanatomy for a given case. This type of information may be useful both inside and outside the hospital setting. Those who may receive this integrated information (with written permission) may include:
   A. Parents.
   B. Patients.
   C. Physicians.

D. School personnel.
E. Social service agencies.
F. Governmental agencies (such as the Social Security Administration).
G. Mental health professionals.
H. All of the above.

References

1. Andelman F, Neufeld MY, Fried I. Contribution of neuropsychology to epilepsy surgery. Isr J Psychiatry Relat Sci. 2004;41(2):125–32.
2. Loring DW. History of neuropsychology through epilepsy eyes. Arch Clin Neuropsychol. 2010;25(4):259–73.
3. Wilson SJ, Baxendale S, Barr W, Hamed S, Langfitt J, Samson S, Watanabe M, Baker GA, Helmstaedter C, Hermann BP, Smith ML. Indications and expectations for neuropsychological assessment in routine epilepsy care: report of the ILAE Neuropsychology Task Force, Diagnostic Methods Commission, 2013–2017. Epilepsia. 2015;56(5):674–81.
4. Shurtleff H. Neuropsychology's role in pediatric epilepsy surgery. J Pediatr Epilepsy. 2017;2017(6):51–61.
5. Chou N, Serafini S, Muh C. Cortical language areas and plasticity in pediatric patients with epilepsy: a review. Pediatr Neurol. 2018;78:3–12.
6. Shurtleff H, Warner M, Poliakov A, Bournival B, Shaw DW, Ishak G, Yang T, Karandikar M, Saneto RP, Browd SR, Ojemann JG. Functional magnetic resonance imaging for presurgical evaluation of very young patients with epilepsy. J Neurosurg Pediatr. 2010;5(5):500–6.
7. Jenkinson M, Beckmann CF, Behrens TE, Woolrich MW, Smith SM. FSL [the FMRIB Software Library]. Neuroimage. 2012;62:782–90.
8. Gleissner U, Kurthen M, Sassen R, Kuczaty S, Elger CE, Linke DB, Urbach H, Helmstaedter C. Clinical and neuropsychological characteristics of pediatric epilepsy patients with atypical language dominance. Epilepsy Behav. 2003;4(6):746–52.
9. Kadis DS, Koji I, Kerr EN, Logan WJ, McAndrews MP, Ayako O, Hirshi O, Rutka JT, Snead OC, Weiss SK, Smith ML. Intrahemispheric reorganization of language in children with medically intractable epilepsy of the left hemisphere. J Int Neuropsychol Soc. 2007;13:505–16.
10. Shurtleff HA, Barry D, Firman T, Warner MH, Aguilar-Estrada RL, Saneto RP, Kuratani JJ, Ellenbogen RG, Novotny EJ, Ojemann JG. Impact of epilepsy surgery on development of preschool children: identification of a cohort likely to benefit from early intervention. J Neurosurg Pediatr. 2015;16(4):383–92.
11. Liégeos F, Connelly A, Helen Cross J, Boyd SG, Gadian DG, Varght-Khadem V, Baldeweg T. Language reorganization in children with early-onset lesions of the left hemisphere: an fMRI study. Brain. 2004;127:1229–36.
12. Yuan W, Szaflarsky JP, Schmithorst VJ, Shapiro M, Byars AW, Strawsburg RH, Holland SK. fMRI shows atypical language lateralization in pediatric epilepsy patients. Epilepsia. 2006;47(3):593–600.
13. Vannest J, Karunanayaka PR, Schmithorst VJ, Szaflarski JP, Holland SK. Language networks in children: evidence from functional MRI studies. Am J Roentgenol. 2009;192(5):1190–6.
14. Hermann B. The effects of localization-related epilepsy on language lateralization and networks. Epilepsy Currents. 2006;6(4):114–6.
15. Kovac S, Möddel G, Reinholz J, Alexopoulos AV, Syed T, Schuele SU, Lineweaver TT, Loddenkemper TT. Memory performance is related to language dominance as determined by the intracarotid amobarbital procedure. Epilepsy Behav. 2009;16:145–9.
16. Eddy CM, Rickards HE, Cavanna AE. The cognitive impact of antiepileptic drugs. Ther Adv Neurol Disord. 2011;4(6):385–407.

17. Mula M. Topiramate and cognitive impairment: evidence and clinical implications. Ther Adv Drug Saf. 2012;3(6):279–89.
18. Shurtleff H, Nixon J, Warner M, Poliakov A, Shaw D, Novotny E, Ojemann J. fMRI temporal activation paradigm for children with epilepsy and/or tumors. Epilepsy Curr. 2015;15(Suppl. 1):520. https://doi.org/10.5698/1535-9597-s1.1.
19. Greicius MD, Krasnow B, Boyett-Anderson JM, Eliez S, Schatzberg AF, Reiss AL, Menon V. Regional analysis of hippocampal activation during memory encoding and retrieval: fMRI study. Hippocampus. 2003;13(1):164–74.
20. Woermann FG, Jokeit H, Luerding R, Freitag H, Schulz R, Guertler S, Okujava M, Wolf P, Tuxhorn I, Ebner A. Language lateralization by Wada Test and fMRI in 100 patients with epilepsy. Neurology. 2003;61(5):699–701.
21. Wang AC, Ibrahim GM, Poliakov AV, Wang PI, Fallah A, Mathern GW, Buckley RT, Collins K, Weil AG, Shurtleff HA, Warner MH, Perez FA, Shaw DA, Wright JN, Saneto RP, Novotny EJ, Lee A, Browd SR, Ojemann JG. Corticospinal tract atrophy and motor fMRI predict motor preservation after functional cerebral hemispherectomy. J Neurosurg Pediatr. 2018;21(1):81–9.

Chapter 12
Alzheimer's Disease and Overview of Dementia

Emily H. Trittschuh and Lucy Wang

Introduction

Dementia is a clinical syndrome characterized by a decline from the baseline in cognitive function and/or behavior and comportment. The decline typically begins insidiously (although many patients or their family members will point to one key event when they first "knew something was wrong"), and changes are progressive. The etiology of the decline is neurodegeneration, with the exact pathological substrate often only determinable after death via brain autopsy and microscopic examination. Clinically, it is important to remember that the conferral of a diagnosis of a specific type of dementia, for example, Alzheimer's disease (AD), is only a "probable" or "possible" diagnosis [1]. Another key clinical requirement for the diagnosis of dementia is that the decline in thinking or behavior must be sufficient to have caused losses in an individual's independence for daily living—the determination of which can range from the obvious, "My wife now takes care of the appointments, medications, finances, and driving," to the less obvious, "My wife keeps our calendar, occasionally reminds me to take my medications, and my son, the accountant, does our taxes…. I'm a great driver—I haven't had any accidents or tickets."

Dementia caused by Alzheimer's disease stands as an exemplar for neurodegenerative diseases of aging for several reasons, foremost of which are: (1) it is the most common cause of sporadic dementia, particularly in adults over age 65 [2], and (2) it is the only dementia etiology for which FDA-approved pharmaceuticals exist and their only possible beneficial effect is to delay clinical progression [3]. Conservative projections for individuals living in the USA with clinical AD by 2050 are over 13 million [2]. Worldwide projections suggest the number of people with AD will triple

E. H. Trittschuh (✉) · L. Wang
Department of Psychiatry and Behavioral Sciences, University of Washington School of Medicine, VA Puget Sound Health Care System, Geriatric Research Education and Clinical Center, Seattle, Washington, USA
e-mail: emily.trittschuh@va.gov

K. M. Sanders (ed.), *Physician's Field Guide to Neuropsychology*,
https://doi.org/10.1007/978-1-4939-8722-1_12

over the next 20 years [4] and these individuals will join the over 80 million people living with dementia by 2040 [5]. The economic impact will be astronomical. As the healthcare community waits, hopes, and prays for the discovery of a disease-modifying intervention, researchers have addressed the question of whether early diagnosis can result in net benefit. The answer is yes; even with existing symptomatic treatments, there is a net benefit gained with early diagnosis [6]. Given the increasing numbers and economic impact, there will be corresponding increasing demands upon frontline medical providers (e.g., primary care) to recognize and initiate workup for suspected cases of dementia.

In Alzheimer's disease, the hallmark neurofibrillary tangles and amyloid plaques were first described by Alois Alzheimer in 1907. Neuropathologists use classification systems to rate and grade the density and distribution of the plaques and tangles before making a pathologic diagnosis of AD. Classic descriptions by Braak and Braak [7] have given way to modern guidelines developed by the National Institute on Aging in conjunction with the Alzheimer's Association [8]. As clinicians, our appreciation of the clinical syndrome of AD is much advanced by an understanding of the underlying pathology and its classic pattern of first appearing in the structures of the medial temporal lobes (MTL), next in heteromodal/association cortices, and often sparing primary cortices until the disease is most advanced. With the structures of the MTL, the hippocampus, entorhinal cortex, and dentate gyrus, being necessary for the creation of new explicit memories, it is not surprising that a pattern of amnesia (rapid forgetting of newly learned material) is one of the first signs of typical Alzheimer's disease dementia, and this is often soon followed by, or detected along with, markers of anomia (word-finding problems) and declines in complex attention (see Jahn [9] for a review).

As you will see in the following chapters, like Alzheimer's disease and dementia, there are other types of dementia which are named after scientists who first identified or published on the pathognomonic pathology (e.g., Lewy body disease), while other dementia syndromes are named for the area of typical initial brain neurodegeneration (e.g., frontotemporal dementia [FTD]). The uniting rule is that all are diagnosed clinically by identifying a syndrome of decline in functions that the affected brain regions (or their projections) support.

The clinical diagnosis of AD relies on a multifaceted approach and a solid/basic understanding of the literature. One important primer is on the distinction between "early onset" and "late onset" terminology versus "early stage" and "late stage." Late onset refers to symptoms appearing after age 65 and is typically associated with "sporadic" AD—for which there is no known genetic mutation or protein synthesis/clearing abnormality. Early onset refers to an age of onset of dementia <65; in these younger adults, AD (followed by FTD) is the most likely etiologies [10]. Early-onset AD is sometimes sporadic but can also be indicative of familial AD, for which there are known dominant genetic mutations: amyloid precursor protein, presenilin 1, and presenilin 2. Cases of early-onset AD make up less than 5% of patients ([11] or [12], for review). Referring to AD as late stage versus early stage should be reserved for when one is commenting on the degree of impairment, likely associated with the degree of pathological burden in the brain.

There are numerous risk factors for the development of Alzheimer's disease (e.g., increasing age and race) as well as resilience factors (e.g., higher years of education), which have been identified. There is only one consistently associated risk gene for late-onset AD: having one or two copies of the apolipoprotein E, e4 allele (ApoE, e4). With a worldwide population frequency of under 14%, having two copies has been associated with an odds ratio of 14.9 of developing AD, while having one copy, paired with the most common allele (e3), is associated with an odds ratio of 3.2 [13]. Genome-wide association studies (GWAS) are breaking ground to identify additional risk genes which might allow researchers to develop more targeted interventions with more personalized applications down the road [12]. Additionally, there is great excitement in the AD community over the relatively recent development of in vivo techniques for identifying and quantifying pathological amyloid and most recently tau pathology in the brain [14]. These types of PET scans will likely become available outside of research when/if a disease-modifying treatment becomes FDA approved. However, for now, the false-positive rates (identifying pathology in individuals *without* clinical evidence of dementia) are untenable in a clinical setting.

Key Point
Neuropsychological evaluation is a safe, economical, reliable, and accurate method for diagnosing early-stage Alzheimer's disease.

Therefore, in support of a thorough medical workup, the neuropsychological evaluation persists as a safe, economical, reliable, and accurate method for diagnosing early AD [15–17]. In addition, while a neuropsychological evaluation is invaluable as part of the dementia workup for primary care providers and other nonspecialist medical providers, we demonstrate in the case example below how there is diagnostic utility even in the context of a geriatric specialist as referring provider. At the Veterans Affairs Puget Sound Health Care System, the Geriatric Research Education and Clinical Center runs an outpatient, consultation-based Memory Disorders Clinic. The patients are veterans of the US Armed Services, and a typical referral is a veteran with medical, and often psychiatric, comorbidities for whom specialty workup is requested.

Dr. Wang is a geriatric psychiatrist in this clinic. Dr. Trittschuh is a clinical neuropsychologist. In this relatively straightforward case example, Dr. Wang completed her consultation first and identified that neuropsychological evaluation would be helpful. In our clinic, some consults are triaged to neuropsychology first, while others typically see psychiatry first. While there is no strict systematic decision tree, older veterans (75+) with Montreal Cognitive Assessment (MoCA) scores <22 and those with psychiatric comorbidities tend to see a psychiatrist first, while younger veterans with higher MoCA scores see Dr. Trittschuh first.

Case Study: Psychiatry MD, Initial Visit

Presenting Problem

Mr. A is a 75-year-old male with a history of chronic post-traumatic stress disorder (PTSD) who was referred for consultation in the Memory Disorders Clinic by his primary care provider due to the veteran and his wife's concerns regarding new memory problems.

History

Mr. A came to the clinic with worries about worsening memory problems. He was also accompanied by his spouse, who expressed equal concern. Both described him having trouble remembering things, a problem that has gradually worsened over the past year. He recently forgot to pay some bills, and was beginning to forget whether he had taken his medications for the day. He used to hold a leadership position in a local chapter of a veteran's service organization but voluntarily stepped down last month because of difficulty completing tasks.

At the time of the visit, he was still driving and denied any problems in this area. He explained that his trouble with the bills was not his fault and that the forgetfulness for medications is due to a recent change in schedule. He continued to do all of his regular chores around the home, such as taking out the garbage and doing the dishes. He continued to be socially active, being highly involved in veteran's advocacy groups and playing golf regularly with friends.

Mr. A also had a long-standing diagnosis of PTSD due to combat exposure in Vietnam. He had a good response to treatment that included psychotherapy and sertraline but still had persistent symptoms including intrusive memories, irritability, exaggerated startle, concentration problems, and difficulty staying asleep. These symptoms had been relatively stable; however, about 6 months ago, he began to notice intrusive memories occurring more frequently and concentration problems worse than before. He otherwise did not have other psychiatric symptoms, such as depressed mood or generalized anxiety. He did not drink or use recreational drugs.

Past Medical History

In addition to PTSD, Mr. A's medical problems included hypertension and low back pain. His hypertension had been well controlled. His medications included a multivitamin, sertraline, hydrochlorothiazide, and naproxen. He was not taking additional over-the-counter medications.

Social History

After his military service, he obtained a college degree in business. He subsequently managed and eventually took over his family business, which remained successful and later transitioned to his children when he retired 5 years prior to evaluation. He had been married twice, divorced once, and had two children from his second marriage. He described his current spouse and his adult children as strongly supportive.

Family History

His mother developed Alzheimer's disease in her late 70s/early 80s. He recalled that her initial symptoms involved forgetting recent conversations and recent events. She died in her late 80s.

Exam

On exam, Mr. A presented as well groomed, and he maintained good eye contact. He described his mood as normal and his affect was full range. His thought processes were logical and linear. He had no tremor or gait abnormalities. Finger-to-nose testing and rapid alternating movements were intact. There was no evidence of focal weakness, and his deep tendon reflexes were symmetric throughout.

He scored 26 out of 30 points on the Montreal Cognitive Assessment (MoCA). He missed four out of five word recall items and only recalled one more when given category and multiple-choice cues.

Labs and Imaging

Based on Mr. A and his spouse's concerns, further workup was pursued. Laboratory studies including a complete blood count (CBC), basic metabolic panel, TSH, and vitamin B12 were all within normal limits. A brain MRI showed mild global atrophy but no evidence of mass or cerebrovascular disease.

Psychiatrist's Impression and Reason for Referral for Neuropsychological Evaluation

Based on the history and medical workup described above, the differential diagnosis for this case includes a mild-versus-major neurocognitive disorder (concern for early AD) and/or a PTSD exacerbation. The patient's and his spouse's report of new-onset, short-term memory deficits with mild impact on his functioning, along with a family history of AD, is concerning for neurocognitive disorder. On the other hand, his worsening PTSD symptoms, which include concentration problems and sleep impairment, can also contribute to cognitive concerns. The history, exam, and laboratory workup excluded other medical or psychiatric causes for his cognitive impairment. MRI findings neither supported nor negated neurodegenerative disease as a possible cause of reported changes.

In addition to the difficulty discerning between Alzheimer's disease versus PTSD, this case is complicated by a relatively strong performance on a cognitive screening measure, the MoCA. For a diagnosis of neurocognitive disorder (AD, in particular), a patient must have impairment on objective cognitive measures and corresponding decline in daily function; the MoCA performance does not meet this standard (refer to pp. X-X, for more information). Due to Mr. A's level of education and high prior level of functioning, it is possible the MoCA alone would not be sensitive enough to detect the cognitive impairment that is currently affecting his day-to-day functioning. Neuropsychological evaluation of cognitive function provides the best method for integrating these factors into the overall impression and detection of objective cognitive impairments.

Therefore, a referral for a neuropsychological evaluation was requested to (1) provide an objective measure of cognitive impairment and (2) determine whether his symptoms meet the criteria for a mild-versus-major neurocognitive disorder (AD) or are better explained by PTSD.

Case Study: Neuropsychological Evaluation

Interview Data

This provider had the electronic medical record notes from Dr. Wang's evaluation. In addition, prior to neuropsychological evaluation, our office mails out three questionnaires: (1) medical history questionnaire; (2) patient symptoms, time course, and activities of daily living questionnaire; and (3) a similar questionnaire for collateral informant to complete (typically a spouse or other close family member). The account provided to Dr. Wang was supported. However, a review of the spouse's questionnaire indicated that she was endorsing more concern than she had before, and follow-up on this during the clinical interview suggested that the first cognitive changes were noted more than a year ago, perhaps as much as 2 years ago. Her responses to the activities of daily living scale were similar to her husband's, but careful querying revealed that while he has not been in any accidents or gotten lost, she is concerned about his driving because he is not keeping up with traffic on the highway and his lane changes are abrupt and often demonstrate lack of awareness of other cars on the road. It came out that their adult daughter does not let the veteran drive his grandson to soccer practice anymore. The veteran vehemently denied that he was having any trouble with driving. If his family members are accurate, his denial could be defensive in nature or perhaps indicative of the loss of insight into one's weaknesses (anosognosia) that is often seen in AD and other dementias.

Other Major Medical/Psychiatric/Neurological History

Sleep was queried specifically to gather more information about the veteran's difficulty staying asleep, and Mrs. A did note that while her husband didn't snore, she felt like he occasionally would gasp awake, but not always endorse nightmare. Querying of daytime fatigue suggested he can fall asleep quite easily if sitting still for more than 30 minutes while reading or watching television. His sleep for the past two nights was typical, and he denied any excessive fatigue on the morning of evaluation. Chronic and/or acute pain was denied by Mr. A, but it is important to query in older adults who often have arthritis or nagging pain from remote injuries or surgery.

Early history reflected an uncomplicated birth, and developmental milestones were reached on time, with no notable childhood illnesses. Academic success in elementary school with poor grades in high school attributed to "not being interested in school." During this time, he played high school football and had his "bell rung" three to five times over the course of 3 years; however, none resulted in loss of consciousness greater than "at most a minute." He denied any physical or cognitive sequelae of these events. He had no other history of head injury. He joined the Army and served for 4 years; in his first 2 years of service, he saw combat. After 2 years, he was referred to officer training and later discharged with a notable history of early advancement. Using the Government Issue (GI) bill, he graduated from a high-tier university with As and Bs.

Behavioral Observations

No evidence for thought disorder, delusions, or auditory/visual hallucinations; no significant hearing or vision problems; gait was unremarkable. Mr. A was cooperative but a little quick to give up—encouragement often elicited more, but not notably so. He seemed acutely aware of his poor performance during the testing and vocalized his frustration with his lack of ability. Later, after testing was completed and we rejoined his wife, he spontaneously commented to her that he had "fun" and "it wasn't too hard."

Neuropsychological Evaluation

My approach to test selection is a flexible one but with the consistent goal of utilizing measures with specificity and sensitivity to detecting the signs of neurodegenerative disease. With Alzheimer's disease being the most common form of dementia in older age, it is common to select measures which will pick up on the earliest symptoms of this disease. Assessments of episodic memory—single trial and multiple trial learning, short-term retrieval, as well as the expected delayed recall—are especially useful. Cuing and recognition facets to a test measure are helpful for discerning whether information learned is lost or simply difficult to retrieve. In addition, testing new learning and memory in verbal and visual modalities, as well as with and without contextual information, also provides valuable information about the integrity (or lack thereof) of the neuroanatomical substrates for memory formation and retrieval. With most of these structures located in the medial temporal lobe (e.g., hippocampus, entorhinal cortex) and the first neuropathological changes associated with Alzheimer's disease having a predilection for this region, poor performance on these tests can be a clue to the neuroanatomical underpinnings. With brain MRI negative except for "mild global atrophy," one must rely on testing the *function* of the structures, rather than looking for structural markers.

Other tests sensitive to early Alzheimer's disease are also based on the earliest stage findings of where neurofibrillary tangles are found; for instance, anomia (difficulty with word retrieval to match a specific stimulus) can be seen early in the course of AD. Other tests are chosen for their sensitivity, for example, visuomotor sequencing (trail making) measures.

Test Results: Summary

Cognitive domain	Measure type	Percentile	Descriptor
Performance validity	Embedded and stand-alone measures	Within normal limits (WNL)	Pass
Premorbid estimate	Word reading	75	Above average
Global measure	100-Point measure	WNL	No dementia
Memory	Story learning	10	Below average
	Story recall	1	Mildly impaired
	Word list learning	15	Below average
	Word list short delay recall	1	Mildly impaired
	Word list long delay recall	2	Mildly impaired
	Word list cued long delay	<1	Impaired
	Word list recognition	1	Mildly impaired
	Word list false positives	<1	Impaired
	Word list repetitions	2	Mildly impaired
	Figure learning total trials	16	Below average
	Figure learning delay	1	Mildly impaired

Cognitive domain	Measure type	Percentile	Descriptor
Attention	Immediate auditory attention	50	Average
	Auditory working memory	25	Average
	Trail making (sequencing only)	84	Above average
	Trail making (sequencing with set-shifting)	25	Average
Language	Naming (60 items)	6	Borderline impaired
	Category fluency	14	Below average
	Phonemic fluency	58	Average
Visuospatial/ construction	Figure copy	WNL	
	Abstract visuomotor construction	75	Above average
	Line orientation	63	Average
Abstraction/ reasoning	Visual	75	Above average
	Verbal	37	Average
Mood	Depression self-report	Mild	Mild depression
	PTSD symptom self-report	Moderate	Moderate PTSD

Neuropsychologist's Impression Based on Formal Testing

With performance validity data supporting my clinical observation that Mr. A was able to put forth good effort on testing (i.e., affective distress did not notably impair his effort), I can proceed with interpretation of testing. Mr. A's score on the premorbid IQ estimate suggested that he has a baseline of at least an "above-average" ability. This is helpful because "setting the bar" of expectation at the standard, 50 percentile, would miss areas of relative decline for this bright veteran. Scores toward the lower end of the below-average range and below are flagged and suspicious as representing areas of decline.

With this approach, one sees evidence of a mild decline in new learning and notable impairments in retention/retrieval. These deficits are not much aided by cuing or recognition formats and are not specific to verbal versus visual modality. In addition, there is evidence for a decline in language measures, most notably for naming and category fluency. As an experienced clinician, this fluency split—with category fluency worse than phonemic fluency—is one I often see in early AD cases.

Other results from the evaluation suggest intact performance; no declines were found for the measures administered in the domains of attention, visuospatial/construction ability, or abstraction/reasoning. Evidence for affective disorder, primarily PTSD symptoms, is present but insufficient to explain the pattern of weaknesses. PTSD has been associated with overall changes in neurocognition in older adults and declines in new learning, but not with language changes or with this degree of retentive memory loss [18].

There is objective evidence of cognitive disorder such that the diagnosis of a neurocognitive disorder is appropriate. The veteran has had mild losses in his daily function which seem to correlate with the onset and described progression in his symptoms, suggesting that criteria for a major neurocognitive disorder are met. The overall pattern of memory performance is strongly suggestive of medial temporal lobe dysfunction, and declines in aspects of language are suggestive of additional temporal lobe involvement (particularly the language network and anterior temporal lobe regions). These findings, combined with symptom onset and history, the veteran's age, and other causes of decline having been ruled out, are strongly supportive of a diagnosis of early dementia, most likely that associated with Alzheimer's disease pathology.

Neuropsychologist's Feedback Session and Recommendations for the Patient

After briefly reviewing the history and neuropsychological findings, I talked to the patient and his wife about how a diagnosis of early-stage dementia, likely Alzheimer's disease, is supported. I always explain the limitations of clinical diagnosis. In addition, I highlight any findings or history which made interpretation challenging or provided for alternative diagnoses. In Mr. A's case, there were none. During feedback, I always provide education regarding the diagnosis, a typed summary of the Impression and Recommendations from my report using lay language, and printed educational materials from third parties. For dementia diagnoses, I often utilize materials developed and shared freely by the Alzheimer's Association.

One addition to the medical recommendations made by Dr. Wang, I suggested that while not a primary cause of the neuropsychological profile above, Mr. A's gasps for air while sleeping might be indicative of sleep apnea. Together with Dr. Wang, we placed a consultation for a sleep study to rule out apnea as a contributing factor. In our feedback session, we reviewed the importance of managing his cerebrovascular risk factors. Positive support was given for his healthy diet, efforts to take medications as prescribed, and engagement in regular exercise.

Twenty minutes of the hour-long neuropsychology feedback session was spent reviewing Mr. A's specific needs for compensatory external memory aids and developing concrete strategies for implementation. In particular, we reviewed how to use a pill box with alarms to help him remain independent for his medications. I presented information on resources through services like speech pathology or occupational therapy should new needs emerge. Given the veteran's possible lack of insight regarding his driving abilities, we provided information on our facility's driver rehabilitation program and a copy of the Hartford publication "At the Crossroads: Family Conversations About Alzheimer's Disease, Dementia & Driving."

Our final recommendation was that we would follow the patient in our clinic over the short term (3 months, Dr. Wang) and long term (12–18 months, Dr. Trittschuh) for monitoring a trial of a cholinesterase inhibitor approved for mild-moderate AD, followed by cognitive monitoring via repeat neuropsychological testing. While repeat neuropsychological evaluation is not often necessary for diagnostic purposes at this point, it can be quite helpful to the medical providers and family for information on the rate of decline, identifying new areas of weakness, and providing additional support to family via caregiving resources and long-term planning.

Key Point
Clinical diagnosis of Alzheimer's disease (or any type of dementia) is a *diagnosis of exclusion*. There are many conditions which can mimic the cognitive and behavioral symptoms and might seem to have corresponding functional decline. However, it might not be dementia and the condition may be treatable.

A last important note about the clinical diagnosis of Alzheimer's disease (or any type of dementia) is that it should always be approached as a diagnosis of exclusion. There are many conditions which can mimic the cognitive and behavioral symptoms and might even seem to have corresponding functional decline. However, it might not be dementia, and the condition may or may not be treatable. The most common syndromes mimicking dementia that I come across include depression, subacute delirium, sleep apnea, post-traumatic stress disorder (PTSD), nutritional deficiencies (e.g., low B12), thyroid disorder, substance use (including medical or recreational cannabis), pain syndromes and the opioids often used in treatment, and problems with prescribed medications (either polypharmacy or over-the-counter medications with anticholinergic effects). A thorough neuropsychological evaluation can be a key part of the diagnostic workup to distinguish among these syndromes.

Further Resources

National Institute on Aging—Alzheimer's disease: https://www.nia.nih.gov/alzheimers

Alzheimer's Association: www.alz.org

The Hartford resources on Driving in Aging and with Dementia: https://www.thehartford.com/resources/mature-market-excellence/publications-on-aging

Chapter Review Questions

1. Alzheimer's disease with symptom onset when the individual is in their early 80s is suggestive of:
   A. Familial AD.
   B. Sporadic AD.

2. Mr. A suffers from PTSD. Which neuropsychological measures helped the neuropsychologist determine that weaknesses on the MoCA were not due to affective distress (select two)?
   A. Trail making test.
   B. Performance validity measures.
   C. PTSD symptom self-report.
   D. Word reading.

3. While the MoCA has three naming items, the current battery utilized a 60-item naming measure. This aided:
   A. Reliability.
   B. Validity.
   C. Specificity.
   D. Sensitivity.

4. Which AD-associated neuropathological change is most closely associated with the symptomatic cognitive pattern?
   A. Neurofibrillary tangles.
   B. Amyloid plaques.

5. Which of the following *must* be present to make a diagnosis of Alzheimer's disease dementia?
   A. Patient is aware of memory loss.
   B. Strong family history of dementia.
   C. Losses of independence in daily function.
   D. No PTSD or other affective disorder.

References

1. McKhann GM, Knopman DS, Chertkow H, Hyman BT, Jack CR Jr, Kawas CH, Klunk WE, Koroshetz WJ, Manly JJ, Mayeux R, Mohs RC, Morris JC, Rossor MN, Scheltens P, Carrillo MC, Thies B, Weintraub S, Phelps CH. The diagnosis of dementia due to Alzheimer's disease: recommendations from the National Institute on Aging-Alzheimer's Association workgroups on diagnostic guidelines for Alzheimer's disease. Alzheimers Dement. 2011;7(3):263–9.
2. Hebert LE, Weuve J, Scherr PA, Evans DA. Alzheimer disease in the United States (2010–2050) estimated using the 2010 census. Neurology. 2013;80(19):1778–83.
3. Zhu CW, Livote EE, Scarmeas N, Albert M, Brandt J, Blacker D, Sano M, Stern Y. Long-term associations between cholinesterase inhibitors and memantine use and health outcomes among patients with Alzheimer's disease. Alzheimers Dement. 2013;9(6):733–40.
4. Wimo A, Jonsson L, Winblad B. An estimate of the worldwide prevalence and direct costs of dementia in 2003. Dement Geriatr Cogn Dis. 2006;21:175–81.
5. Ferri CP, Prince M, Brayne C, Brodaty H, Fratiglioni L, Ganguli M, Hall K, Hasegawa K, Hendrie H, Huang Y, Jorm A, Mathers C, Menezes PR, Rimmer E, Scazufca M, Alzheimer's Disease International. Global prevalence of dementia: a Delphi consensus study. Lancet. 2005;366(9503):2112–7.
6. Barnett JH, Lewis L, Blackwell AD, Taylor M. Early intervention in Alzheimer's disease: a health economic study of the effects of diagnostic timing. BMC Neurol. 2014;14:101.

7. Braak H, Braak E. Neurofibrillary changes confined to the entorhinal region and an abundance of cortical amyloid in cases of presenile and senile dementia. Acta Neuropathol. 1990;80:479–86.
8. Montine TJ, Phelps CH, Beach TG, Bigio EH, Cairns NJ, Dickson DW, Duyckaerts C, Frosch MP, Masliah E, Mirra SS, Nelson PT, Schneider JA, Thal DR, Trojanowski JQ, Vinters HV, Hyman BT, National Institute on Aging; Alzheimer's Association. National Institute on Aging-Alzheimer's Association guidelines for the neuropathologic assessment of Alzheimer's disease: a practical approach. Acta Neuropathol. 2012;123(1):1–11.
9. Jahn, H., Memory Loss in Alzheimer's disease. Dialogues in Clinical Neuroscience, 2013; 15(4): 445–454.
10. Harvey RJ, Skelton-Robinson M, Rossor MN. The prevalence and causes of dementia in people under the age of 65 years. J Neurol Neurosurg Psychiatry. 2003;74:1206–9.
11. Giri M, Zhang M, Lü Y. Genes associated with Alzheimer's disease: an overview and current status. Clin Interv Aging. 2016;11:665–81.
12. Ballard C, Gauthier S, Corbett A, Brayne C, Aarsland D, Jones E. Alzheimer's disease. Lancet. 2011;377(9770):1019–31.
13. Farrer LA, Cupples LA, Haines JL, Hyman B, Kukull WA, Mayeux R, Myers RH, Pericak-Vance MA, Risch N, van Duijn CM. Effects of age, sex, and ethnicity on the association between apolipoprotein E genotype and Alzheimer disease. A meta-analysis. APOE and Alzheimer Disease Meta Analysis Consortium. JAMA. 1997;278(16):1349–56.
14. Cho H, Choi JY, Hwang MS, Kim YJ, Lee HM, Lee HS, Lee JH, Ryu YH, Lee MS, Lyoo CH. In vivo cortical spreading pattern of tau and amyloid in the Alzheimer disease spectrum. Ann Neurol. 2016;80(2):247–58.
15. Pasquier F. Early diagnosis of dementia: neuropsychology. J Neurol. 1999;246(1):6–15.
16. Salmon DP, Bondi MW. Neuropsychological assessment of dementia. Annu Rev Psychol. 2009;60:257–82.
17. Sano M. Neuropsychological testing in the diagnosis of dementia. J Geriatr Psychiatry Neurol. 2006;19(3):155–9.
18. Schuitevoerder S, Rosen JW, Twamley EW, Ayers CR, Sones H, Lohr JB, Goetter EM, Fonzo GA, Holloway KJ, Thorp SR. A meta-analysis of cognitive functioning in older adults with PTSD. J Anxiety Disord. 2013;27(6):550–8.

Chapter 13
Posterior Cortical Atrophy

Ernest Y. S. Fung and Mark O. Herring

Introduction

Posterior cortical atrophy (PCA) is a relatively rare neurodegenerative syndrome marked by prominent disturbance in visuoperceptual and visuospatial functioning. Its prevalence and incidence rates are unknown [1]. There has been increased awareness of this condition among the general public, with the diagnosis made by British author Sir Terry Pratchett (1948–2015). He was quite open about his journey with the disease, making several documentaries and appearing on a number of radio programs. He was initially misdiagnosed, which is typical with the challenges of making this diagnosis. This condition was also written about by American neurologist/author Dr. Oliver Sacks in his 2010 book, *The Mind's Eye*, in which he describes this condition in one of his case reports.

In clinical settings, presenting complaints from patients with differential diagnosis of PCA often involve disturbance in activities of daily living, such as difficulties recognizing familiar routes, reading maps, or locating and organizing objects in the environment. They may report recent history of fender benders or more serious car accidents. Reading may have become challenging because of its visuospatial component, but verbal comprehension likely remains intact. In a recent study, patients with PCA were found to be more severely impaired in everyday skills and self-care (majority associated with visuoperceptual and visuospatial impairments) than their Alzheimer's disease (AD) counterparts, while more AD patients showed high levels of impairment in stereotypic and motor behaviors, but they maintained motivation to keep in contact with friends or family [2].

E. Y. S. Fung (✉)
Atlanta Neuropsychology, LLC, NP Neuropsychology, LLC, Atlanta, GA, USA
e-mail: ef@ernestfung.com

M. O. Herring
Oregon Neurology Associates, Springfield, OR, USA
e-mail: Mherring@Oregonneurology.com

K. M. Sanders (ed.), *Physician's Field Guide to Neuropsychology*,
https://doi.org/10.1007/978-1-4939-8722-1_13

Clinical diagnostic criteria of PCA were previously proposed by Mendez et al. [3] and Tang-Wai et al. [4]. Crutch et al. [5] noted that misdiagnosis of PCA is common because of "its relative rarity and variable presentation, but also because patients frequently first seek the opinion of an ophthalmologist who may note normal eye examinations by their usual tests but may not appreciate cortical brain dysfunction." Presentation of prominent anxiety and distress related to the individual's awareness of the extent of cognitive dysfunction, combined with the rarity of the syndrome, may inadvertently mislead clinicians into considering the possibility of psychogenic or conversion disorders.

Given the challenges in recognizing this disease and the need to raise awareness, an international working party comprising representatives from 23 institutions and 9 countries gathered in Vancouver, Canada, in July 2012 just prior to the Alzheimer's Association International Conference to address definitions and diagnostic criteria for this rare condition. These experienced researchers and clinicians ultimately formed the Posterior Cortical Atrophy Professional Interest Area Group for further collaborative work, which resulted in the recent publication of the first, three-level, classification framework of the condition [6].

Key Point

Three-level consensus classification framework of posterior cortical atrophy [6]:

Classification level 1: Core features of the PCA clinico-radiological syndrome.
Classification level 2: Classification of PCA-pure and PCA-plus.
Classification level 3: Diagnostic criteria for disease-level descriptions.

For full listing of the features for each classification level, please refer to Appendix 1.

Even though a proportion of PCA cases have been associated with dementia with Lewy bodies, corticobasal degeneration, or prion-associated diseases [7, 8], it has most often been conceptualized and classified as the atypical, nonamnestic, or posterior variant of AD. Its earlier age of onset of around 60 years [9] might be consistent with atypical AD, where patients show a similar pattern of high cortical binding on amyloid PET imaging and analogous changes in CSF level of amyloid beta 42, total tau, and phosphorylated tau [5]. However, there are notable differences in their neuropathology. It is widely known that typical AD is associated with hippocampal atrophy and dysfunction, but in cases of PCA, atrophy has been found in parietal, occipital, and occipitotemporal regions [10], as well as right hemisphere [11]. Hypometabolism was observed in posterior regions and frontal eye fields in a PCA group [12]. In comparison studies, patients with typical AD showed greater atrophy in the left hippocampus than those with PCA, while greater atrophy was noted in the right visual association cortex in cases of PCA than patients with typical

AD [13]. Higher levels of aggregation of neurofibrillary tangles and neuritic plaques have been found in the occipital and parietal cortices of PCA patients in contrast to the mediotemporal cortices of typical AD patients [14]. Apart from cortical pathology, white matter degeneration has been noted in atypical AD, including PCA [15].

Consistent with their neuroanatomical correlates, there are significant differences between PCA and typical AD in their effects on neurocognitive and functional performance.

In PCA, the progression of pathology usually involves worsening of visuospatial skills, while memory functions are relatively preserved during the beginning stages of the disease. Patients suspected of typical AD present with prominent memory difficulties for both visual and verbal information. Visual memory in patients with PCA might be impaired, but it is more likely associated with visuoperceptual and visuospatial processing difficulties, negating their abilities to encode accurately and effectively. Typical AD may have associated visuospatial difficulties, but their level of impairment is relatively milder than the prominent memory deficits, which are not the most salient presenting problems. Furthermore, patients with typical AD often present with executive dysfunction, such as deficits in reasoning, cognitive flexibility, and problem-solving, and their level of insight into their cognitive difficulties is usually impaired. In contrast, patients with PCA are more likely to have adequate or intact insight owing to their relatively preserved frontal/executive networks.

Neuropsychiatric disturbance is usually not an accompanying diagnostic feature for PCA. However, patients' relatively intact insight often leads to adjustment and emotional difficulties, such as depression and anxiety, which would present additional challenges in coping.

Of note, similar to patients in the initial stages of typical AD, individuals suspected of PCA based on disturbance in functional performance may not have positive/remarkable neuroimaging when they are first referred for evaluation. Their laboratory test results may be normal and not indicative of any particular underlying neuropathological or infectious disease processes. Genetic testing has not been utilized in diagnosis, although evidence for genetic risk factors has been provided [16].

There is limited specific information regarding treatment for this condition, but given the overlap with typical AD pathology, in the majority of patients, it is reasonable to initiate a trial of an acetylcholinesterase inhibitor. Other medications, depending upon associated symptoms, can also be considered such as antidepressants for mood disturbance associated with adjustment difficulties. Efforts to improve functional performance, such as use of reading aids to increase reading accuracy [17], would assist with adjustment. Given the early preservation of other abilities, such as language, memory, and insight, participation in physical and social activities, psychotherapy, and/or occupational and physical therapy may play a role in improving quality of life.

The disturbance in neurologic presentation, neurocognitive skills, and psychological functioning in any neurologic disorder highlights the importance of multidisciplinary collaboration in diagnosis and management. PCA's symptom constellation particularly calls for neurologists and neuropsychologists working together in differential diagnosis. The following is a case study on how these two disciplines came together during the assessment of a patient with suspected PCA.

Key Point
"When I need to do a Mini Mental Status Examination with a patient, sometimes the reason for their cognitive impairment is clear. However, most of the time, I do think about if he/she should also be seen by neuropsychology for assessment to clarify the extent and etiology of impairment or functional changes. Careful testing is essential to help sort out complex and at times overlapping syndromes and bring us closer to at least a reasonable working diagnosis."—Mark O. Herring, MD.

Case Study

The patient was a 58-year-old Caucasian woman with complaints of visual and mathematical problems. MRI performed around the time of the neurologic and neuropsychological evaluations revealed hyperintense T2 and FLAIR signal foci likely due to mild microvascular ischemic disease, but it was otherwise unremarkable.

History

The patient's early developmental history was reportedly unremarkable. She had a history of adrenal insufficiency which was reportedly treated successfully by naturopathic medications. She reported history of Lyme disease and celiac disease. She was asymptomatic at the time of the evaluation. Her family medical history was reportedly remarkable for diabetes mellitus II (paternal grandfather), astrocytoma (mother), heart disease (mother and brothers), and phlebitis (father).

The patient underwent psychotherapeutic treatment in the late 1990s to address bereavement and work-related stress. She denied history of psychopharmacological treatment. Her family psychiatric history was reportedly remarkable for bipolar disorder (paternal uncle). She denied history of significant use of alcohol, tobacco products, or recreational substances.

She completed 16 years of formal education. She graduated from university with a Bachelor's degree in accounting. She worked as a Certified Public Accountant until 5 years before the evaluation when she and her husband relocated to a different city. She was unemployed at the time of the evaluation. She had been looking after three vegetable gardens totaling 2000 square feet. She denied major difficulties in managing her vegetables but reported feeling "scattered and fragmented by all the chores." She was not planning to return to work.

Physician's Impression prior to Neuropsychological Testing

When I first saw the patient, she was able to provide very clear information on her problems, including recollections of details of previous office-based mental status testing. Her premorbid functioning was quite high and she previously had a high-level job. She began noticing symptoms in her late 40s or early 50s which included inability to calculate, trouble driving, misperceptions, and special challenges when driving in construction zones in the rain and in the dark. She had difficulty reacting to road signs and was getting lost. She had trouble reading phone numbers, tracking when reading (going from line to line), filling out forms, locating items, and playing Scrabble. She complained of difficulty focusing, slowness in her activities of daily living, and decline in her problem-solving ability. She reported preservation of other skills such as "the ability to argue well." She felt she no longer could work in accounting. She admitted to experiencing anxiety because of the problems she had observed.

Prior to seeing me for consultation, she was seen by her naturopathic physician for Lyme disease, roundworm, and tapeworm. She was also treated with bioequivalent hormones to aid in preventing Alzheimer's disease. She did have an eye exam, which resulted in prescription and use of glasses, but that did not help her visual symptoms. She initially had a relatively normal neurologic exam. Laboratory workup was remarkable only for elevated B6 level, which was felt to be secondary to her multiple supplements, including "brain enhancing" supplements that she was taking.

Neuropsychological testing was ordered because data on her neurocognitive functioning, especially information on the decline of her visuospatial abilities, would greatly assist in guiding diagnosis and treatment. Given unremarkable neuroimaging, we needed neuropsychology's input to localize pathologies. We also needed to rule out possibility of a psychogenic disorder.

> **Key Point**
> Neuropsychological evaluation is in a unique position to assess a patient's visuospatial and other neurocognitive abilities to guide diagnosis and treatment.

Neuropsychological Evaluation

Interview data: The patient stated that she had been experiencing significant problems in the visuospatial realm. She reported scanning difficulty that had led to frequent challenges in locating objects in the environment ("it is like I don't even see certain things!"). She had experienced challenges in painting and telling time from an analog clock. In addition, she reported visual memory problems, specifically, difficulties remembering where objects had been placed. She denied difficulties remembering verbally-mediated materials, such as conversations and instructions.

She denied forgetting her appointments, but her husband explained that she often required reminders to remember her appointments. He had also observed reduced level of endurance and more difficulties performing complicated or multi-step tasks.

With regard to day-to-day activities, the patient reported significant difficulties with driving, marked by problems in reading street signs and locating traffic lights. Consequently, she had limited her driving to familiar and short-distance routes. She denied difficulties in cooking, but her husband reported previous incidents of her leaving the stove on unattended. While they denied her having difficulties in managing finances, her husband stated he had taken over bill payments because it had become a time-consuming endeavor for her as she had difficulties placing information accurately on checks. She reportedly was not encountering difficulties in managing her medications.

While the patient shared that she began to experience cognitive difficulties during her 40s, her husband noticed a decline approximately 3 years prior to the evaluation after he returned from an extended leave. She denied noticing any possible precipitating medical and psychological factors. As a result of her difficulties, she reported increased levels of anxiety and frustration. Her husband added that her performance likely worsened when she felt anxious.

The patient reported a history of nightmares and hypnopompic hallucinations since her early 40s. She described a recent incident during which she woke up at night, looked out of the window, and saw "little pigs in the bushes." Her husband reported the frequency of her nighttime visual hallucination to be approximately once per month. She denied ongoing difficulties in sleep initiation or maintenance. She did not report changes in her olfactory functioning.

Behavioral observations: The patient's affect and behaviors were appropriate. She was occasionally tearful when discussing her difficulties. She required use of reading glasses. She utilized her right (dominant) hand for all motorically-mediated tasks. Abnormal movements, such as tremor and myoclonus, were not observed. Her speech was fluent with no evidence of word-finding difficulty or paraphasias. Her verbal comprehension was intact, although she often required repetition of test instructions of visuospatial tasks. Her thought processes were linear, logical, and goal-directed.

Throughout the testing session, she was easily engaged and cooperative. She did not exhibit distractibility. She worked at a slow to medium pace. She was persistent in her test-taking approach. On a task that required her to mark her answers on a bubble sheet, she was unaware of the erroneous placements of some of her responses, and she ultimately required a writer's assistance in going over those items with her and marking the necessary corrections. Her insight into her difficulties was good.

Approach to test selection: Given the referral question, a flexible, diagnostically driven approach was taken. Her initial signs of visuospatial difficulties led to a more extensive use of measures tapping into her visuoperceptual and visuospatial abilities. Instruments assessing domains other than her visuospatial skills were also administered to enable ruling in/out other potential neurologic disorders.

Test results: Consistent with difficulties noted by her and Dr. Herring, formal neurocognitive testing revealed prominent visuospatial deficits. Her visuoperception and visual scanning speed were severely impaired. Her speed of processing visual stimuli was moderately to severely impaired. Her visuoconstruction was moderately impaired. Her visual reasoning skills were mildly impaired. Her visual memory was marked by moderately impaired encoding and recall, with evidence of loss of previously learned information over time. Her visuospatial difficulties likely affected her performance on an unstructured problem-solving task that contained a significant visual component. Her completion time on a divided attention task was slow because of visual scanning impairment, but she did not make errors while following two sets of information concurrently. Her test responses did not reveal evidence of unilateral neglect/inattention.

In other domains, her basic auditory attention and working memory performance were average. Her language functions were generally intact, but her ability to verbally produce items from a specific category (in this case, animals) within a specific amount of time was moderately impaired. Her verbal memory was characterized by low average encoding and low average to average recall, likely below expectation. Her abstract verbal reasoning was superior. Motor testing demonstrated qualitatively weaker performance for her left hand, taking into account the effects of hand dominance.

She endorsed mild levels of anxiety and depression, likely associated with her insight into her problems.

Neuropsychologist's Impression Based on Formal Testing

The patient's significant deficits in the visuospatial realm suggested primary involvement of posterior cortical areas, with possibly more significant contributions from her right hemisphere, likely consistent with PCA. Her experience of visual hallucination raised the question of dementia with Lewy bodies. However, her prominent and circumscribed visually mediated deficits were much more impaired than the extent of the visuospatial difficulties often associated with dementia with Lewy bodies. Furthermore, there were no reports of Parkinsonian features, symptoms suggestive of REM sleep behavior disorder, or fluctuations in attention and arousal during the day, which are often-observed associated symptoms of dementia with Lewy bodies. Of note, approximately 25% of patients who met criteria for PCA reported occurrence of visual hallucinations [4]. Contributions associated with neuropsychological sequelae of Lyme disease, which primarily involve frontal systems dysfunction [18], appeared unlikely. Even though she endorsed mild levels of depressive and anxiety symptoms, emotional or psychological factors were not significant contributors to her deficits. Further decline in her functioning was felt to be likely.

Her relatively intact insight and verbal memory, within the setting of PCA, are consistent with what had previously been suggested [1]. Her nonspecific and unremarkable brain imaging may not necessarily indicate absence of neuropathology, as many patients with a suspected neurodegenerative disorder, such as AD, may present with unremarkable MRI or CT scans, especially during the initial stages of the disease.

Her prominent visuospatial deficits had negatively affected, and would likely continue to impact, her performance in instrumental activities of daily living. Furthermore, her difficulties would likely attenuate her ability to adapt and independently devise compensatory strategies, which would make ongoing adjustment and coping more difficult, especially taking into account her high premorbid level of intellectual functioning. It was felt that she would require increasing level of supervision over time as her condition would likely continue to worsen and she would find any task with a visuospatial component challenging.

Neuropsychologist's Recommendations for the Patient

It was recommended that she refrain from operating any motorized vehicles under any circumstances, regardless of travel distance.

She was encouraged to continue to participate and perform instrumental activities of daily living, but secondary to her prominent visuospatial deficits; she would likely require increasing level of supervision over time.

She was encouraged to consider participation in psychotherapy to assist with coping and adjustment, especially as she would likely continue to experience decline in her functioning.

She was encouraged to continue to consult with Dr. Herring for further evaluation and management of her neurologic condition. In addition, a referral to neuro-ophthalmology was recommended to assist in differential diagnoses such as ruling out Balint's syndrome.

Retesting in approximately 1–2 years was recommended to clarify differential diagnosis considerations.

Post-assessment Updates

She was subsequently referred to a tertiary care center, where a neuro-ophthalmologist and a neurologist, who is a specialist in neurocognition, ultimately made the diagnosis of PCA, noting the visuospatial deficits revealed by the neuropsychological evaluation and a 10-year-plus history of visuospatial difficulties including a self-diagnosis of prosopagnosia. Another MRI was performed, which was unremarkable. PET study documented abnormally low radiotracer uptake within the occipital and posterior parietal cortex bilaterally (right greater than left, consistent with neuropsychological data). CSF was remarkable for elevated phosphorylated tau levels. Prion diseases, such as Creutzfeldt-Jakob disease, were ruled out given the time course.

The patient subsequently demonstrated a left homonymous hemianopsia and had complaints of increasing visual difficulties, memory problems, trouble with facial recognition, irritability, emotional lability, and depression. She reported that her handwriting looked like dots and made no sense to her. She declined trials of acetylcholinesterase inhibitors. She noted progressively worsening sensitivity to light and sound and noted that food "felt different." She reached a point where she could no longer write checks. She could not read her own (or other's) handwriting.

Her husband graciously provided information on her end-stage presentation:

Her visuoperception continued to decline and she reportedly had approximately 25% of her vision left by the end of her life. She continued to have worsening visual processing problems. Her processing speed was significantly reduced.

Beyond the visuospatial realm, she was able to understand concepts, but she would require numerous repetitions to "get it." She suffered from word-finding difficulty. Her memory was said to be quite intact, even during the late stage of her illness.

From a physical standpoint, she began to have balance problems over time. She showed difficulties controlling movement in her arms and legs. She evidenced mild jerks towards the end of her life. She suffered from reduced sense of smell.

Emotionally, she experienced more difficulties controlling her emotions. She evidenced increased agitation. She seemed unwilling to face her diagnosis until 1.5 years after she underwent neuropsychological evaluation.

She eventually decided to pursue physician-assisted suicide in Switzerland and ultimately passed away 2 years after her neuropsychological evaluation, with friends and family by her bedside.

Further Resources

Due to the rarity of the syndrome, the patient's husband encountered difficulties obtaining information on the disorder and seeking peer support from other patients and their family members. He eventually became a member of a closed worldwide Facebook support group, which reportedly has been a much-valued source of information and support. It currently has more than 400 members. Access is granted by searching for "posterior cortical atrophy awareness" on the Facebook page and contacting the group directly.

In the United States, Alzheimer's Association offers disease information and local support groups. Patients and family members are encouraged to contact their local chapter, even if the primary diagnosis is a dementing disorder other than Alzheimer's disease. Their information can be found on their website (http://www.alz.org).

In London, United Kingdom, University College London Dementia Research Centre runs a support group for patients and their families who have been affected by PCA (http://www.raredementiasupport.org/pca/).

Chapter Review Questions

1. It is important to consider referral for neuropsychological testing when:
   A. Patients present with unexplained difficulties in navigating their familiar environments, such as bumping into things or having difficulty locating objects.
   B. Patients have difficulties in safely operating a motor vehicle within the setting of intact physical functioning.
   C. Patients have difficulties in safely operating a motor vehicle within the setting of intact physical functioning.
   D. A and B.

2. Apart from AD, what other neuropathological processes have been linked to PCA?
   A. Corticobasal degeneration, mild traumatic brain injury/concussion, and prion disease.
   B. Corticobasal degeneration, prion disease, and metabolic encephalopathy.
   C. Dementia with Lewy bodies, corticobasal degeneration, and prion disease.
   D. Dementia with Lewy bodies, prion disease, and frontotemporal dementia.

3. In PCA patients, their level of insight:
   A. Is severely impaired and they do not appreciate the scope of their functional difficulties.
   B. Is likely more intact than that of patients with AD.
   C. Is reduced because of their posterior cortical dysfunction.
   D. Is not usually associated with their level of adjustment and coping.

4. True/False: Visuospatial difficulties in PCA can affect a patient's ability to adapt and formulate compensatory strategies.

5. Neuroimaging studies during early part of the PCA disease process:
   A. Would reveal prominent atrophy in occipital and parietal lobes.
   B. May be unremarkable.
   C. Is currently a biomarker for PCA.

6. A collaborative approach involving multiple disciplines in diagnosing PCA:
   A. Would enhance diagnostic accuracy and enable more appropriate recommendations for patients and families.
   B. May increase likelihood of misdiagnosis of conversion disorder.
   C. May not add value in PCA differential diagnosis.
   D. Prolongs the diagnostic process unnecessarily.

Appendix 1 [6]

Core Features of the PCA Clinico-radiological Syndrome (Classification Level 1)

Clinical, cognitive, and neuroimaging features are rank ordered in terms of (decreasing) frequency at first assessment, as rated by online survey participants.

Clinical Features
Insidious onset
Gradual progression
Prominent early disturbance of visual +/– other posterior cognitive functions

Cognitive Features
At least three of the following must be present as early or presenting features +/– evidence of their impact on activities of daily living:

Space perception deficit
Simultanagnosia
Object perception deficit
Constructional dyspraxia
Environmental agnosia
Oculomotor apraxia
Dressing apraxia
Optic ataxia
Alexia
Left/right disorientation
Acalculia
Limb apraxia (not limb-kinetic)
Apperceptive prosopagnosia
Agraphia
Homonymous visual field defect
Finger agnosia

All of the following must be evident:

Relatively spared anterograde memory function
Relatively spared speech and nonvisual language functions
Relatively spared executive functions
Relatively spared behavior and personality

Neuroimaging

Predominant occipitoparietal or occipitotemporal atrophy/hypometabolism/hypoperfusion on MRI/FDG-PET/SPECT

Exclusion Criteria

Evidence of a brain tumor or other mass lesion sufficient to explain the symptoms
Evidence of significant vascular disease including focal stroke sufficient to explain the symptoms
Evidence of afferent visual cause (e.g., optic nerve, chiasm, or tract)
Evidence of other identifiable causes for cognitive impairment (e.g., renal failure)

Classification of PCA-Pure and PCA-Plus (Classification Level 2)

PCA-Pure

Individuals must fulfill the criteria for the core clinico-radiological PCA syndrome (level 1) and not fulfill core clinical criteria for any other neurodegenerative syndrome.

PCA-Plus

Individuals must fulfill the criteria for the core clinico-radiological PCA syndrome (level 1) and also fulfill core clinical criteria for at least one other neurodegenerative syndrome, such as dementia with Lewy bodies (DLB).

Following the diagnostic criteria proposed by the DLB consortium [19], individuals must exhibit two or more core features of DLBs (list A) or one or more core features (list A) and one or more suggestive features (list B):

A. Core features

- Fluctuating cognition with pronounced variations in attention and alertness
- Recurrent visual hallucinations that are typically well formed and detailed
- Spontaneous features of parkinsonism

B. Suggestive features

- Rapid eye movement (REM) sleep behavior disorder
- Severe neuroleptic sensitivity
- Low dopamine transporter uptake in basal ganglia demonstrated by SPECT or PET imaging

Corticobasal Syndrome (CBS)

Following the modified CBS criteria proposed by [20], a diagnosis of probable CBS requires asymmetric presentation of two of the following:

(a) Limb rigidity or akinesia
(b) Limb dystonia
(c) Limb myoclonus

plus two of the following:

(d) Orobuccal or limb apraxia
(e) Cortical sensory deficit
(f) Alien limb phenomena (more than simple levitation)

Possible corticobasal syndrome may be symmetric and requires presentation of one of a–c plus one of d–f.

Diagnostic Criteria for Disease-Level Descriptions (Classification Level 3)

PCA-AD

Following International Working Group (IWG2) [21], the classification of PCA-AD (and, by extension, of IWG2's broader category of "atypical AD") requires fulfillment of the PCA syndrome (classification level 1) plus in vivo evidence of Alzheimer's pathology (at least one of the following):

- Decreased $A\beta_{1-42}$ together with increased T-tau and/or P-tau in CSF
- Increased tracer retention on amyloid PET
- Alzheimer's disease autosomal-dominant mutation present (in *PSEN1*, *PSEN2*, or *APP*)

If autopsy confirmation of AD is available, the term definite PCA-AD would be appropriate.

PCA-LBD

Molecular biomarkers for LBD are currently unavailable; therefore, an in vivo diagnosis of PCA-LBD cannot be assigned at present. For individuals who are both classified as PCA-mixed by virtue of fulfilling DLB clinical criteria and shown to be AD-biomarker negative, the term probable PCA-LBD may be appropriate. If autopsy confirmation of LBD is available, the term definite PCA-LBD would be appropriate. Other disease-level classifications may also be appropriate for individuals with mixed or multiple pathologies (e.g., PCA-AD/LBD).

PCA-CBD

Molecular biomarkers for CBD are currently unavailable; therefore, an in vivo diagnosis of PCA-CBD cannot be assigned at present. For individuals who are both classified as PCA-mixed by virtue of fulfilling CBS criteria and shown to be AD-biomarker negative, the term probable PCA-CBD may be appropriate. If autopsy confirmation of CBD is available, the term definite PCA-CBD would be appropriate.

PCA-Prion

There are a number of promising biomarkers for prion disease (e.g., [22–24]), but these have yet to be incorporated into diagnostic criteria. Pending this process, an in vivo diagnosis of PCA-prion may be feasible. If autopsy confirmation of prion disease is available or a known genetic form of prion disease has been determined, the term definite PCA-prion would be appropriate.

From: Crutch SJ, Schott JM, Rabinovici GD, et al. Consensus classification of posterior cortical atrophy [6].

References

1. Crutch SJ, Lehmann M, Schott JM, Rabinovici GD, Rossor MN, Fox NC. Posterior cortical atrophy. Lancet Neurol. 2012;11(2):170–8.
2. Shakespeare TJ, Yong KX, Foxe D, Hodges J, Crutch SJ. Pronounced impairment of everyday skills and self-care in posterior cortical atrophy. J Alzheimers Dis. 2015;43(2):381–4.
3. Mendez MF, Ghajarania M, Perryman KM. Posterior cortical atrophy: clinical characteristics and differences compared to Alzheimer's disease. Dement Geriatr Cogn Disord. 2002;14(1):33–40.
4. Tang-Wai DF, Graff-Radford NR, Boeve BF, et al. Clinical, genetic, and neuropathologic characteristics of posterior cortical atrophy. Neurology. 2004;63(7):1168–74.
5. Crutch SJ, Schott JM, Rabinovici GD, et al. Shining a light on posterior cortical atrophy. Alzheimers Dement. 2013;9(4):463–5.
6. Crutch SJ, Schott JM, Rabinovici GD, et al. Consensus classification of posterior cortical atrophy. Alzheimers Dement. 2017;13(8):870–84.
7. Renner JA, Burns JM, Hou CE, McKeel DW, Storandt M, Morris JC. Progressive posterior cortical dysfunction: a clinicopathologic series. Neurology. 2004;63(7):1175–80.
8. Tang-Wai DF, Josephs KA, Boeve BF, Dickson DW, Parisi JE, Petersen RC. Pathologically confirmed corticobasal degeneration presenting with visuospatial dysfunction. Neurology. 2003;61(8):1134–5.
9. Ropper AH, Samuels MA, Klein J. Adams and Victor's principles of neurology. 10th ed. New York: McGraw-Hill Education Medical; 2014.
10. Lehmann M, Crutch SJ, Ridgway GR, et al. Cortical thickness and voxel-based morphometry in posterior cortical atrophy and typical Alzheimer's disease. Neurobiol Aging. 2011;32(8):1466–76.
11. Migliaccio R, Agosta F, Rascovsky K, et al. Clinical syndromes associated with posterior atrophy: early age at onset AD spectrum. Neurology. 2009;73(19):1571–8.

12. Nestor PJ, Caine D, Fryer TD, Clarke J, Hodges JR. The topography of metabolic deficits in posterior cortical atrophy (the visual variant of Alzheimer's disease) with FDG-PET. J Neurol Neurosurg Psychiatry. 2003;74(11):1521–9.
13. Whitwell JL, Jack CR, Kantarci K, et al. Imaging correlates of posterior cortical atrophy. Neurobiol Aging. 2007;28(7):1051–61.
14. Hof PR, Vogt BA, Bouras C, Morrison JH. Atypical form of Alzheimer's disease with prominent posterior cortical atrophy: a review of lesion distribution and circuit disconnection in cortical visual pathways. Vision Res. 1997;37(24):3609–25.
15. Caso F, Agosta F, Mattavelli D, et al. White Matter Degeneration in Atypical Alzheimer Disease. Radiology. 2015;277(1):162–72.
16. Schott JM, Crutch SJ, Carrasquillo MM, et al. Genetic risk factors for the posterior cortical atrophy variant of Alzheimer's disease. Alzheimers Dement. 2016;12(8):862–71.
17. Yong KX, Rajdev K, Shakespeare TJ, Leff AP, Crutch SJ. Facilitating text reading in posterior cortical atrophy. Neurology. 2015;85(4):339–48.
18. Westervelt HJ, McCaffrey RJ. Neuropsychological functioning in chronic Lyme disease. Neuropsychol Rev. 2002;12(3):153–77.
19. IG MK, Dickson DW, Lowe J, Emre M, O'Brien JT, Feldman H, Cummings J, Duda JE, Lippa C, Perry EK, Aarsland D, Arai H, Ballard CG, Boeve B, Burn DJ, Costa D, Del Ser T, Dubois B, Galasko D, Gauthier S, Goetz CG, Gomez-Tortosa E, Halliday G, Hansen LA, Hardy J, Iwatsubo T, Kalaria RN, Kaufer D, Kenny RA, Korczyn A, Kosaka K, Lee VM, Lees A, Litvan I, Londos E, Lopez OL, Minoshima S, Mizuno Y, Molina JA, Mukaetova-Ladinska EB, Pasquier F, Perry RH, Schulz JB, Trojanowski JQ, Yamada M, Consortium on DLB. Diagnosis and management of dementia with Lewy bodies: third report of the DLB Consortium. Neurology. 2005;65:1863–72.
20. Armstrong MJ, Litvan I, Lang AE, Bak TH, Bhatia KP, Borroni B, Boxer AL, Dickson DW, Grossman M, Hallett M, Josephs KA, Kertesz A, Lee SE, Miller BL, Reich SG, Riley DE, Tolosa E, Tröster AI, Vidailhet M, Weiner WJ. Criteria for the diagnosis of corticobasal degeneration. Neurology. 2013;80:496–503.
21. Dubois B, Feldman HH, Jacova C, Hampel H, Molinuevo JL, Blennow K, DeKosky ST, Gauthier S, Selkoe D, Bateman R, Cappa S, Crutch S, Engelborghs S, Frisoni GB, Fox NC, Galasko D, Habert MO, Jicha GA, Nordberg A, Pasquier F, Rabinovici G, Robert P, Rowe C, Salloway S, Sarazin M, Epelbaum S, de Souza LC, Vellas B, Visser PJ, Schneider L, Stern Y, Scheltens P, Cummings JL. Advancing research diagnostic criteria for Alzheimer's disease: the IWG-2 criteria. Lancet Neurol. 2014;13:614–29.
22. CD1 O, Bongianni M, Tonoli G, Ferrari S, Hughson AG, Groveman BR, Fiorini M, Pocchiari M, Monaco S, Caughey B, Zanusso G. A test for Creutzfeldt-Jakob disease using nasal brushings. N Engl J Med. 2014;371(6):519–29.
23. Jackson GS, Burk-Rafel J, Edgeworth JA, Sicilia A, Abdilahi S, Korteweg J, Mackey J, Thomas C, Wang G, Mead S, Collinge J. A highly specific blood test for vCJD. Blood. 2014;123(3):452–3.
24. McGuire LI, Peden AH, Orrú CD, Wilham JM, Appleford NE, Cbiol GM, Andrews M, Head MW, Caughey B, Will RG, Knight RSG, Green AJE. RT-QuIC analysis of cerebrospinal fluid in sporadic Creutzfeldt-Jakob disease. Ann Neurol. 2012;72(2):278–85.

Chapter 14
Dementia with Lewy Bodies

Jacqueline Phillips-Sabol and Dimitrios A. Nacopoulos

Introduction

Dementia with Lewy bodies (DLB) is a type of dementia that falls under the heading of atypical parkinsonian/movement disorders or "Parkinson's Plus" disorders, referring to findings that patients with Parkinson's Plus syndromes have movement symptoms (parkinsonism) "plus" other symptoms. This fascinating group of movement disorders, which have cognitive symptoms that progress into dementias, includes, in addition to DLB, such disorders as cortical-basal ganglionic degeneration (CBD), progressive supranuclear palsy (PSP), and multiple system atrophy (MSA). These syndromes can be difficult to distinguish from one another, especially in earlier or prodromal stages. In addition, DLB is most often misdiagnosed as Parkinson's disease (PD) when abnormalities of movement are present and due to the fact that, to many physicians, the movement symptoms of DLB may look similar to PD and may respond to dopaminergic medications. However, these medications can cause significant psychiatric side effects not seen in early treatment of PD with dopaminergic medications. Although DLB is typically ranked as the second or third most common type of dementia, depending on the source [1], DLB continues to be a lesser-known type of dementia in comparison to Alzheimer's disease (AD) and vascular dementia (VaD).

J. Phillips-Sabol (✉)
Neuropsychology Speciality and Consultants, Erie, PA, USA
e-mail: DrSabol@NPSpecialty.com

D. A. Nacopoulos
Department of Neurology, UPMC School of Medicine, Pittsburgh, PA, USA

K. M. Sanders (ed.), *Physician's Field Guide to Neuropsychology*,
https://doi.org/10.1007/978-1-4939-8722-1_14

Overview of Dementia with Lewy Bodies

Dementia with Lewy bodies tends to present (as with other dementias) between the ages of 60 and 80, but it can occasionally present earlier. The progression tends to be more rapid than that of Alzheimer's disease, with an average survival of approximately 8 years. Diagnosis of DLB can be challenging due to the presence of movement symptoms and cognitive symptoms. It is not uncommon for the disorder to be misdiagnosed as Parkinson's disease (PD) or Parkinson's disease with dementia (PDD), especially when movement symptoms are prominent. DLB can sometimes be misdiagnosed as another type of dementia, such as Alzheimer's disease (AD), especially when the patient's cognitive symptoms are more prominent and movement symptoms are either not tested or very subtle during motor exam. "Memory problems" are a frequent complaint of patients and family members who are not familiar with the possible reasons that deficits in other cognitive domains, such as attention or comprehension, may seem like memory difficulty to them, leading them to explain many different cognitive symptoms as "memory problems" to providers. This contributes to inaccurate overdiagnosis of AD.

The name "Dementia with Lewy Bodies" refers to the pathology of DLB in which Lewy bodies are observed in the cortical and subcortical regions of the brain [2, 3]. Patients with DLB demonstrate various neuropsychological difficulties and psychiatric symptoms. However, greater difficulty is typically seen on measures of visual processing, attention, and some areas of executive function, with typical memory being less affected [4, 5]. Parahippocampal and temporal lobe Lewy bodies typically correlate with greater cognitive dysfunction. Diffusion tensor imaging (DTI) studies have demonstrated that patients with DLB tend to have decreased integrity of white matter in areas that correlate well with the pattern of cognitive deficits, including in the occipitoparietal and frontal white matter connections [6, 7]. In addition, the degree of change in neurotransmitters, including acetylcholine and dopamine, impacts cognitive function and psychiatric features. Decreased cerebral blood flow has been associated with correlating cognitive deficits [8]. Core diagnostic features of DLB, in addition to cognitive decline/dementia, include a triad of symptoms that can appear in DLB, in addition to other suggestive/supportive symptoms. This triad consists of spontaneous parkinsonism, cognitive fluctuations, and hallucinations. While knowledge of these features is helpful and the features have high specificity for DLB, they have low sensitivity, with many patients with DLB being misdiagnosed because a clinician may only be looking for a combination of the core features for diagnosis. Many clinicians rely on visual hallucinations for diagnosis, and the issue of cognitive fluctuations is difficult to conceptualize or quantify [9]. Cases of DLB are often misdiagnosed when visual hallucinations are not apparent. Recent revision of the criteria for the diagnosis of DLB [10] added REM sleep behavior disorder (RBD) to the core symptoms. Cognitive decline/dementia (not necessarily with prominent memory involvement) is an essential feature for the diagnosis of DLB. Cognitive declines in DLB may occur prior to other symptoms being present/apparent. The cognitive pattern of DLB, as identified during neuropsychological evaluation, increases correct diagnosis. Patients with DLB have a pattern of visuospatial deficits, especially for visuoconstructional tasks; difficulty with working memory and complex attention; memory declines that are not as severe as Alzheimer's disease but are below expectation; slowed processing speed (especially on tasks requiring visual processing); and executive dysfunction. Patients with DLB tend to have difficulty with cognitive flexibility, such as is required in switching between two different sets. Relatively speaking, language functions may remain reasonably intact until late in the disease [11].

Misdiagnosis of DLB with subsequent treatment with the inappropriate medications can have severe and even life-threatening consequences in patients with DLB. Dopaminergic medications used to treat PD can cause serious exacerbations of psychotic symptoms, while typical and some atypical antipsychotics used to treat delusions and hallucinations can cause severe, sometimes life-threatening exacerbations of motor symptoms in DLB. Treatment of hallucinations and psychosis in dementia with Lewy bodies may sometimes only safely respond to particular atypical antipsychotics, including quetiapine and clozapine, although evidence is mixed on efficacy [12]. A newer non-dopaminergic medication called pimavanserin, which is a serotonergic medication, is likely safe in dementia with Lewy bodies and PDD [13], but efficacy studies are lacking. The cognitive profile of DLB can be difficult to distinguish from AD and PDD, especially on basic screening measures. Patients started on anticholinesterase inhibitors may experience a dramatic response due to a significant brain cholinergic deficit in dementia with Lewy bodies, a response that should raise suspicion clinically of DLB rather than Alzheimer's dementia [14]. A diagnostic test of dopaminergic function can be pursued with functional brain imaging testing. Dopamine transporter scan (DaT scan) can reflect a deficit in the dopaminergic uptake signal in the caudate and putamen, indicating a degenerative dopaminergic process assisting in differentiating DLB from some other types of dementia [10]. However, specificity of DaT scan is not as helpful in differentiating dementia with Lewy bodies from Parkinson's disease, as both have a loss of dopamine signal. Bilateral putaminal loss is generally thought to be reflective of DLB [10]. Patients with cognitive complaints should routinely undergo neuropsychological evaluation by neuropsychologists with sufficient experience in differential diagnosis of dementias and DLB.

Purpose of the Neuropsychological Evaluation

Neuropsychologists conduct a detailed assessment of cognitive functioning in cognitive domains, such as attention, language, memory, visuospatial ability, and executive functioning. These tests are designed to evaluate the functional integrity of different brain areas and different brain processes. These processes interact with each other and affect one another. For example, poor attention may appear to the patient, to the family members, and to the treating physician to be a memory-based dementia. When significant attentional difficulties are identified during testing, treatments and strategies recommended to improve attention typically assist in improving memory also. Difficulties with language are also frequently misattributed to memory problems. Just as an MRI may be performed in order to determine if brain areas *look* the way they are supposed to look, neuropsychological assessment determines if brain areas are *actually functioning* the way they should be. Because information from neuropsychological assessment provides an "active" picture of how the brain is functioning, and many people continue to be able to function normally despite the finding of some abnormalities on their brain MRI, neuropsychological findings with valid results trump imaging findings. It is also known that neuropsychological testing frequently identifies abnormalities prior to changes showing up on MRIs. Patients with significant pathology on brain MRI may show minimal decline in cognitive and functional ability. Neuropsychological evaluation includes an in-depth interview of symptoms and the timeline of symptom presentation and neurobehavioral observations (which may include an in-depth structured neurobehavioral examination of cognitive processes and brain areas required for things such as complex movements, which assist in building hypotheses regarding etiology), followed by formal standardized testing of cognitive abilities. The neuropsychologist comprehensively examines the cognitive, neurobehavioral, and psychiatric profile to determine which etiology/etiologies the pattern of cognitive and neurological symptoms best fits and identifies the most likely diagnosis/diagnoses. Treatments and interventions are recommended to the referring physician and to the patient and family members. The cognitive pattern also assists in determining the patient's ability to safely perform everyday tasks, such as driving, working, or managing medications. Comorbid contributors, such as a mood disorder or monetary secondary gain, are also evaluated and taken into consideration.

Neurology Case Presentation

Referral (Initial)

Patient: 69-year-old, right-handed male
Education: Master of Business Administration; Occupation: Retired accountant
Presenting problem: Reported cognitive decline. Patient presented with his wife, who requested evaluation by a neurologist.

History

The patient's spouse reported significant confusion after a recent colonoscopy that was performed secondary to severe constipation. He had significant anxiety following this procedure and believed that there was another family living with them when they returned home from the test. He was also somewhat slower to respond during conversation. These were new issues but resolved back to baseline after several weeks. He is reportedly able to perform activities of daily living, such as managing a checkbook, although it is more difficult. He is able to do yard work and continues to be able to operate a riding lawn mower. The patient's wife expressed some concern regarding his driving ability, such as not being able to park between the lines in their church parking lot. The patient and his wife have noticed some memory decline. The patient denied getting lost while driving.

The patient's wife stated that he is becoming more isolated in his activities and is more anxious around a group of long-standing friends and at family functions. His wife stated that at times her husband appears withdrawn and quieter than usual, but this fluctuates. The patient's wife also reported that at times he is somewhat obsessed with the thought of mice he has reportedly seen in different rooms of the house (patient's wife has not seen mice or any evidence of them). The patient's health was otherwise in good condition, and he was not taking any other medications. His wife reported some sleep changes, stating that her husband has been thrashing in his sleep during dreams. The patient endorsed some mild problems with balance and mobility (which he felt were age-related), including trouble getting out of a chair. His wife also stated that when they visited their daughter in Orlando, he was slow and lingered behind the rest of the family at the amusement park. He denied any falls.

Past Medical History

The patient suffered a back injury during military service in Vietnam, which resulted in mild intermittent periods of lower back pain. Additionally, he has a history of mild hypertension, which has improved in the past few years without medications. He has taken over-the-counter medications in the past for occasional seasonal allergies, but these reportedly made him sleepy and mentally confused.

Social History

The patient is a 69-year-old retired accountant who owned an accounting firm. He has an MBA and is a certified public accountant. After serving in the military, he went to college and married at age 26. He has three adult children and five grandchildren. He denies significant alcohol intake ("only on special occasions") and reports nicotine/smoking use for 2 years during the time of his military service. He denied prior or current substance abuse.

Family History

There is a family history of cardiac disease in the patient's father. No significant neurological history in the family was endorsed.

Neurological Exam and Findings

- The patient appeared in good physical health, was not obese, and participated in the exam. He had normal vital signs. His mood was normal, but his affect was mildly flat at times.
- He had some difficulty with executive function on Montreal Cognitive Assessment (MoCA), including a poorly drawn cube, and some mild difficulty in understanding the correct placement of hands on a clock, but with prompting, he self-corrected. Slowness in repetition was noted, but language was fluent. He had mild inattentiveness on serial 7s, missing one of the numbers in sequence. He was able to recall 4 of 5 items from memory. His total MoCA score was 26 out of 30.
- Physical exam demonstrated slight stiffness in the muscles of the neck and arms bilaterally with some failure to relax.
- A very slight positional tremor was noted in the right hand with arms outstretched.
- He had slight slowness in movement during hand opening and closing bilaterally. He had normal reflexes and normal strength.
- Sensation was preserved.
- His gait was slightly slowed and somewhat stiff with decreased stride length, turn was en bloc and slightly unsteady, but he walked independently without difficulty.

Labs and Imaging

- Based on his testing and examination, workup included vitamin B12 serum levels, TSH, and free T4, which were all normal.
- His MRI brain study demonstrated normal age-related atrophic changes, minimally more prevalent in the temporoparietal and parahippocampal/hippocampal regions, but not impressively so. No significant white matter disease noted and no acute processes.

Physician's Impression and Referral for Neuropsychological Testing

Given the clinical history and medical examination, the differentials included mild cognitive impairment; pseudodementia secondary to mood disorder, such as depression or anxiety; or another neurodegenerative condition, such as Alzheimer's dementia, dementia with Lewy bodies, or frontotemporal dementia (FTD). Given the patient's history of exacerbation of cognitive dysfunction with medication, there was also consideration of normal cognitive function with cognitive side effects from medication. The patient also has poor sleep, and this was viewed as a possible contribution to the presentation of perceived cognitive impairment.

Given the difficulties in biomarkers for determining differentiation of cognitive impairment as a result of true degeneration versus pseudodementia as a result of a mood disorder, a neuropsychological evaluation was recommended. The differentiation of types of dementia was also a factor in referral for neuropsychological assessment, given that the patient did not have the typical profile of pronounced difficulty with short-term memory recall observed in Alzheimer's dementia. The patient only demonstrated mild executive-type difficulties on mental status exam.

Given the presence of reported memory problems, an acetylcholinesterase inhibitor was initiated. Clonazepam was prescribed for the sleep issues.

Physician Perspective

> **Key Point**
> In-office mental status screening is not sufficient to distinguish between neurodegenerative syndromes or to acquire a detailed profile of cognitive functioning and ability.

The patient's score on the Montreal Cognitive Assessment was not reflective of significant cognitive decline despite significant cognitive complaints by the patient and his wife. Scores on in-office screening measures may lead physicians to false conclusions as to whether cognition is intact or not. Physicians have a limited amount of time in which to obtain background information and perform medical exams and mental status screening. When there is cause for cognitive concern, the standard of care is referral for neuropsychological evaluation.

> **Key Point**
> Neuropsychological evaluation provides a much more intensive and detailed assessment of cognitive functioning with testing of cognitive ability than what is capable during medical provider office visits. Neuropsychologists evaluate differences in cognitive patterns and neurobehavioral presentations in order to determine probable etiologies of cognitive decline and provide impressions to the referring physician, with appropriate recommendations. Cognitive issues are explained in detail to the patient and family members.

Neuropsychological Assessment

Chief Complaints and Interview Information

The patient was interviewed with his wife, who assisted in providing historical information. The couple reported that the patient began having difficulty approximately 2 years prior to evaluation. However, the patient had a period of worsening cognitive status following a recent medical procedure during which he was under light sedation. He slowly returned to baseline. The patient's wife reported that her husband was recently unable to count out $0.60 worth of change (patient is a retired accountant). He has been managing the checkbook, but it has become more difficult for him, and she is concerned that he may be making mistakes. There has been some reported memory decline, which has been progressive. The patient is sometimes repeating questions and information from day to day. The patient was recently put on Exelon by the neurologist due to memory concerns, and the patient and his wife stated that it was noticeably helpful. The patient endorsed increasing word-finding problems, and this was occasionally observed during interview. The patient reported that he also finds it more difficult to plan things step by step and is deferring decision making to his wife.

With regard to instrumental activities of daily living, the patient is still driving, and he and his wife stated that he has had some difficulty with accurately parking the car and staying squarely in his lane while driving. He denied becoming lost or disoriented while driving. He no longer drives at night. As noted, the patient is having some difficulty making correct change, and there has been a decline in his ability to do projects around the home as well. His wife assists in managing his medications. The patient has been involved in several hobbies in the past, including golfing and fishing, but his activities have decreased significantly, and he has less desire to engage in social events. The patient is clumsier with a tendency to run into door frames or knock things over. Although he is reportedly independent in basic activities of daily living, his wife reported that she now has to cue him to take showers.

Key Point
At this point in the history, it is readily apparent how easily DLB can be misdiagnosed as other types of dementia. Patients coming from primary care physicians or general neurologists typically have referral information containing some of the above-noted symptoms.

The patient also reported changes in motor function. There have been no falls, but near falls were reported. He and his wife reported intermittent right-hand tremor, which is most pronounced in an action state. Mild bilateral action tremor was noted on fine motor tasks during testing such as placing pegs. A very mild resting tremor was noted in the patient's right hand during interview. The patient endorsed that it is more difficult for him to speak. He also reportedly becomes light-headed when he stands up, and he is slower to rise from a chair.

Key Point
The previous paragraph illustrates typical referral information contained in neurological exams and also illustrates how patients with DLB can easily be misdiagnosed with PD or essential tremor (ET).

With regard to his personality and emotional functioning, the patient and his wife reported that there has been a significant change in the patient's personality. His wife stated that he used to be very social and is no longer "outgoing." He is also more withdrawn and more emotional and tearful. The patient's wife also reported significant fluctuations in her husband's state, reporting that at times he appears almost stuporous and other times he is mostly himself. The patient has also had a new onset of anxiety, which is most pronounced at night. He has had one panic attack. The patient and his wife noted that the patient's mood and fluctuations have improved since the patient was prescribed Exelon by the referring neurologist. The patient has a history of vivid dreaming but more recently developed REM behavior disorder. The patient's wife reported that this has improved since initiation of Klonopin. The patient denied being depressed but stated that he feels more emotional in general and gets frustrated when he cannot do things.

Key Point
The preceding paragraph notes symptoms that might typically accompany a referral from psychiatry and features mood symptoms and personality changes that might be mistaken for depression or anxiety, and other features that might be misdiagnosed as frontotemporal dementia (FTD), including requiring cues to shower.

There is a reported recent history of visual illusions/hallucinations that occur both during the night and in the day. The patient reported that he will wake up in the middle of the night and "see a small child floating in the air or sitting in the chair." After his recent medical procedure, he believed that another family was living in the home, but this resolved. Although these hallucinations could be hypnopompic, both the patient and his wife reported that the patient appears to be fully awake during these events and even reaches for the person. The patient has more definitive visual hallucinations during the day where he sees spiders and bugs crawling on the curtains and blinds, but he realizes that they are not real. He also frequently thinks that he sees mice out of the corner of his eye and is somewhat overly focused on the possibility of mice in the house. The patient also complained of hallucinations where the tiles on the floor rise up to shoulder level and he can see the subfloor underneath the tiles. There are significant cognitive fluctuations and inertia which have decreased since the patient was prescribed Exelon, which both patient and wife stated has been helpful. He denied suicidal ideation, intent, or plan.

Key Point

The preceding paragraph features symptoms that are easily confused for psychosis due to other etiologies, which could lead to treatment with a typical or atypical neuroleptic, possibly leading to dangerous or life-threatening side effects in patients with DLB. It is not uncommon for DLB patients who present to emergency departments or provider's offices to be administered antipsychotic medications, especially when these symptoms are prominent and upsetting and lead patients and family members to emphasize these symptoms while not mentioning other symptoms that may be important for differential diagnosis.

Neurobehavioral Exam and Behavioral Observations: The patient was casually dressed and appropriately groomed. He was alert and oriented to person, place, date, and time. His speech was spontaneous, fluent, and goal-directed but lacked significant reciprocity and was somewhat soft. Mild word-finding difficulties were noted. Comprehension appeared intact. Mild cogwheel rigidity in the upper extremities was present and increased with augmentation (R > L). There was retropulsion and anteropulsion with slight tugs. Gait was observed to be slowed, with mild en bloc turning. There was mildly decreased arm swing bilaterally (R > L). There was a glabellar reflex, but no other frontal release signs. The patient had difficulty with three-step hand sequences bilaterally, and mild oral-motor apraxia was observed. The patient had mild hypomimia and mildly decreased blink, but mood was reported as generally "improved" since his primary care physician recently prescribed Effexor. There were frequent instances of perseverations and intrusions during testing, and the patient utilized relatively simple strategies to solve problems. The patient was mildly slow to respond to questions and requests.

Test Selection: Tests were selected to narrow and rule out several neurodegenerative processes, including atypical parkinsonian syndromes.

Test Results

The patient had deficits in several cognitive domains. Intellectual functioning was average, with lower scores on nonverbal IQ subtests than verbal subtests.

Attention was variable, with simple auditory attention and tasks involving visuomotor number sequencing mildly below expectation, while attentional ability to rapidly read simple words, identify colors, or arrange number sequences was impaired.

Significant visuoconstructional deficits were noted on a task requiring the patient to draw a clock and copy geometric designs. The designs were highly distorted. The clock was distorted as well, and the patient incorrectly drew pentagons that intersected. The patient's clock face did not improve after observing the examiner draw a clock. The patient also had difficulty on a task reproducing three-dimensional designs using blocks. Processing speed was slow overall but worse for tasks requiring visual processing. A test of moving discs on pegs to match a picture was performed very slowly, and the patient had difficulty with more complex constructions.

Verbal memory testing was mildly below expectation. The patient's ability to recall words on a list was low average and the patient made word intrusions from another word list while recalling the learned word list. Visual memory for geometric figures was at the low end of low average for designs he had viewed six times. These scores are below expectation for age, education, and occupation, but are not impaired.

Language abilities were mildly below expectation. The patient was able to name objects but had mild word-finding difficulty with occasional paraphasias during verbal interactions. Ability to rapidly name words from a category was also mildly below expectation.

Very mild depression and anxiety were reported on mood measures and were not considered to have affected cognitive scores.

Neuropsychological Profile of Dementia with Lewy Bodies

The pathology in DLB reflects a greater degree and likelihood of Lewy bodies in cortical areas versus Lewy bodies primarily within the brain stem, as in Parkinson's disease (PD) and Parkinson's disease with dementia (PDD). While it would seem logical, the degree of cortical Lewy body pathology does not seem to correlate well with the degree of cognitive deficits or dementia. Research tends to support that cognitive symptoms and degree of dementia worsen as the load of parahippocampal Lewy body densities increases [3]. Cognition is also significantly affected in patients with DLB by reductions in cortical acetylcholine and with the presence of hallucinations [15].

The pattern of cognitive deficits in DLB is fairly distinct, with visuoconstructional and attentional declines being quite prominent. As noted earlier, memory decline is present, but memory difficulty is not as pronounced as in Alzheimer's disease (AD) and is related more to attentional and other dysfunctions than the typical severe encoding deficits observed in AD. Memory deficits tend to worsen as the disorder progresses. It should be noted that DLB and AD pathology can be present in the same patient, which is not uncommon. Language, such as naming and verbal fluency, may be well preserved in the initial stages of the disorder but decline as DLB progresses. Visual hallucinations/illusions are a common feature, but the disorder has a tendency to be misdiagnosed when hallucinations are not present but movement symptoms are. Another early feature is REM behavioral disorder (RBD).

As noted in key criteria of the disorder, RBD is common in DLB, but it is not uncommon in other movement disorders. DLB and Parkinson's disease with dementia (PDD) tend to have a very similar cognitive profile once dementia has developed. However, it is generally accepted that DLB is not diagnosed unless significant cognitive declines/dementia develop within the first 12 months (debate regarding relevant time period continues) after the emergence of movement symptoms [11]. PDD tends to not develop until well into the course of PD. Patients with PD who develop dementia in less than 10 years tend to have more of a resemblance to DLB. Hallucinations are often the telltale sign of DLB while hallucinations are generally not present in PD until increasing amounts of dopaminergic medications are required. Hallucinations are not uncommon in PDD, most likely due to the spread of Lewy body pathology and the necessary use of dopaminergic medications to control severe Parkinson's symptoms.

Neuropsychological Impressions

The neurocognitive symptom presentation and profile are most consistent with dementia with Lewy bodies [5, 11]. The patient's most prominent declines were in the areas of visuoperceptual/visuoconstructional skills and decreased attention, with memory and language mildly below expectation but more preserved. Slowed processing speed was noted, both in responding to interview questions and on testing. Executive issues were noted on testing and on neurobehavioral planning of three-step motor commands in addition to difficulty with attention and mental tracking. There is evidence of cognitive declines combined with motor issues, as identified by the neurologist on neurological exam and during the neurobehavioral exam. Psychiatric symptoms were also consistent with DLB, including new onset of hallucinations and mood symptoms. The patient was embarrassed to talk about the visual hallucinations and stated that the extent of the hallucinations had not previously been disclosed. The patient demonstrates the classic DLB triad of parkinsonism, cognitive fluctuations, and hallucinations [16], in addition to the core feature of RBD. Significant improvement of both behavioral (hallucinations) and cognitive (fluctuations and attention/memory) symptoms with the initiation of rivastigmine is more specific to DLB than to AD or other dementias. Rivastigmine is quite helpful [17] to the point of being almost diagnostic of the disorder in some cases because the deficit of acetylcholine in DLB is more pronounced than in other dementias, including Alzheimer's dementia [14], for which the medication was originally developed. McKeith et al. [18] found that cognitive and behavioral symptoms of DLB responded well to rivastigmine, with more than half the sample experiencing nearly complete resolution of psychotic symptoms. More than 63% of patients with dementia with Lewy bodies improved a minimum of 30% compared to baseline. Attention and reaction time also improved significantly [19].

Collaborative Discussion

Dementia with Lewy bodies (DLB) can be among the most difficult of dementias for physicians to recognize. Office mental status exams and other brief bedside measures are not effective in differentiating between DLB and other types of dementias [20]. Often this is a diagnosis for which only neurologists who specialize in movement disorders have significant familiarity. When movement disorder specialists suspect DLB (as with other dementias), a referral for neuropsychological evaluation with a neuropsychologist familiar with DLB is standard of care. As previously noted, given the complexity of cognitive, psychiatric, and movement symptoms, the disorder is easily misdiagnosed, and treatment with the wrong medications can lead to serious side effects. In this case, although the patient presented with mild parkinsonian symptoms and cognitive decline, the pattern of cognitive decline required identification while taking the other symptoms into account as well. It is noted that movement symptoms can occur in other types of dementia, including frontotemporal dementias.

Key Point
Neuropsychological evaluation assisted in accurate diagnosis and confirmed treatment with appropriate medication. As an added diagnostic step, a (dopamine transporter) DaT scan was ordered by the neurologist following neuropsychological evaluation. The DaT scan was consistent with probable Lewy body disease.

Rivastigmine is the first-line treatment for patients with DLB. DLB patients commonly have symptoms of both parkinsonism and hallucinations. However, they are exquisitely sensitive to dopaminergics and other medications used to treat Parkinson's disease, especially to amantadine, anticholinergics, and dopamine agonists. Although levodopa may improve movement symptoms, there is a pronounced risk of a resulting exacerbation of psychotic symptoms [21, 22]. In addition, if psychotic symptoms are treated with typical or even some atypical antipsychotics, it can lead to severe muscular rigidity, with the inability to move and possible life-threatening neuroleptic malignant syndrome [1].

Fortunately, treatment with rivastigmine frequently improves cognitive and psychotic symptoms. If psychotic symptoms remain, a very small amount of quetiapine or clozapine can be added because they have the best extrapyramidal side-effect profile, with less of a tendency to aggravate parkinsonism. Clozapine requires regular blood monitoring and remains controversial due to risk of agranulocytosis, although this risk is very low [1]. Pimavanserin, a newer agent, can also be added with relative safety. If motor symptoms are significant, very small amounts of levodopa can be added and gradually increased, while observing for worsening of psychiatric symptoms [23, 24].

Recommendations

1. Given the presence of impaired visuoperceptual processing on neuropsychological testing, in addition to slowed processing speed and difficulty parking and maintaining his lane, the neuropsychologist recommended that the patient stop driving. It is often helpful for the neuropsychologist to remove driving privileges based on testing than for family members or physicians to make this very difficult call, which relates significantly to most patients' identity and independence and can cause animosity towards family members.
2. This patient had comorbid anxiety and depression, which were of new onset. These mood changes are often part of the prodromal DLB and other movement disorders and dementias, and results should not be attributed to "pseudodementia," unless this diagnosis is made by a neuropsychologist. Effexor was helpful in relieving symptoms of depression and anxiety, and was also helpful because it is considered an "activating" antidepressant.
3. Extra time should be permitted to complete tasks and formulate responses. Carpets/area rugs should be removed secondary to visuoperceptual deficits and a history of near falls. Furniture should be removed from walking paths in the house. The patient should also avoid the use of power tools and climbing on ladders.
4. Notes, alarms, reminders, and calendars will assist with memory decline. Finances should be handled jointly between the patient and his wife. It is recommended that a pillbox be utilized for medication management.
5. Remaining physically, socially, and cognitively active is important in managing the rate of progression in dementias.
6. The patient will require regular follow-up with a neurologist for appropriate medication management and will require neuropsychological re-evaluation to evaluate progression with appropriate recommendations for family members and referral sources.

Chapter Review Questions

1. Key symptoms of dementia with Lewy bodies include:
   A. Fluctuations in cognition.
   B. Severe memory decline.
   C. Difficulty drawing things correctly/visuoperceptual deficits.
   D. A and C.

2. Dementia with Lewy bodies may be easily confused with:
   A. Parkinson's disease.
   B. A psychiatric disorder.
   C. Vascular dementia.
   D. All of the above.
   E. A and B.

3. Correct diagnosis with the aid of neuropsychological assessment is particularly important in dementia with Lewy bodies because:
   A. Misdiagnosis can lead to severe and possibly life-threatening side effects as a result of treatment with medications to treat hallucinations.
   B. Misdiagnosis based on the presence of Parkinson-like movement symptoms can lead to treatment with drugs that severely increase psychiatric symptoms.
   C. Misdiagnosis frequently delays treatment with medications that can very significantly improve, but not reverse progression of, psychosis and cognition.
   D. All of the above.

References

1. Baskys A. Lewy body dementia: the litmus test for neuroleptic sensitivity and extrapyramidal symptoms. J Clin Psychiatry. 2004;65(Suppl 11):16–22.
2. Fujishiro H, Ferman TJ, Boeve BF, Smith GE, Graff-Radford NR, Uitti RJ, Wszolek ZK, Knopman DS, Petersen RC, Parisi JE, Dickson DW. Validation of the neuropathologic criteria of the third consortium for dementia with Lewy bodies for prospectively diagnosed cases. J Neuropathol Exp Neurol. 2008;67(7):649–56.
3. Harding AJ, Halliday GM. Cortical Lewy body pathology in the diagnosis of dementia. Acta Neuropathol. 2001;102:355–72.
4. Ferman TJ, Smith GE, Boever BF, Graff-Radford NR, Lucas JA, Knopman DS, Petersen RC, Ivnik RJ, Wszolek Z, Uitti R, Dickson DW. Neuropsychological differentiation of dementia with Lewy bodies from normal aging and Alzheimer's disease. Clin Neuropsychol. 2006;20:623–36.
5. Metzler-Baddeley C. A review of cognitive impairments in dementia with Lewy bodies relative to Alzheimer's disease and Parkinson's disease with dementia. Cortex. 2007;43(5):583–600.
6. Bozzali M, Falini A, Cercignani M, Baglio F, Farina E, Alberoni M, et al. Brain tissue damage in dementia with Lewy bodies: an in vivo diffusion tensor MRI study. Brain. 2005;128:1595–604.
7. Watson R, Blamire AM, Colloby SJ, Wood JS, Barber R, He J, O'Brien JT. Characterizing dementia with Lewy bodies by means of diffusion tensor imaging. Neurology. 2012;79:906–14.
8. Oda H, Yamamoto Y, Maeda K. Neuropsychological profile of dementia with Lewy bodies. Psychogeriatrics. 2009;9(2):85–90.
9. Lee DR, McKeith I, Mosimann U, Ghosh-Nodial A, Grayson L, Wilson B, Thomas AJ. The dementia cognitive fluctuation scale, a new psychometric test for clinicians to identify cognitive fluctuations in people with dementia. Am J Geriatr Psychiatry. 2014;22(9):926–35.
10. McKeith IG, et al. Diagnosis and management of dementia with Lewy bodies: fourth consensus report of the DLB Consortium. Neurology. 2017;89(1):88–100.
11. Troster A. Neuropsychological characteristics of dementia with Lewy bodies and Parkinson's disease with dementia: differentiation, early detection, and implications for "mild cognitive impairment" and biomarkers. Neuropsychol Rev. 2008;18:103–19.
12. Zesiewicz TA, Baker MJ, Dunne PB, et al. Diffuse Lewy body disease. Curr Treat Options Neurol. 2001;3:507–18.
13. Boot BP. Comprehensive treatment of dementia with Lewy bodies. Alzheimers Res Ther. 2015;7(1):45.
14. Shimada H, et al. Dementia with Lewy bodies can be well-differentiated from Alzheimer's disease by measurement of brain acetylcholinesterase activity-a [11C]MP4A PET study. Int J Geriatr Psychiatry. 2015;30(11):1105–13.

15. Samuel W, Alford M, Hofstetter CR, Hansen L. Dementia with Lewy bodies versus pure Alzheimer disease: differences in cognition, neuropathology, cholinergic dysfunction, and synaptic density. J Neuropsychol Exp Neurol. 1997;56:499–508.
16. McKeith IG. Consensus guidelines for the clinical and pathological diagnosis of dementia with Lewy bodies (DLB): report of the consortium on DLB international workshop. J Alzheimers Dis. 2006;9:417–23.
17. Mori E, Ikeda M, Kosaka K. Donepezil for dementia with Lewy bodies: a randomized, placebo-controlled trial. Ann Neurol. 2012;72(1):41–52.
18. McKeith I, Del Ser T, Spano P, Emre M, Wesnes K, Anand R, Speigel R. Efficacy of rivastigmine in dementia with Lewy bodies: a randomized, double-blind, placebo controlled international study. Lancet. 2000;356:2031–3036.
19. Ikeda M, Mori E, Kosaka K, Iseki E, Hashimoto M, Matsukawa N, Matsuo K, Nakagawa M. Long-term safety and efficacy of donepezil in patients with dementia with Lewy bodies: results from a 52-week, open-label, multicenter extension study. Dement Geriatr Cogn Disord. 2013;36(3-4):229–41.
20. Zupancic M, Mahajan A, Handa K. Dementia with Lewy bodies: diagnosis and management for primary care providers. Prim Care Companion CNS Disord. 2011;13(5)
21. Goldman JG, Goetz CG, Brandabur M, Sanfilippo M, Stebbins GT. Effects of dopaminergic medications on psychosis in dementia with Lewy bodies. Mov Disord. 2008;23:2248–50.
22. Molloy S, McKeith IG, O'Brien JT, Burn DJ. The role of levodopa in the treatment and management of dementia with Lewy bodies. J Neurol Neurosurg Psychiatry. 2005;76:1200–3.
23. Lucetti C, Logi C, Del Dotto P, Berti C, Ceravolo R, Balduci F, Bonucelli U. Levodopa response in dementia with Lewy bodies: a 1-year follow-up study. Parkinsonism Relat Disord. 2010;16:522–626.
24. Molloy S, McKeith IG, O'Brien JT, Burn JD. The role of levodopa in the management of dementia with Lewy bodies. J Neurol Neurosurg Psychiatry. 2005;76:1200–3.

Chapter 15
Amyotrophic Lateral Sclerosis

Jonathan S. Katz and Susan C. Woolley

Neurologist Perspective

Clinical management of an amyotrophic lateral sclerosis (ALS) patient is complex and requires attention to many different factors. Ideally, patients are managed within the setting of a multidisciplinary clinic. The medical needs evolve as the weakness spreads throughout the upper and lower limbs, the trunk, and the bulbar and respiratory muscles. As a result, patients seek interventions from a number of different specialists in pulmonary medicine, speech and augmentative communication, physical therapy, occupational therapy, nutrition, and neurology. Although ALS was once considered a purely neuromuscular condition, it is now accepted that approximately half of patients exhibit at least mild cognitive or behavioral changes, while up to 15% meet criteria for frontotemporal dementia (FTD) [1].

The presence of any significant dementia will affect disease management. First of all, neurologists trained in neuromuscular disease do not practice behavioral neurology routinely, and it is not unusual that extramotor symptoms or signs are overlooked. The identification of cognitive and behavioral syndromes requires a baseline level of suspicion grounded simply on the underlying incidence, combined with either a formal approach to screening patients or access to expert neuropsychological consultation. Accurate assessment of FTD symptoms in ALS patients may be hampered by physical disabilities, especially when ALS affects speech, which can make certain behavioral observations difficult. Those with bulbar involvement cannot be properly assessed for anomia, changes in fluency, or agrammatisms that would point to the onset of aphasia. Similarly, a patient with any significant paralysis may not exhibit the disinhibited or stereotypical behaviors that are part of FTD.

J. S. Katz · S. C. Woolley (✉)
Forbes Norris Center, California Pacific Medical Center, Sutter Pacific Medical Foundation, San Francisco, CA, USA
e-mail: Katzjs@cpmcri.org; Woolles@sutterhealth.org

K. M. Sanders (ed.), *Physician's Field Guide to Neuropsychology*,
https://doi.org/10.1007/978-1-4939-8722-1_15

In our ALS clinic, the biggest clues about FTD come from family members and caregivers and from historical findings about the patient's behaviors prior to ALS. It is not uncommon that ALS patients presenting with clear-cut FTD have failed to receive the diagnosis, and it is the diagnosis of ALS that gives the biggest clue that FTD may also be present. Some of these patients were referred for psychiatric care prior to the ALS diagnosis, presumably suffering from a mood disorder. In others, it is not uncommon to receive reports of substance abuse, arrests, divorces, or work issues that had occurred in the year or two prior to the onset of weakness. When patients are diagnosed with ALS, it is not uncommon for family members to communicate for them during appointments, especially when speech is involved. Clinicians may assume that bulbar symptoms have progressed to the point of complete disability, despite showing little clinical involvement of the tongue or throat. Unless it is directly sought, aphasia arising from PNFA (progressive non-fluent aphasia) pathology or profound apathy can be overlooked.

Patients and family members rarely complain directly of symptoms associated with milder forms of cognitive impairment (ALSci). They may be unaware that cognition or behavior can be affected in ALS and may not report symptoms. If they have noticed symptoms, it is common to attribute them to the ALS itself. Diminished verbal fluency is difficult to assess without a systematic method like neuropsychological testing, especially when patients use augmentative communication devices and communicate very slowly to begin with. Other patients will complain of difficulty with memory or thinking speed, which can be attributed to medication side effects, sleep deficits, CO_2 retention, or mood alterations.

To address these concerns, our neuromuscular clinic has adapted the practice of screening patients when there is any suspicion of cognitive impairment (ALSci) or dementia, using the ALS Cognitive Behavioral Screen (ALS CBS) [2]. The ALS CBS is a highly accurate, ALS-specific screen for FTD. This type of approach has been recommended in recent ALS practice parameters [3]. ALS-FTD patients require a different approach than simple ALS cases. They tend to have poor survival outcomes [4] and, not surprisingly, decreased compliance with therapeutic recommendations [5]. They also fail to participate in planning, leaving the caregivers to make decisions for them. Elamin and colleagues [4] determined that even mild executive dysfunction, not meeting frank criteria for dementia, is also a negative prognostic indicator. Perhaps the most important reason to diagnose FTD in a patient with ALS is to educate family members about the process of decision making and remind them that the patient is not capable. A diagnosis also allows the care team to temper aggressive interventions accordingly. Since apathy is a common component of FTD, families often take solace in knowing that the patient usually does not worry about dying the same way as patients without cognitive impairment.

Testing cognition in ALS can be subject to a number of confounds unique to the disease. Aside from typical factors, like limited education or reduced English proficiency, ALS patients routinely suffer from respiratory compromise, motor weakness, dysarthria, and fatigue. On a practical level, even relatively low scores on a screening measure must be interpreted with these variables in mind. When the ALS portion of the disease is relatively mild and patients do very poorly on cognitive or behavioral screening, there is increased confidence in making a diagnosis at the bedside. When the scores are intermediate or when the confounding variables are confusing, we favor referral for more definitive neuropsychological testing to provide diagnostic clarity. Comprehensive neuropsychological testing is also ideal, so specific tests can be selected to minimize demands on either motor or speech abilities, as needed.

Neuropsychological assessment requires careful consideration of the motor disturbance inherent in ALS, which may impact motor spontaneity, speech output, and emotional reactivity. Therefore, referral should ideally be made to a clinician with expertise in ALS, and if not available, neuropsychologists in movement disorder clinics (i.e., Huntington's disease, multiple sclerosis, Parkinson's disease) may have the most appropriate experience in test selection with consideration of neuromuscular involvement.

Review of the Literature

Evidence from pathological, genetic, neuropsychological, and neuroanatomical studies supports the notion that ALS and FTD reflect the same underlying disease [6]. Depending on the spread of pathology through the nervous system, patients express clinical symptoms of ALS, FTD, or both. Reports are mixed with regard to the most common types of FTD seen in ALS. One study found that the behavioral variant of FTD is most common in ALS [7], while other studies suggest that language-based dementia (i.e., PNFA) is more prominent [1, 8]. Delusions appear to be common in patients diagnosed with ALS-FTD [9].

International consensus criteria were recently revised to guide the diagnosis of frontotemporal syndromes in ALS [6]. Behavioral variant FTD diagnosis in ALS is primarily based on the Rascovsky criteria [10]. Many ALS patients do not fulfill the criteria for FTD yet exhibit changes in personality, social comportment, or behavior. ALS patients who demonstrate two or more distinct behavioral abnormalities, which are not better explained by psychological reactions or premorbid characteristics, are diagnosed with behavioral impairment (ALSbi). Patients with cognitive impairment (ALSci) are diagnosed through neuropsychological assessment, when scores on two or more distinct executive or language measures fall at or below the 5th percentile based on demographically corrected norms. Recent studies suggest that language impairment occurs at the same rate, if not more frequently, as executive dysfunction [11].

Cognitive deficits in ALS are characterized primarily by deficits in verbal fluency, which occur independently of dysarthria or other weakness [12]. Cognitive dysfunction in ALS is not associated with the site of motor onset but does have a moderate association with the presence of dysarthria, even when motor speed and speech rate are controlled for [13]. Verbal fluency deficits have been extensively researched, and neuroanatomical correlates localize to the dorsolateral prefrontal cortex [14]. Other forms of executive dysfunction in ALS include impaired set shifting or cognitive flexibility. Up to half of patients are found to have a mild form of cognitive dysfunction upon direct neuropsychological assessment [1, 7].

The most common behavioral abnormality detected in ALS patients is apathy [15–17]. Many ALS patients without FTD exhibit significant apathy that is not fully explained by the degree of motor weakness or respiratory compromise. Apathy scores correlate with anterior cingulate changes but not with physical disability [18] or depression [15]. Other common behavioral symptoms include self-centeredness and reduced empathy for others [19]. Mild neurobehavioral symptoms may develop prior to motor symptoms in ALS [20]. While behavioral change may be pervasive in ALS, mild behavioral symptoms may not impact survival, in contrast to the effect of mild executive impairment and ALS-FTD.

Assessment of psychiatric history in ALS patients is important for differentiating between apathy and depression. Perhaps surprisingly, clinically significant depression is not prevalent in ALS [21], but a systematic diagnostic interview is needed to identify cases of clinically significant depression. Caregivers, and physicians without experience in ALS, often misdiagnose fatigue or apathy as a mood disorder, and, as a result, there are probably many more ALS patients taking antidepressants than those who have actual depression. Alternatively, disinhibition is another common manifestation of FTD and may be misdiagnosed as bipolar disorder or other forms of mania. In these instances, a detailed neuropsychological interview can clarify whether behaviors previously classified as hypomanic are better attributed to the progressive orbitofrontal pathology of FTD. In an FTD cohort, somatic delusions and associated repetitive behaviors are strongly associated with the C9orf mutation [22], which is the most common genetic form of ALS-FTD.

For patients with ALS-FTD, it is more common for FTD to start before ALS. This has been attributed to the fact that patients die faster from ALS, so there is simply less time for a second disease to develop. The interval between the onset of FTD and the diagnosis of ALS in one cohort was less than 2 years [16]. Another group found this duration can average more than 7 years [23]. Median survival from disease onset for ALS-FTD patients was estimated at 2 years [4] to 2.4 years [16]. This is much shorter than the survival rates for bvFTD without ALS (7.6 years on average) [24] and up to a year shorter than ALS patients without cognitive or behavioral disorders [4]. Non-demented patients with executive dysfunction also have shorter survival compared to ALS patients without cognitive impairment [4].

Neuropsychology Case Example

Identifying Information and Reason for Referral: Mrs. O is a 76-year-old, widowed, Caucasian female referred for neuropsychological assessment. Testing was requested to clarify the working diagnosis of dementia, occurring in the context of ALS. A question was raised by her family about her relative capacity to manage financial and legal decisions of a dependent adult son. A screening exam had found that she had difficulty following even simple commands and that she could not complete simple saccades or antisaccades.

A year prior to this referral, she was evaluated by a neuromuscular specialist. During the interview, she nodded yes when asked if the year was 1998 (in 2013). Six months prior to the current assessment, she was asked to write the year and initially wrote *19204* and then *2007*. When given a multiple choice format, she incorrectly selected *2005*.

Mrs. O was unaware of the reason for the assessment, although she nodded affirmatively to her daughter that she understood. Her family members reported that she was "fine" cognitively and that she had been evaluated by both a psychiatrist and psychologist at unspecified times in the past without receiving a diagnosis. Her daughter reported that she makes decisions well. For example, she recently chose a carpet for her home and had helped select a new car. However, when the family was asked for specifics about how she made these selections, the answers were wanting. Her daughter stated that Mrs. O uses a letter board to communicate but had left it in the car. Mrs. O did not naturally gravitate toward using the substitute board that was provided to her during testing, nor did she spontaneously use the provided pen and paper.

Medical History: The patient first developed dysarthria in 2011, which progressed over time. She also eventually developed extremity weakness, diffuse spasticity, and hyperreflexia. A diagnosis of ALS was made in December 2013. Electromyography and nerve conduction studies showed rare fasciculations and fibrillation potentials with chronic neurogenic abnormalities, suggestive of ALS. Forced vital capacity (FVC) could not be obtained due to moderate oropharyngeal dysphagia and cognitive deficits, but she denied respiratory symptoms. Other medical history included rheumatoid arthritis, chronic pain, urinary incontinence, urinary tract infections, and multiple falls. She took multiple medications, including three with potential influence on cognition: valium, Norco, and methadone.

Physician Perspective: *The family asked me to sign a document confirming the patient's capacity to manage the financial and legal affairs of her dependent son. This patient had undergone cognitive screening prior to the referral, but her "advanced ALS" made it impossible to administer all screen items, and a total score was never calculated.*

It was evident that the family did all communicating for the patient, despite having access to an augmentative communication board. She showed an obvious lack of initiative related to communication, and on direct examination she was not able to complete three part commands. She also did not comprehend a simple screening task like saccades and antisaccades. These observations provided a strong suggestion that cognitive impairment was present and that her observed difficulties should not be attributed to her speech problems alone. Once discussed, the family was surprised at the notion that impairments were present and insisted that the patient was cognitively intact. They had never been informed that dementia could occur in the setting of ALS. From my perspective, however, the poor showing on screening called for a formal neuropsychological assessment to ensure that there was dementia on top of her motor and speech disability. A formal diagnosis could then be used to help educate the family about the nature of her deficits. Since I was asked to sign a legal document related to her competency, which would have real repercussions for her family, I felt a more direct approach to cognitive assessment was required.

Neuropsychologist Perspective: *This referral was not straightforward because the disease had progressed to a point where standard testing was no longer feasible. Typically, the benefit of neuropsychological assessment lies in the utility of age and education-based norms to clarify the level of impairment.*

A flexible approach was used, which included taking additional time to repeat questions and tasks to assess the patient's response consistency and reliability. The multidisciplinary ALS clinic setting where screening is usually performed is rushed, which therefore did not allow for this type of repetitive questioning. The evaluation also sought to characterize her capacities qualitatively in order to provide concrete examples of her difficulties to the family and to encourage awareness of deficits.

Multiple factors needed to be considered in this case. Despite having ALS, because of her advanced age, Alzheimer's disease and vascular dementia belonged on the differential. The median age of onset for ALS patients is in the late 50s or early 60s, when the wider differential diagnoses do not come into play. The patient could not tolerate neuroimaging due to severe sialorrhea and subsequent risk of choking. While she took several medications which could slow cognition, it seemed unlikely that side effects explained the consistent history of repeated problems with orientation and language that were noted since the diagnostic visit. A mood disorder was not considered because she was not tearful or despondent and because clinically significant depression is not common in ALS.

Behavioral Observations and Mental Status: Mrs. O arrived on time for her appointment accompanied by her daughter, K. She was alert, cooperative, and oriented only to the city. She was casually dressed and well groomed. She was confined to a wheelchair. Motor movements were limited, and manual dexterity was severely compromised by arthritis. She drooled coffee from her mouth which stained her sweater, and sialorrhea was evident throughout most of the interview. She did not reach for nearby tissues or use a provided towel to manage this. Her eye contact was good. Speech was notable mainly for infrequent, non-comprehensible monosyllabic utterances. Despite prompts, she did not spontaneously use a letter board or pencil/paper. Her range of affect was clearly reduced, although she generally smiled and was pleasant. There was no evidence of pseudobulbar affect. Her thought processes and content could not be assessed due to limited communication.

Orientation and Memory: She was not oriented to the year. When provided with a written multiple choice format, she selected 2012 (correct: 2014). She thought the current month was January (correct: August). She indicated that her age was 70, although she was 76. She correctly selected the city where the evaluation took place from a list of four cities. Formal assessment of memory was not completed given her inability to follow simple commands, language deficits, and inability to copy simple designs.

Expressive Language: Her daughter reported that she could use a letter board to communicate, but it was not brought to the examination. When she was encouraged to use a replica, she did not use it. She also failed to use a pencil and paper that was provided. During the 2-h examination, she only wrote one word spontaneously, which was a repetition of a word stated by the examiner. The word was nearly illegible. Her signature was also illegible. She could spell only the simplest words. For some words, she substituted a synonym or a semantically associated word. For example, when asked to spell candy, she wrote *baby math.* When asked to spell big, she wrote *huge.*

Receptive Language: Auditory comprehension was impaired, primarily due to slowed processing speed. She was fairly accurate in identifying letters, colors, and words presented verbally. She could identify written letters and words, although reading comprehension of phrases was variable. She could not respond to the written instruction of *Your Signature:________*, but she could read and respond to the written instruction of *Please Sign Your Name.* On the BDAE, her score on a measure of picture-word matching was markedly impaired (4/10). This suggested semantic breakdown and/or impaired spelling.

Executive Functioning: She stopped at "O" when she was asked to write the alphabet. When asked to draw the face of a clock, she drew an actual face. Her second attempt was markedly impaired: she wrote 4321 in the clock face. Saccades were also impaired and she was not able to voluntarily direct her gaze to the right. She could not complete 3-step commands and was inconsistent with 1- and 2-step commands.

She revealed apraxia with natural gestures (show how you would indicate that you felt cold or if it was too noisy), suggesting difficulty with nonverbal expression of personal feelings or sensations. Her performance on this task, when compared to a cohort of aphasic patients, was impaired (3rd percentile). For conventional gestures (i.e., saluting), she scored in the average range (30th percentile) for patients with aphasia.

In terms of judgment, she had poor awareness by essentially pouring coffee into her mouth despite her obvious inability to swallow. After it spilled onto her sweater and lap, she continued to try to drink it, still without success. She did not clean herself and sat through the remaining examination with soaked clothes.

Visuospatial Reasoning: Her ability to think abstractly on a nonverbal task of reasoning (WASI-II Matrix Reasoning) was impaired (<1st percentile).

Numerical Reasoning: Mrs. O could accurately identify numbers but was impaired on the WIAT-II Numerical Reasoning subtest (<1st percentile). Performance on this type of pencil and paper mathematical test correlates with financial competence and the ability to manage finances.

Psychiatric Presentation: Mrs. O was not depressed, anxious, psychotic, or behaviorally inappropriate.

Conclusions: Diagnostically, dementia seemed clear, although characterizing the type was difficult. Her deficits were global, but ALS-FTD seemed most likely. The comprehensive deficits suggested a complicated and advanced dementia, despite the family's insistence that she was intact cognitively.

Clinical Recommendations: The patient and family were both advised that she could not effectively manage her son's financial and legal matters. We also recommended that Mrs. O receive a Durable Power of Attorney (DPOA), which had not yet been established. Supervision was recommended whenever she ate or drank due to risk of choking. Our observations led to further discussions of stuffing her mouth with food, which her caregiver endorsed enthusiastically. This behavior is common in FTD and supported our recommendations for supervision. Deficits in language and communication were also discussed, and the family was advised to pose yes/no questions. The family and caregiver were also educated about receptive language difficulties and problems with response consistency. The augmentative communication specialist on the multidisciplinary care team was informed that low-tech devices would be best for this patient, along with training of caregivers for effective communication and patient limitations.

A provisional diagnosis of ALS-FTD was discussed with the patient, her daughter, and the primary caregiver. This was based on the profound language and behavioral changes discovered on testing. We instructed them about the progressive and untreatable nature of the disease. Because of the dementia, the patient did not express any reaction to the diagnosis, nor did she react when examples of her deficits were explained. She did not ask any questions and made no attempt to communicate or refute the deficits described. We told the family that this behavior probably represented a combination of her comprehension problems, impaired insight, and apathy, as opposed to the ALS. The daughter inquired about her mother's life expectancy and took some comfort in hearing that some of the same deficits, especially apathy, documented during testing would make it easier for Mrs. O to cope with disease progression and ultimately with death. The testing ultimately served as both a formal way to make a diagnosis of dementia and as an informal way for the family members to see the cognitive aspects of a disease they presumed had only motor manifestations.

Impact of Subsequent Interventions: The multidisciplinary treatment team was informed about her cognitive status, which helped them adjust their approach to communication and the level of recommended intervention. She had limited follow-up with the clinic following the assessment, although the family communicated some concern about her breathing difficulty.

Collaborative Issues: Key Points

In ALS, motor disease (weakness, dysarthria) confounds the utility of traditional cognitive screens, making the referral to neuropsychology more relevant.

Neuropsychologists are uniquely trained to identify cognitive and behavioral deficits, and therefore provide unique support for the practice of neuromuscular physicians.

Neuropsychologists select and administer tests with high reliability and validity to differentiate symptoms of weakness, apathy, depression, fatigue, and pseudobulbar affect in ALS patients. This is essential for accurate differential diagnosis for extramotor disease manifestations.

When motor manifestations are relatively mild and patients do poorly on cognitive or behavioral screening, there is increased confidence in making a diagnosis at the bedside. When the scores are intermediate or when the confounding variables are confusing, referral for more definitive neuropsychological testing is favored to provide diagnostic clarity.

Detection of ALS-FTD helps the treatment team to adjust recommendations and inform the patients and family about the expected course. It is not uncommon that ALS patients presenting with clear-cut FTD have failed to receive the diagnosis, and it is the diagnosis of ALS that gives the biggest clue that FTD may also be present.

ALS patients with concomitant FTD have significantly shorter survival time from symptom onset than ALS patients without dementia. However, ALS patients with mild executive dysfunction, not meeting criteria for dementia, also have significantly shorter survival. Without accurate neuropsychological diagnosis, discussion about prognosis may be incomplete or inaccurate.

More attention is now being paid to psychiatric symptoms in ALS patients to help with neuropsychological diagnosis. A history of psychosis and/or somatic delusions is associated with the C9orf72 mutation, which is the most common genetic form of ALS-FTD. ALS patients suffering from fatigue or apathy may be misdiagnosed with depression. Disinhibition may be incorrectly misdiagnosed as bipolar disorder or other forms of mania when it actually represents a symptom of FTD. In these instances, a detailed neuropsychological interview can clarify whether aberrant behaviors are explained by respiratory or motor weakness, frontal lobe changes, reactive depression, or chronic mental illness.

Caregivers and patients may be unaware of the cognitive and behavioral manifestations of ALS, and education about these symptoms can impact medical decision making and coping. Perhaps the most important reason to diagnose FTD in a patient with ALS is to educate family members that the patient's capacity to make complex medical decisions is compromised.

Apathy is a common component of FTD. Families can take solace in knowing that the patient usually does not worry about dying the same way as patients without cognitive impairment. However, apathy also makes it more difficult to understand a patient's perspective on dying and desired level of intervention.

Chapter Review Questions

1. How common is FTD in ALS?
   A. 50%.
   B. 40%.
   C. 15%.
   D. 20%.

2. Which condition is more common, behavioral variant FTD or PNFA in ALS patients?
   A. Behavioral variant.
   B. PNFA.
   C. Neither, the prevalence is equivalent.
   D. Semantic dementia.

3. How common is cognitive impairment in ALS?
   A. 15%.
   B. 50%.
   C. 75%.
   D. 35%.

4. What are the most common behavioral abnormalities seen in non-demented ALS patients?
   A. Apathy.
   B. Disinhibition.
   C. Overeating.
   D. Stealing and hoarding.

5. Does executive dysfunction impact survival even if an ALS patient is not demented?
   A. No, only dementia impacts survival in ALS.
   B. Yes, it reduces survival by 2 months.
   C. Yes, it reduces survival similar to dementia.
   D. This has not been studied.

References

1. Ringholz GM, Appel SH, Bradshaw M, Cooke NA. Prevalence and patterns of cognitive impairment in sporadic ALS. Neurology. 2005;65(4):586–90.
2. Woolley SC, York MK, Moore DH, et al. Detecting frontotemporal dysfunction in ALS: utility of the ALS Cognitive Behavioral Screen (ALS-CBS™). Amyotroph Lateral Scler. 2010;11(3):303–11.
3. Miller RG, Jackson C, Kasarskis EJ, et al. Practice parameter update: the care of the patient with amyotrophic lateral sclerosis: multidisciplinary care, symptom management, and cognitive/behavioral impairment (an evidence-based review): report of the Quality Standards Subcommittee of the American Academy of Neurology. Neurology. 2009;73(15):1227–33.
4. Elamin M, Phukan J, Bede P, et al. Executive dysfunction is a negative prognostic indicator in patients with ALS without dementia. Neurology. 2011;76(14):1263–9.
5. Olney RK, Murphy J, Forshew D, et al. The effects of executive and behavioral dysfunction on the course of ALS. Neurology. 2005;65(11):1774–7.
6. Strong MJ, Abrahams S, Goldstein LH, et al. Amyotrophic lateral sclerosis-frontotemporal spectrum disorder (ALS-FTSD): revised diagnostic criteria. Amyotroph Lateral Scler. 2017;18(3-4):153–74. https://doi.org/10.1080/21678421.2016.1267768.
7. Lomen-Hoerth C, Murphy J, Langmore S, Kramer JH. Are amyotrophic lateral sclerosis patients cognitively normal? Neurology. 2003;60(7):1094–7.

8. Rakowicz WP, Hodges JR. Dementia and aphasia in motor neuron disease: an underrecognised association? J Neurol Neurosurg Psychiatry. 1998;65(6):881–9.
9. Lillo P, Garcin B, Hornberger M, Bak TH, Hodges JR. Neurobehavioral features in frontotemporal dementia with amyotrophic lateral sclerosis. Arch Neurol. 2010;67(7):826–30.
10. Rascovsky K, Hodges JR, Knopman D, Mendez MF, Kramer JH, Neuhaus J, et al. Sensitivity of revised diagnostic criteria for the behavioural variant of frontotemporal dementia. Brain. 2011;134:2456–77.
11. Taylor LJ, Brown RG, Tsermentseli S, et al. Is language impairment more common than executive dysfunction in amyotrophic lateral sclerosis? J Neurol Neurosurg Psychiatry. 2013;84(5):494–8.
12. Abrahams S, Leigh PN, Harvey A, Vythelingum GN. Verbal fluency and executive dysfunction in amyotrophic lateral sclerosis. Neuropsychologia. 2000;38:734–47.
13. Sterling LE, Jawaid A, Salamone AR, et al. Association between dysarthria and cognitive impairment in ALS: a prospective study. Amyotroph Lateral Scler. 2010;11(1-2):46–51.
14. Abrahams S, Goldstein LH, Simmons A, et al. Word retrieval in amyotrophic lateral sclerosis; a functional magnetic resonance imaging study. Brain. 2004;127(7):1507–17.
15. Grossman AB, Woolley-Levine S, Bradley WG, Miller RG. Detecting neurobehavioral changes in amyotrophic lateral sclerosis. Amyotroph Lateral Scler. 2007;8:56–61.
16. Lillo P, Mioshi E, Zoing MC, Kiernan MC, Hodges JR. How common are behavioral changes in amyotrophic lateral sclerosis? Amyotroph Lateral Scler. 2011;12(1):45–51.
17. Mioshi E, Hsieh S, Caga J, et al. A novel tool to detect behavioural symptoms in ALS. Amyotroph Lateral Scler Frontotemporal Degener. 2014;15(3-4):298–304.
18. Woolley SC, Zhang Y, Schuff N, Weiner MW, Katz JS. Neuroanatomical correlates of apathy in ALS using 4 Tesla diffusion tensor MRI. Amyotroph Lateral Scler. 2011;12:52–8.
19. Gibbons ZC, Richardson A, Neary D, Snowden JS. Behaviour in amyotrophic lateral sclerosis. Amyotroph Lateral Scler. 2008;9:67–74.
20. Mioshi E, Caga J, Lillo P, et al. Neuropsychiatric changes precede classic motor symptoms in ALS and do not affect survival. Neurology. 2014;82(2):149–55.
21. Taylor L, Wicks P, Leigh PN, Goldstein LH. Prevalence of depression in amyotrophic lateral sclerosis and other motor disorders. Eur J Neurol. 2010;17:1047–53.
22. Snowden JS, Rollinson S, Thompson JC, et al. Distinct clinical and pathological characteristics of frontotemporal dementia associated with C9ORF72 mutations. Brain. 2012;135:693–708.23.
23. Murphy JM, Henry RG, Langmore S, Kramer JH. Continuum of frontal lobe impairment in amyotrophic lateral sclerosis. Arch Neurol. 2007;64:530–4.
24. Garcin B, Lillo P, Hornberger M, et al. Determinants of survival in behavioral variant frontotemporal dementia. Neurology. 2009;73(20):1656–61.

Chapter 16
Vascular Cognitive Impairment

Felicia C. Goldstein and Ihab Hajjar

Introduction

Vascular cognitive impairment (VCI) is an umbrella term introduced in the 1990s to describe the impact of vascular disease on cognitive functioning, ranging from mild deficits to dementia. The case we present in this chapter demonstrates the value of neuropsychological testing in identifying the subtle cognitive deficits associated with VCI and the role of such testing in differential diagnosis and treatment recommendations.

Referral

Patient: A 62-year-old, African American female
Education: High school degree
Occupation: Retired clerical worker

Reason for Referral: Neurological and cognitive deficits were not apparent during the patient's clinical exam. However, her subjective cognitive complaints prompted a referral for an in-depth neuropsychological assessment to determine whether objective impairments were present and, if so, their etiology.

F. C. Goldstein (✉) · I. Hajjar
Department of Neurology, Emory University School of Medicine, Atlanta, GA, USA
e-mail: fgoldst@emory.edu

K. M. Sanders (ed.), *Physician's Field Guide to Neuropsychology*,
https://doi.org/10.1007/978-1-4939-8722-1_16

Case Presentation

This patient presented with subjective complaints of a 3- to 4-year history of memory loss (e.g., forgetting names, misplacing items), occasional topographic confusion, and poor attention. She stated that she had experienced difficulty recalling the details of training seminars at work, and she was "just forgetting a lot." Around this time, the patient also reported the onset of depression and anxiety, the latter associated with her fear of making work-related mistakes. Currently, she stated that she uses strategies (i.e., checklists) to help her remember everything she needs to do. She denied any difficulties with instrumental activities of daily living such as cooking, driving, managing finances, and organizing and taking her medications.

Neurological Exam and Findings

- Neurological exam was normal with the exception of mild difficulty with tandem gait. Heart sounds were normal. Carotid arteries were normal without bruits. No pedal edema was seen.
- MRI brain scan demonstrated areas of moderately increased T2 signal in the periventricular subcortical white matter. There was also an elongated area of increased T2 signal in the left external capsule. Parahippocampal gyrus did not demonstrate any evidence to suggest volume loss. The findings were interpreted as consistent with subcortical ischemic vascular disease (SIVD).
- Medical history included benign essential hypertension, diabetes mellitus, and hyperlipidemia. The patient was taking amlodipine, metformin, omeprazole, and simvastatin.
- Social history was significant for past cigarette smoking but none in the past year. The patient drank 2–3 glasses of wine a week.
- Family history was significant for heart disease, hypertension, and stroke. There was no known history of Alzheimer's disease or other dementias.
- The Mini-Mental State Examination (MMSE) score was 26/30 points, interpreted as being in the low average range.

The Physician Perspective

This case illustrates a common scenario in patients with mild VCI. Subjective cognitive complaints may be present; yet, the neurological examination and performance on a mental status screen are normal. Brief cognitive screening instruments such as the MMSE that do not adequately address executive functioning can miss subtle deficits in these patients, erroneously leading the clinician to assume that cognitive functioning is within normal limits.

Key Point
The Neuropsychological Working Group of the vascular cognitive impairment workshop sponsored by the National Institute for Neurological Disorders and Stroke (NINDS) and the Canadian Stroke Network (CSN) recommends the Montreal Cognitive Assessment (MoCA) [1] over the MMSE [2] for screening purposes [3]. The MoCA has been found to be more sensitive than the MMSE to VCI due to the inclusion of several items evaluating executive functioning, such as set shifting and working memory (short version of Trails B, Digits Backwards), divergent thinking (timed word fluency), and reasoning and conceptualization (similarities, clock drawing). Traditional interpretation of MoCA results is based upon the summed points across all items, with a maximum of 30 points. Recently, Julayanont and colleagues developed MoCA Index scores for the domains of memory, executive function, visuospatial, language, attention, and orientation [4]. However, the incremental validity of the subscales versus the total MoCA score has not been investigated for patients with vascular cognitive impairment.

VCI Overview

The term "vascular cognitive impairment" was introduced by Vladimir Hachinski in the mid-1990s to describe a continuum of cognitive impairments assumed to be caused by cerebrovascular diseases [5]. These range from mild deficits (vascular cognitive impairment-no dementia, or VCIND) that do not significantly impact daily functioning to severe deficits (vascular dementia, or VaD) resulting in a loss of independence in performing instrumental activities. A third category of mixed dementia is also included in the spectrum of VCI to recognize its tremendous overlap with other neurodegenerative diseases, most commonly Alzheimer's disease (VaD/AD).

Subcortical ischemic vascular disease (SIVD), as manifested by our patient, is the most common cause of VCI [6]. Advances in neuroimaging, especially magnetic resonance imaging, in the late 1980s led to the appreciation that cerebral white matter damage, microbleeds, and lacunar infarcts in the absence of large vessel strokes can produce subtle or no neurologic deficits. Occlusion of the arteries leads to acute ischemic injury and results in lacunar infarcts (<1.5 cm in diameter) that are most prevalent in the deeper parts of the brain, including the basal ganglia, thalamus, and brain stem. White matter changes can typically be seen as hyperintensities on T2-weighted MRI or flow-attenuated inversion recovery (FLAIR) imaging, a finding on neuroimaging referred to as leukoaraiosis. Narrowing and occlusion of the arteries and resulting hypoperfusion can also lead to incomplete infarction of the deep white matter near the brainstem and in the centrum semiovale, a large region of white matter in the dorsal core of the frontal and parietal lobes [7]. Silent infarcts that lack clinically overt stroke-like symptoms typically go unnoticed by the patient and during the neurologic examination, and these are the risk factors for future strokes and cognitive decline. Community-based studies of the elderly population indicate a prevalence of silent infarcts ranging from 8% to 28% [8]. Increasing age is a risk factor for "silent" cerebral infarction, with an estimated prevalence of <8% in 30–49-year-olds to >15% in persons aged 70–89 years [9].

Diagnosis of VCI

Clinical guidelines for VCI proposed by the American Heart Association/American Stroke Association (AHA/ASA) [10] take into account both the severity of cognitive deficits (mild impairment to dementia) and the relationship between these deficits and a vascular etiology (from a possible to a probable association). The diagnosis of mild cognitive impairment (MCI) requires impairment in at least one cognitive domain that either does not or only minimally disrupts instrumental activities of daily living (IADLs), whereas the diagnosis of dementia requires impairments in two or more cognitive domains with a corresponding decline in the ability to perform IADLs. In both cases, any changes in IADLs cannot be due to motor and/or sensory deficits caused by a vascular event (e.g., inability to drive due to hemiparesis or hemianopsia). The classification of a possible versus a probable vascular etiology depends on the degree of certainty that there is a temporal relationship between vascular disease and the onset of cognitive deficits, as well as an absence of other nonvascular cognitive causes. The requirement that there be an established temporal relationship between a vascular event and the onset of cognitive impairment to diagnose probable VCI is often difficult to determine because, as previously noted, older adults can sustain silent strokes that do not result in obvious overt symptoms. To be diagnosed as having possible VCI, the AHA/ASA guidelines require that there is no clear relationship between vascular disease and the onset of cognitive impairments, and imaging data are unavailable to document the presence of vascular disease. In addition, the clinician may determine that there are other neurodegenerative conditions, such as Alzheimer's disease that contribute to the cognitive impairments.

Key Point

The American Heart Association/American Stroke Association defines VCI as "a syndrome with evidence of clinical stroke or subclinical vascular brain injury and cognitive impairment affecting at least one cognitive domain" [10].

The MD Perspective

Value of Requesting a Neuropsychological Evaluation

Neuropsychological testing is valuable in detecting areas of cognitive impairment that can be overlooked in a busy clinical practice when only brief bedside screening is performed. Although screening measures such as the MoCA are useful for providing a global index of overall cognitive status, they are not meant to be a substitute for a neuropsychological evaluation. The full evaluation elucidates the etiology for these impairments by analyzing both the pattern of strengths and weaknesses across domains and the qualitative characteristics of performance. It is on the basis of these patterns that the neuropsychologist can help determine the likely etiology.

Key Point
Neuropsychological findings correlate with real-world functioning and can be useful in predicting success in carrying out IADLs such as driving and medication management. The neuropsychological assessment can also determine whether there are non-neurologic explanations for a patient's subjective complaints. For example, the issue of effort may come up when a relatively young patient stops working due to subjective complaints; yet, there are few objective findings to support their claim. In addition, the contribution of comorbid depression can be evaluated.

Neuropsychological Testing

Neuropsychologists conduct a detailed assessment of cognitive domains including attention, language, memory, visuospatial ability, and executive functioning. Similar to an MRI brain scan, information is provided about the integrity of different brain regions. However, the neuropsychological evaluation goes a step further by providing information about how these disruptions impact the patient's behavior.

Key Point
Patients with VCI due to cerebral small vessel disease frequently display a neuropsychological profile characterized by slow processing speed and impaired executive functioning. Although learning of new information may be poor, patients show evidence for some retention of this material after a delay, in contrast to those with MCI due to Alzheimer's disease [11–13].

Executive Functioning: The "executive functions" refer to complex behaviors including motivation and self-awareness, planning, execution of a strategy, and self-monitoring of performance. Executive functioning deficits are associated with increased white matter abnormalities in nondemented adults as well as in persons with vascular comorbidities [14, 15]. The clinical syndrome of SIVD is commonly associated with a dysexecutive pattern. Our patient demonstrated impairments in aspects of executive functioning involving planning, organization, and conceptual ability. On a clock drawing task, she drew the numbers in the correct order but they were not correctly spaced on the right side of the circle. She was also unable to set the hands to indicate the requested time. Her performance on a problem-solving task requiring her to generate hypotheses and to shift response sets based on the examiner's feedback was moderately severely impaired. She made excessive perseverative responses and only obtained three correct card sorts in 64 trials. On another task, her copy of a complex figure was poor. Although she was able to recognize and draw details of the figure, she did not maintain the gestalt, and her drawing was highly disorganized.

Information Processing Speed: Slow processing speed is a common feature of SIVD, reflecting the impact of disruptions in cerebral white matter integrity. White matter pathways include projection fibers that transmit sensory and motor information to and from the cortex, commissural fibers that act via the corpus callosum to allow communication between the cerebral hemispheres, and association fibers that connect cortical areas. Destruction of these myelinated tracts can disrupt communication between cortical structures and functional connectivity of those structures despite normal cortical and subcortical gray matter [16, 17]. Measures that require rapid responding are therefore especially sensitive to SIVD. Our patient was mildly slow in alternating between numbers and letters, and she made a sequencing error. Timed generation of words beginning with specific letters was low average (letter fluency).

Memory: The pattern of memory performance in patients with SIVD is typically characterized by slow encoding of information, with some savings over time as well as a benefit from cues [12]. On a list learning procedure requiring her to encode 16 words over 5 trials, our patient exhibited a relatively flat learning curve until the fifth trial (trials 1–5 recall: 1, 5, 3, 5, and 8 words), but she retained 5 words after 25 minutes (63% retention). When given a memory task that did not require her to impose any organizational strategies (paragraph recall), our patient demonstrated average immediate recall, with 30-minutes delayed recall in the superior range (80% retention of details). With recognition cues, she correctly answered 23/30 questions about the stories. While her recall of designs and their placement on a page were moderately severely impaired, she benefited from recognition cues and correctly identified all six shapes and made only one false alarm error.

Effort Testing: The inclusion of formal performance validity tests (PVTs) as routine components of neuropsychological assessment protocols is a recommended practice [18]. PVTs may be either stand-alone measures that are explicitly included to evaluate the validity of performance or embedded measures in which scores are derived from existing neuropsychological measures. Our patient was applying for disability benefits, and while there were no obvious signs that she was faking her symptoms for monetary gain, validity measures were administered to rule out poor effort. She performed within normal limits on both free standing and embedded measures.

Additional Findings: Other cognitive domains, including language, visuospatial abilities, and attention, were intact.

Emotional Functioning: Our patient completed the Minnesota Multiphasic Personality Inventory-2. Her elevated clinical scales suggested a great deal of emotional turmoil, including feelings of nervousness, hopelessness, sadness, and pessimism, consistent with some of the core features of depression.

Collaborative Discussion

Objective findings from the neuropsychological evaluation confirmed our patient's subjective cognitive complaints and were useful in providing information for the referring physician concerning etiology as well as recommendations for treatment and follow-up, as discussed below.

We diagnosed our patient as having vascular cognitive impairment-no dementia based on her neuropsychological profile, neuroimaging findings, and independence in performing IADLs. Alzheimer's disease was excluded as a likely etiology due to her relatively intact recall and recognition memory as well as her preserved language and visuospatial abilities. While this clinical impression was reassuring to our patient, it was recommended that she be followed with a repeat evaluation in 1 year to monitor her cognitive functioning and the possibility of coexisting AD. A mixed etiology is not uncommon, with brain autopsy series indicating that at least one-third of patients have both cerebral infarcts and AD pathology [19, 20]. Diabetes and hypertension, especially in midlife, increase the risk of cognitive decline and age-related neurodegenerative conditions such as Alzheimer's disease (AD) [21–24].

The importance of achieving good control of her vascular comorbidities was emphasized to our patient. Clinical guidelines for the treatment of hypertension proposed by the Eighth Joint National Committee in 2014 recommend a target BP of <150/<90 mmHg in persons who are 60 years and older [25]. However, recent studies suggest the neuroprotective value of even lower BP values. The Systolic Blood Pressure Intervention Trial (SPRINT) was terminated due to the unequivocal conclusion in persons 50 years and older that a target BP of 120 mmHg results in a significant reduction in cardiovascular events and death compared to a target systolic pressure of 140 mmHg. Cognitive benefits of BP values <140 and <150 mmHg in older adults have been demonstrated as well [26, 27], including persons who have mild cognitive impairment [23].

Our patient exhibited depressive symptoms and evidence of experiencing significant emotional stress. She had difficulty performing her job duties and was applying for disability benefits. In addition to her reactive depression due to significant life changes, we also felt that her vascular disease could be contributing to her mood disorder. Cerebrovascular disease is a risk factor for the onset of late-life depression, occurring de novo in persons who are in their 50s and 60s. Vascular depression is associated with an increase in the severity of white matter hyperintensities, and the severity of depression has been linked to a disruption of white matter tracts in the frontosubcortical and limbic regions. These, in turn, result in a cognitive profile of executive dysfunction and slow processing speed [28, 29]. We recommended that our patient be seen by a psychiatrist to determine whether pharmacological management would be beneficial. We also recommended that she be seen by a clinical psychologist skilled in using a cognitive behavioral approach involving teaching her strategies for managing her stress.

Finally, lifestyle modifications were recommended for our patient including the importance of engaging in physical exercise. Studies and meta-analytic reviews have reported that physical activity protects against cognitive decline associated with normal aging, while also lowering the risk of MCI and dementia [30–35]. Investigators have demonstrated a positive benefit of aerobic exercise on vascular function, including both reduced endothelial dysfunction and arterial stiffness [36, 37]. In addition, there is evidence that episodic memory and executive functioning are especially benefitted by engagement in aerobic exercise [30, 34].

Key Point

The US Department of Health and Human Services guidelines recommend that healthy older adults should engage in either 150 minutes a week of moderately intense aerobic activity or 75 minutes of vigorous intensity activities for at least 10 minutes at a time to garner significant health benefits. It is also recommended that less vigorous activity such as muscle strengthening exercises should be done more than twice a week.

Chapter Review Questions

1. The Montreal Cognitive Assessment (MoCA) is recommended as a screening tool for vascular cognitive impairment over the Mini-Mental State Exam because the MoCA is:
   A. More sensitive to language functioning.
   B. Shorter to administer in a busy clinic.
   C. Easier to administer by clinicians.
   D. More sensitive to executive functioning.

2. What are the American Heart Association/American Stroke Association criteria for diagnosing someone with probable vascular cognitive impairment? Possible vascular cognitive impairment?

3. The key difference between diagnosing someone with mild cognitive impairment and dementia involves:
   A. The severity of cognitive deficits.
   B. Whether or not the patient is independent in performing instrumental activities of daily living.
   C. Whether the patient is <65 years old versus 65 years and older.
   D. None of the above.

4. What are the most common cognitive deficits that occur in patients with vascular cognitive impairment? How does the pattern of memory performance typically differ from patients with Alzheimer's disease?
5. How can the neuropsychological evaluation assist in identifying contributing causes of a patient's cognitive impairments and help guide treatment recommendations?

References

1. Nasreddine ZS, Phillips NA, Bedirian V, Charbonneau S, Whitehead V, Collin I, Cummings JL, Chertkow H. The Montreal Cognitive Assessment, MoCA: a brief screening tool for mild cognitive impairment. J Am Geriatr Soc. 2005;53:695–9.
2. Folstein MF, Folstein MF, McHugh PR. Mini-mental state: a practical method for grading the cognitive state of outpatients for the clinician. J Psychiatr Res. 1975;12:189–98.
3. Hachinski V, Iadecola C, Petersen RC, Breteler MM, Nyenhuis DL, Black SE, Powers WJ, DeCarli C, Merino JG, Kalaria RN, et al. National Institute of Neurological Disorders and Stroke-Canadian Network Vascular Cognitive Impairment Harmonization Standards. Stroke. 2006;37:2220–41.
4. Julayanont P, Brousseau M, Chertkow H, Phillips NA, Nasreddine ZS. Montreal cognitive assessment memory index score (MoCA-MIS) as a predictor of conversion from mild cognitive impairment to Alzheimer's disease. J Am Geriatr Soc. 2014;62:679–84.
5. Hachinski VC, Bowler JV. Vascular dementia. Neurology. 1993;43:2159–60.
6. Pantoni L. Cerebral small vessel disease: from pathogenesis and clinical characteristics to therapeutic challenges. Lancet Neurol. 2010;9(7):689–701.
7. Fisher CM. Lacunes: small, deep cerebral infarcts. Neurology. 1965;6(7):611–9.
8. Vermeer SE, Longstreth WTJ, Koudstaal PJ. Silent brain infarcts: a systematic review. Lancet Neurol. 2007;6(7):611–9.
9. Das RR, Seshadri S, Beiser AS, Kelly-Hayes M, Au R, Himali JJ, Kase CS, Benjamin EJ, Polak JF, O'Donnell CJ, et al. Prevalence and correlates of silent cerebral infarcts in the Framington Offspring Study. Stroke. 2008;39(11):2929–35.
10. Gorelick PB, Scuteri A, Black SE, DeCarli C, Greenberg SM, Iadecola C, Launer LJ, Laurent S, Lopez OL, Nyenhuis D, et al. Vascular contributions to cognitive impairment and dementia: a statement for healthcare professionals from the American Heart Association/American Stroke Association. Stroke. 2011;42:2672–713.
11. Reed BR, Mungas DM, Kramer JH, Ellis W, Vinters HV, Zarow C, Jagust WJ, Chui HC. Profiles of neuropsychological impairment in autopsy-defined Alzheimer's disease and cerebrovascular disease. Brain. 2007;130((Pt 3)):731–9.
12. Vasquez BP, Zakzanis KK. The neuropsychological profile of vascular cognitive impairment not dementia: a meta-analysis. J Neuropsychol. 2015;9(1):109–36.
13. Nyenhuis DL, Gorelick PB, Geenen EJ, Smith CA, Gencheva E, Freels S, deToledo-Morrell L. The pattern of neuropsychological deficits in vascular cognitive impairment-no dementia (Vascular CIND). Clin Neuropsychol. 2004;18(1):41–9.
14. Raz N, Rodrigue KM, Acker JD. Hypertension and the brain: vulnerability of the prefrontal regions and executive functions. Behav Neurosci. 2003;117(6):1169–80.
15. Saxby BK, Harrington F, McKeith IG, Wesnes K, Ford GA. Effects of hypertension on attention, memory, and executive function in older adults. Health Psychol. 2003;22(6):587–91.
16. Filley CM. White matter: organization and functional relevance. Neuropsychol Rev. 2010;20(2):158–73.
17. Filley CM, editor. The behavioral neurology of white matter. 2nd ed. New York: Oxford University Press; 2012.

18. Bush SS, Ruff RM, Troster AI, Barth JT, Koffler SP, Pliskin NH, Reynolds CR, Silver CH. Symptom validity assessment: practice issues and medical necessity NAN policy & planning committee. Arch Clin Neuropsychol. 2005;20(4):419–26.
19. Attems J, Jellinger KA. Converging pathogenic mechanisms in vascular and neurodegenerative dementia. Stroke. 2014;34:335–7.
20. Schneider JA, Arvanitakis Z, Bang W, Bennett DA. Mixed brain pathologies account for most dementia cases in community-dwelling older persons. Neurology. 2007;69:2197–204.
21. Dore GA, Elias MF, Robbins MA, Elias PK, Nagy Z. Presence of the APOE e4 allele modifies the relationship between type 2 diabetes and cognitive performance: the Maine-Syracuse Study. Diabetologia. 2009;52:2551–60.
22. Elias MF, Davey A. Midlife blood pressure, amyloid-beta, and risk for Alzheimer disease: one more reason to treat hypertension. Hypertension. 2012;59(4):771–2.
23. Goldstein FC, Levey AI, Steenland K. High blood pressure and cognitive decline in mild cognitive impairment. J Am Geriatr Soc. 2013;61:67–73.
24. Shah NS, Vidal JS, Masaki K, Petrovich H, Ross GW, Tilley C, DeMattos RB, Tracy RP, White LR, Launer LJ. Midlife blood pressure, plasma beta-amyloid, and the risk for Alzheimer disease: the Honolulu Asia Aging Study. Hypertension. 2012;59(4):780–6.
25. James PA, Oparil S, Carter BL, Cushman WC, Dennison-Himmelfarb C, Handler J, Lackland DT, LeFevre ML, MacKenzie TD, Ogedegbe O, et al. Evidence-based guideline for the management of high blood pressure in adults: report from the panel members appointed to the Eighth Joint National Committee (JNC-8). JAMA. 2014;311(5):507–20.
26. Goldstein FC, Hajjar IM, Dunn CB, Levey AI, Wharton W. The relationship between cognitive functionining and the JNC-8 guidelines for hypertension in older adults. J Gerontol Ser A: Biol Sci Med Sci. 2017;72(1):121–6.
27. Hajjar I, Rosenberger KJ, Kulshreshtha A, Ayonayon HN, Yaffe K, Goldstein FC. Association of JNC-8 and SPRINT systolic blood pressure levels with cognitive function and related racial disparity. JAMA Neurol. 2017;72(10):1199–205.
28. Alexopoulos GS, Meyers BS, Young RC, Campbell S, Silbersweig D, Charlson M. 'Vascular depression' hypothesis. Arch Gen Psychiatry. 1997;54(10):915–22.
29. Vu NQ, Aizenstein HJ. Depression in the elderly: brain correlates, neuropsychological findings, and role of vascular lesion load. Curr Opin. 2013;26(6):656–61.
30. Colcombe S, Kramer AF. Fitness effects on the cognitive function of older adults: a meta-analytic study. Psychol Sci. 2003;14:125–30.
31. Geda YE, Roberts RO, Knopman DS, Christianson TJH, Pankratz VS, Ivnik RJ, Boeve BF, Tangalos EG, Petersen RC, Rocca WA. Physical exercise, aging, and mild cognitive impairment: a population-based study. Arch Neurol. 2010;67(1):80–6.
32. Hamer M, Chida Y. Physical activity and risk of neurodegenerative disease: a systematic review of prospective evidence. Psychol Med. 2009;39:3–11.
33. Middleton LE, Barnes DE, Lui LY, Yaffe K. Physical activity over the life course and its association with cognitive performance and impairment in old age. J Am Geriatr Soc. 2010;58:1322–6.
34. Smith PJ, Blumenthal JA, Hoffman BM, Cooper H, Strauman TA, Welsh-Bohmer K, Browndyke JN, Sherwood A. Aerobic exercise and neurocognitive performance: a meta-analytic review of randomized controlled trials. Psychosom Med. 2010;72(3):239–52.
35. Sofi F, Valecchi D, Bacci D, Abbate R, Gensini GF, Casini A, Macchi C. Physical activity and risk of cognitive decline: a meta-analysis of prospective studies. J Intern Med. 2011;269:107–17.
36. Feairheller DL, Diaz KM, Kashem MA, Thakkar SR, Veerabhadrappa P, Sturgeon KM, Ling C, Williamson ST, Kretzschmar J, Lee H, et al. Effects of moderate aerobic exercise training on vascular health and blood pressure in African Americans. J Clin Hypertens. 2014;16:504–10.
37. Nualnim N, Parkhurst M, Dhindsa T, Tarumi T, Vavrek J, Tanaka H. Effects of swimming training on blood pressure and vascular function in adults >50 years of age. Am J Cardiol. 2012;109(7):1005–10.

Chapter 17
Right Middle Cerebral Artery Stroke in a Male of Prime Working Age

Karen M. Sanders and William Likosky

Introduction

This case is an example of a right middle cerebral artery infarct in a young man, Mr. Young. His notable motor improvement and persistence of good language skills raised unique questions to his medical team regarding potential to resume normal activities and his failure to do so. Were his deficits amenable to specific rehabilitation modalities? Issues concerning ability to live independently, vocational planning, completion of schooling, and driving were on the minds of the patient and the family, as well as his professional caregivers. Neuropsychological testing was used to help determine ability to complete these tasks.

Key Questions

1. *How does neuropsychological testing help determine the potential for successful functioning in the community, considering the unique strengths and weaknesses in the neuropsychological profile?*
2. *What is the unique contribution of neuropsychology to the treatment of this patient?*

K. M. Sanders (✉)
Department of Psychiatry and Behavioral Sciences, University of Washington School of Medicine, Seattle, WA, USA

W. Likosky
Department of Neurology, University of California at San Francisco/Fresno, Fresno, CA, USA

K. M. Sanders (ed.), *Physician's Field Guide to Neuropsychology*,
https://doi.org/10.1007/978-1-4939-8722-1_17

Key Points
In right middle cerebral artery (RMCA) neurocognitive disability occurs with regularity. It can be missed as it does not present with loss of speech or language abilities. In dominant hemisphere extensive stroke, it is readily apparent that the individual has incurred a significant disabling condition. The presence of a speech abnormality and hemiparesis is very much on the surface. In nondominant hemisphere infarcts, especially those in which the individual's moderate-to-excellent motor recovery occurs and speech is not impaired, cognitive impairment may be more subtle. And yet, the impairment often alters impairment of functional skills involved in vocational ability and independence. The case below describes such an example and explores how one may assess such patients.

Background Epidemiology and Demographics

Referral

Patient: Right-handed 40-year-old male
Education: Bachelor's degree
Occupation: Sales

Although improvements in acute stroke care have occurred in recent years, often decreasing long-term morbidity, these unfortunately apply only to a minority of patients. Acute stroke therapies which have had greater press have limited applicability as they must be applied in a very short window after stroke onset; overall they provide a modest benefit. Most stroke patients have alteration in function following their acute illness. **Although not widely known, a third of stroke patients are less than 65 years of age** [1]. Stroke in these age groups often dramatically changes the lives of patients at a time when financial, occupational, and parental responsibilities are greatest; hence, much attention has been directed to the residual treatment needs of stroke patients. As our population ages, a larger portion of persons fall into higher-risk stroke categories. It should also be noted that stroke is not randomly distributed; rather, persons in lower socioeconomic groups are at a higher risk. These persons may need special help in recuperation from stroke. With the advances in, and availability of, potentially helpful new techniques for rehabilitation, medical practitioners can impact patient lives to a greater extent (see [2], p. 333). Reason for referral: There were multiple reasons for the initiation of neurocognitive testing (e.g., why now, what happened). Is Mr. Young safe to live alone? Can he drive, work, and make personal medical decisions? A major consideration is his ability to return to high-level occupational duties. If all clinical signs have substantially improved, does this mean Mr. Young's neurocognitive functioning has fully recovered? Are his problems functioning secondary to clinical depression alone and hence amenable to treatment with medication and/or counseling? What is the long-term prognosis as it pertains to potential independence?

Neurological Exams and Findings

Outlined below are the physician's steps in diagnosis and pattern of thinking (e.g., physician's medical concerns, cognitive concerns, treatment needs, and medical data):

- Mr. Young presented to the hospital with a sudden-onset stroke in the context of a severe gastrointestinal disturbance, suggesting an acute viral infection with dehydration. His family found him "down" after he did not respond to a phone call.
- The time of the last known normal as well as the onset of the stroke was unclear (perhaps 12 or more hours earlier); hence, he was not a candidate for a clot lysis or the use of a retrieval procedure.
- On admission he was severely hypernatremic with evidence of renal decompensation—both compatible with dehydration. He was initially admitted to the neurologic intensive care unit encephalopathic with confusion, disorientation, and agitation. He had an initial moderately severe left hemiparesis and sensory deficit. His exam did not reveal evidence for retinal vascular disease to suggest a more pervasive atherosclerotic cause. Initial CT imaging confirmed the clinical impression of stroke.
- Laboratory testing demonstrated a striking electrolyte disturbance with hypernatremia and impaired renal function. In the intensive care setting, he was treated for dehydration and evaluated for a clotting disorder, which was not found.
- His early neurological exams revealed a diminished level of awareness, disturbed speech fluency, a dense left motor weakness, and a marked diminished reception to sensory stimuli, such as a pinprick or light touch. He had a gaze preference to the right. He did not blink to left-sided visual stimuli.
- His imaging did demonstrate a large right middle cerebral artery territory infarct. As it evolved a moderate amount of swelling took place which slowly resolved. At its maximum he had a herniation of brain tissue from the right hemisphere to the left of 9.5 mm. Additionally, he demonstrated a small amount of hemorrhagic transformation, which is common in large infarcts. There was no evidence for a vascular dissection, tumor, patent foramen ovale, or pervasive clotting disorder. The imaging did not present evidence for earlier stroke or leukomalacia.
- His cardiac evaluation focusing on potential for embolic disease was negative.
- His ultrasound studies of extracranial and intracranial vascular structures were normal.
- An MR angiogram demonstrated an occlusion of his right middle cerebral artery.
- His major conventional risk factors for stroke and vascular disease were modest with tobacco abuse, mild hypertension, and overweight status.
- Evaluation for evidence of prior clinical stroke or silent infarcts was negative. The cause of his stroke remained unclear but was thought to be a transient clotting disorder.

- Family history was positive for hypertension, stroke, high cholesterol, and diabetes. The patient has a younger sister with hypertension.
- His past medical history was significant for prior mild depression. He did not have a significant alcohol history and did not use illicit substances.
- His medical condition and encephalopathy rapidly improved. He lived alone and was not able to make a transition to home self-care so was temporarily placed in a nursing facility. During that stay, his hemiparesis and sensory deficits improved substantially.

Recovery Course

- He received follow-up neurological care at a local hospital-based stroke clinic. In the clinic he demonstrated a slow and substantial improvement in strength on the left side. He had continued difficulties with tasks requiring fine motor skills. He had increased reflexes on the affected side and diminished fine motor usage. His sensory deficits passed. **Subtle abnormalities surfaced as the major deficits waned**. He was noted to have a left-sided neglect and difficulty coping with his illness. He had a mild depression with rumination. Over time, the energetic aspects waned and he was apathetic.
- A CT scan revealed findings compatible with early stroke in the right external capsule at the level of the lateral ventricles in the right frontal lobe. There was evidence of diffuse loss of gray junction involving the right middle cerebral artery distribution associated with a 3-mm midline shift at the interventricular septum.
- Carotid Doppler and transcranial Doppler (TCD) of the basilar and vertebral arteries were unremarkable. There was no other evidence of mass hemorrhage or mass effect.
- The patient had a neurological impact from his stroke similar to others with non-dominant hemisphere middle cerebral artery infarcts. His speech was mildly slowed and slurred, but he did not have problems with understanding or making himself understood. He had an initially very dense motor and sensory abnormality on the right side; in most instances the sensory abnormality passes rather rapidly, as did his. His motor deficit slowly improved but had not returned to normal. The greatest impact was in fine motor movements on the left side, with his hand motion more severely affected than shoulder or leg movements. His visual impairment improved in that he could see objects in the left field, but a neglect of objects on his left side persisted.

Need for Neuropsychological Evaluation from a Medical Perspective

As he improved, a number of long-term issues arose within the context of a young man who had been fully productive prior to his stroke. He was a man without a home support network, although family was nearby and medical caregivers thought he would potentially be able to return to gainful employment. The practical question regarding safety to drive arose in the context of considering his visual neglect.

Additionally, we needed to assess the degree to which depression played a role in his illness as this was also important. The depression he manifested appeared not out of context in his situation, suggesting apathy might be the dominant issue. He did not feel able to return to gainful employment. With time, he had improvement in mood and was able to initiate self-improvement strategies, which included tapering of cigarette abuse, weight loss, and social engagements, but was unable to return to work. The self-management activities were associated with substantial improvement of mood. A lingering apathy remained. Overall, his functional impairment seemed in excess of his motor, sensory, mood, and linguistic capabilities. Especially early in his course, these raised the questions as to why he was not progressing better functionally and whether mood disturbance played a role in this.

The following questions were a concern when referring for neuropsychological testing:

1. To what degree are depression and apathy impairing his function?
2. To what degree does he manifest hemineglect and would that interfere with more complex tasks such as driving?
3. Does he have significant executive dysfunction, and can that explain his inability to regain self-management skills and return to employment, apathy?
4. To what degree does he have cognitive dysfunction and how does that interfere with a return to work?
5. What aspects of his status are amenable to therapy that may improve function? What would those activities be?

Key Point

In this case, mood and motor and sensory deficits improved, but Mr. Young remained apathetic and hesitant to return to work.

Is the apathy due to depression or is it neurocognitive in nature?

If it is neurocognitive in nature, what is his cognitive profile and how can the patient be helped?

Is there cognitive impairment beyond the noticeable apathy? How can this be described and what is the underlying mechanism neurologically?

Neuropsychological Testing

Neuropsychological testing revealed positive areas of functioning, including normal language functioning, superior verbal intellectual functioning, simple and complex attention tasks within normal limits, and immediate and delayed auditory memory within normal limits. All items of validity showed adequate engagement. Areas of difficulty included below-average visual reasoning, visual attention tasks, visual tracking, and visual distraction tests. Immediate and delayed visual memory was significantly impaired. There was significant impairment in areas of visual construction, trouble with constructional apraxia, and difficulty with integration and analysis of nonverbal material. There was significant difficulty with adaptive problem-solving, including maintaining a shifting of set, nonverbal abstract reasoning, below-average conceptual formation and proverbs, and difficulty with organization and planning. Mr. Young had difficulty with visual tracking and sequencing. He had continued difficulty with depression, most likely also organic in nature as well as in reaction to his situation. Mr. Young's impairments on this NP evaluation are even more striking considering his high cognitive reserve.

Findings were consistent with a right middle cerebral artery stroke, including poor visual memory, poor visual-spatial functioning, poor visual reasoning, and especially poor executive functioning. Executive functioning issues may have added to safety concerns, especially in the independent activities of daily living and in his ability to move back to a management position in his vocation.

Recommendations included continued medical, neurological, and physiatry follow-up, as well as continued psychiatric follow-up. Continued cognitive rehabilitation, including occupational, physical, and speech therapy, was appropriate to increase independence. The patient was advised to consider a vocational intervention with a vocational expert to work out an appropriate employment situation with job coaching and proper accommodation and support. Repeat neuropsychological testing in 12 months was recommended, as well as an on-the-road driving test to review safety on the road.

Neuropsychological Theory by Functional Domain in RMCA: Evidence-Based Literature

Overview

The following summarizes major studies in evidence-based medicine (EBM) in RMCA integrated with the cognitive domain as in the case of Mr. Young.

Typical NP findings center around visuospatial and visual memory deficits [3]; however, executive functioning issues are also quite common. Because language and verbal IQ are not impacted in most cases, patients are often mistakenly thought to be fully functioning. Even if neglect and walking have recovered in RMCA patients, they often have cognitive deficits that limit them in successful vocational goals, family needs, and general safety issues (e.g., driving).

Overall, RMCA stroke involves neglect or anosognosia. Both right hemisphere strokes and right frontal strokes can cause neglect. Stroke in the anterior communicating artery territory can also cause neglect. Other avenues of disruption can include deep subcortical strokes in the right hemisphere, including the striatum, deep white matter, posterior internal capsule, and thalamus. When ascending and descending pathways are disrupted, SPECT scans often show hypoperfusion in the right parietal lobe. Festa notes that mechanisms of hemineglect include altered sensation, disordered body schema, disordered attention, unilateral hypokinesia, and motor akinesia [4].

Anosognosia, or lack of awareness of deficits on the part of the patient, in any cognitive domain increases risk of accidents, medication errors, difficulty following medical regimes, understanding complex information, and making clear decisions.

Neuropsychological Findings Specific to Mr. Young

(a) General ability

Verbal IQ was within normal limits (in fact, well above average) and similar to Mr. Young's expected premorbid levels. Perceptual reasoning is often impacted, as was demonstrated in Mr. Young's test findings. Of note, his Wechsler Adult Intelligence Scale-Fourth Edition (WAIS-IV) Similarities score was lower than expected, demonstrating some concrete thinking. It may be lower related to frontal decline with special change in R frontal (see Executive functioning section below).

It is important to note that cognitive reserve, especially in the case of Mr. Young, is a factor in realizing the extent of cognitive change after a stroke. The Mini-Mental Status Exam (MMSE) does not take this into account and misses significant cognitive decline. Mr. Young's cognitive abilities needed to be compared to others of his age and educational and occupational ability. IQ testing, as well as norm-referenced neuropsychological testing stratified by age, education, gender, and, at times, race, helps to identify individuals with higher cognitive reserve (see Table 17.1).

Table 17.1 General ability

General ability	Scaled score (SS)	St score	Index score	Range
WTAR		St Sc = 101		Average
WAIS-4				
Verbal comprehension			116	High average
Perceptual reasoning			75	Borderline
Working memory			128	Superior
Processing speed			74	Borderline
FSIQ			97	Average
Verbal comprehension subtests				
Similarities	8			Average
Vocabulary	13			High average
Information	18			Very superior
Perceptual reasoning subtests				
Block design	5			Borderline
Matrix reasoning	6			Low average
Visual puzzles	6			Low average
Working memory subtests				
Digit span	13 (9F; 8B)			High average
Arithmetic	17			Very superior
Processing speed subtests				
Coding	7			Low average
Symbol search	3			Moderately impaired
	SS=10 ± 10			
	St Sc/Index Sc = 100 ± 15			

(b) Visuospatial ability

Visuospatial impairment is often most pronounced in RMCA, including topographic orientation, constructional abilities, trouble with spatial orientation, route-finding, safety concerns, hemi-inattention, poststroke delirium, constructional apraxia, spatial topographic impairment, motor impersistence, R-hemisphere language/communication problems, short-term memory issues, bilateral syndrome, and prosopagnosia. Anosognosia should be assessed in any patient with right hemisphere damage—it is as essential as neglect and issues of extinction [5]. Vossel et al. [5] emphasize the assessment treatment of anosognosia as it relates to adult daily living (ADL) skills and safety.

Even neuroimaging is showing promise in establishing evidence of real neurocognitive underpinnings of the subtle issues in RMCA, especially regarding visuospatial deficits, even when it is believed the patient has "recovered." Interesting research in rehabilitation techniques using neuroimaging has begun to demonstrate the complex circuitry involved in motor tasks that depend on R-hemispheric regions (e.g., superior parietal areas, secondary motor cortices, primary sensory cortex, and cerebellum) [6, 7].

Acalculia (acquired trouble with math), often a parietal lobe issue, can be impaired by lesions in either the right or left parietal area and may be the result of trouble with mental rotation [8]. Asada et al. [8] discuss the influence of parietal lobe damage in math manipulation (an imagery-bound task) (see Table 17.2).

(c) Learning and memory

Verbal memory is often quite good but visual memory poor in RMCA. This is evident in the case of Mr. Young. His visual memory is quite poor and the direct result of visuospatial injury. However, even his auditory memory for complex novel material (supraspan verbal memory; see Table 17.3) was inefficient and likely the result of decreased organization in the frontal lobe. Poor visual memory and inefficient memory will likely challenge him in the pursuit of complex vocational tasks and complex independent adult daily living tasks (e.g., finances, medical decisions, follow-through with medical regimens).

(d) Executive functioning

Executive functioning includes dorsolateral findings, apathy [9], anosognosia, lack of initiation, poor impulse control, trouble with complex attention, poor multitasking sequencing, personality change, and lack of emotional awareness, among other issues.

Table 17.2 Visual-spatial functioning

	Scaled score	Percentile	Range
CFT copy		<1	Impaired
Block design	5		Borderline
Matrix reasoning	6		Low average
Visual puzzles	6		Low average
	SS = 10 ± 3		

Table 17.3 Memory

Memory	Scaled score	T score	Z scores	Range
WMS-4				
Verbal memory subtests				
Logical memory I	18			Very superior
Logical memory II	18			Very superior
Visual memory subtests				
Visual reproduction I	1			Impaired
Visual reproduction II	6			Low average
CVLT-2 (St)				
Trial 1			–0.5	Average
Trial 5			0.5	Average
Long delay free recall			0.5	Average
Total		53		Average
Visual memory subtests				
CFT immediate		20		Impaired
CFT delay		<20		Impaired
CFT recognition		<20		Impaired
	SS = 10 ± 3			
	T = 50 ± 10			
	2 Scores = 0.0 ± 1.0			

Trouble with dorsolateral function is frequent in RMCA and causes more safety issues and impairment in adult daily living skills (ADLs) than does memory disorder alone. Impairment in executive functioning (EF) can disrupt everyday functioning, complex work environments, and academic success.

1. *Multitasking, organization, planning, sequencing, and problem-solving*: Executive functioning circuitry is highly sensitive to brain impairment of any kind. This includes RMCA. The "CEO" or "conductor" of the brain is essential to everyday functioning, safety, and ability to fully function vocationally. Regarding right frontal lobe impairment, Robinson makes the case that numerous functions may be affected and can include design fluency, gesture fluency, and ideational fluency [10]. In the case of Mr. Young, all these arenas of function were crucial to his independence, safety, and future well-being.
2. *Abstract reasoning*: Murphy et al. [11] addressed the influence of right frontal impairment on "proverb interpretation" (p. 1). They found that processing of proverbs may take place in the right medial and left lateral frontal areas. Mr. Young had difficulty on both fluid IQ measures of proverbs (Similarities and D-KEFS Proverbs).
3. *Planning in the natural environment*: Goel et al. [12] found that patients with right prefrontal cortex impairment tend to make less accurate and slower conclusions when surveying information due to poor exploration of all data that might influence a situation.

4. *Emotional regulation and synthesis*: Frontal lobe lesions are noted for trouble with apathy and poor ability to utilize and regulate empathy. **This is a true neurocognitive deficit and not just a symptom of clinical depression**. Caeiro et al. [13] reviewed the literature in this area and concluded that apathy is very prevalent in frontal lobe stroke and is even more frequent than depression. Apathy can worsen depression symptoms and certainly impact daily functioning in the home and work environment. Leigh et al. [14] discusses the fact that empathy is often disrupted in frontal lobe damage and is involved in circuitry throughout the brain ("amygdala, prefrontal cortex, cingulate gyrus, temporal-parietal junction, orbitofrontal gyrus, anterior insula, anterior cingulate cortex, etc."). The type of empathy involved impairs affective regulation and understanding. This is very debilitating for the patient and even more disturbing for the family and caregivers. This phenomenon is separate from clinical depression etiology and not willful. In cases such as this, neuropsychotherapy and rehabilitation are very important for the patient and the family (see Judd and Backhaus chapters in Part 3 of this volume).

In addition to traditional neuropsychological assessment tools used by trained neuropsychologists, the Frontal Assessment Battery is sometimes used [15]. This tool is designed to assess both cognitive and behavioral domains through several brief tests and shows promise in detecting changes in right frontal impairment. Domains tested include "conceptualization and abstract reasoning, lexical verbal fluency and mental flexibility, motor programming and executive control of action, self-regulation and resistance to interference, inhibitory control, and environmental autonomy." Researchers have used this assessment along with the MoCA and have found it to capture the frontal lobe issues more readily. **Still, when trying to make decisions about returning to work, a comprehensive NP battery with assessment of cognitive reserve (general ability and IQ) is essential** (see Table 17.4).

(e) Language

Language, though traditionally thought to be unchanged in RMCA, can be disrupted even in dominant right handers in 20% of RMCA cases. Also, the understanding of nuance, emotional inflection, and emotional content is regulated by the right hemisphere (see Table 17.5).

Table 17.4 Executive functioning

	T score	Scaled score	Percentile	Range
Wisconsin card sort			1/6 Categories (2–5 ‰)	Borderline
Category test	19			Impaired
D-KEFS tower		8		Average
Tower achievement		9		Average
Multiple choice		9		Average
	SS = 10 ± 3			
	T = 50 ± 10			

Table 17.5 Language

	T score	Range
Boston naming test	52	Average
Aphasia screen	No errors/100% correct	Average
Letter fluency (FAS)	41	Low average
Semantic fluency (Animals)	47	Average
	T = 50 ± 10	

Table 17.6 Attention

Attention/processing speed	Scaled score	Index	Range
Digit span	(9F; 8B) SS = 14		High average
Arithmetic	17		Very superior
Coding	8		Average
Symbol search	4		Borderline
Working memory		131	Very superior
Processing speed		79	Borderline
	SS = 10 ± 3		
	Index = 1000 ± 15		

(f) Emotional functioning

Mr. Young did have a history of depression. Increased depression is often a symptom of stroke. Clinical depression cannot explain his other neurocognitive findings on this exam, but certainly exacerbated his ability to recover. Treatment was suggested and sought and eventually did decrease excess disability related to clinical depression. Medication and psychosocial support were vital in his overall recovery.

(g) Attention/speed of processing

Slowed processing and difficulty with visual attention were evident, as would be expected. Attention and slowed processing alone can cause significant daily interference. This finding further complicated Mr. Young's neuropsychological picture (see Table 17.6).

In summary, this neuropsychological testing informed Mr. Young and his caregivers that he will most likely have neurocognitive trouble in day-to-day life and on a functional basis in these areas: recognizing he has impairment (anosognosia), planning ahead, initiating behavior (even with resolution of depression), sequencing, visual scanning, searching, and attending to things visually (e.g., playing sports, driving, walking into unfamiliar environments). Executive functioning and visuospatial impairment will likely create an inability to cope with complex demands. The assistance of a vocational rehabilitation specialist is critical for those desiring to remain employed (see Chap. 31 in this book).

Discussion with Evidenced-Based Citations

Key Question

1. *Is Mr. Young fully recovered if all neurological signs are resolved?*

The neurological exam and mini-mental status can easily miss impairments found in RMCA, which involves more than neglect and simple visuospatial problems. When language is fine, cognitive dysfunction in RMCA can easily go unnoticed and lead to poor medical outcomes, safety issues, loss of employment, and failure in academics. This case illustrates how the integration of neuroimaging, neurology, and neuropsychology offer a rich and comprehensive brain-related functional picture. Tanner et al. also demonstrated the integration of neuropsychology and brain imaging [16].

Neuropsychological testing data add diagnostic clarity and ability to track neurocognitive functions, as in the example of dressing therapy. Walker et al. discussed targeted dressing therapy treatment (targeted coordinated movement for dressing) from specific NP assessment [17]. The NP test highlighted certain cognitive problems that were placed in a routine treatment regime for dressing. The formalized treatment was statistically more robust for RMCA patients than standard OT dressing therapy. In this study, targeted therapy for dressing guided by neuropsychological assessment in RMCA strokes was more effective than standard occupational therapy for dressing.

Neuropsychological testing is also important for designing patient and family interventions. Providing this early diagnostic information helps full recovery. Knowing all cognitive issues helps more complete recovery and prevents job loss, lowered self-esteem, etc. Whenever possible, patients are assisted and accommodated for return to work. If not possible, structured meaningful activity is designed by skilled vocational rehabilitation professionals (certified rehabilitation counselors). In a 2-year follow-up study for first ever stroke, Turunen [18] found that "Long-lasting cognitive impairment was common even after good neurological recovery. An early neuropsychological evaluation is essential in evaluating cognitive dysfunction and need for rehabilitation."

Chapter Review Questions

1. True/False: Beyond the clinical signs of RMCA (neglect, etc.), there are no cognitive deficits.

2. MMSE misses what potential neurocognitive deficits in RMCA?
   A. Subtle and complex visuospatial dysfunction.
   B. Executive functioning, inefficient memory and learning, slowed attention, and cognitive reserve.
   C. Depression.
   D. Comparisons of test performance against age, education, and occupation.
   E. All of the above.

3. True/False: Once neglect has recovered, there may still be some visuospatial deficits.

4. Safety in the home and in the environment can be assessed by:
   A. OT.
   B. Neuropsychology, physical therapy, and OT in combination.
   C. Neurology.

References

1. Freburger JK, Holmes GM, Ku LJ, Cutchin MP, Heatwole-Shank K, Edwards LJ. Disparities in post-acute rehabilitation care for stroke: an analysis of the state inpatient databases. Arch Phys Med Rehabil. 2011;92(8):1220–9.
2. Ricker J, DeLuca J, Frey S. On the changing roles of neuroimaging in rehabilitation science. Brain Imaging Behav. 2014;8(3):333–4.
3. Crouse EM, Roper BL. Large right hemisphere stroke. In: Morgan JE, Baron IS, Ricker JH, editors. Casebook of clinical neuropsychology. New York: Oxford Press. p. 2011.
4. Festa J, Lazar R, editors. Neurovascular neuropsychology. New York: Springer; 2009.
5. Vossel S, Weiss P, Eschenbeck P, Fink GR. Anosognosia, neglect, extinction and lesion site predict impairment of daily living after right-hemispheric stroke. Cortex. 2013;49(7):1782–9.
6. Chen P, Goedert KM, Shah P, Foundas AL, Barrett AM. Integrity of medial temporal structures may predict better improvement of spatial neglect with prism adaptation treatment. Brain Imaging Behav. 2014;8(3):346–58.
7. Wittenberg GF, Lovelace CT, Foster DJ, Maldjian JA. Functional neuroimaging of dressing-related skills. Brain Imaging Behav. 2014;8(3):335–45.
8. Asada T, Takayama Y, Oita J, Fukuyama H. Effects of mental rotation on acalculia: differences in the direction of mental rotation account for the differing characteristics of acalculia induced by right and left hemispheric brain injury. Neurocase. 2014;20(2):163–74.
9. Lara C, Ferro J, Costa J. Apathy secondary to stroke: a systematic review and meta-analysis. Cerebrovasc Dis. 2013;35(1):23–39.
10. Robinson G, Shallice T, Bozzali M, Cipolotti L. The differing roles of the frontal cortex in fluency tests. Brain. 2012;135(7):2202–14.
11. Murphy P, Shallice T, Robinson G, et al. Impairments in proverb interpretation following focal frontal lobe lesions. Neuropsychologia. 2013;51(11):2075–86.
12. Goel V, Vartanian O, Bartolo A, et al. Lesions to right prefrontal cortex impair real-world planning through premature commitment. Neuropsychologia. 2013;51(4):713–24.
13. Caeiro L, Ferro JM, Costa J. Apathy secondary to stroke: a systemic review and meta-analysis. Cerebrovasc Dis. 2013;35(1):23–39.
14. Leigh R, Oishi K, Hsu J, et al. Acute lesions that impair affective empathy. Brain. 2013;136:2539–49.
15. DuBois B, Slachevsky A, Litvan I, Pillon B. The FAB: a frontal assessment battery at bedside. Neurology. 2000;55(11):1621–6.
16. Tanner JJ, Mellott EM, Dunne EM, Price CC. Integrating neuropsychology and brain imaging for a referral of possible pseudodementia: a case report. Clin Neuropsychol. 2015;29(2):272–92.
17. Walker M, Sunderland A, Fletcher-Smith J, et al. The DRESS trial: a feasibility randomized controlled trial of a neuropsychological approach to dressing therapy for stroke patients. Clin Rehabil. 2012;26(8):675–85.
18. Turunen KEA, Laari SPK, Kauranen TV, et al. Domain-specific cognitive recovery after first-ever stroke: a 2-year follow-up. J Int Neuropsychol Soc. 2018;24:117–27.

Chapter 18
Deep Brain Stimulation for Parkinson's Disease

Cynthia S. Kubu, Michal Gostkowski, Joseph Rudolph, and Sean Nagel

Introduction

More than 100,000 individuals have had deep brain stimulation (DBS), and most of those have had DBS for the treatment of tremor or motor symptoms of Parkinson's disease (PD) [1]. DBS was initially approved by the FDA in 1997 for the treatment of tremor, and in 2002, it was approved for the treatment of motor symptoms of PD. DBS involves the implantation of an electrode into specific brain regions. The most common targets for the treatment of motor symptoms of PD include the subthalamic nucleus (STN), globus pallidus interna (GPi), and ventral intermediate (VIM) nucleus of the thalamus. The electrode is connected, via a cable tunneled underneath the skin, to an internal pulse generator (IPG, similar to a cardiac pacemaker) typically placed in the chest. The stimulation parameters of the DBS electrode can be changed via the IPG by an external programming device. DBS is advantageous over previously used lesion procedures (e.g., thalamotomy, pallidotomy) due to the ability to change parameters to maximize benefit and minimize side effects and its theoretically reversible nature. In most cases, the patient's ability to control the stimulation parameters is limited, and the patient relies on a clinician with expertise in programming to adjust the stimulator settings. DBS is highly effective in treating many of the motor symptoms of PD in well-selected patients [2–4]. Selection of patients who are candidates for DBS includes consideration of cognitive and neurobehavioral function. Consequently, several groups have argued

C. S. Kubu (✉) · M. Gostkowski
Center for Neurological Restoration, Cleveland Clinic, Cleveland, OH, USA
e-mail: kubuc@ccf.org

J. Rudolph · S. Nagel
Center for Neurological Restoration, Neurologic Institute, Cleveland Clinic, Cleveland, OH, USA

K. M. Sanders (ed.), *Physician's Field Guide to Neuropsychology*,
https://doi.org/10.1007/978-1-4939-8722-1_18

that neuropsychologists should be integral members of DBS teams [5, 6]. This chapter provides a rationale for inclusion of neuropsychologists on DBS teams and illustrative case examples.

Rationale

In his famous 1817 essay on the shaking palsy, James Parkinson argued that the "senses and intellect are uninjured" [7]. Two hundred years later, there are now ample data that Parkinson was wrong in his assertion. Non-motor symptoms, including neurocognitive and neurobehavioral symptoms, are very common in PD and may be more disabling for some patients than the cardinal features of tremor, rigidity, akinesia, and postural instability [8].

This is not surprising given the underlying neuropathology of PD. PD is a synucleinopathy characterized by Lewy neurites and Lewy bodies present throughout multiple brain regions. Braak and colleagues elegantly demonstrated in a large autopsy series how PD is a multisystem disease that progresses over six stages [9]. Stages 1 and 2 are characterized by pathological changes in the dorsal motor nucleus of the vagus nerve, medulla oblongata/pontine tegmentum, and anterior olfactory structures. Changes in the substantia nigra and basal forebrain regions along with the anterior Ammon's horn become apparent in Stages 3 and 4. It is at this stage that clinical symptoms of PD become evident. Stages 5 and 6 are characterized by cortical changes including regions of the anterior cingulate cortex, insula, and other limbic regions. Due to these structural pathological changes, multiple neurotransmitters systems are impacted including dopaminergic, cholinergic, and serotonergic.

In addition to neuropathological changes characteristic of PD, Alexander, DeLong, and Strick's discussion of cortico-striato-thalamo-cortical circuits provides a neuroanatomical framework for understanding the types of cognitive and behavioral symptoms one might expect to see in the context of PD [10]. In their seminal paper, Alexander, DeLong, and Strick postulated the existence of five segregated, parallel circuits that originated in discrete regions of the frontal lobe (i.e., supplementary motor area [SMA], frontal eye fields, dorsolateral prefrontal cortex [DLPFC], anterior cingulate cortex [ACC], and orbitofrontal cortex [OFC]). The circuits travel to different regions within the basal ganglia and then to the thalamus before returning to the cortical region of origin. Damage anywhere along those circuits could give rise to symptoms that might be seen with dysfunction involving the cortical region of origin. Dysfunction in the SMA network is implicated in the pathophysiology of PD, and different nodes in the network are targets for neurosurgical treatment of motor symptoms of PD. The DLPFC, ACC, and OFC networks are of special interest to neuropsychologists, and dysfunction in these networks is associated with executive cognitive and limbic symptoms. These networks are closely situated in the basal ganglia, particularly in the subthalamic nucleus.

Neurocognitive and neurobehavioral symptoms may arise in patients with PD due to the underlying pathophysiology of the disease and treatment side effects, including medication and surgical treatments. The typical cognitive symptoms associated with idiopathic PD include slowed psychomotor processing speed, decreased verbal fluency, executive cognitive impairments (i.e., impairments on tests assessing problem-solving, planning, mental flexibility, response inhibition), memory retrieval inefficiencies, and, later in the disease, visuospatial and visuoconstructional impairments [11]. PD is associated with a sixfold higher prevalence of dementia than the normal population with a point prevalence of 25–30% [12]. Most patients will develop dementia if they survive more than 10 years following diagnosis [12]. Cognitive changes may also occur as a function of medication side effects including dopamine agonists or anticholinergics. In addition, neurosurgical treatments may theoretically impact cognitive function due to either direct impact on cognitive networks or non-specific effects associated with other surgical variables (e.g., anesthesia).

Neuropsychiatric symptoms are also common in PD. This is not surprising given what is known about the underlying functional neuroanatomy and neuropathology of the disease. Dysthymia and depression are very common with estimates ranging from 40% to 70% of patients meeting criteria for dysthymia and up to 50% of those meeting formal diagnostic criteria for depression [8, 13–15]. Anxiety is also very common and may co-occur with depression (up to 40% of patients). Anxiety may be more common when patients with PD are in the "off" state. Apathy is the third most common neuropsychiatric symptom in PD with estimates up to 30% of patients [8, 14, 16]. Hallucinations and delusions may occur in the context of PD due to neuropathological changes in limbic regions or as a side effect of medications [17]. Common clinical lore holds that the hallucinations associated with PD are "benign" and typically include seeing small children or animals; however, this does not always hold true, and some patients experience much more disturbing hallucinations. The hallucinations can be visual, auditory, or, more rarely, haptic. Delusional thinking may also occur due to medication side effects or as a function of the underlying disease. PD may also be associated with dopamine dysregulation syndrome which is characterized by dopaminergic medication misuse/abuse [18]. Patients will resist efforts to reduce their medications, may self-medicate, and/or hoard their medications. Other symptoms of this disorder include walkabouts and impulse control disorders (e.g., hypersexuality, gambling, impulse shopping, gorging of sweets, etc.). The syndrome has typically been associated with young men, but women and older patients may also demonstrate symptoms. Often reduction of dopaminergic medications (particularly dopamine agonists) will result in the reduction of symptoms. Patients with PD may also demonstrate punding—stereotyped aimless, repetitive motor acts such as assembling and dissembling items or arranging and rearranging items. This is a relatively rare symptom and associated with dopamine dysregulation. More rarely, we have observed patients with other kinds of repetitive behaviors, such as trichotillomania or picking that may increase risk of infection in the context of neurosurgical treatments for motor symptoms of PD [19]. Finally, there has been some debate in the literature regarding the possibility of increased suicidal risk associated with DBS [20]; however, other groups have not found that to be the case [21].

Neuropsychological assessments composed of detailed testing and a careful clinical interview provide critical data that contribute to determinations regarding a patient's candidacy for DBS as well as identify potential risk factors. Exclusion criteria for DBS include severe cognitive impairment; severe depression, including suicidal ideation; psychotic symptoms; and other severe psychiatric symptoms (e.g., substance abuse) [22]. Dementia is typically viewed to be a contraindication for DBS. In addition, evidence of milder neuropsychological impairments prior to surgery is significantly related to greater postoperative confusion, longer hospital stays, and postoperative declines in verbal memory and may be associated with diminished benefit on functional and quality-of-life measures [23–26]. Similarly, neuropsychiatric symptoms identified via testing or in detailed clinical interviews, such as anxiety, compulsive picking, impulse control symptoms, and personality characteristics (e.g., factors associated with noncompliance), may be associated with increased risk in the context of DBS [19–21, 27–29].

Consequently, neuropsychologists are typically key members of DBS teams. There are four primary goals of the preoperative neuropsychological assessment: (1) assessment of cognitive function and identification of any potential cognitive factors that might impact care, (2) assessment of neuropsychiatric function and identification of any factors that might impact care, (3) assessment of family support for the decision to pursue DBS, and (4) identification of patients' and family members' goals and expectations for surgery [6, 29, 30]. These data are highly relevant to the most common ethical challenges in DBS including challenges surrounding risk/benefit assessments, determinations regarding inclusion/exclusion, autonomy, and patient benefit/quality of life [29].

Key Point

The neuropsychologist's role in evaluating DBS candidates is not limited to cognitive testing but includes evaluation of neuropsychiatric function, social support, and expectations for DBS.

Case 1

Mr. X is a 62-year-old, right-handed gentleman who completed 12 years of formal education followed by some college-level courses. He worked as a delivery man. Mr. X initially observed left fifth finger trembling about 5 years ago while playing drums in a band. He was diagnosed with PD within a year or two. Mr. X's symptoms progressed over time, and he presented to our team for consideration of DBS.

Neuropsychological Evaluation: Mr. X completed a standard neuropsychological assessment including a semi-structured interview designed to address the four goals listed above. His stated goals were to reduce his tremor, lessen his fatigue, improve his ambition, and reduce his medications. His long-term girlfriend was very supportive of his decision and eager to "have the old Mike back." Her goals include increased energy.

Mr. X's medical history was otherwise remarkable for borderline diabetes, hypertension, hypothyroidism, tonsillectomy, cardiac catheterizations, and chronic knee and back pain. Mr. X described poor sleep. His primary care physician (PCP) had prescribed anxiety medications for years that he took on an as needed basis. Both Mr. X and his partner described an increase in anxiety over the past few years. Mr. X's family history was remarkable for substance abuse, anxiety, and stroke. He stopped smoking in 1995 and reported a 3.0 ppd. habit prior to that. Mr. X also stopped drinking alcohol 3 years ago. He described some bouts of heavy drinking prior to that. Mr. X attributed fatigue and dyskinesias to his current medication regimen; his partner added that anxiety and panic attacks appear to be related to his medications as well. Mr. X lives with his partner, A, of 6 years. He described their relationship as very good.

On functional inquiry, Mr. X endorsed mild, relative declines in his memory, attention, thinking speed, planning, and word finding abilities. He described more marked problems with his handwriting and occasional speech difficulties characterized by hoarseness and slight stammering. No significant sensory difficulties or changes were endorsed. Mr. X described poor sleep that he attributed to back pain. His appetite varies, and his weight has reflected that variability. Mr. X endorsed a mild decline in his interest in music but denied any other indications of anhedonia. Libido is reduced, and the couple also described mildly diminished initiative. Mr. X denied significant changes in his personality over the course of his illness, whereas his partner described a mild decline in his sense of humor. In general, the couple characterized his mood as a mix of anxious and frustrated. On direct questioning, Mr. X endorsed a history of panic attacks, REM behavior disorder symptoms, increased picking behaviors, questionable punding, and a mild increase in obsessional thinking. The cognitive test data are summarized in Table 18.1.

Neuropsychologist's Perspective: Mr. Mike X is a 62-year-old, right-handed gentleman whose neuropsychological assessment was most remarkable for the neuropsychiatric findings with indications in the interview of REM behavior disorder symptoms, panic attacks, picking behaviors, questionable punding, and increased obsessional thinking. Mr. X endorsed moderate psychological distress characterized by symptoms of anxiety and depression, per his responses on self-report questionnaires. The cognitive data were largely unremarkable with the exception of a borderline impaired score on a measure of problem-solving with evidence of mild perseveration. This latter finding is very consistent with his diagnosis of PD. Mr. X and his partner were able to articulate generally reasonable goals for DBS, and he reported good support in his decision to pursue surgery. Prior to surgery, formal mental health assessment and treatment, including both behavioral and pharmacological approaches, were recommended with close follow-up by Mr. X's mental health team after surgery. His history of anxiety and panic attacks should be considered when planning for his surgery. In addition, continued monitoring of his other neurobehavioral symptoms as outlined above was recommended.

Key Point
Sometimes the most important findings in the neuropsychological assessment are the neurobehavioral symptoms.

Table 18.1 Summary of neuropsychological test scores

	Patient X	Patient Z
Global cognition function		
Dementia rating scale, total score	Raw = 141, SS = 12	Raw = 141, SS = 12
Wechsler abbreviated scale of intelligence, FSIQ	103	109
VIQ	102	114
PIQ	103	103
Psychological function		
Beck depression inventory	Raw = 22	Raw = 7
Beck anxiety inventory	Raw = 20	Raw = 3
Attention, working memory, processing speed, executive cognitive		
Wechsler memory scale-III, digit span	ACSS = 11	ACSS = 14
Wechsler memory scale-III, letter number sequencing	ACSS = 12	ACSS = 13
Symbol digit modalities test (oral version)	Standard score = 101	Standard score = 87
D-KEFS Stroop, color	SS = 14	SS = 12
D-KEFS Stroop, word	SS = 15	SS = 12
D-KEFS Stroop, inhibition	SS = 12	SS = 13
D-KEFS Stroop, inhibition/switching	SS = 12	SS = 13
WCST, categories	Raw = 1, 6th %ile	Raw = 6, >16th%ile
WCST, trials to first category	Raw = 12, >16th %ile	Raw = 12, >16th %ile
WCST, perseverative errors	Raw = 42, SS = 78	Raw = 7, SS = 110
WCST, set failures	Raw = 0, >16th%ile	Raw = 2, 11–15th %ile
Language		
WRAT-4: Reading	SS = 99	SS = 107
WASI, vocabulary	T = 50	T = 58
WASI, similarities	T = 53	T = 60
Boston naming test	Raw = 57, SS = 12	Raw = 58, SS = 8
Controlled oral word association test	SS = 10	SS = 11
Semantic word fluency	SS = 8	SS = 6
Visuospatial and visuoconstructional		
WASI, block design	T = 47	T = 46
WASI, matrix reasoning	T = 58	T = 59
Judgment of line orientation	SS = 13	SS = 13
Memory		
WMS-III: Logical memory I	SS = 13	SS = 4
WMS-III: Logical memory II	SS = 13	SS = 4
Rey auditory verbal learning test, trial I	SS = 7	SS = 10
Rey auditory verbal learning test, learning over trials	SS = 10	SS = 9
Rey auditory verbal learning test, list B	SS = 7	SS = 8
Rey auditory verbal learning test, immediate recall	SS = 11	SS = 7
Rey auditory verbal learning test, delayed recall	SS = 10	SS = 7
Rey auditory verbal learning test, delayed recognition	SS = 10	SS = 10

Note: *WASI* Wechsler Abbreviated Scale of Intelligence, *WMS-III* Wechsler Memory Scale-III, *WCST* Wisconsin Card Sorting Test, *D-KEFS* Delis-Kaplan Executive Function System. Mayo Older Adult Normative Sample (MOANS) norms were used to determine scale scores (SS) for the following tests: Boston Naming Test, Controlled Oral Word Association Test, Semantic Word Fluency Test, Judgment of Line Orientation Test, and Rey Auditory Verbal Learning Test. All other tests were scored and normed per the recommendations in the test manual

Neurologist's Perspective: Mr. X developed tremor in the left hand and arm 5 years ago. There was not much rigidity at the time, but he did have trouble with fine motor movements. These symptoms interfered with his activities including his ability to play drums. Mr. X also described shuffling gait but only near the end of the day. The only major non-motor features of PD he reported early in his illness were mild forgetfulness and occasional nocturia. Mr. X's condition was complicated by preexisting back pain that interfered with his sleep as well. He was put on carbidopa-levodopa and rasagiline, and while he benefitted from the medicine, he also developed dyskinesias.

Over the course of his disease, Mr. X experienced clear declines in balance and tremor and worsening medication side effects. Although the levodopa-carbidopa controlled his tremor so that he could continue to play drums, he clearly had dyskinesias and significant OFF periods. Pramipexole helped manage the wearing OFF and the tremor; amantadine was added a little later to help with the dyskinesias.

Mr. X eventually retired from his band due to difficulty with carrying the drum set (he was still able to play). He continued to worsen, particularly with respect to dyskinesias, energy, cognition, and mood. Stopping the pramipexole helped his cognition improve, but it also resulted in less control of motor symptoms. Finally, approximately 4 years into his diagnosis, he agreed to undergo an interdisciplinary evaluation to assess his candidacy for DBS. From a neurological perspective, Mr. X was a good candidate for DBS since his primary symptoms were motor features, most specifically tremor, that were clearly levodopa-responsive. His levodopa challenge scores (OFF-ON testing) were 30 and 11, respectively, indicating an improvement of almost 66%.

Key Point

One of the most important tests to evaluate candidacy for DBS for the treatment of motor symptoms of PD includes the OFF/ON medication test. Patients complete a standardized motor evaluation (Unified Parkinson's Disease Rating Scale – Part III, motor subtest) in the effective OFF medication state (i.e., 12 h with no PD medication). They are then provided with a higher dose of their dopaminergic medication and reassessed using the same scale. A robust response to dopaminergic medication is viewed as a good predictor of response to DBS (with the possible exception of tremor symptoms).

Neurosurgeon's Perspective: In many centers, asleep surgery and awake surgery are offered depending on the patient's age, comorbidities, target, and surgeon preference. In some cases, when awake mapping is planned, significant brain shift is expected following CSF loss during the awake testing and implantation of the first lead. This could lead to errors in targeting the second side. Brain atrophy, which increases with age, will often lead to increase in brain shift. To minimize this risk, the surgeon may elect to stage the surgery over several weeks: implantation of one lead following by implantation of the contralateral side and then insertion of the pulse generator.

Mr. X, like many patients who elect to proceed with the evaluation for DBS, is in his seventh decade of life and will likely have brain atrophy. He also has several comorbidities that could increase his risk for a poor outcome with surgery, and each would factor into the decision on how to best proceed in his case. These variables, coupled with the patient's anxiety, suggest that a staged bilateral implant may be the best alternative in this case. Although the surgeries are relatively short and the estimated blood loss in total is usually less than 100 cm^3, repeat surgery over a short period of time will stress even the most fit individual. In most cases, patients considering DBS are in their sixth, seventh, or eighth decade. The specter of multiple surgeries may loom large in the patient's mind and might exacerbate any underlying psychological or psychiatric diagnoses as well as exhaust the patient's physiological reserves.

Mr. X's history of high blood pressure could compromise the safe insertion of the DBS lead in the operating room. Strict systolic parameters are intended to reduce the risk of hemorrhage. A labile blood pressure reading may prolong the surgery as anesthesia works to correct this, especially during the electrophysiologic testing. These will generally compound the stress on the patient that spreads to the surgical team, exacerbating the problem especially in a watchful patient with anxiety.

Mr. X's anxiety is another neurosurgical concern. The stereotactic frame that is secured to the bed, sterile draping, and intraoperative imaging all contribute to the patient's correct perception that they are enclosed and restrained which may magnify anxiety. The patient's back pain, a frequent complaint in those with PD, also tends to be amplified when fixed to the operative bed.

Finally, there are few surgical procedures that place such high demand on patient cooperation under such unfavorable circumstances as awake intraoperative testing. Patients are educated preoperatively about the expectations, but this may only elicit feelings of dread. It is expected that the patient will remain calm and cooperative during the awake testing with the realization that there is a probe actively advancing through their brain tissue. Psychologists are not uncommonly included in the OR team to soothe the patient's anxiety and offer concrete relaxation techniques [31]. In some patients with severe anxiety, asleep DBS may be the only safe option.

Infection of a DBS system, though quite uncommon, remains a relevant concern that frequently requires explant of some or all components of the system. This risk is increased in patients with diabetes. In addition, picking behavior, especially when severe, is a relative contraindication. This will not only delay incisional healing but under some circumstances contribute to hardware erosion and eventual device explantation. In some situations, when it is not controlled, a lesional procedure such as gamma knife or MR-guided high-frequency ultrasound may be the more advisable surgery.

Team Decision and Outcome: Mr. X was judged to be a reasonable candidate for DBS and was offered staged, bilateral surgery. Prior to surgery, he was instructed to follow through with the team's clinical health psychologist for mental health treatment as part of his perioperative care plan. Mr. X also agreed to participate in a clinical research study using a new electrode. He underwent placement of a left STN electrode followed by placement of a right STN lead 2 weeks later.

He recently came in for his third programming session and stated that things were going well and he was returning to his normal activities. Mr. X was able to reduce his medication intake and described less dyskinesias. He has continued to experience medication fluctuations and reported one fall since the last visit (i.e., he slipped on ice when going up the stairs outside). Although his tremor is significantly reduced, Mr. X's biggest complaint is persistent thumb and first finger tremor (as opposed to the whole hand shaking).

Case 2

Mr. Z is a 67-year-old, right-handed, married gentleman who completed 16 years of formal education followed by 1 year of graduate school. He worked primarily as a high school math teacher and retired about 4 years ago. Mr. Z described the onset of left-hand and foot tremor about 13 years ago and more recent right-hand tremor. Mr. Z presented to our team for consideration of DBS.

Neuropsychological Evaluation: Mr. Z completed a standard assessment with a semi-structured interview designed to address the four goals outlined above. Mr. Z's goals were to live a relatively normal life and improve his quality of life. Specifically, he indicated that his goals for DBS were to reduce his back pain, tremor, rigidity, and medication burden. His wife was very supportive of his decision to consider surgery and shared his goals.

Mr. Z's medical history was otherwise remarkable for three surgeries in the late 1960s to treat colitis, ileostomy, revision of the stoma site for his ileostomy, bladder surgery, and tonsillectomy. He had a presumed TIA following the bladder surgery characterized by kaleidoscopic visual phenomena and loss of vision. Mr. Z had been hospitalized for kidney stones and was treated for hyperlipidemia. He reported chronic low back pain. There was no history of mental health difficulties or treatment. Mr. Z's family neurological medical history was remarkable for questionable depression and late-life tremor in his father. Mr. Z denied tobacco, alcohol, and illicit drug use. Mr. Z questioned if blurred vision and poor sleep might be related to his current medication regimen and also reported dyskinesias. At the time of the evaluation, Mr. Z was living with his wife of almost 40 years. He described their relationship and his relationships with other family members and friends as very good.

Mr. Z completed the interview assessing his perception of his cognitive abilities with his wife. The couple described occasional problems with his thinking speed as a function of his medication status, and his wife noted occasional problems with remembering to take his medications as required. Very mild declines in word finding were noted as well as intermittent difficulties maintaining his train of thought. No other cognitive difficulties or changes were endorsed. Mr. Z described his speech as softer and less clear. Handwriting is impaired. Mr. Z denied concerns with his driving but will have his wife drive longer distances due to his rigidity. Vision was described as slightly blurry and hearing reduced but corrected with hearing aids.

Mr. Z noted a diminished sense of smell. Senses of taste and touch were described as intact. Mr. Z described a disrupted sleep schedule and is up often during the night; nonetheless, he typically awakens feeling rested. No concerns were raised regarding appetite. Mr. Z denied anhedonia and characterized his initiative as strong. His wife agreed with his assessment. In addition, the couple has observed an increase in libido. Mr. Z and his wife denied changes in his personality over the course of his illness and characterized his mood as primarily good. On direct questioning, they described an increase in vivid dreams, and Mr. Z occasionally experiences a "sense of presence" but no frank hallucinations. See Table 18.1 for the cognitive data.

Neuropsychologist's Perspective: The assessment findings were essentially unremarkable except for impairments on a story memory test. The story memory findings are somewhat atypical for PD especially in the context of Mr. Z's other test scores; however, his performance on the word list learning test was within normal limits. It was recommended that Mr. Z be monitored for impulse control symptoms over time in light of the history of increased libido. Mr. Z stated reasonable goals for surgery, and it appeared that he had good support with his decision to consider DBS.

Neurologist's Perspective: Mr. Z reported that his initial symptom of Parkinson's disease was left-leg tremor. One year later, he developed a similar rest tremor in the left arm. He was placed on carbidopa/levodopa and selegiline which was quickly discontinued by his neurologist and replaced with ropinirole 4 mg four times a day. There was marginal improvement to this tremor with this change. It appears that this outside neurologist revised his diagnosis from Parkinson's disease to essential tremor and placed the patient on primidone 150 mg three times a day and atenolol 25 mg twice a day. The ropinirole was continued at 4 mg four times daily, and the patient reported the development of mild impulse control disorder related to hypersexuality. After 2 years, the patient developed right hemisomal rest tremor. The patient was restarted on levodopa, and after 8 years, he had developed disabling peak-dose dyskinesias. The patient presented for deep brain surgery evaluation after 12 years of Parkinson's disease with the following unorthodox regimen of carbidopa/levodopa/entacapone 25/100/200 mg six times daily, ropinirole 4 mg four to six times daily, and rasagiline 0.5 mg twice a day.

He underwent DBS patient screening. His OFF/ON testing went from 31 to 9 with the development of dyskinesia. This patient was deemed a reasonable candidate for deep brain stimulation given his history of PD, robust response on the OFF/ON testing, and stated goals to reduce tremor, improve his ON time duration, improve his peak-dose dyskinesias, and reduce medication burden.

Neurosurgeon's Perspective: Mr. Z's onset and progression of PD are very typical of patients referred for DBS. With age, as the list of medical conditions expands into most organ systems, the preoperative workup and optimization process may demand additional testing and consultations to ensure that the risks are appropriately addressed and ameliorated where possible. Fortunately, there are very few absolute contraindications to DBS surgery. Many patients are either on antiplatelet or anticoagulation therapy. It is almost mandatory; these are stopped for the insertion of the leads and microelectrode recording if planned. Surgeon preference, based on research, experience, and often anecdotal reports, will inform the decision when to restart these medications but is usually taken on a case-by-case basis. Patients are however at elevated risk of a potentially catastrophic event when these medications are stopped. Additional counseling is essential. In patients deemed very high risk, these medications may be resumed during the battery implantation.

As there are two targets that have shown effectiveness with DBS surgery for PD, the globus pallidus internus and the subthalamic nucleus, a patient's memory or verbal skills that may be susceptible to worsening could influence this choice. The STN, in particular, is associated with reduced verbal fluency. The clinical significance of this worsening, however, may be less obvious to the patient. Impulse control symptoms, such as increased libido, most often reflect fluctuations in dopamine levels and may be further disrupted with DBS. These risks should be conveyed to the patient, spouse, or other family members. Although we now have decades of data from which to explore long-term changes in personality and motivational states, a predictable understanding is still beyond our grasp.

Team Decision and Outcome: The team wanted more information regarding Mr. Z's reported TIA. Those details were obtained from the patient, and an MRA of the head and neck was ordered to evaluate for stenosis to determine if he could go off his antiplatelet medication around the time of surgery. The discussion also focused on the memory findings; the patient and his partner denied significant memory difficulties in his daily life, and the formal testing did not indicate frank memory impairments on all tests. It was also possible that Mr. Z's medication burden may have contributed to his poor score on the story memory test.

Mr. Z ultimately received bilateral STN stimulation which was very effective in reducing his tremor. His levodopa burden was slightly reduced to five times daily, and his rasagiline was unchanged. The biggest change was with ropinirole which was reduced to 2 mg four times daily. Mr. Z recently returned for his third programming session. He reported a 70% improvement in his motor symptoms despite reducing his dopaminergic medications. Mr. Z reported a reduction in dyskinesias as well as fewer hallucinations and REM behavior disorder symptoms (i.e., vivid dreams) since surgery. Mr. Z described mild difficulties maintaining his train of thought which were present prior to his surgeries and may have worsened slightly since. He will complete a postoperative neuropsychological assessment approximately 6 months following his initial surgery.

Chapter Review Questions

1. PD results in a cognitive pattern characterized by:
   A. Prominent memory impairments.
   B. Early signs of visuospatial dysfunction.
   C. Slowed processing speed and executive cognitive impairments.
   D. Generally normal function.

2. Neurobehavioral symptoms are common in PD and can include which of the following:
   A. Depression.
   B. Anxiety.
   C. Apathy.
   D. Hallucinations.
   E. All of the above.

3. Which of the following is not one of the goals of a preoperative neuropsychological evaluation?
   A. Determination regarding candidacy for DBS.
   B. Evaluation of cognitive status and potential risk factors.
   C. Evaluation of neurobehavioral status and potential risk factors.
   D. Assessment of patient's goals and expectations for DBS.

References

1. Medtronic website. https://www.medtronicdbs.com/why-dbs/innovation-leader/index.htm. Accessed 14 Feb 2018.
2. Benabid AL, Chabardes S, Mitrofanis J, et al. Deep brain stimulation of the subthalamic nucleus for the treatment of Parkinson's disease. Lancet Neurol. 2009;8(1):67–81.
3. Deuschl G, Schade-Brittinger C, Krack P, et al. A randomized trial of deep-brain stimulation for Parkinson's disease. N Engl J Med. 2006;355:896–908.
4. Weaver FM, Follett I, Stern M, et al. Bilateral deep brain stimulation vs. best medical therapy for patients with advanced Parkinson disease: a randomized controlled trial. JAMA. 2009;301(1):63–73.
5. Lang AE, Houeto J-L, Krack P, et al. Deep brain stimulation: preoperative issues. Mov Disord. 2006;21(Suppl 14):S171–96.
6. Rezai AR, Machado A, Deogaonkar M, Azmi H, Kubu CS, Boulis N. Surgery for movement disorders. Neurosurgery. 2008;62(Suppl2):809–38.
7. Parkinson J. An essay on the shaking palsy. 1817. J Neuropsychiatry Clin Neurosci. 2002;14(2):223–36.
8. Pandya M, Kubu C, Giroux M. The many faces of Parkinson's disease: not just a movement disorder. Cleve Clin J Med. 2008;75(12):856–64.
9. Braak H, Bohl JR, Muller CM, Rub U, de Vos RAI, Del Tredici K. Stanley Fahn lecture 2005: The staging procedure for the inclusion body pathology associated with sporadic Parkinson's disease reconsidered. Mov Disord. 2006;21(12):2042–50.
10. Alexander GE, De Long MR, Strick PL. Parallel organization of functionally segregated circuits linking basal ganglia and cortex. Annu Rev Neurosci. 1986;9:357–81.
11. Lezak MD. Neuropsychological assessment. 3rd ed. New York: Oxford University Press; 1995.
12. Aarsland D, Creese B, Politis M, Chaudhuri KR, Ffytech DH, Weintraub D, Ballard C. Cognitive decline in Parkinson disease. Nat Rev Neurol. 2017;13(4):217–31.
13. Aarsland D, Larsen JP, Lim NG, Janvin C, Karlsen K, Tandberg E, Cummings JL. Range of neuropsychiatric disturbances in patients with Parkinson's disease. J Neurol Neurosurg Psychiatry. 1999;67:492–6.

14. Lichter DG, Cummings JL. Frontal-subcortical circuits in psychiatric and neurological disorders. New York: Guilford Press; 2001.
15. Miyasaki JM, Shannon K, Voon V, Ravina B, Kleiner-Fisman G, Anderson K, Shulman LM, Gronseth G, Weiner WJ. Practice parameter: evaluation and treatment of depression, psychosis, and dementia in Parkinson disease (an evidence based review). Neurology. 2006;66:996–1002.
16. Kirsch Darrow L, Fernandez HF, Marsiske M, Okun MS, Bowers D. Dissociating apathy and depression in Parkinson disease. Neurology. 2006;67(1):33–8.
17. Fenelon G, Mahieux F, Huon R, Ziegler M. Hallucinations in Parkinson's disease. Prevalence, phenomenology and risk factors. Brain. 2000;123:733–45.
18. Weintraub D, Koester J, Potenza MN, Siderowf AD, Stacy M, Voon V, Whetteckey J, Wunderlich GR, Lang AE. Impulse control disorder in Parkinson disease. A cross-sectional study of 3090 patients. Arch Neurol. 2010;67(5):589–95.
19. Machado AG, Hiremuth GK, Salazar F, Rezai AR. Fracture of subthalamic nucleus deep brain stimulation hardware as a result of compulsive manipulation: case report. Neurosurgery. 2005;57(6):E1318.
20. Voon V, Krack P, Lang AE, et al. A multicenter study on suicide outcomes following subthalamic stimulation for Parkinson disease. Brain. 2008;131:2720–8.
21. Weintraub D, Duda JE, Carlson K, et al. Suicide ideation and behaviours after STN and GPi DBS surgery for Parkinson's disease: results from a randomized, controlled trial. J Neurol Neurosurg Psychiatry. 2013;84(10):1113–8.
22. Defer GL, Widner H, Marie RM, Remy P, Levivier M. Core assessment program for surgical interventional therapies in Parkinson's disease (CAPSIT-PD). Mov Disord. 1999;14:572–84.
23. Abboud H, Floden D, Thompson NR, Genc G, Oravivattanakul S, Alsallom F, et al. Impact of mild cognitive impairment on outcome following deep brain stimulation surgery for Parkinson's disease. Parkinsonism Relat Disord. 2015;21(3):249–53.
24. Mikos A, Pavon J, Bowers D, Foote KD, Resnick AS, Fernandez HH, et al. Factors related to extended hospital stays following deep brain stimulation for Parkinson's disease. Parkinsonism Relat Disord. 2010;16(5):324–8.
25. Pilitsis JG, Rezai AR, Boulis NM, Henderson JM, Busch RM, Kubu CS. A preliminary study of transient confusional states following bilateral subthalamic stimulation for Parkinson's disease. J Stereot Funct Neurosurg. 2005;8:67–70.
26. Yaguez L, Costello A, Moriarty J, Hulse N, Selway R, Clough C, Samuel M, Keyoumars A. Cognitive predictors of cognitive change following bilateral subthalamic nucleus deep brain stimulation in Parkinson's disease. J Clin Neurosci. 2014;21:445–50.
27. Ford PJ, Boulis NM, Montgomery EB, Rezai AR. A patient revoking consent during awake craniotomy: an ethical challenge. Neuromodulation. 2007;10(4):329–32.
28. Kasemsuk C, Oyama G, Hattori N. Management of impulse control disorders with deep brain stimulation: a double edged sword. J Neurol Sci. 2017;37:63–8.
29. Kubu CS, Ford PJ. Clinical ethics in DBS. Arch Clin Neuropsychol. 2017;32:829–39.
30. Ford PJ, Kubu CS. Stimulating debate: ethics in a multidisciplinary functional neurosurgery committee. J Med Ethics. 2006;32(2):106–9.
31. Broer K, Chapin JS, Kubu CS. Counselor trainees in the operating room. Counseling Today. 2008. 44–7.

Chapter 19
Huntington's Disease Case Study

Karen M. Sanders and Daniel J. Burdick

Huntington's disease (HD) is a devastating and complex disease that deeply impacts patients and their families. Changes in basic health, cognition, and personality tax patients, families, and caregivers. A team approach involving neuropsychologists and medical providers offering comprehensive evaluation and treatment in collaboration with patients and families enhances care of those with Huntington's disease (HD).

Introduction

This is a longitudinal case example of HD using serial neuropsychological (NP) and neurological evaluations (with frequent MRI). The patient and family were persistent in their continued concern about diagnosis, prognosis, and need for planning and understanding. There was no clinically obvious caudate atrophy in the neuroradiological findings. However, there was early decline in neurocognitive function on serial neuropsychological evaluations (the sixth vital sign – see Preface).

Key Questions:

1. *Does Mr. Hunt have HD? He had early cognitive symptoms, no clinically detected caudate atrophy for years, early motor signs were not considered to be HD by the initial clinicians, and symptoms were considered too late for typical onset by the initial clinicians.*

K. M. Sanders (✉)
Department of Psychiatry and Behavioral Sciences, University of Washington School of Medicine, Seattle, WA, USA

D. J. Burdick
EvergreenHealth Neurosciences Institute, Kirkland, WA, USA

Department of Neurology, University of Washington School of Medicine, Seattle, WA, USA

K. M. Sanders (ed.), *Physician's Field Guide to Neuropsychology*,
https://doi.org/10.1007/978-1-4939-8722-1_19

Key Point
This case study helps to demonstrate the value of NP testing in HD. NP testing is norm-referenced, comprehensive, highly reliable, and valid [1] and is unique and highly useful in the multidisciplinary diagnosis and treatment of HD. It also highlights the crucial element of collaboration not only between MD and NP but with the patient and family for information vital to diagnosis and treatment planning.

When Mr. and Mrs. Hunt first saw the neuropsychologist, they were both concerned and frustrated with a change in his physical and cognitive functioning, and they wanted answers and help. Even though he had some physical signs and there was a strong family history, they had been told he did not have HD, but no genetic testing was done until the later visit with a movement disorder neurologist. He was told he was past the typical age of onset and that his MRI showed no caudate atrophy; therefore, he likely did not have HD. They wanted to know why he had mild personality, cognitive, and physical changes, and though the neuropsychologist could not examine or diagnose the physical issues of HD, she could examine personality and cognitive changes relative to possible HD. The rich HD neuropsychology research demonstrated early change in cognitive functioning, prior to physical changes. What was interesting in this case was the later age of onset and Mr. Hunt's high cognitive reserve.

The couple persisted through four neuropsychology evaluations over 7 years and sought continued advice regarding diagnosis, treatment issues, and impact on not only their lives but the lives of their family members. The patient and family were invested in understanding the medical, neuropsychological, and functional changes and became key members of the collaborative team.

Key Point
Neuropsychological assessment can identify HD up to 15 years [3] prior to detectable motor symptoms. Neurocognitive deficits develop before movement symptoms in a high percentage of HD patients. Early diagnosis of HD is important for planning treatment, helping with family needs, and addressing issues related to vocational ability, driving, and planning for future medical decisions.

Neurological evaluation was essential in defining and diagnosing key anatomical neurological changes. NP testing was a key part of the overall diagnostic picture from pre-diagnosis to follow-up and through the course of disease progression.

Neuropsychological data clearly documented change early in the course of the disease and illustrated classic neurocognitive changes across testing periods. It is well known [2] that fronto-striatal/fronto-subcortical changes manifest in behavioral changes and the test data in this case supported this pattern.

In this case, a low cytosine-adenine-guanine (CAG) repeat would explain the onset, course, and variation in clinical signs with this man. Mr. Hunt was evaluated over the course of 7 years by general neurologists, during which there was no clear determination of HD. In early neurological exams, he was considered too old for an onset of HD, which is typically considered between 30 and 40 years of age [4]. It was also noted that he had no positive MRI findings. HD gene testing was not pursued until his initial evaluation by a movement disorders neurologist (Dr. Burdick).

The standard of practice and supporting research in HD holds that CAG repeats plus motor signs is the standard mode for diagnosis. This case had a positive CAG repeat (found in 2013) without significant caudate/putamen atrophy on MRI and gradual cognitive decline in fronto-subcortical areas.

Key Concern: *It is at this point that early NP testing with identification of cognitive change would help the family with planning, decisions about genetic testing, implementation of psycho-education and support, continued enriched environment, and other medical interventions.*

Referral

Patient: 74-year-old male (in 2013 – age 67 at first evaluation in 2006)
Education: Bachelor's degree
Occupation: Retired computer science expert

Reason for referral: Mr. Hunt had symptoms of involuntary movements beginning around 2006, as well as some irritability and mild cognitive impairment (MCI), even as early as 2006. He had an initial neurology exam at that time with referral for his first neuropsychological exam.

Neurological Exams and Findings

Case Presentation

Mr. Hunt, a 74-year-old right-handed man with a family history of Huntington's disease (HD), was referred to our movement disorders center in 2013 with a 7-year history of involuntary movements. These movements had begun as intermittent jerks in his hands but had progressed significantly to become constant, flowing, random, and fully involuntary movements of all extremities and trunk. The movements led him to spill drinks and knock over objects, were not associated with a premonitory sensation, and were never suppressible. Prior neurological evaluation had discounted HD on the basis of his age (67 at the time). A second neurological opinion in 2011 cited a lack of caudate atrophy on MRI to discount HD and reported the movements were distractible, concluding that he had a tic disorder.

Over the same time period, Mr. Hunt began having mood changes, with increasing irritability. To address this, he underwent neuropsychological evaluation in 2006, 2007, and 2008, which found progressive deficits in executive function and visuospatial skills.

Past medical history included hypothyroidism, hyperlipidemia, and benign prostatic hypertrophy. Medications included atorvastatin, citalopram, doxazosin, and levothyroxine.

Family history was notable for the presence of HD in Mr. Hunt's paternal grandfather, who died in his mid-50s with chorea and dementia, and his paternal aunt, who died in her 60s with HD. His father died at 51 with renal failure, with no evidence of chorea, and he had one paternal uncle who died in WWII in his 20s with no evidence of chorea. He had two adult children and five grandchildren, ranging in age from 6 to 22.

Neurological examination was notable for constant, flowing, random movements of all extremities, both proximal and distal, and occasionally his trunk, consistent with generalized chorea. The tone was normal. He had slight bradykinesia on finger tapping bilaterally. Strength was normal. Cranial nerves were normal except for impaired initiation of saccades, requiring a head thrust, and motor impersistence of tongue protrusion, which could be held for no more than 5 s. Sensory exam revealed impaired vibratory sensation distal to the ankles bilaterally. Deep tendon reflexes were brisk, 3+, throughout. The plantar response was extensor on the right and flexor on the left. He had no dysmetria. Gait had a dancing quality, and he was unable to perform tandem gait.

A brain MRI in 2011 showed extensive leukoaraiosis, global atrophy with ex vacuo ventriculomegaly, and no focal caudate atrophy.

Based on his chorea on exam and his family history of HD, the clinical impression was of probable Huntington's disease. The diagnosis was confirmed by DNA testing, showing CAG repeats of 40 (allele 1) and 19 (allele 2).

Discussion

Key Point
Several significant points are made by this case: neuropsychological evaluation helped in diagnosis and in anticipating problems (e.g., driving); age of onset is highly variable; CAG is correlated with age of onset; lack of caudate atrophy does not rule out HD.

Huntington's disease (HD) is an autosomal dominant heredodegenerative disease that produces cognitive, psychiatric, and motor abnormalities. Age of onset is typically in the 40s or 50s but can range from childhood to the 90s and is closely correlated with the size of the genetic abnormality, the CAG repeat number. Prevalence estimates vary by methodology, but those relying on genetic testing in Europe, Australia, and North America have generally found prevalence rates of 5–7 per 100,000, with a meta-analysis of these studies arriving at an overall prevalence of 5.7 per 100,000 [4]. Because of genetic founder effects, though, HD is unevenly distributed across the globe, with much lower prevalence in Asia (0.4 per 100,000) [4] and with some regions (Moray Firth in Scotland, Lake Maracaibo in Venezuela) having rates as high as 500–700 per 100,000 [5].

Clinical onset is defined by the appearance of motor abnormalities. Chorea, defined as rapid, random, flowing, dance-like movements, is the most common motor abnormality in adult-onset HD. However, other motor abnormalities, such as dystonia, ataxia, and myoclonus, can also be present in HD. Often, people with HD are not aware of the abnormal movements. Indeed, in the case of Mr. Hunt, it was his wife who brought the movements to his attention. Even when mild, chorea can cause difficulty with manual dexterity, gait impairment, and social isolation.

Although HD onset is defined by motor signs, it is not uncommon for neuropsychiatric symptoms to precede the clinical diagnosis of HD. Cognitive and psychiatric symptoms in prodromal HD are incompletely understood, but evidence suggests that deficits in memory and executive function occur in prodromal and early HD and are sufficient to cause clinically significant impairment in 8–14% of patients [6]. Indeed, among those who have not yet manifested motor signs of HD, those who are closest to the predicted age of onset based on CAG repeat number show the greatest impairment in the greatest number of cognitive domains, though detectable differences from non-carriers may be present at least a decade before motor onset [7].

In this case, Mr. Hunt had undergone serial neuropsychological testing that demonstrated increasing visuospatial and executive dysfunction, both not uncommon in early or prodromal HD. This did contribute to the clinical suspicion of HD and, in addition to the motor abnormalities, prompted the decision to pursue confirmatory genetic testing.

HD Genetics

> **Key Point**
> For anyone considering HD gene testing, genetic counseling is an important pre-requisite. The European Huntington's Disease Network has established guidelines for counseling prior to predictive genetic testing for HD [8].

HD is caused by a triplet expansion in a gene on the short arm of chromosome 4. The gene, located at 4p16.3 [9, 10], encodes the protein huntingtin, the function of which is unknown. At the 5′ end of this gene, an abnormal expansion of the sequence cytosine-adenine-guanine (CAG) confers HD [11]. The normal repeat size is between 10 and 26. The signs and symptoms of HD are fully penetrant when the CAG repeat number equals or exceeds 40 [12]. With a CAG repeat size of 36–39, the gene has reduced penetrance, affecting some individuals but not others [13]. A CAG repeat size between 27 and 35 is considered an intermediate allele. This allele size is believed to produce a normal phenotype, although some have found behavioral abnormalities in those with intermediate alleles and have suggested a low penetrance in this group [14]. Notably, the intermediate allele is unstable, and carriers of this allele may pass down an allele that has expanded into the unequivocally abnormal region, resulting in offspring who will be affected by HD [15, 16].

The CAG repeat size is closely linked with age of onset. Generally, the greater the CAG repeat size, the younger the age of onset [17, 18], a finding that has been consistent across numerous studies. Indeed, the age of onset can be predicted with a small standard deviation for larger repeat numbers, though below a CAG repeat length of 42, the confidence interval of the prediction widens [19]. CAG expansion size is also inversely correlated with prognosis, with greater CAG size being correlated with faster accumulation of neurologic signs, motor impairment, cognitive impairment, and disability [20].

In the case of Mr. Hunt, when he was 67 years old he was told that his symptoms could not be due to HD because he was past the typical age of onset for the disease. However, age of onset for HD with shorter CAG repeat lengths can extend well into the 80s. With the knowledge that Mr. Hunt has 40 CAG repeats, we can in retrospect say that onset at age 67 would be not at all unusual; an individual with 40 CAG repeats has an approximately 70% chance of manifesting HD by age 70 and a 97% chance by age 85, meaning that more than a quarter of people with a repeat length of 40 will have onset after age 70 [21].

HD Imaging

Atrophy of the caudate is a consistently demonstrated finding in early and presymptomatic HD [22, 23] and may prove to be a useful biomarker to assess progression in presymptomatic HD. As with age of onset, caudate atrophy is inversely correlated with CAG expansion size [22]. However, to assess caudate atrophy in premanifest or early HD, careful volumetric analysis – that is, a software-based assessment of a region's volume relative to normal values – must be performed [24], and early atrophy may not be apparent on simple visual inspection in a typical clinical setting. This was seen in the case of Mr. Hunt, who has a relatively small CAG expansion size, who was in an early stage of HD, and for whom volumetric analysis of the caudate was not performed on his routine clinical brain MRI. Before Mr. Hunt's referral to our movement disorders center, an earlier neurologist's opinion had relied on this negative result to exclude the diagnosis of HD.

> **Key Point**
> For reasons that this case illustrates, genetic testing has replaced brain imaging in the clinical diagnosis of HD. Even so, brain MRI remains an important tool in the evaluation of chorea generally and may be used to exclude structural causes of chorea.

Neurologist Perspective of Neuropsychological Consult

Neuropsychological assessment early in the course of HD can provide valuable information. In Mr. Hunt's case, the progressive loss of executive function and visuospatial ability found on his neuropsychological assessment, when considered in conjunction with his movement disorder, supported the decision to obtain diagnostic testing for HD. Cognition has been shown to decline in prodromal HD, with greater change as motor onset approaches [21], but with changes evident on sensitive testing at least 10 years before motor onset [12].

Neuropsychological Testing Input

Neuropsychological testing is used in this case to contrast Mini-Mental State Examination (MMSE)/Montreal Cognitive Assessment (MoCA) [25, 26] screening results with NP, to demonstrate the influence of cognitive reserve, and to discuss the typical fronto-striatal cognitive pattern in HD and the typical psychiatric and behavioral changes. All data is integrated with NP theory and evidence-based literature.

Clinical Findings and History Beginning in 2006

Mr. Hunt received a full battery of neuropsychological testing conducted in four sessions over the course of 7 years. Serial NP testing revealed continued potential for depression, which is a classic Huntington's symptom and frequently involves an increased potential for suicidal ideation or intent and sometimes impulsivity and frontal lobe decline. Mr. Hunt had no history of suicidal ideation or intent in the past or at the time of evaluation. Suicide potential was to be watched closely by family and professional caregivers and eventually augmented through genetic counseling and other counseling endeavors and through Huntington's disease support groups at the hospital. His wife was coached about HD and received support for her caregiver stress. Eventually, family genetic counseling and more specific interventions were included.

Serial neuropsychological testing revealed consistent impairment in areas of executive functioning (EF). EF dysfunction may have further interfered with his memory functioning, by creating lack of structure and inefficiency in learning. He developed difficulty with social comportment, initiation of conversation, and reduced self-awareness. This may reveal some classic executive functioning decline. It is also very interesting to note that Mr. Hunt developed more cognitive symptoms and mild emotional symptoms early along with some classic HD motor symptoms. As mentioned above, caudate atrophy was not found on visual MRI examination, until 2013.

Neuropsychological Theory by Cognitive Domain

A few relevant evidence-based research articles are reviewed below as they relate to the case of Mr. Hunt. This data demonstrates the fronto-subcortical test pattern typical of HD with preserved language functioning, inefficient memory dysfunction, and greater difficulty in areas of executive functioning, complex attention, slowed processing, and subtle visual-spatial issues [27]. Of note, the type of memory deficit common in HD is that of deficiencies in forming categories and organization secondary to poor executive functioning. The episodic memory is generally intact. Trouble with episodic memory is often a hallmark of amnestic memory disorders (e.g., Alzheimer's). Depression (including suicide potential) and obsessive-compulsive psychological symptoms are common in HD as in many other diagnoses.

In the case of Mr. Hunt, cognitive reserve may have pushed the onset to later in his life along with typical cognitive issues found in shorter CAG.

Data from the PREDICT-HD study [28] found that HD individuals have non-amnestic mild cognitive impairment (MCI) in at least one domain, usually processing speed, and sometimes more. Duff claims that a case can be made for MCI in prodromal HD.

In addition to CAG and atrophy issues already mentioned, there are several other etiologies thought responsible for onset or progression of HD. These include positron emission tomography (PET) in relation to episodic memory [29]; hypoperfusion [30]; fMRI findings of lower activity in the cerebellum, prefrontal lobe, right thalamus, and parietal lobe [31]; white matter disease [32–34]; and BOLD changes [35].

Biomarkers and neurocognitive testing patterns have been shown to detect HD in early stages, as much as 15 years prior to onset and before signs of motor dysfunction [2].

The following sections explain neurocognitive changes over four testing dates with the most salient domains described first and in successive order of impairment. NP testing clearly identifies subtle changes in the fronto-striatal pattern and follows neuroanatomical/neurochemical changes in the disease course.

Cognitive Screens/General Ability/Cognitive Reserve

Certainly, Mr. Hunt had undetected and minimal caudate or putamen atrophy and was late onset.

Table 19.1 General ability

Year	2006	2007	2008	2013
MMSE	26	25	22	–
WTAR				St Score = 101
MDRS	SS = 14 (High Avg)	SS = 13 (High Avg)	SS = 11 (Avg)	SS = 8 (Avg)
WAIS/Vocabulary	SS = 12 (Avg)	SS = 12 (Avg)		
WAIS/Similarities	SS = 13 (High Avg)	SS = 14 (High Avg)	SS = 16 (Very Superior)	SS = 10 (Avg)
WAIS/Comp.	SS = 13 (High Avg)	SS = 13 (High Avg)	SS = 13 (High Avg)	SS = 12 (Avg)
WAIS/Block Design	SS = 11 (Avg)	SS = 10 (Avg)	SS = 9 (Avg)	SS = 8 (Avg)
WAIS/Matrix				SS = 8 (Avg)
	SS = 10 ± 3			
	T = 50 ± 10			
	St Score = 100 ± 15			
	WAIS-3 (2006-08)			
	WAIS-4 (2013)			
	MMSE Total = 30			

He may be a good example of the benefits of cognitive reserve (high intelligence, education, and occupational attainment – see glossary) and enriched environment.

Mr. Hunt demonstrated general ability (IQ) in the high average range with notable achievements in occupation. He also maintained active involvement in his community and continued to learn to the best of his ability. His cognitive reserve was identified by higher IQ estimates. Global neurocognitive functions declined independently and not until the last two exams due to effects of HD progression. Thus, general ability (IQ) is independent of other neurocognitive functions that decline in HD. Screens miss cognitive reserve, and subtle neurocognitive changes are not detected until later in the disease.

Mr. Hunt's general ability test results: (Table 19.1)

Cognitive reserve or general ability has been shown to protect against or delay the onset in cognitive decline in many diseases. The MMSE and MoCA do not calculate general ability or IQ estimate. NP testing and education/occupation are used to establish general ability (IQ). Issues of cognitive reserve were important in the case of Mr. Hunt and crucial to accurate assessment and diagnosis. Bonner-Jackson [36] discusses a cognitive reserve hypothesis in relation to HD clinical signs. The rate of cognitive decline and caudate/putamen volume loss has been shown to be slower in HD patients with high cognitive reserve.

Zhang et al. [37] discuss the use of a CAP (CAG age product: score or formula that factors in variables of CAG repeats and age). A discussion of CAP can be found in Harrington [38]. Troster [2] summarized the Harrington findings listing six neurocognitive domains that are impaired in the prodromal HD stage as found by CAP. It is possible to determine years to diagnosis with these neurocognitive factors as well.

Global functioning as shown on the MMSE did not decline until later in Mr. Hunt's disease course. Mr. Hunt's Dementia Rating Scale (DRS) total scores declined over time but did not decline to less than 140 until the 2008 testing. At this point, there can be concerns about driving and other activities of daily living.

As is clear with Mr. Hunt, cognitive reserve may preserve some cognitive functions and even relate to less atrophy, even though there can be subtle fronto-subcortical findings related to the striatal network.

Executive Functioning/Complex Attention

The neurological changes listed below reveal some classic executive functioning impairments. Mr. Hunt had evidence of executive dysfunction, including fronto-striatal cognitive issues of poor sequencing, planning, and problem-solving. Behavior change (orbitofrontal/anterior cingulate forms of executive function) was not noted by the family or by Mr. Hunt but may have begun to emerge later in the disease.

Mr. Hunt and his family complained of issues with poor organization, perseveration, impulsivity, and judgment. Mr. Hunt's test results showed that complex attention and switching abilities were gradually affected as evidenced by impairment on tests such as the Wisconsin Card Sorting Test (WCST) [39], Delis-Kaplan Executive Function System (D-KEFS) inhibition [40], and Switching and Copy of Rey Complex Figure Test (RCFT) [41]. Mr. Hunt was fully aware of these executive functioning issues which demonstrates that anosognosia (lack of awareness of deficit) is not a typical feature of HD.

Mr. Hunt's EF test results: (Table 19.2).

There are three types of executive function, dorsolateral, orbitofrontal, and anterior cingulate, all affected differently in HD as compared to other diseases.

Dorsolateral frontal issues were evident in areas of severely disorganized Rey-Osterrieth complex figure, difficulty with planning ahead, inefficient moves and problem-solving, mildly impaired hypothesis formation with significant evidence of perseveration, and trouble with initiating tasks and complex attention.

Orbitofrontal decline was gathered through collateral interview and self-report inventories and demonstrated issues with social comportment, including impulse control, observation, and adjustment of appropriate behavior.

Anterior cingulate cortex is involved in regulating emotions, both initiation and inhibition of behavior. Impairment may involve apathy, abulia, or akinetic mutism. Some inhibition was noticed in Mr. Hunt's behavior.

Table 19.2 Executive functioning

Year	2006	2007	2008	2013
WCST/Cat	3/6	D/C 0/6	1/6	4/6
WCST/Pers	T = 42 (Low Avg)	D/C	T = 39 (Low Avg)	T = 41 (Low Avg)
Trials B	T = 40 (Low Avg)	T = 44 (Avg)	T = 35 (Borderline)	T = 42 (Low Avg)
RCFT/Copy	>16 Percentile (Above Avg)	<1 Percentile (Impaired)	<1 Percentile (Impaired)	<1 Percentile (Impaired)
FAS/LF	T = 44 (Avg)	T = 30 (Borderline)	T = 41 (Low Avg)	T = 30 (Borderline)
D-KEFS/TOWER	–	–	–	SS = 11 (Avg)
	SS = 10 ± 3			
	T = 50 ± 10			
	Stan Sc = 100 ± 15			

Impairments in any of these functions can be signs of fronto-subcortical pattern typical with Huntington's disease. Fronto-striatal and fronto-subcortical dementia in HD is a top-down/bottom-up functioning neuropsychological theory. This process, labeled "the vertically-organized brain," is discussed comprehensively by Koziol [42]. This can explain reward-driven, frontally mediated, and refined complex executive functions.

Thus, fronto-subcortical circuitry is compromised early in HD and is a significant cognitive dysfunction. This subtlety is often overlooked or undetected as it is not a frank memory deficit nor is it detected in global functioning screening tools. **The fronto-subcortical cognitive changes are independent of psychiatric changes. This cognitive change in executive functioning was apparent even before motor and neurological signs (classic neurology exam).**

Regarding NP tests specifically, Ho et al. found the most change in verbal fluency, object recall, and Stroop tests in short time intervals (within 1 year) [43], but with WCST there is not much change in shorter intervals of time. Papp noted that HD has minimal changes over short time periods in other areas of cognition [44]. Further, Papp and Nicoll [45] discuss EF in relation to speed and efficiency of planning (Tower Test [40]) and prospective memory (Memory for Intentions Test) in more refined issues with fronto-subcortical process. Prospective memory is used constantly in planning and executing future events with environmental context in mind [46].

Table 19.3 Attention

Year	2006	2007	2008	2013
Trials A	T = 41 (Low Avg)	T = 35 (Borderline)	T = 50 (Avg)	T = 43 (Avg)
Trials B	T = 30 (Borderline)	T = 44 (Avg)	T = 35 (Borderline)	T = 42 (Low Avg)
Digit Span	SS = 7 (Low Avg)	SS = 9 (Avg)	SS = 7 (Low Avg)	SS = 7 (Low Avg)
SDMT/Wr	–	–	–	SS = 1 (Impaired)
SDMT/Oral	–	–	–	SS = 8 (Avg)
D-KEFS/In	–	–	–	SS = 1 (Impaired)
D-KEFS/SW	–	–	–	S = 7 (Low Avg)
	SS = 10 ± 3			
	T = 50 ± 10			

Integration of Neuropsychology and Neuroanatomy/Neurotransmitters in Executive Function (EF)

Structural and neurotransmitter system changes occur in HD and drive the EF dysfunction discussed above. Striatal structures are responsible for automatic functions and routines, and the health of striatal structures is related to neurotransmitter levels, specifically GABA [42, 47]. When the striatal structures decline, there is less regulation of these automatic functions; thus, even simple tasks of attention can become impaired. Some research indicates that this type of cognitive change may occur early in the disease. All contribute to difficulty with coordinating movements and sequenced and integrated executive tasks (inhibition, impulsivity, judgment, slowed processing, and trouble with fronto-striatal communication circuits).

Attention: Slowed Processing as Basic Type of EF

Mr. Hunt demonstrated slowed processing on many tasks (see Table 19.3).

Attention is a basic building block of executive functioning. Duff [25] stresses that attention and executive functioning problems in HD are very predictive of HD cognitive decline. Dysfunction in HD involves fronto-subcortical circuitry driving the change in cognitive functioning. Cognitive dysfunction in HD is a major biomarker, and behavior changes are not related to purely psychiatric cause (e.g., depression, anxiety).

A decrease in performance on MMSE serial sevens is common in HD. Peavy [48] discusses that decreased motor skills lead to mental slowing causing the HD patient to compensate with other brain circuitry to accomplish the same task, thus leading to slowed processing. The Symbol Digit Modalities Test [49] is frequently used in HD research, as it contrasts oral vs. written coding speed, parsing out the motor factor. It is particularly sensitive to detecting early signs of change in attention even in asymptomatic HD carriers.

Key Point
Executive functioning difficulties can be more problematic in ways than simple memory difficulties, and increased structure involving prompts and cues in the environment are crucial. Neuropsychological testing is specific enough to identify executive functioning, whereas the MMSE and cognitive screens routinely miss this functional domain. This is an important finding for Huntington's disease, and an ability to track this over time is critical.

Memory

Mr. Hunt had inefficient memory with preserved semantic/episodic memory performance, typical for a fronto-striatal neurocognitive picture in HD (see Table 19.4).

The type of memory deficit in HD is found in some key patterns [50]:

- Inefficient memory (non-amnestic/cortical) is common in HD and is secondary to motor slowing/processing and impaired executive functioning changes (organization of new data).

Table 19.4 Memory

Year	2006	2007	2008	2013
LMI	SS = 8 (Avg)	SS = 10 (Avg)	SS = 12 (Avg)	SS = 9 (Avg)
LMII	SS = 9 (Avg)	SS = 12 (Avg)	SS = 12 (Avg)	SS = 11 (Avg)
VisRep I	SS = 14 (High Avg)	S = 17 (Very Sup)	SS = 16 (Very Sup)	SS = 14 (High Avg)
VisRep II	SS = 13 (High Avg)	S = 16 (Very Sup)	S = 14 (High Avg)	SS = 16 (Very Sup)
RCFT Im	T = 71 (Very Sup)	T = 39 (Low Avg)	T = 63 (High Avg)	T = 24 (Impaired)
RCFT Delayed	T = 66 (Superior)	T = 41 (Low Avg)	T = 73 (Very Sup)	T = 23 (Impaired)
RCFT Recog	T = 49 (Avg)	T = 26 (Impaired)	T = 49 (Avg)	T = 44 (Avg)
CVLT-2(SF) T1	−1.0 (Low Avg)	−0.5 (Avg)	−0.5 (Avg)	−2.5 (Impaired)
CVLT-2(SF) T4	−1.5 (Borderline)	0.5 (Avg)	−1.0 (Low Avg)	−1.0 (Low Avg)
CVLT-2(SF) Total	T = 46 (Avg)	T = 48 (Avg)	T = 53 (Avg)	T = 42 (Low Avg)
CVLT-2(SF) LDFR	−1.0 (Low Avg)	−1.0 (Low Avg)	−1.0 (Low Avg)	−1.5 (Borderline)
CVLT-2(SF) Recog	0.0 (Avg)	0.0 (Avg)	−1.5 (Borderline)	−1.0 (Low Avg)
	SS = 10 ± 3			
	T = 50 ± 10			
	Z Scores 0.0 ± 1.0			

Semantic/episodic memory and delayed recall are preserved until late in HD; the MMSE and MoCA do not pick up on subtle inefficient memory changes and have limited ability to fully document subtle EF changes. In contrast, AD patients have more trouble with delayed memory (an amnestic picture), learning, language, and problem-solving than those with HD. Memory can be more impaired later in the course of HD. AD and HD have different neuroanatomical and biochemical etiology. HD is fronto-striatal and AD is hippocampal and entorhinal related. Hippocampal decline often relates to episodic memory decline (stories in context), whereas fronto-striatal decline results in inefficient memory (organization of serial list learning).

Language

Mr. Hunt's language functioning was intact as seen in Table 19.5.

Language functioning in HD remains generally within normal limits in HD, but speech can be slow and labored. Sometimes mutism evolves. Aphasia and agnosia are not a part of HD until late stage. HD patients are slow to interact due to fronto-subcortical issues but totally understand their environment. To facilitate communication, "talking mats" may be useful [51].

Visuospatial Functioning

Mr. Hunt had subtle visuospatial impairment as seen in Table 19.6.

Table 19.5 Language

Year	2006	2007	2008	2013
BNT	T = 48 (Average)	T = 52 (Average)	T = 60 (High Average)	T = 50 (Average)
Letter Fluency	T = 44 (Average)	T = 30 (Borderline)	T = 41 (Low Average)	T = 30 (Borderline)
Animals Cat	T = 35 (Borderline)	T = 44 (Average)	T = 41 (Low Average)	T = 30 (Borderline)
	T = 50 ± 10			

Table 19.6 Visuospatial

Year	2006	2007	2008	2013
JOLO	–	–	–	SS = 10 (Average)
RCFT Copy	>16 Percentile (Above Avg)	<1 Percentile (Impaired)	2–5 Percentile (Borderline)	<1 Percentile (Impaired)
	SS = 10 ± 3			

Findings of constructional apraxia in HD are more common than in AD. Motor symptoms of HD can interfere with visuospatial functions [27]. Mr. Hunt began to have trouble with visuospatial functioning later in the disease, around 2013.

Motor

Mr. Hunt demonstrated slowed motor speed, a common finding in HD. Subtle motor signs were evident to the NP examiner as early as 2006, and comments were made to the original neurologist. Mr. Hunt had clear movement chorea problems early on. There was clear evidence of involuntary movement problems rather than voluntary. By 2013, Mr. Hunt had trouble swallowing and had noticeable chaotic jerking [52].

Psychological

Psychiatric (and cognitive) changes can occur before motor signs are present. Mr. Hunt did not endorse depression per self-report and clinical interview, perhaps because he began medication for depression prior to the 2006 evaluation. Obsessive-compulsive features can be common along with trouble comprehending emotions. Psychosis and behavioral change are common. With Mr. Hunt, a lack of emotional awareness was most notable.

Mr. Hunt's psychological test results can be seen in Table 19.7.

Pre-manifest HD and manifest HD patients can have trouble with recognition of negative emotions [53]. They have trouble with identification of emotions and social cues even though they understand emotions, and there is a breakdown in identification of facial cues.

Interestingly, lack of awareness has been correlated with WCST failure to maintain set. This is not the same as anosognosia.

Validity Indicators

Sometimes, test validity (performance validity and symptom validity tests [PVT/SVT]) can be impaired by difficulty in volition (fronto-subcortical) but is not considered evidence of poor motivation. It is considered a biological symptom of HD neurological change. Some experts have argued that PVT/SVT are not always appropriate in dementia evaluation [54]. One PVT was given to the patient in 2013.

Functional Evaluation

The family did not endorse frontal lobe dysfunction on the Frontal Systems Behavior Scale (FrSBe) [55], a functional survey of executive functioning.

Table 19.7 Emotional

Year	2006	2007	2008	2013
GDS	Mild 2	2	2	Mild 4

Conclusions regarding Clinical Findings

It is well established that decreased neurocognitive functioning in HD is the result of changes in the fronto-subcortical areas and basal ganglion. Research continues to suggest white matter changes, atrophy of striatal systems, and global atrophy as the underlying neuropathology that explains this decline. Classic literature reviews are available regarding the neuropsychology of HD [21, 54].

Collaborative Questions and Discussion with Evidence-Based Citations

We have established in this case study that cognitive reserve is one reason for delay, especially in caudate atrophy, illustrating the need for NP testing to detect and test for cog reserve (IQ vs. other) [25, 56]. Cognitive decline can begin as early as 15 years prior to motor diagnosis (traditional HD diagnosis). Haaland et al. [27] discuss the last 30 years and the next 30 years in the research and treatment of HD and indicate that cognitive neuroscience will be clearly a part of coordination with neuroimaging and other medical specialties. A thorough neurological exam with volumetric analysis of the caudate can also indicate change in late onset. In this case of Mr. Hunt, a more refined caudate analysis was likely related to the late-onset HD. Other neurochemical and neuroanatomical etiologies have been proposed as discussed above.

Treatment Concerns and Recommendations

Neuropsychological testing guiding treatment and recommendations:

- Diagnostic clarity and ability to track neurocognitive biomarkers of HD.
- Important patient and family interventions.
- Early diagnostic identification of HD can potentially aid in minimizing disease effects [35].

Neuropsychological testing results help to direct treatment and recommendations for further cognitive stimuli on the level of complex occupational/volunteer and/or educational pursuits in the community. Complex environments have been shown effective in rehab settings. Koffler [57] discusses the latest evidence-based rehabilitation research including the idea of enriched environments. Higher cognitive reserve may have some relation to better lifestyle habits.

After the 2013 NP evaluation, advice was given for continued follow-through with psychiatric support, including cognitive intervention for executive functioning with occupational therapy, follow-through with a Huntington's support group for the family, social work intervention in the community for help with community resources, continued monitoring for depression and suicidal thoughts or intent, and an on-the-road driving test to assess for safety on the road, as well as having other activities of daily living possibly assessed by occupational therapy, and someone to monitor his medications and make sure he avoids mistakes due to his frontal lobe organizational difficulties. Continued structured programming in a daily activity would be helpful for him, and use of the buddy system in his community so he does not get lost would be quite helpful.

Of special note, in 2013, Mr. Hunt and his family were referred for genetic counseling as they began to consider the CAG test. They were concerned about family response to the knowledge of genetic potential and plans for further pregnancies.

Medical treatment of HD remains purely symptomatic. When the chorea produces functional impairment, it may be treated with a dopamine-depleting agent such as reserpine, tetrabenazine, or deutetrabenazine or it may be treated with a dopamine-receptor-blocking agent such as haloperidol, risperidone, or fluphenazine.

Psychiatric complications such as depression, anxiety, and irritability may be treated with the usual anti-depressants, including selective serotonin reuptake inhibitors (SSRIs) (e.g., sertraline, citalopram, fluoxetine, paroxetine) and serotonin-norepinephrine reuptake inhibitors (SNRIs) such as venlafaxine. Psychosis can be managed with either typical antipsychotics (listed above) or atypical antipsychotics such as olanzapine, ziprasidone, and aripiprazole. The risk of suicide is high among people with HD and must be screened for regularly, particularly in adolescent patients, for whom SSRIs may increase the risk of suicide (not just for those with HD).

Cognitive symptoms may benefit from acetylcholinesterase inhibitors such as donepezil, rivastigmine, or galantamine.

While currently approved treatments for HD provide improvement in symptoms, the possibility of treating the underlying pathology may be drawing closer. In December 2017, Ionis Pharmaceuticals issued a press release indicating positive results from their Phase 1/2a trial of Ionis-HTTRx [58]. This antisense oligonucleotide binds to messenger RNA and prevents the translation of the mutant huntingtin protein. According to the press release, results of the Phase 1/2a trial showed that Ionis-HTTRx was safe and tolerable and demonstrated a dose-dependent reduction in huntingtin. What effect this has on the clinical progression of HD will be the subject of future trials, but if this proceeds through FDA approval, it is presumed that it would be the first disease-modifying treatment for HD. Of note, the results of the Ionis Phase 1/2a trial have not been presented in a peer-reviewed forum as of this writing.

Chapter Review Questions

1. It is important to use NP testing when:
   A. There is concern about depression only.
   B. Helping with medical treatment planning and decisions.
   C. Helping with family dynamics and planning issues.
   D. All of the above.

2. Using only screens such as MMSE/MoCA can miss:
   A. Fronto-subcortical signs.
   B. High vs. low education or cognitive reserve.
   C. Subtle change over time.
   D. All of the above.

3. Neurocognitive issues in HD begin:
   A. Early before CAG (subtle change).
   B. Late—after obvious movement disorder.
   C. Around the age of onset (some literature indicates significant change related to biomarkers).
   D. Never.

4. Cognitive and behavioral decline can:
   A. Be a factor in determining overall diagnosis.
   B. Be related to family distress.
   C. Predict nursing home placement or need for extra help in the home.
   D. All of the above.

5. True/False: Psychiatric issues are common in HD.

6. Early onset with no caudate atrophy:
   A. Is common.
   B. Is rare.
   C. Can exist in the context of cognitive reserve.
   D. Is a biomarker for HD.
   E. C and D.

7. Comprehensive work-up for HD should include:
   A. Neurology only.
   B. Neurology and genetic testing (when and if the patient is ready).
   C. Neuropsychology and patient and family psychoeducational support.
   D. All of the above.

References

1. Braun M, Tupper D, Kaufman P, et al. Neuropsychological assessment: a valuable tool in the diagnosis and management of neurological, neurodevelopmental, medical, and psychiatric disorders. Cogn Behav Neurol. 2011;24(3):107.
2. Troster A, editor. Clinical neuropsychology and cognitive neurology of Parkinson's disease and other movement disorders. New York, NY: Oxford University Press; 2015.
3. Paulsen JS, Langbehn DR, Stout JC, et al PREDICT-HD Investigators and Coordinators of the Huntington Study Group. Detection of Huntington's disease decades before diagnosis: the PREDICT-HD study. J Neurol Neurosurg Pyschiatry 2008;79:874-880.
4. Pringsheim T, Wiltshire K, Day L, et al. The incidence and prevalence of Huntington's disease: a systematic review and meta-analysis. Mov Disord. 2012;27(9):1083–91.
5. Harper PS. The epidemiology of Huntington's disease. Hum Genet. 1992;89:365–76.
6. Vaccarino AL, Sills T, Anderson K, et al. Assessment of cognitive symptoms in prodromal and Huntington disease. PLoS Curr. 2011;25(3):RRN 1250.
7. Stout JC. (2011). Neurocognitive signs in prodromal Huntington disease. Neuropsychology. 2011;25(1):1–14.
8. MacLeod R, Tibben A, Frontali M, et al. Recommendations for the predictive genetic test in Huntington's disease. Clin Genet. 2013;83:221–31.
9. Bates GP, MacDonald ME, Baxendale S, et al. Defined physical limits of the Huntington disease gene candidate region. Am J Hum Genet. 1991;49:7–16.
10. Wexler NS, Rose EA, Housman DE. Molecular approaches to hereditary diseases of the nervous system. Annu Rev Neurosci. 1991;14:503–29.
11. The Huntington's Disease Collaborative Research Group. A novel gene containing a trinucleotide repeat that is expanded and unstable on Huntington's disease chromosomes. Cell. 1993;72:971–83.
12. Kremer B, Goldberg P, Andrew SE, et al. A worldwide study of the Huntington's disease mutation: the sensitivity and specificity of measuring CAG repeats. N Engl J Med. 1994;330:1401–6.
13. Rubinsztein DC, Leggo J, Coles R, et al. Phenotypic characterization of individuals with 30-40 CAG repeats in the Huntington disease (HD) gene reveals HD cases with 36 repeats and apparently normal elderly individuals with 36-39 repeats. Am J Hum Genet. 1996;59:16–22.
14. Killoran A, Biglan KM, Jankovic J, et al. Characterization of the Huntington intermediate CAG repeat expansion phenotype in PHAROS. Neurology. 2013;80:2022–7.
15. Maat-Kievet A, Losekoot M, Van den Boer-Van den Berg H, et al. New problems in testing for Huntington's disease: the issue of intermediate and reduced penetrance alleles. J Med Genet. 2001;38:E12.
16. Potter NT, Spector EB, Prior TW. Technical standards and guidelines for Huntington disease testing. Genet Med. 2004;6:61–5.
17. Duyao M, Ambrose C, Myers R, et al. Trinucleotide repeat length instability and age of onset in Huntington's disease. Nat Genet. 1993;4:387–92.
18. Brinkman RR, Mezei MM, Theilman J, Almqvist E, Hayden MR. The likelihood of being affected with Huntington disease by a particular age, for a specific CAG size. Am J Hum Genet. 1997;60:1202–10.
19. Langbehn DR, Brinkman RR, Falush D, et al. A new model for prediction of the age of onset and penetrance for Huntington's disease based on CAG length. Clin Genet. 2004 Apr;65(4):267–77.
20. Rosenblatt A, Kumar BV, Mo A, et al. Age, CAG repeat length, and clinical progression in Huntington's disease. Mov Disord. 2012;27(2):272–6.
21. Aylward EH, Nopoulos PC, Ross CA, et al. Longitudinal change in regional brain volumes in prodromal Huntington disease. J Neurol Neurosurg Psychiatry. 2011;82:405–10.
22. Dominguez DJF, Egan GF, Gray MA, et al. Multi-modal neuroimaging in premanifest and early Huntington's disease: 18-month longitudinal data from the IMAGE-HD study. PLoS One. 2013;8(9):e74131.

23. Aylward EH, Rosenblatt A, Field K, et al. Caudate volume as an outcome measure in clinical trials for Huntington's disease: a pilot study. Brain Res Bull. 2003;62:137–41.
24. Paulsen JS, Smith MM, Long JD. Cognitive decline in prodromal Huntington disease: implications for clinical trials. J Neurol Neurosurg Psychiatry. 2013;84(11):1233–9.
25. Folstein MF, Folstein SE, McHugh PR. "Mini-mental state". A practical method for grading the cognitive state of patients for the clinician. J Psychiatr Res. 1975;12(3):189–98.
26. Nasreddine ZS, Phillips NA, Bedirian V, et al. The Montreal Cognitive Assessment, MoCA: a Brief Screening Tool for Mild Cognitive Impairment. J Am Geriatr Soc. 2005;53(4):695–9.
27. Haaland KY, Dum RP, Mutha PK, Strick PL, Troster AI. The neuropsychology of movement and movement disorders: neuroanatomical and cognitive considerations. J Int Neuropsychol Soc. 2017;23:768–77.
28. Duff K, Paulsen JS, Mills J, et al; PREDICT-HD Investigators and Coordinators of the Huntington Study Group. Mild cognitive impairment in prediagnosed Huntington disease. Neurology. 2010;75(6):500-507.
29. Montoya A, Price BH, Menear M, Lepage M. Brain imaging and cognitive dysfunctions in Huntington's disease. J Psychiatry Neurosci. 2006;31(1):21–9.
30. Chen JJ, Salat DH, Rosas HD. Complex relationships between cerebral blood flow and brain atrophy in early Huntington's disease. Neuroimage. Jan 2018;59(2):1043–51.
31. Paradiso S, Turner BM, Paulsen JS, Jorge R, Ponto LL, Robinson RG. Neural bases of dysphoria in early Huntington's disease. Psychiatry Res. 2008;162(1):73–87.
32. Alosco ML, Gunstad J, Jerskey BA, et al. The adverse effects of reduced cerebral perfusion on cognition and brain structure in older adults with cardiovascular disease. Brain Behav. 2013;3(6):626–36.
33. Beglinger LJ, Nopoulos PC, Jorge RE, et al. White matter volume and cognitive dysfunction in early Huntington's disease. Cogn Behav Neurol. 2005;18:102–7.
34. McColgan P, Seunarine KK, Gregory S, et al. Topological length of white matter connections predicts their rate of atrophy in premanifest Huntington's disease. JCI Insight. 2017;2(8):e92641.
35. Dominguez JF, Poudel G, Stout J, et al. Longitudinal changes in the fronto-striatal network are associated with executive dysfunction and behavioral dysregulation in Huntington's disease: 30 months IMAGE-HD data. Cortex. 2017;92:139–49.
36. Bonner-Jackson A, Long JD, Westerveld H, et al. Cognitive reserve and brain reserve in prodromal Huntington's disease. J Int Neuropsychol Soc. 2013;19:739–50.
37. Zhang Y, Long JD, Mills JA, Warner JH, Lu W, Paulsen; and PREDICT-HD Investigators and Coordinators of the Huntington Study Group. Indexing disease progression at study entry with individuals at risk for Huntington disease. Am J Med Genet B Neuropsychiatr Genet. 2011;156(7):751-763.
38. Harrington DL, Smith MM, Zhang Y, Carlozzi NE, Paulsen JS; PREDICT-HD Investigators of the Huntington Study Group. Cognitive domains that predict time to diagnosis in prodromal Huntington disease. J Neurol Neurosurg Psychiatry. 2012;83:612-619.
39. Heaton RK, Chelune GJ, Talley JL, Kay GG, Curtis G. Wisconsin card sort test: manual, revised and expanded. Psychological Assessment Resources; 1993.
40. Delis DC, Kaplan E, Kramer JH. Delis-Kaplan Executive Function System (D-KEFS) Examiner's Manual. San Antonio, TX: The Psychological Corporation; 2001.
41. Meyers JE, Meyers K. RCFT: Rey complex figure test and recognition trial, professional manual. Psychological Assessment Resources; 1995.
42. Koziol LF, Budding DE. Subcortical structures and cognition: implications for neuropsychological assessment. New York, NY: Springer; 2009.
43. Ho AK, Sahakian BJ, Brown RG, et al. Profile of cognitive progression in early Huntington's disease. Neurology. 2003;61:1702–6.
44. Papp KV, Snyder PJ, Mills JA, et al. Measuring executive dysfunction longitudinally and in relation to genetic burden, brain volumetrics, and depression in prodromal Huntington disease. Arch Clin Neuropsychol. 2013;28:156–68.

45. Nicoll DR, Pirogovsky E, Woods SP, et al. "Forgetting to remember" in Huntington's disease: a study of laboratory, semi-naturalistic, and self-perceptions of prospective memory. J Int Neuropsychol Soc. 2014;20:192–9.
46. Raskin S. Memory for Intentions Screening Test: psychometric properties and clinical evidence. Brain Impairment. 2009;10(1):23–33.
47. Strange PG. Brain biochemistry and brain disorders. Oxford: Oxford University Press; 1992.
48. Peavy GM, Jacobson MW, Goldstein JL, et al. Cognitive and functional decline in Huntington's disease: dementia criteria revisited. Mov Disord. 2010;25(9):1163–9.
49. Smith A. Symbol digit modalities test manual. Western Psychological Services; 1982.
50. Paulsen JS, Butters N, Sadek JR, et al. Distinct cognitive profiles of cortical and subcortical dementia in advanced illness. Neurology. 1995;45(5):951–6.
51. Ferm U, Sahlin A, Sundin L, Hartelius L. Using Talking Mats to support communication in personals with Huntington's disease. Int J Lang Commun Disord. 2010;45(5):523–36.
52. Snowden JS, Craufurd D, Thompson J, Neary D. Psychomotor, executive, and memory function in preclinical Huntington's disease. J Clin Exp Neuropsychol. 2002;24(2):133–45.
53. Snowden JS, Austin NA, Sembi S, Thompson JC, Craufurd D, Neary D. Emotion recognition in Huntington's disease and frontotemporal dementia. Neuropsychologia. 2008;46(11):2638–49.
54. Grace J, Mallory P. FrSBe, Frontal Systems Behavior Scale: professional manual. Psychological Assessment Resources; 2001.
55. Lezak MD, Howieson DB, Bigler ED, Tranel D. Neuropsychological assessment: 5th edition. Oxford Press; 2012.
56. Stern Y. Cognitive reserve. Neuropsychologica. 2009;47(10):2015–28.
57. Koffler S, Morgan J, Baron IS, Greiffenstein MF. (eds) Neuropsychology: science and practice, I. Oxford Press; 2013.
58. Ionis Pharmaceuticals (2017). Dose-dependent reductions of mutant huntingtin protein observed; Ionis earns $45 million license fee. Press release of 11 December 2017. ir.ionispharma.com/news-releases. Accessed 25 Jan 2018.

Chapter 20
Traumatic Brain Injury: Sports Concussion

David B. Coppel and Stanley A. Herring

Introduction

In the last decade, sports concussion has emerged as a focus within sports medicine and general public health concerns. It has been discussed within the context of mild traumatic brain injury and triggered the interest and involvement of clinicians and researchers in many fields including neuroscience, neuropsychology, rehabilitation medicine, sports medicine, neurosurgery, neurology, pediatrics, and clinical psychology. Based on the physical, cognitive, and emotional aspects of concussion, and their impact on patients' lives, the educational, political, and legal systems have become involved in developing policy. Practice guidelines have been developed and modified over time as more evidence-based research is completed. The context of sports involvement is crucial to understanding the complexities of the impact on a concussed athlete, just as the military context is crucial for understanding the impact of concussions sustained from war zone blasts. Both neuropsychologists and medical providers are typically involved in the evaluation and management of sports concussion, which makes their collaboration and communication paramount to good patient care. Neuropsychologists can provide data regarding neurocognitive functions which may have been impacted by concussion, as well as the psychosocial and emotional factors that may impact persistent symptom reporting and the patients' general adjustment and ability to function in school, sports, or life.

D. B. Coppel (✉)
Department of Neurological Surgery, UW Medicine Sports Concussion Program, University of Washington School of Medicine, Seattle, WA, USA
e-mail: dcoppel@neurosurgery.washington.edu; dcoppel@uw.edu

S. A. Herring
Department of Rehabilitation Medicine, University of Washington School of Medicine, Seattle, WA, USA

K. M. Sanders (ed.), *Physician's Field Guide to Neuropsychology*,
https://doi.org/10.1007/978-1-4939-8722-1_20

Definition

The definition of sports concussion continues to be refined as clinical observations and scientific research progress. The most commonly employed definition is the one developed at the Fifth International Conference on Concussion in Sport held in Berlin, October 2016 [1]. The document produced at that consensus meeting defines sports concussion as follows:

Sports-related concussion (SRC) is a traumatic brain injury induced by biomechanical forces. Several common features that may be utilized in clinically defining the nature of a concussive head injury include:

- SRC may be caused by a direct blow either to the head, face, neck, or elsewhere on the body with an impulsive force transmitted to the head.
- SRC typically results in the rapid onset of short-lived impairment of neurological function that resolves spontaneously. However, in some cases, signs and symptoms evolve over a number of minutes to hours.
- SRC may result in neuropathological changes, but the acute clinical signs and symptoms largely reflect a functional disturbance rather than a structural injury and, as such, no abnormality is seen on standard structural neuroimaging studies.
- SRC results in a range of clinical signs and symptoms that may or may not involve loss of consciousness. Resolution of the clinical and cognitive features typically follows a sequential course. However, in some cases symptoms may be prolonged.

The clinical signs and symptoms cannot be explained by drug, alcohol, or medication use, other injuries (such as cervical injuries, peripheral vestibular dysfunction, etc.), or other comorbidities (e.g., psychological factors or coexisting medical conditions).

At the Berlin meeting, there was emphasis placed on noting that a concussion is indeed a brain injury and, although most concussions have a favorable prognosis, all brain injuries should be taken seriously.

Epidemiology

It has been estimated that between 1.1 million and 1.9 million sports and recreation concussions occur annually in the United States in children aged <18 years. This demonstrates how remarkably commonly this injury occurs [2]. It has been suggested that there is a "concussion crisis" with a rapidly increasing rate of concussions; however, it is likely that to a significant degree, it is the rate of reporting concussions which has increased rather than the frequency of the injury itself [3–5]. Further emphasizing this point, even though the reported rate of sports concussions has risen, there has not been a corresponding reported increase in the catastrophic brain injuries related to sports [6].

Thirty percent of all concussions in youth between the ages of 5 and 19 are sports-related [7] and account for 5–18% of all sports-related injuries in high school and collegiate athletes [8–10]. While the highest number of concussions occur in high school and college football, concussions are common in wrestling, girls' and boys' soccer, and girls' basketball [6]. Indeed, the rate of concussions is higher in collegiate women's soccer than in collegiate football [9].

Pathophysiology

Concussions occur due to forces applied to the brain, and while these forces may be linear or angular, currently the threshold of these forces needed to produce a concussion is unknown. Based on animal modeling, when sufficient force is applied to the brain, there is disruption of the normal metabolism in the area of the brain affected; a neurometabolic cascade of events is triggered [11–13]. This brain impairment has been described as largely functional (see definition above), but advanced imaging techniques have demonstrated some cases of microscopic axonal damage [6, 14]. In order to re-establish homeostasis after a concussion, energy (glucose) is required and must be delivered via cerebral blood flow. However, the injured part of the brain has decreased blood flow creating a fuel supply/demand mismatch [11, 12, 15]. Until this mismatch is corrected and normal brain metabolism returns, the brain remains vulnerable to repeat impacts [12, 13, 15–20]. This underscores the importance of full recovery before suffering another concussive injury. Experimental work has also shown that when part of the brain has been concussed, it is less responsive to physiological activation [11, 13]. Clinically, this finding helps explain why physical and cognitive activities after a concussion may not be as well tolerated and, if pursued too soon and too aggressively, may delay recovery.

The brains of young people may demonstrate these pathophysiological changes to a greater degree explaining why they often take longer than adults to recover from a concussion and why they may be particularly susceptible to the effects of a second concussion while still symptomatic from the first one [13].

Diagnosis

Diagnosis of concussion revolves around eliciting the mechanism of injury, resulting symptoms, and a focused physical and neurological examination. Ultimately this diagnosis remains a clinical one [14] and is dependent upon the knowledge, experience, and skill of the healthcare provider. Concussion diagnosis can be challenging requiring a structured approach and careful consideration of other potential injuries and issues.

While headache is the most common symptom of a concussion [21, 22], concussions can be quite variable in their presentation. Initial concussion symptoms can be grouped into three categories, cognitive, somatic, and affective, with a fourth category, sleep disturbance, added after the first day (see Table 20.1) [23].

It is important to ask about symptoms in each category as concussion presentation is quite variable between patients and within the same patient suffering a repeat injury. Use of a concussion symptom checklist can be helpful. It is also pertinent to realize that these symptoms are non-specific and associated with many other conditions (e.g., fatigue, dehydration, depression) and careful questioning is necessary. Along with a disciplined review of symptoms, a standardized approach to the patient should continue.

Key Point

An initial focused physical and neurological examination to assess for more significant neurological injury or concomitant injuries such as cervical spine injury is important. The presence of significant cervical pain and limited range of motion or deteriorating mental status, severe or persisting headache, repeated emesis, and asymmetry of cranial nerve or limb motor/sensory examination are examples of findings that would warrant immediate transport via ambulance. Barring such findings, a sideline or initial office examination should proceed. Evaluating the athlete in four domains—orientation, concentration, memory, and balance—is a cornerstone of this examination.

Table 20.1 Selected acute and delayed signs and symptoms suggestive of concussion

Cognitive	Somatic	Affective	Sleep disturbances
Contusion	Headache	Emotional lability	Trouble falling asleep
Anterograde amnesia	Dizziness	Irritability	Sleeping more than usual
Retrograde amnesia	Balance disruption	Fatigue	Sleeping less than usual
LOC	Nausea/Vomiting	Anxiety	
Disorientation	Visual disturbances (photophobia, blurry/double vision)	Sadness	
Feeling "in a fog," "zoned out"	Phonophobia		
Vacant stare			
Inability to focus			
Delayed verbal and motor responses			
Slurred/Incoherent speech			
Excessive drowsiness			

Many tools are available with varying sensitivity and specificity [6] and may be more valuable if there is baseline data for comparison. A widely utilized tool containing a symptom checklist and tests for these four domains is the Sideline Concussion Assessment Tool version 5 (SCAT5) [24] which is free to be downloaded (see Appendix 1). Patricios and Makdissi [25] have described the role of medical providers to "evaluate the history, consider confounding variables (modifying factors), perform general, systemic and functional examinations, order and interpret appropriate investigations and repeat this process as necessary, to determine the best course of action for the patient."

Neuropsychological consultation and testing has been utilized for decades in the diagnosis and management of traumatic brain injury and increasingly with sports concussion. Neuropsychological assessment provides "performance-based" age-normed data regarding neurocognitive functions, in contrast to self-report appraisals about cognitive functions [26].

Key Point

Neuropsychological testing in sports concussion typically focuses on areas of functioning most often impacted by concussion (e.g., processing, attention/concentration, learning, and memory) and is often structured as neurocognitive screenings; serial testing over the course of recovery may be indicated to track improvement over time.

Many athletic teams utilize a preseason or baseline testing approach in which non-concussed athletes are tested and the results are used as a comparison marker for recovery if they sustain a concussion. Neuropsychologists may be involved in the preseason or baseline testing and/or the follow-up to a concussion testing and evaluation. Neuropsychological evaluation typically involves a clinical interview with the athlete, self-report questionnaires or symptom checklists, neurocognitive testing, and, if indicated, assessment of psychosocial and emotional factors [27].

Key Point

McCrea [28] described a biopsychosocial model in which the roles of neuropsychologists include monitoring for psychosocial factors that may negatively impact the patient's natural recovery, using psychological techniques to treat the interfering psychosocial factors and providing comprehensive education about the expected recovery and outcomes from concussion.

Neuropsychological or neurocognitive testing for sports concussion has included in-person testing and/or computerized neurocognitive testing. While traditional in-person paper-and-pencil testing continues to be utilized in the evaluation of sports concussion, computerized neurocognitive testing has grown exponentially over the last decade and appears to be the predominant testing modality at all levels of sports (youth, high school, college, and professional) and other activities (military). Resch, McCrea, and Cullum [29] review computerized testing in sports and note a number of advantages including the ability to baseline test groups of athletes, wide availability via Internet and other platforms, ease of administration, access to alternate test forms to reduce practice effects, and creation of centralized data repositories for access by users. The computerized testing platforms vary in their recommendation for a neuropsychologist to interpret the results, with some indicating that best practices involve the use of a neuropsychologist for interpretation of test results and others suggesting it is a go-no go result not needing a neuropsychologist. The psychometric aspects of the computerized tests have been scrutinized and found wanting according to some researchers and adequate according to other data. While computerized testing has a number of advantages, there are a number of notable limitations such as the absence of any auditory processing or auditory memory tasks. In addition, the memory tests are typically structured as recognition memory tasks not recall memory tasks. With mild traumatic brain injury (mTBI), recognition memory typically remains intact, while recall memory is more likely compromised, so computerized testing may not pick up on recall deficits. Other limitations of computerized testing include no opportunities for neurobehavioral observations or direct information about attention/distraction, problem solving, or effort behavior.

The use of baseline computerized testing to provide a comparison marker for subsequent post-concussion test performances has become a common approach in the evaluation and management of sports concussion. The value of baseline testing is directly related to the reliability and stability of the test results to depict non-concussed performance. Thus, management of a concussion is based on the approach that recovery or readiness to return to play or start the return-to-play protocol occurs when an athlete has returned to baseline neurocognitive performance level (or above) and endorses no symptoms (or is at baseline symptom-level endorsement). Providers must determine if return to baseline levels (after presumed declined levels due to concussion) is due to actual recovery or increased effort on follow-up in order to return to play. Conversely, providers must determine if the lack of return to baseline performance (and/or symptom endorsement) is due to ongoing brain injury or the contributions of other factors.

As with other testing, baseline computerized testing may be influenced by testing environment distractions (typically baseline testing is done in a group setting, and follow-up testing is done individually), sleep the night before, caffeine consumption, general stress, and variable motivation and effort (level of effort can vary from a relatively meaningless baseline marker to a performance that could influence the decision to return to play).

Key Point

Neuropsychological testing should not be used as a stand-alone measure to make the diagnosis of concussion, and the same is true for all of the other components of the examination. Even if neuropsychological testing returns to baseline, the patient can still be concussed. There is no single "concussion test" and clinical acumen remains the key. It should also be remembered that concussion signs and symptoms can evolve over minutes to hours limiting the sensitivity of an immediate post-injury assessment and dictating the importance of observation and serial evaluations and collaborative provider care.

Management

In the case of a suspected concussion, there is no same day return to play for athletes at any level of competition [14]. Most sports concussions have a favorable prognosis with 80–90% of patients reporting recovery in 7–10 days with younger athletes sometimes feeling better more slowly [14]. There are modifiers that can prolong recovery (see Table 20.2) [23], and recognizing and discussing these modifiers with the patient and family is an important part of the management plan.

With or without modifiers being present, each concussion is unique and must be managed as such. Predicting recovery to be in a certain number of days or weeks at the onset of management is unwise. Concussions are not managed by a calendar, rather by the patient reaching milestones on a path of supervised return to activity and sports.

The initial treatment for an acute concussion is rest, both physical and relative cognitive rest [1]. If there is too much physical or cognitive activity and the concussion symptoms are exacerbated, recovery can be delayed. It is important for the patient and family to understand that the rest should be relative, not absolute. Strict rest versus limited rest for the first 5 days after a concussion has been associated with a worse outcome [30], with a negative affect symptom reporting. In some instances, the physical and cognitive rest or restriction management approach can have iatrogenic consequences; when athletes are unable to practice, they are often deprived of a coping outlet and/or access to social support; some feel a degree of

Table 20.2 Risk factors that may prolong or complicate recovery from concussion

Factors	Modifier
Concussion history	Total number, proximity, severity (duration)
Symptoms	Total number, severity (intensity and especially duration)
Signs	Prolonged LOC (>1 minutes)
Susceptibility	Concussions occurring with lower impact magnitude and/or requiring longer recovery
Age	Youth and adolescent athletes may recover more slowly
Preexisting conditions	Migraine, depression, anxiety/panic attacks, attention deficit/hyperactivity disorder, learning disabilities

physical, cognitive, or emotional vulnerability and can experience challenges or threats to self-esteem, identity, and future plans or goals. It is important to understand that concussion may initially be metabolic brain alteration but over time is typically experienced more within the psychological aspect of neuropsychology.

It is also important for patients and parents to understand that if some physical or cognitive activity does cause a transient increase in symptoms that there is no further brain damage being done. It can be difficult for athletes (and parents) to understand that the initial causal factors (mTBI) of their concussion symptoms may not be the determining factors/causes of prolonged symptoms or symptoms re-emerging at a later date. Often it is the stress of returning to schoolwork or assignments that generates some tension and mimics post-concussion symptoms, not that the brain injury is ongoing. Ongoing headaches can be especially frustrating and negatively impact cognitive functioning; for example, it is hard to concentrate with a significant headache, which can impact encoding of information and, ultimately, storing and retrieving of information (memory complaints). If persistent headache is the sole or even predominant symptom in cases of prolonged recovery, consideration for the development of a post-traumatic headache disorder (or exacerbation of a preexisting headache disorder) should be considered before labeling the patient as having post-concussive syndrome [6].

After the initial rest period when the patient is at his/her usual baseline, the next milestone to be reached concerns the return to learn [31] process. The patient needs to progress to where he/she is performing all schoolwork, homework, and after-school activities with the usual amount of effort without causing symptoms [32] (see Return to Learn section). Subsequently, as the final milestone, the patient needs to complete a multiday medically supervised graduated return-to-play program without return of any symptoms (see Table 20.3 and Appendix 1). Return-to-play

Table 20.3 Graduated return-to-sport strategy

	Exercise step	Functional exercise at each step	Goal of each step
1.	Symptom-limited activity	Daily activities that do not provoke symptoms	Gradual reintroduction of work/school activities
2.	Light aerobic exercise	Walking or stationary cycling at slow to medium pace. No resistance training	Increase heart rate
3.	Sport-specific exercise	Running or skating drills. No head impact activities	Add movement
4.	Non-contact training drills	Harder training drills, e.g., passing drills. May start progressive resistance training	Exercise, coordination, and increased thinking
5.	Full contact practice	Following medical clearance, participate in normal training activities	Restore confidence and assess functional skills by coaching staff
6.	Return to play/sport	Normal gameplay	

In this example, it would be typical to have 24 h (or longer) for each step of the progression. If any symptoms worsen while exercising, the athlete should go back to the previous step. Resistance training should be added only in the later stages (Stage 3 or 4 at the earliest)

Written clearance should be provided by a healthcare professional before return to play/sport as directed by local laws and regulations clearance given by a licensed healthcare provider is now mandated by law in all 50 states and the District of Columbia. The specifics of which healthcare providers can provide this clearance vary by state. There is no one specialty that is uniquely qualified to make this decision, and there are some states where neuropsychologists are included as those can assume this role.

Key Point
The collaboration of providers is crucial for the return-to-play decision regardless of who takes responsibility by law or regulation. Input from providers to be integrated can include radiological findings (ruling out catastrophic concerns), medical test results (other concomitant medical issues), symptom checklist progression, balance test results, neurocognitive test results, training room results, school performance, general observed behavioral patterns, and psychological status. These areas provide the opportunity to collaborate and provide customized or individualized care to the concussed patient.

In cases of persistent concussion symptoms, it is important to note that often these symptoms are non-specific and other conditions should be investigated which may have preceded the concussion, occurred in conjunction with the concussion or now be present as a result of the concussion. As examples, concern for structural lesions may warrant the use of neuroimaging, and persistent dizziness or vertigo should have a thorough investigation. Also, it is essential to consider psychological issues, especially depression and anxiety [1]. Neuropsychological assessment can be very valuable in helping to sort out ongoing cognitive injury from symptoms due primarily to psychological sources. Because of the complexities of these cases, when concussion recovery falls outside the usual time parameters (more than 10 days) and signs and symptoms remain significant or are escalating, consideration for referral to multidisciplinary center specializing in concussion/brain injury care should be strongly considered [1]. In athletes with prolonged recovery from concussion, the contributory role of psychosocial and emotional factors such as depressive mood or anxiety or stress factors is well supported [33]. The neuropsychologist may be particularly helpful in the assessment and management of the athletes with a prolonged recovery. Prolonging factors can include depression, anxiety, frustration, anger, sleep disturbance, symptom vigilance, sense of loss, identity concerns (athletic or academic), psychosocial issues emerging from family, friends/teammates, and coaches, and school stress (being out of school or the making up and keeping up with assignment stress). Psychological or psychiatric consultation may be indicated to deal with these typically secondary factors. Providers with knowledge of the athletes and the athletic subculture, such as clinical or counseling sport psychologists, may be particularly helpful with these patients.

Premature Return to Play

There are short-term risks with premature return to play including the rare occurrence of second impact syndrome (SIS). SIS occurs when an athlete returns to play while still symptomatic from a concussion and sustains a second blow (often minor) followed by collapse within several seconds to minutes [34]. There is the rapid onset of massive malignant brain edema with or without a small subdural hematoma. Marked increased intracranial pressure and uncal herniation ensue usually resulting in death or severe residual brain injury. While there has been some controversy as to whether SIS is due to receiving a second blow to the brain versus being due to a different diffuse cerebral swelling syndrome described in children [35–37], the association of this tragic event with returning to play while still symptomatic from a concussion dictates the absolute need for complete treatment of the initial concussion [6].

Even if an athlete does not suffer catastrophic SIS injury, premature return to play can have significant consequences. Resumption of physical and cognitive activities too soon can exacerbate concussion signs and symptoms prolonging recovery. Young athletes are also students, and premature return to play with resulting persistence of these signs and symptoms affects not only sports participation but important activities such as schoolwork, homework, driver's education, and college aptitude testing.

Return to Learn

While the majority of concussions do not require a structured return-to-learn protocol, some individuals are best supported by a gradual return-to-learn strategy [38]. This often allows for the reduction of symptoms which are exacerbated from academic involvements. Post-concussion symptoms such as headaches, difficulty with concentration and attention, problems with new learning, and fatigue can all create challenges and difficulties for students' school performances.

Generally, concussed students may benefit from a short period of reduced academic activity (or temporary accommodations), followed by a gradual return to full academic activities. Progression with cognitive activity should be on an "as tolerated" basis. Strategies for gradual return for school are included in Table 20.4 and the SCAT5 and Child SCAT5 (see Appendices 1 and 2).

Long-Term Consequences of Concussion

While most concussions resolve fairly quickly as noted above, there are long-term concerns regarding this injury, especially for those athletes who have had more exposure to head trauma over time. Depression, mild cognitive impairment, and

Table 20.4 Graduated return-to-school strategy

	Mental activity	Activity at each step	Goal of each step
1.	Daily activities that do not give the athlete symptoms	Typical activities that the athlete does during the day as long as they do not increase symptoms (e.g., reading, texting, screen time). Start with 5–15 minutes at a time and gradually build up	Gradual return to typical activities
2.	School activities	Homework, reading, or other cognitive activities outside of the classroom	Increase tolerance to cognitive work
3.	Return to school part-time	Gradual introduction of schoolwork. May need to start with a partial school day or with increased breaks during the day	Increase academic activities
4.	Return to school full-time	Gradually progress school activities until a full day can be tolerated	Return to full academic activities and catch up on missed work

Concussion may affect the ability to learn at school. The athlete may need to miss a few days of school after a concussion. When going back to school, some athletes may need to go back gradually and may need to have some changes made to their schedule so that concussion symptoms do not get worse. If a particular activity makes symptoms worse, then the athlete should stop that activity and rest until symptoms get better. To make sure that the athlete can get back to school without problems, it is important that the healthcare provider, parents, caregivers, and teachers talk to each other so that everyone knows what the plan is for the athlete to go back to school
Note: If mental activity does not cause any symptoms, the athlete may be able to skip step 2 and return to school part-time before doing school activities at home first

chronic traumatic encephalopathy (CTE) are three diagnoses that are frequently mentioned in this context.

In surveys of retired professional athletes, there is some evidence linking the number of concussions to the risk of developing depression. There are much less data available connecting the number of concussions to suicidal thoughts and behaviors [39]. Also in research involving retired professional athletes, there is evidence linking concussions to cognitive decline, especially in the areas of memory and processing speed. While the results of research in this area of cognition are mixed, more studies than not report development of problems [39]. It is important to avoid generalizing this mental health and cognitive impairment data to male and female athletes at all levels of play. Long-term prospective, population-based studies are needed, with greater inclusion of other potential factors which influence cognitive outcomes (e.g., substance use/abuse, psychiatric history (treated or untreated), learning disabilities, or attention deficit disorder).

CTE is a progressive neurodegenerative tauopathy, with associated clinical, behavioral, and neuropathological findings. Currently the only way to diagnosis CTE is at autopsy which does not allow for assigning causation to this disease nor can incidence and prevalence be determined. CTE does appear to be associated with head trauma but does not appear to correlate with the number of recorded concussions. There may be other factors (e.g., genetic, substance use, total burden of head trauma) that are contributors to an individual's specific risk given the large number of athletes competing in collision and contact sports and the small number of cases reported [6, 40]. As with depression and mild cognitive impairment, there is the need for prospective, longitudinal, population-based studies to better understand the risk for developing CTE. This is an important area that deserves further study.

While there remains much to learn about the long-term mental health, cognitive, and neurodegenerative consequences of concussions, there is no harm in taking steps now to prevent unnecessary head contact in sports. Education for athletes, parents, coaches, administrators, and healthcare providers raises awareness and knowledge about concussion [41] and training and conditioning of athletes may be helpful as well. Fair play [42] and rules enforcement along with practice and game modifications [43] are important interventions as well.

Case Example

Referral

John is a 17-year, 7-month-old male who was referred by his family physician for sports concussion evaluation/consultation. He sustained a sports-related concussion while playing soccer 4 weeks ago. His sports concussion had been managed by his family physician for 3 weeks with minimal improvement in self-reported symptoms, until his referral to the Sports Concussion Clinic. John is an elite-level soccer player with a scholarship offer to college for soccer. Referral to neuropsychologist was triggered by John's ongoing cognitive complaints and concern about future school functioning, along with his apparent anxiety. Prolonged cognitive issues and/or emotional factors are typical factors in referral to neuropsychologist in the clinic. John was seen by sports medicine provider/physiatrist for an initial intake evaluation, which included history of concussions and symptom/recovery course, general medical history, administration of Sports Concussion Assessment Tool-3 (SCAT3), and collateral information from parents. As part of the initial intake with the physician, sports neuropsychologist/sports psychologist was introduced and was briefly involved in the information gathering portion; a subsequent clinical interview and neuropsychological testing appointment were set up.

Case Presentation

John's recent concussion occurred during a soccer game when he was kicked in the left ear/side of the head and fell to the grass field; he reported a possible brief loss of consciousness but has poor memory for the time period 10 minutes before and after the injury. He was observed to have shallow breathing and some leg twitching for a period of time post-injury. He was transported to the emergency room and evaluated; CT scan was within normal limits. John was discharged and told to follow up with his primary care physician. Initial symptoms included headache and fogginess for 2 days, nausea for 1 day, photosensitivity, increased irritability, and slowed processing. John's primary care physician recommended he stay out of school for 1 week and restrict his screen time (computer, phone). He was also encouraged to have cognitive rest. When John returned to school 1 week later, he reported difficulty processing information and comprehending in a number of classes and was worried about falling behind in his schoolwork. Ten days post-injury, John chose to jog for 15 minutes without symptoms emerging and felt encouraged but continued to describe not feeling normal and having times of poor focus and concentration, memory lapses, and worry. Given John's ongoing reported symptoms, his family physician referred him to the Sports Concussion Clinic.

John's medical history was negative for birth trauma or developmental delay. He reports no history of diagnosed learning disabilities/difficulties or attention deficit disorder, and family history is negative for these conditions. He reports no history of headache condition/migraine; family history was positive for migraine on maternal side. John has no pre-injury history of vision or hearing problems and no history of non-sports-related head trauma. He reports no alcohol or drug use. John's history is positive for seeing a counselor over the past 4 months for self-described family and relationship issues. He reported no history of suicidal ideation or attempts. Family history is reportedly negative for known major mental or emotional disorders. John is a senior in high school and reported that he has maintained his strong 3.5 GPA; he does describe some apprehension about falling behind in school and concern over future cognitive dysfunction. Information obtained follows the SCAT5 athlete background areas.

Medical Evaluation

The clinic medical examination revealed a normal neurological examination for cranial nerve, reflex, sensation, motor, and balance testing. SCAT5 performance appeared adequate with some struggle on digits backward noted. John reported sleep onset problems that were associated with mental activation/worry. Appetite, energy, and libido were described as normal. Cognitive symptoms reported included slowed processing, poor attention, and reports of forgetfulness. Emotional symptoms were described as some increased tension and worry. He describes three prior sports-related concussions all in soccer, occurring 2, 3, and 5 years ago. John described increased concern over having a total of three or four concussions (he does not count the one from 2 years ago), having heard from his medical providers, and read on a sports concussion-related Internet blog that three or more concussions lead to significant brain damage and related problems. He is very anxious about future concussions and shares his apprehension about continuing in soccer at the next level but is torn due to scholarship offers. MRI was completed and was within normal limits.

Neuropsychological Evaluation

Computerized neurocognitive testing (ImPACT) was completed through his high school and included a baseline test and one post-injury follow-up test. The post-injury follow-up test revealed his relatively high symptom endorsement (number and severity). Verbal and visual memory composite test scores and visual-motor speed composite test scores were not significantly reduced from baseline levels; reaction time composite measure was slower than baseline.

John's neuropsychological evaluation included a clinical interview (history and background and more expanded exploration/clarification of symptoms) and neuropsychological testing. The clinical interview revealed that while he had no diagnosed ADD, he did have noted attention and focus issues in middle school that were described within the context of anxiety. John offers that he is a better visual learner than verbal-auditory learner. John described counseling over the past 4 months related to conflicts within his family and disrupted relationships with his peers/teammates.

John's current symptoms were explored further, and he revealed recurrent thoughts about brain damage and his future, and he described the occurrence of "panic-like" episodes. He also expressed concern that cognitive activity would be harm his brain and, as a result, had reduced his cognitive effort in school and on assignments during this recovery time. He described becoming hypervigilant to any perceived cognitive slippage/inefficiencies, and these observations are proof of decline and ongoing brain-related concussion symptoms.

John completed a 60-minute neuropsychological screening battery and performed in the high average or above ranges on all measures. Effort measures reflected normal effort. Measures included visual sequencing/visual scanning, visual and auditory attention and processing, visual search and attention, visual-motor and visual-oral coding, word retrieval, visual design learning and memory, and verbal-auditory learning and memory (word list). Self-report measures of anxiety and depression reflected moderately severe anxiety level and mild depressive symptom level.

Results

Testing results did not reveal evidence of significant neurocognitive impairment. While these test results were reassuring, John still described significant anxiety, distraction, and slowed processing. Medical provider and neuropsychologist discussed findings with John and his parents. Based on available research of aggregated data, he was noted to be at a statistically increased risk for having another concussion and possibly longer recovery times based on his prior history of concussions; however, his personal risk was unknown. This concussion, in and of itself, from a medical and neuropsychological perspective, would not necessarily warrant retirement. However, his decision was based on psychosocial factors. It was recommended that John return to the clinic for counseling related to his anxiety-related concerns and his future sports issues.

Follow-Up

John returned and was seen for counseling over the next 2 months. He was seen by the neuropsychologist, who is also a clinical and sports psychologist. A general cognitive-behavioral approach was utilized and focused on his anxiety responses and rumination/catastrophizing about brain damage. A discussion regarding his ideas about what had happened in his brain allowed for reeducative moments. Discussions regarding other potential influences on his thinking and emotions such as psychosocial/interactions and sleep proved to be very helpful in shifting away from attributions to brain injury. It was also revealed that he had similar overresponding patterns with other injuries in the past. John became comfortable providing his usual level of cognitive exertion in school and felt his cognitive functioning had normalized. He questioned his commitment to soccer and his scholarship options. He gradually reduced his concern and anxiety and increased engagement in physical and mental activities; these activities were experienced as helping to reduce anxiety and an indication of normalcy. Significant family conflict developed as parents shared that without the scholarship their financial situation would become very difficult. John continued to question his desire/motivation for soccer, his soccer future, and the scholarship options; he described thinking about discontinuing soccer as the potential loss of a dream, but he had other interests he wanted to pursue. John's parents subsequently sought second and third opinions regarding John's soccer risk/future and became frustrated with the range of opinions (return to soccer to retirement). John was feeling better overall in terms of anxiety and worry about his neurocognitive functioning. He decided to decline his soccer opportunity and obtained cross-country scholarship. John and his parents returned to their previous individual and family counseling.

Key Points

1. Neuropsychological consultation/referral can provide information regarding patient's emotional and psychosocial status that may be making a further contribution to their reported neurocognitive difficulties, beyond the concussive event.
2. The integration of medical, neurocognitive performance patterns, and psychosocial/emotional factors is the added value of neuropsychological consultation.
3. With sports concussion patients, collaboration and communication with the medical provider are crucial; ideally, neuropsychologist should be initially presented as part of the evaluation/treatment team.
4. Neuropsychological test data can be collected sequentially to track recovery. It can provide reassurance to patients or help direct interventions needed.

Chapter Review Questions

1. Neuropsychological testing for sports concussion:
   A. Is the only measure needed to make a concussion diagnosis.
   B. Can be helpful in sorting out cognitive injury from symptoms primarily due to psychological sources.
   C. Typically involves a full academic evaluation.
   D. Provides performance-based age-normed data regarding neurocognitive functions.
   E. B and D.

2. In cases of persistent or prolonged concussion symptoms:
   A. Athletes typically have to retire from all sports.
   B. Athletes should jump back into their sport at full participation level if they want to.
   C. Athletes should reduce their cognitive activity to help the brain heal.
   D. Psychosocial and emotional factors such as depression and anxiety play a role in recovery.

3. Chronic traumatic encephalopathy (CTE):
   A. Has a high incidence and prevalence in contact sports.
   B. Is associated with the number of documented concussions an athlete has experienced.
   C. Needs prospective longitudinal studies to better understand this disease.
   D. Is now reliably diagnosed antemortem.

Appendix 1

SCAT5©

SPORT CONCUSSION ASSESSMENT TOOL — 5TH EDITION
DEVELOPED BY THE CONCUSSION IN SPORT GROUP
FOR USE BY MEDICAL PROFESSIONALS ONLY

supported by

FIFA® FEI

Patient details

Name:____________________

DOB: ____________________

Address:____________________

ID number: ____________________

Examiner:____________________

Date of Injury:____________________ Time: ____________________

WHAT IS THE SCAT5?

The SCAT5 is a standardized tool for evaluating concussions designed for use by physicians and licensed healthcare professionals[1]. The SCAT5 cannot be performed correctly in less than 10 minutes.

If you are not a physician or licensed healthcare professional, please use the Concussion Recognition Tool 5 (CRT5). The SCAT5 is to be used for evaluating athletes aged 13 years and older. For children aged 12 years or younger, please use the Child SCAT5.

Preseason SCAT5 baseline testing can be useful for interpreting post-injury test scores, but is not required for that purpose. Detailed instructions for use of the SCAT5 are provided on page 7. Please read through these instructions carefully before testing the athlete. Brief verbal instructions for each test are given in italics. The only equipment required for the tester is a watch or timer.

This tool may be freely copied in its current form for distribution to individuals, teams, groups and organizations. It should not be altered in any way, re-branded or sold for commercial gain. Any revision, translation or reproduction in a digital form requires specific approval by the Concussion in Sport Group.

Recognise and Remove

A head impact by either a direct blow or indirect transmission of force can be associated with a serious and potentially fatal brain injury. If there are significant concerns, including any of the red flags listed in Box 1, then activation of emergency procedures and urgent transport to the nearest hospital should be arranged.

Key points

- Any athlete with suspected concussion should be REMOVED FROM PLAY, medically assessed and monitored for deterioration. No athlete diagnosed with concussion should be returned to play on the day of injury.
- If an athlete is suspected of having a concussion and medical personnel are not immediately available, the athlete should be referred to a medical facility for urgent assessment.
- Athletes with suspected concussion should not drink alcohol, use recreational drugs and should not drive a motor vehicle until cleared to do so by a medical professional.
- Concussion signs and symptoms evolve over time and it is important to consider repeat evaluation in the assessment of concussion.
- The diagnosis of a concussion is a clinical judgment, made by a medical professional. The SCAT5 should NOT be used by itself to make, or exclude, the diagnosis of concussion. An athlete may have a concussion even if their SCAT5 is "normal".

Remember:

- The basic principles of first aid (danger, response, airway, breathing, circulation) should be followed.
- Do not attempt to move the athlete (other than that required for airway management) unless trained to do so.
- Assessment for a spinal cord injury is a critical part of the initial on-field assessment.
- Do not remove a helmet or any other equipment unless trained to do so safely.

1

Name: ____________________

DOB: ____________________

Address: ____________________

ID number: ____________________

Examiner: ____________________

Date: ____________________

IMMEDIATE OR ON-FIELD ASSESSMENT

The following elements should be assessed for all athletes who are suspected of having a concussion prior to proceeding to the neurocognitive assessment and ideally should be done on-field after the first first aid / emergency care priorities are completed.

If any of the "Red Flags" or observable signs are noted after a direct or indirect blow to the head, the athlete should be immediately and safely removed from participation and evaluated by a physician or licensed healthcare professional.

Consideration of transportation to a medical facility should be at the discretion of the physician or licensed healthcare professional.

The GCS is important as a standard measure for all patients and can be done serially if necessary in the event of deterioration in conscious state. The Maddocks questions and cervical spine exam are critical steps of the immediate assessment; however, these do not need to be done serially.

STEP 1: RED FLAGS

RED FLAGS:

- Neck pain or tenderness
- Double vision
- Weakness or tingling/ burning in arms or legs
- Severe or increasing headache
- Seizure or convulsion
- Loss of consciousness
- Deteriorating conscious state
- Vomiting
- Increasingly restless, agitated or combative

STEP 2: OBSERVABLE SIGNS

Witnessed ☐ Observed on Video ☐

Lying motionless on the playing surface	Y	N
Balance / gait difficulties / motor incoordination: stumbling, slow / laboured movements	Y	N
Disorientation or confusion, or an inability to respond appropriately to questions	Y	N
Blank or vacant look	Y	N
Facial injury after head trauma	Y	N

STEP 3: MEMORY ASSESSMENT MADDOCKS QUESTIONS[2]

"I am going to ask you a few questions, please listen carefully and give your best effort. First, tell me what happened?"

____

____

Mark Y for correct answer / N for incorrect

What venue are we at today?	Y	N
Which half is it now?	Y	N
Who scored last in this match?	Y	N
What team did you play last week / game?	Y	N
Did your team win the last game?	Y	N

Note: Appropriate sport-specific questions may be substituted.

STEP 4: EXAMINATION GLASGOW COMA SCALE (GCS)[3]

Time of assessment			
Date of assessment			
Best eye response (E)			
No eye opening	1	1	1
Eye opening in response to pain	2	2	2
Eye opening to speech	3	3	3
Eyes opening spontaneously	4	4	4
Best verbal response (V)			
No verbal response	1	1	1
Incomprehensible sounds	2	2	2
Inappropriate words	3	3	3
Confused	4	4	4
Oriented	5	5	5
Best motor response (M)			
No motor response	1	1	1
Extension to pain	2	2	2
Abnormal flexion to pain	3	3	3
Flexion / Withdrawal to pain	4	4	4
Localizes to pain	5	5	5
Obeys commands	6	6	6
Glasgow Coma score (E + V + M)			

CERVICAL SPINE ASSESSMENT

Does the athlete report that their neck is pain free at rest?	Y	N
If there is NO neck pain at rest, does the athlete have a full range of ACTIVE pain free movement?	Y	N
Is the limb strength and sensation normal?	Y	N

In a patient who is not lucid or fully conscious, a cervical spine injury should be assumed until proven otherwise.

OFFICE OR OFF-FIELD ASSESSMENT

Please note that the neurocognitive assessment should be done in a distraction-free environment with the athlete in a resting state.

STEP 1: ATHLETE BACKGROUND

Sport / team / school: ___

Date / time of injury: ___

Years of education completed: ___

Age: ___

Gender: M / F / Other

Dominant hand: left / neither / right

How many diagnosed concussions has the athlete had in the past?: ___

When was the most recent concussion?: ___

How long was the recovery (time to being cleared to play) from the most recent concussion?: ___ (days)

Has the athlete ever been:

Hospitalized for a head injury?	Yes	No
Diagnosed / treated for headache disorder or migraines?	Yes	No
Diagnosed with a learning disability / dyslexia?	Yes	No
Diagnosed with ADD / ADHD?	Yes	No
Diagnosed with depression, anxiety or other psychiatric disorder?	Yes	No

Current medications? If yes, please list:

___

___

___

___

___

___

Name: ___

DOB: ___

Address: ___

ID number: ___

Examiner: ___

Date: ___

2

STEP 2: SYMPTOM EVALUATION

The athlete should be given the symptom form and asked to read this instruction paragraph out loud then complete the symptom scale. For the baseline assessment, the athlete should rate his/her symptoms based on how he/she typically feels and for the post injury assessment the athlete should rate their symptoms at this point in time.

Please Check: ☐ **Baseline** ☐ **Post-Injury**

Please hand the form to the athlete

	none	mild		moderate		severe	
Headache	0	1	2	3	4	5	6
"Pressure in head"	0	1	2	3	4	5	6
Neck Pain	0	1	2	3	4	5	6
Nausea or vomiting	0	1	2	3	4	5	6
Dizziness	0	1	2	3	4	5	6
Blurred vision	0	1	2	3	4	5	6
Balance problems	0	1	2	3	4	5	6
Sensitivity to light	0	1	2	3	4	5	6
Sensitivity to noise	0	1	2	3	4	5	6
Feeling slowed down	0	1	2	3	4	5	6
Feeling like "in a fog"	0	1	2	3	4	5	6
"Don't feel right"	0	1	2	3	4	5	6
Difficulty concentrating	0	1	2	3	4	5	6
Difficulty remembering	0	1	2	3	4	5	6
Fatigue or low energy	0	1	2	3	4	5	6
Confusion	0	1	2	3	4	5	6
Drowsiness	0	1	2	3	4	5	6
More emotional	0	1	2	3	4	5	6
Irritability	0	1	2	3	4	5	6
Sadness	0	1	2	3	4	5	6
Nervous or Anxious	0	1	2	3	4	5	6
Trouble falling asleep (if applicable)	0	1	2	3	4	5	6

Total number of symptoms:	of 22
Symptom severity score:	of 132
Do your symptoms get worse with physical activity?	Y N
Do your symptoms get worse with mental activity?	Y N
If 100% is feeling perfectly normal, what percent of normal do you feel?	

If not 100%, why?

___

___

___

Please hand form back to examiner

3

STEP 3: COGNITIVE SCREENING

Standardised Assessment of Concussion (SAC)[4]

Name:
DOB:
Address:
ID number:
Examiner:
Date:

ORIENTATION

What month is it?	0	1
What is the date today?	0	1
What is the day of the week?	0	1
What year is it?	0	1
What time is it right now? (within 1 hour)	0	1
Orientation score		of 5

IMMEDIATE MEMORY

The Immediate Memory component can be completed using the traditional 5-word per trial list or optionally using 10-words per trial to minimise any ceiling effect. All 3 trials must be administered irrespective of the number correct on the first trial. Administer at the rate of one word per second.

Please choose EITHER the 5 or 10 word list groups and circle the specific word list chosen for this test.

I am going to test your memory. I will read you a list of words and when I am done, repeat back as many words as you can remember, in any order. For Trials 2 & 3: I am going to repeat the same list again. Repeat back as many words as you can remember in any order, even if you said the word before.

List	Alternate 5 word lists					Score (of 5) Trial 1	Trial 2	Trial 3
A	Finger	Penny	Blanket	Lemon	Insect			
B	Candle	Paper	Sugar	Sandwich	Wagon			
C	Baby	Monkey	Perfume	Sunset	Iron			
D	Elbow	Apple	Carpet	Saddle	Bubble			
E	Jacket	Arrow	Pepper	Cotton	Movie			
F	Dollar	Honey	Mirror	Saddle	Anchor			
			Immediate Memory Score					of 15
			Time that last trial was completed					

List	Alternate 10 word lists					Score (of 10) Trial 1	Trial 2	Trial 3
G	Finger Candle	Penny Paper	Blanket Sugar	Lemon Sandwich	Insect Wagon			
H	Baby Elbow	Monkey Apple	Perfume Carpet	Sunset Saddle	Iron Bubble			
I	Jacket Dollar	Arrow Honey	Pepper Mirror	Cotton Saddle	Movie Anchor			
			Immediate Memory Score					of 30
			Time that last trial was completed					

CONCENTRATION

DIGITS BACKWARDS

Please circle the Digit list chosen (A, B, C, D, E, F). Administer at the rate of one digit per second reading DOWN the selected column.

I am going to read a string of numbers and when I am done, you repeat them back to me in reverse order of how I read them to you. For example, if I say 7-1-9, you would say 9-1-7.

Concentration Number Lists (circle one)					
List A	List B	List C			
4-9-3	5-2-6	1-4-2	Y	N	0
6-2-9	4-1-5	6-5-8	Y	N	1
3-8-1-4	1-7-9-5	6-8-3-1	Y	N	0
3-2-7-9	4-9-6-8	3-4-8-1	Y	N	1
6-2-9-7-1	4-8-5-2-7	4-9-1-5-3	Y	N	0
1-5-2-8-6	6-1-8-4-3	6-8-2-5-1	Y	N	1
7-1-8-4-6-2	8-3-1-9-6-4	3-7-6-5-1-9	Y	N	0
5-3-9-1-4-8	7-2-4-8-5-6	9-2-6-5-1-4	Y	N	1
List D	List E	List F			
7-8-2	3-8-2	2-7-1	Y	N	0
9-2-6	5-1-8	4-7-9	Y	N	1
4-1-8-3	2-7-9-3	1-6-8-3	Y	N	0
9-7-2-3	2-1-6-9	3-9-2-4	Y	N	1
1-7-9-2-6	4-1-8-6-9	2-4-7-5-8	Y	N	0
4-1-7-5-2	9-4-1-7-5	8-3-9-6-4	Y	N	1
2-6-4-8-1-7	6-9-7-3-8-2	5-8-6-2-4-9	Y	N	0
8-4-1-9-3-5	4-2-7-9-3-8	3-1-7-8-2-6	Y	N	1
		Digits Score:			of 4

MONTHS IN REVERSE ORDER

Now tell me the months of the year in reverse order. Start with the last month and go backward. So you'll say December, November. Go ahead.

Dec - Nov - Oct - Sept - Aug - Jul - Jun - May - Apr - Mar - Feb - Jan	0 1
Months Score	of 1
Concentration Total Score (Digits + Months)	of 5

4

STEP 4: NEUROLOGICAL SCREEN

See the instruction sheet (page 7) for details of test administration and scoring of the tests.

Can the patient read aloud (e.g. symptom check-list) and follow instructions without difficulty?	Y	N
Does the patient have a full range of pain-free PASSIVE cervical spine movement?	Y	N
Without moving their head or neck, can the patient look side-to-side and up-and-down without double vision?	Y	N
Can the patient perform the finger nose coordination test normally?	Y	N
Can the patient perform tandem gait normally?	Y	N

BALANCE EXAMINATION

Modified Balance Error Scoring System (mBESS) testing[5]

Which foot was tested (i.e. which is the non-dominant foot) ☐ Left ☐ Right

Testing surface (hard floor, field, etc.) __________

Footwear (shoes, barefoot, braces, tape, etc.) __________

Condition	Errors
Double leg stance	of 10
Single leg stance (non-dominant foot)	of 10
Tandem stance (non-dominant foot at the back)	of 10
Total Errors	of 30

Name: __________

DOB: __________

Address: __________

ID number: __________

Examiner: __________

Date: __________

5

STEP 5: DELAYED RECALL:

The delayed recall should be performed after 5 minutes have elapsed since the end of the Immediate Recall section. Score 1 pt. for each correct response.

Do you remember that list of words I read a few times earlier? Tell me as many words from the list as you can remember in any order.

Time Started

Please record each word correctly recalled. Total score equals number of words recalled.

____

____

____

Total number of words recalled accurately: ____ or of 10

6

STEP 6: DECISION

Domain	Date & time of assessment:		
Symptom number (of 22)			
Symptom severity score (of 132)			
Orientation (of 5)			
Immediate memory	of 15 of 30	of 15 of 30	of 15 of 30
Concentration (of 5)			
Neuro exam	Normal Abnormal	Normal Abnormal	Normal Abnormal
Balance errors (of 30)			
Delayed Recall	of 5 of 10	of 5 of 10	of 5 of 10

Date and time of injury: __________

If the athlete is known to you prior to their injury, are they different from their usual self?
☐ Yes ☐ No ☐ Unsure ☐ Not Applicable
(If different, describe why in the clinical notes section)

Concussion Diagnosed?
☐ Yes ☐ No ☐ Unsure ☐ Not Applicable

If re-testing, has the athlete improved?
☐ Yes ☐ No ☐ Unsure ☐ Not Applicable

I am a physician or licensed healthcare professional and I have personally administered or supervised the administration of this SCAT5.

Signature: __________

Name: __________

Title: __________

Registration number (if applicable): __________

Date: __________

SCORING ON THE SCAT5 SHOULD NOT BE USED AS A STAND-ALONE METHOD TO DIAGNOSE CONCUSSION, MEASURE RECOVERY OR MAKE DECISIONS ABOUT AN ATHLETE'S READINESS TO RETURN TO COMPETITION AFTER CONCUSSION.

CLINICAL NOTES:

Name: ____________
DOB: ____________
Address: ____________
ID number: ____________
Examiner: ____________
Date: ____________

CONCUSSION INJURY ADVICE

(To be given to the person monitoring the concussed athlete)

This patient has received an injury to the head. A careful medical examination has been carried out and no sign of any serious complications has been found. Recovery time is variable across individuals and the patient will need monitoring for a further period by a responsible adult. Your treating physician will provide guidance as to this timeframe.

If you notice any change in behaviour, vomiting, worsening headache, double vision or excessive drowsiness, please telephone your doctor or the nearest hospital emergency department immediately.

Other important points:

Initial rest: Limit physical activity to routine daily activities (avoid exercise, training, sports) and limit activities such as school, work, and screen time to a level that does not worsen symptoms.

1) Avoid alcohol
2) Avoid prescription or non-prescription drugs without medical supervision. Specifically:
   a) Avoid sleeping tablets
   b) Do not use aspirin, anti-inflammatory medication or stronger pain medications such as narcotics
3) Do not drive until cleared by a healthcare professional.
4) Return to play/sport requires clearance by a healthcare professional.

Clinic phone number: ____________

Patient's name: ____________

Date / time of injury: ____________

Date / time of medical review: ____________

Healthcare Provider: ____________

Contact details or stamp

INSTRUCTIONS

Words in *Italics* throughout the SCAT5 are the instructions given to the athlete by the clinician

Symptom Scale

The time frame for symptoms should be based on the type of test being administered. At baseline it is advantageous to assess how an athlete "typically" feels whereas during the acute/post-acute stage it is best to ask how the athlete feels at the time of testing.

The symptom scale should be completed by the athlete, not by the examiner. In situations where the symptom scale is being completed after exercise, it should be done in a resting state, generally by approximating his/her resting heart rate.

For total number of symptoms, maximum possible is 22 except immediately post injury, if sleep item is omitted, which then creates a maximum of 21.

For Symptom severity score, add all scores in table, maximum possible is 22 x 6 = 132, except immediately post injury if sleep item is omitted, which then creates a maximum of 21x6=126.

Immediate Memory

The Immediate Memory component can be completed using the traditional 5-word per trial list or, optionally, using 10-words per trial. The literature suggests that the Immediate Memory has a notable ceiling effect when a 5-word list is used. In settings where this ceiling is prominent, the examiner may wish to make the task more difficult by incorporating two 5-word groups for a total of 10 words per trial. In this case, the maximum score per trial is 10 with a total trial maximum of 30.

Choose one of the word lists (either 5 or 10). Then perform 3 trials of immediate memory using this list.

Complete all 3 trials regardless of score on previous trials.

"I am going to test your memory. I will read you a list of words and when I am done, repeat back as many words as you can remember, in any order." The words must be read at a rate of one word per second.

Trials 2 & 3 MUST be completed regardless of score on trial 1 & 2.

Trials 2 & 3:

"I am going to repeat the same list again. Repeat back as many words as you can remember in any order, even if you said the word before."

Score 1 pt. for each correct response. Total score equals sum across all 3 trials. Do NOT inform the athlete that delayed recall will be tested.

Concentration

Digits backward

Choose one column of digits from lists A, B, C, D, E or F and administer those digits as follows:

Say: *"I am going to read a string of numbers and when I am done, you repeat them back to me in reverse order of how I read them to you. For example, if I say 7-1-9, you would say 9-1-7."*

Begin with first 3 digit string.

If correct, circle "Y" for correct and go to next string length. If incorrect, circle "N" for the first string length and read trial 2 in the same string length. One point possible for each string length. Stop after incorrect on both trials (2 N's) in a string length. The digits should be read at the rate of one per second.

Months in reverse order

"Now tell me the months of the year in reverse order. Start with the last month and go backward. So you'll say December, November ... Go ahead"

1 pt. for entire sequence correct

Delayed Recall

The delayed recall should be performed after 5 minutes have elapsed since the end of the Immediate Recall section.

"Do you remember that list of words I read a few times earlier? Tell me as many words from the list as you can remember in any order."

Score 1 pt. for each correct response

Modified Balance Error Scoring System (mBESS)[5] testing

This balance testing is based on a modified version of the Balance Error Scoring System (BESS)[5]. A timing device is required for this testing.

Each of 20-second trial/stance is scored by counting the number of errors. The examiner will begin counting errors only after the athlete has assumed the proper start position. The modified BESS is calculated by adding one error point for each error during the three 20-second tests. The maximum number of errors for any single condition is 10. If the athlete commits multiple errors simultaneously, only one error is recorded but the athlete should quickly return to the testing position, and counting should resume once the athlete is set. Athletes that are unable to maintain the testing procedure for a minimum of five seconds at the start are assigned the highest possible score, ten, for that testing condition.

OPTION: For further assessment, the same 3 stances can be performed on a surface of medium density foam (e.g., approximately 50cm x 40cm x 6cm).

Balance testing – types of errors

1. Hands lifted off iliac crest
2. Opening eyes
3. Step, stumble, or fall
4. Moving hip into > 30 degrees abduction
5. Lifting forefoot or heel
6. Remaining out of test position > 5sec

"I am now going to test your balance. Please take your shoes off (if applicable), roll up your pant legs above ankle (if applicable), and remove any ankle taping (if applicable). This test will consist of three twenty second tests with different stances."

(a) Double leg stance:

"The first stance is standing with your feet together with your hands on your hips and with your eyes closed. You should try to maintain stability in that position for 20 seconds. I will be counting the number of times you move out of this position. I will start timing when you are set and have closed your eyes."

(b) Single leg stance:

"If you were to kick a ball, which foot would you use? [This will be the dominant foot] *Now stand on your non-dominant foot. The dominant leg should be held in approximately 30 degrees of hip flexion and 45 degrees of knee flexion. Again, you should try to maintain stability for 20 seconds with your hands on your hips and your eyes closed. I will be counting the number of times you move out of this position. If you stumble out of this position, open your eyes and return to the start position and continue balancing. I will start timing when you are set and have closed your eyes."*

(c) Tandem stance:

"Now stand heel-to-toe with your non-dominant foot in back. Your weight should be evenly distributed across both feet. Again, you should try to maintain stability for 20 seconds with your hands on your hips and your eyes closed. I will be counting the number of times you move out of this position. If you stumble out of this position, open your eyes and return to the start position and continue balancing. I will start timing when you are set and have closed your eyes."

Tandem Gait

Participants are instructed to stand with their feet together behind a starting line (the test is best done with footwear removed). Then, they walk in a forward direction as quickly and as accurately as possible along a 38mm wide (sports tape), 3 metre line with an alternate foot heel-to-toe gait ensuring that they approximate their heel and toe on each step. Once they cross the end of the 3m line, they turn 180 degrees and return to the starting point using the same gait. Athletes fail the test if they step off the line, have a separation between their heel and toe, or if they touch or grab the examiner or an object.

Finger to Nose

"I am going to test your coordination now. Please sit comfortably on the chair with your eyes open and your arm (either right or left) outstretched (shoulder flexed to 90 degrees and elbow and fingers extended), pointing in front of you. When I give a start signal, I would like you to perform five successive finger to nose repetitions using your index finger to touch the tip of the nose, and then return to the starting position, as quickly and as accurately as possible."

References

1. McCrory et al. Consensus Statement On Concussion In Sport - The 5th International Conference On Concussion In Sport Held In Berlin, October 2016. British Journal of Sports Medicine 2017 (available at www.bjsm.bmj.com)
2. Maddocks, DL; Dicker, GD; Saling, MM. The assessment of orientation following concussion in athletes. Clinical Journal of Sport Medicine 1995; 5: 32-33
3. Jennett, B., Bond, M. Assessment of outcome after severe brain damage: a practical scale. Lancet 1975; i: 480-484
4. McCrea M. Standardized mental status testing of acute concussion. Clinical Journal of Sport Medicine. 2001; 11: 176-181
5. Guskiewicz KM. Assessment of postural stability following sport-related concussion. Current Sports Medicine Reports. 2003; 2: 24-30

CONCUSSION INFORMATION

Any athlete suspected of having a concussion should be removed from play and seek medical evaluation.

Signs to watch for

Problems could arise over the first 24-48 hours. The athlete should not be left alone and must go to a hospital at once if they experience:

- Worsening headache
- Drowsiness or inability to be awakened
- Inability to recognize people or places
- Repeated vomiting
- Unusual behaviour or confusion or irritable
- Seizures (arms and legs jerk uncontrollably)
- Weakness or numbness in arms or legs
- Unsteadiness on their feet.
- Slurred speech

Consult your physician or licensed healthcare professional after a suspected concussion. Remember, it is better to be safe.

Rest & Rehabilitation

After a concussion, the athlete should have physical rest and relative cognitive rest for a few days to allow their symptoms to improve. In most cases, after no more than a few days of rest, the athlete should gradually increase their daily activity level as long as their symptoms do not worsen. Once the athlete is able to complete their usual daily activities without concussion-related symptoms, the second step of the return to play/sport progression can be started. The athlete should not return to play/sport until their concussion-related symptoms have resolved and the athlete has successfully returned to full school/learning activities.

When returning to play/sport, the athlete should follow a stepwise, **medically managed exercise progression, with increasing amounts of exercise.** For example:

Graduated Return to Sport Strategy

Exercise step	Functional exercise at each step	Goal of each step
1. Symptom-limited activity	Daily activities that do not provoke symptoms.	Gradual reintroduction of work/school activities.
2. Light aerobic exercise	Walking or stationary cycling at slow to medium pace. No resistance training.	Increase heart rate.
3. Sport-specific exercise	Running or skating drills. No head impact activities.	Add movement.
4. Non-contact training drills	Harder training drills, e.g., passing drills. May start progressive resistance training.	Exercise, coordination, and increased thinking.
5. Full contact practice	Following medical clearance, participate in normal training activities.	Restore confidence and assess functional skills by coaching staff.
6. Return to play/sport	Normal game play.	

In this example, it would be typical to have 24 hours (or longer) for each step of the progression. If any symptoms worsen while exercising, the athlete should go back to the previous step. Resistance training should be added only in the later stages (Stage 3 or 4 at the earliest).

Written clearance should be provided by a healthcare professional before return to play/sport as directed by local laws and regulations.

Graduated Return to School Strategy

Concussion may affect the ability to learn at school. The athlete may need to miss a few days of school after a concussion. When going back to school, some athletes may need to go back gradually and may need to have some changes made to their schedule so that concussion symptoms do not get worse. If a particular activity makes symptoms worse, then the athlete should stop that activity and rest until symptoms get better. To make sure that the athlete can get back to school without problems, it is important that the healthcare provider, parents, caregivers and teachers talk to each other so that everyone knows what the plan is for the athlete to go back to school.

Note: If mental activity does not cause any symptoms, the athlete may be able to skip step 2 and return to school part-time before doing school activities at home first.

Mental Activity	Activity at each step	Goal of each step
1. Daily activities that do not give the athlete symptoms	Typical activities that the athlete does during the day as long as they do not increase symptoms (e.g. reading, texting, screen time). Start with 5-15 minutes at a time and gradually build up.	Gradual return to typical activities.
2. School activities	Homework, reading or other cognitive activities outside of the classroom.	Increase tolerance to cognitive work.
3. Return to school part-time	Gradual introduction of schoolwork. May need to start with a partial school day or with increased breaks during the day.	Increase academic activities.
4. Return to school full-time	Gradually progress school activities until a full day can be tolerated.	Return to full academic activities and catch up on missed work.

If the athlete continues to have symptoms with mental activity, some other accomodations that can help with return to school may include:

- Starting school later, only going for half days, or going only to certain classes
- More time to finish assignments/tests
- Quiet room to finish assignments/tests
- Not going to noisy areas like the cafeteria, assembly halls, sporting events, music class, shop class, etc.
- Taking lots of breaks during class, homework, tests
- No more than one exam/day
- Shorter assignments
- Repetition/memory cues
- Use of a student helper/tutor
- Reassurance from teachers that the child will be supported while getting better

The athlete should not go back to sports until they are back to school/learning, without symptoms getting significantly worse and no longer needing any changes to their schedule.

© Concussion in Sport Group 2017

Appendix 2

Child SCAT5©

SPORT CONCUSSION ASSESSMENT TOOL
FOR CHILDREN AGES 5 TO 12 YEARS
FOR USE BY MEDICAL PROFESSIONALS ONLY

supported by

FIFA® FEI

Patient details

Name: ______________________

DOB: ______________________

Address: ______________________

ID number: ______________________

Examiner: ______________________

Date of Injury: ______________ Time: ______________

WHAT IS THE CHILD SCAT5?

The Child SCAT5 is a standardized tool for evaluating concussions designed for use by physicians and licensed healthcare professionals[1].

If you are not a physician or licensed healthcare professional, please use the Concussion Recognition Tool 5 (CRT5). The Child SCAT5 is to be used for evaluating Children aged 5 to 12 years. For athletes aged 13 years and older, please use the SCAT5.

Preseason Child SCAT5 baseline testing can be useful for interpreting post-injury test scores, but not required for that purpose. Detailed instructions for use of the Child SCAT5 are provided on page 7. Please read through these instructions carefully before testing the athlete. Brief verbal instructions for each test are given in italics. The only equipment required for the tester is a watch or timer.

This tool may be freely copied in its current form for distribution to individuals, teams, groups and organizations. It should not be altered in any way, re-branded or sold for commercial gain. Any revision, translation or reproduction in a digital form requires specific approval by the Concussion in Sport Group.

Recognise and Remove

A head impact by either a direct blow or indirect transmission of force can be associated with a serious and potentially fatal brain injury. If there are significant concerns, including any of the red flags listed in Box 1, then activation of emergency procedures and urgent transport to the nearest hospital should be arranged.

Key points

- Any athlete with suspected concussion should be REMOVED FROM PLAY, medically assessed and monitored for deterioration. No athlete diagnosed with concussion should be returned to play on the day of injury.
- If the child is suspected of having a concussion and medical personnel are not immediately available, the child should be referred to a medical facility for urgent assessment.
- Concussion signs and symptoms evolve over time and it is important to consider repeat evaluation in the assessment of concussion.
- The diagnosis of a concussion is a clinical judgment, made by a medical professional. The Child SCAT5 should NOT be used by itself to make, or exclude, the diagnosis of concussion. An athlete may have a a concussion even if their Child SCAT5 is "normal".

Remember:

- The basic principles of first aid (danger, response, airway, breathing, circulation) should be followed.
- Do not attempt to move the athlete (other than that required for airway management) unless trained to do so.
- Assessment for a spinal cord injury is a critical part of the initial on-field assessment.
- Do not remove a helmet or any other equipment unless trained to do so safely.

1

Name: ______________________

DOB: ______________________

Address: ______________________

ID number: ______________________

Examiner: ______________________

Date: ______________________

IMMEDIATE OR ON-FIELD ASSESSMENT

The following elements should be assessed for all athletes who are suspected of having a concussion prior to proceeding to the neurocognitive assessment and ideally should be done on-field after the first first aid / emergency care priorities are completed.

If any of the "Red Flags" or observable signs are noted after a direct or indirect blow to the head, the athlete should be immediately and safely removed from participation and evaluated by a physician or licensed healthcare professional.

Consideration of transportation to a medical facility should be at the discretion of the physician or licensed healthcare professional.

The GCS is important as a standard measure for all patients and can be done serially if necessary in the event of deterioration in conscious state. The cervical spine exam is a critical step of the immediate assessment, however, it does not need to be done serially.

STEP 1: RED FLAGS

RED FLAGS:

- Neck pain or tenderness
- Double vision
- Weakness or tingling/ burning in arms or legs
- Severe or increasing headache
- Seizure or convulsion
- Loss of consciousness
- Deteriorating conscious state
- Vomiting
- Increasingly restless, agitated or combative

STEP 2: OBSERVABLE SIGNS

Witnessed ☐ Observed on Video ☐

Lying motionless on the playing surface	Y	N
Balance / gait difficulties / motor incoordination: stumbling, slow / laboured movements	Y	N
Disorientation or confusion, or an inability to respond appropriately to questions	Y	N
Blank or vacant look	Y	N
Facial injury after head trauma	Y	N

STEP 3: EXAMINATION GLASGOW COMA SCALE (GCS)[2]

Time of assessment			
Date of assessment			
Best eye response (E)			
No eye opening	1	1	1
Eye opening in response to pain	2	2	2
Eye opening to speech	3	3	3
Eyes opening spontaneously	4	4	4
Best verbal response (V)			
No verbal response	1	1	1
Incomprehensible sounds	2	2	2
Inappropriate words	3	3	3
Confused	4	4	4
Oriented	5	5	5
Best motor response (M)			
No motor response	1	1	1
Extension to pain	2	2	2
Abnormal flexion to pain	3	3	3
Flexion / Withdrawal to pain	4	4	4
Localizes to pain	5	5	5
Obeys commands	6	6	6
Glasgow Coma score (E + V + M)			

CERVICAL SPINE ASSESSMENT

Does the athlete report that their neck is pain free at rest?	Y	N
If there is NO neck pain at rest, does the athlete have a full range of ACTIVE pain free movement?	Y	N
Is the limb strength and sensation normal?	Y	N

In a patient who is not lucid or fully conscious, a cervical spine injury should be assumed until proven otherwise.

OFFICE OR OFF-FIELD ASSESSMENT
STEP 1: ATHLETE BACKGROUND

Please note that the neurocognitive assessment should be done in a distraction-free environment with the athlete in a resting state.

Sport / team / school: ______________________

Date / time of injury: ______________________

Years of education completed: ______________________

Age: ______________________

Gender: M / F / Other

Dominant hand: left / neither / right

How many diagnosed concussions has the athlete had in the past?: ______________________

When was the most recent concussion?: ______________________

How long was the recovery (time to being cleared to play) from the most recent concussion?: ______________________ (days)

Has the athlete ever been:

Hospitalized for a head injury?	Yes	No
Diagnosed / treated for headache disorder or migraines?	Yes	No
Diagnosed with a learning disability / dyslexia?	Yes	No
Diagnosed with ADD / ADHD?	Yes	No
Diagnosed with depression, anxiety or other psychiatric disorder?	Yes	No

Current medications? If yes, please list: ______________________

STEP 2: SYMPTOM EVALUATION

The athlete should be given the symptom form and asked to read this instruction paragraph out loud then complete the symptom scale. For the baseline assessment, the athlete should rate his/her symptoms based on how he/she typically feels and for the post injury assessment the athlete should rate their symptoms at this point in time.

To be done in a resting state

Please Check: ☐ **Baseline** ☐ **Post-Injury**

Name: ______
DOB: ______
Address: ______
ID number: ______
Examiner: ______
Date: ______

2

Child Report[3]

	Not at all/ Never	A little/ Rarely	Somewhat/ Sometimes	A lot/ Often
I have headaches	0	1	2	3
I feel dizzy	0	1	2	3
I feel like the room is spinning	0	1	2	3
I feel like I'm going to faint	0	1	2	3
Things are blurry when I look at them	0	1	2	3
I see double	0	1	2	3
I feel sick to my stomach	0	1	2	3
My neck hurts	0	1	2	3
I get tired a lot	0	1	2	3
I get tired easily	0	1	2	3
I have trouble paying attention	0	1	2	3
I get distracted easily	0	1	2	3
I have a hard time concentrating	0	1	2	3
I have problems remembering what people tell me	0	1	2	3
I have problems following directions	0	1	2	3
I daydream too much	0	1	2	3
I get confused	0	1	2	3
I forget things	0	1	2	3
I have problems finishing things	0	1	2	3
I have trouble figuring things out	0	1	2	3
It's hard for me to learn new things	0	1	2	3
Total number of symptoms:			of 21	
Symptom severity score:			of 63	
Do the symptoms get worse with physical activity?			Y	N
Do the symptoms get worse with trying to think?			Y	N

Overall rating for child to answer:

	Very bad										Very good
On a scale of 0 to 10 (where 10 is normal), how do you feel now?	0	1	2	3	4	5	6	7	8	9	10

If not 10, in what way do you feel different?:

Parent Report

The child:

	Not at all/ Never	A little/ Rarely	Somewhat/ Sometimes	A lot/ Often
has headaches	0	1	2	3
feels dizzy	0	1	2	3
has a feeling that the room is spinning	0	1	2	3
feels faint	0	1	2	3
has blurred vision	0	1	2	3
has double vision	0	1	2	3
experiences nausea	0	1	2	3
has a sore neck	0	1	2	3
gets tired a lot	0	1	2	3
gets tired easily	0	1	2	3
has trouble sustaining attention	0	1	2	3
is easily distracted	0	1	2	3
has difficulty concentrating	0	1	2	3
has problems remembering what he/she is told	0	1	2	3
has difficulty following directions	0	1	2	3
tends to daydream	0	1	2	3
gets confused	0	1	2	3
is forgetful	0	1	2	3
has difficulty completing tasks	0	1	2	3
has poor problem solving skills	0	1	2	3
has problems learning	0	1	2	3
Total number of symptoms:				of 21
Symptom severity score:				of 63
Do the symptoms get worse with physical activity?			Y	N
Do the symptoms get worse with mental activity?			Y	N

Overall rating for parent/teacher/coach/carer to answer

On a scale of 0 to 100% (where 100% is normal), how would you rate the child now?

If not 100%, in what way does the child seem different?

3

STEP 3: COGNITIVE SCREENING

Standardized Assessment of Concussion - Child Version (SAC-C)[4]

IMMEDIATE MEMORY

The Immediate Memory component can be completed using the traditional 5-word per trial list or optionally using 10-words per trial to minimise any ceiling effect. All 3 trials must be administered irrespective of the number correct on the first trial. Administer at the rate of one word per second.

Please choose EITHER the 5 or 10 word list groups and circle the specific word list chosen for this test.

I am going to test your memory. I will read you a list of words and when I am done, repeat back as many words as you can remember, in any order. For Trials 2 & 3: I am going to repeat the same list again. Repeat back as many words as you can remember in any order, even if you said the word before.

List	Alternate 5 word lists					Score (of 5) Trial 1	Trial 2	Trial 3
A	Finger	Penny	Blanket	Lemon	Insect			
B	Candle	Paper	Sugar	Sandwich	Wagon			
C	Baby	Monkey	Perfume	Sunset	Iron			
D	Elbow	Apple	Carpet	Saddle	Bubble			
E	Jacket	Arrow	Pepper	Cotton	Movie			
F	Dollar	Honey	Mirror	Saddle	Anchor			
				Immediate Memory Score		of 15		
				Time that last trial was completed				

List	Alternate 10 word lists					Score (of 10) Trial 1	Trial 2	Trial 3
G	Finger	Penny	Blanket	Lemon	Insect			
	Candle	Paper	Sugar	Sandwich	Wagon			
H	Baby	Monkey	Perfume	Sunset	Iron			
	Elbow	Apple	Carpet	Saddle	Bubble			
I	Jacket	Arrow	Pepper	Cotton	Movie			
	Dollar	Honey	Mirror	Saddle	Anchor			
				Immediate Memory Score		of 30		
				Time that last trial was completed				

Name: ______________________

DOB: ______________________

Address: ______________________

ID number: ______________________

Examiner: ______________________

Date: ______________________

CONCENTRATION

DIGITS BACKWARDS

Please circle the Digit list chosen (A, B, C, D, E, F). Administer at the rate of one digit per second reading DOWN the selected column.

I am going to read a string of numbers and when I am done, you repeat them back to me in reverse order of how I read them to you. For example, if I say 7-1-9, you would say 9-1-7.

Concentration Number Lists (circle one)					
List A	List B	List C			
5-2	4-1	4-9	Y	N	0
4-1	9-4	6-2	Y	N	1
4-9-3	5-2-6	1-4-2	Y	N	0
6-2-9	4-1-5	6-5-8	Y	N	1
3-8-1-4	1-7-9-5	6-8-3-1	Y	N	0
3-2-7-9	4-9-6-8	3-4-8-1	Y	N	1
6-2-9-7-1	4-8-5-2-7	4-9-1-5-3	Y	N	0
1-5-2-8-6	6-1-8-4-3	6-8-2-5-1	Y	N	1
7-1-8-4-6-2	8-3-1-9-6-4	3-7-6-5-1-9	Y	N	0
5-3-9-1-4-8	7-2-4-8-5-6	9-2-6-5-1-4	Y	N	1
List D	List E	List F			
2-7	9-2	7-8	Y	N	0
5-9	6-1	5-1	Y	N	1
7-8-2	3-8-2	2-7-1	Y	N	0
9-2-6	5-1-8	4-7-9	Y	N	1
4-1-8-3	2-7-9-3	1-6-8-3	Y	N	0
9-7-2-3	2-1-6-9-	3-9-2-4	Y	N	1
1-7-9-2-6	4-1-8-6-9	2-4-7-5-8	Y	N	0
4-1-7-5-2	9-4-1-7-5	8-3-9-6-4	Y	N	1
2-6-4-8-1-7	6-9-7-3-8-2	5-8-6-2-4-9	Y	N	0
8-4-1-9-3-5	4-2-7-3-9-8	3-1-7-8-2-6	Y	N	1
		Digits Score:			of 5

DAYS IN REVERSE ORDER

Now tell me the days of the week in reverse order. Start with the last day and go backward. So you'll say Sunday, Saturday. Go ahead.

Sunday - Saturday - Friday - Thursday - Wednesday - Tuesday - Monday	0 1
Days Score	of 1
Concentration Total Score (Digits + Days)	of 6

4

STEP 4: NEUROLOGICAL SCREEN

See the instruction sheet (page 7) for details of test administration and scoring of the tests.

Can the patient read aloud (e.g. symptom check-list) and follow instructions without difficulty?	Y	N
Does the patient have a full range of pain-free PASSIVE cervical spine movement?	Y	N
Without moving their head or neck, can the patient look side-to-side and up-and-down without double vision?	Y	N
Can the patient perform the finger nose coordination test normally?	Y	N
Can the patient perform tandem gait normally?	Y	N

BALANCE EXAMINATION

Modified Balance Error Scoring System (BESS) testing[5]

Which foot was tested (i.e. which is the non-dominant foot) ☐ Left ☐ Right

Testing surface (hard floor, field, etc.) ____________

Footwear (shoes, barefoot, braces, tape, etc.) ____________

Condition	Errors	
Double leg stance	of 10	
Single leg stance (non-dominant foot, 10-12 y/o only)	of 10	
Tandem stance (non-dominant foot at back)	of 10	
Total Errors	5-9 y/o of 20	10-12 y/o of 30

Name: ____________

DOB: ____________

Address: ____________

ID number: ____________

Examiner: ____________

Date: ____________

5

STEP 5: DELAYED RECALL:

The delayed recall should be performed after 5 minutes have elapsed since the end of the Immediate Recall section. Score 1 pt. for each correct response.

Do you remember that list of words I read a few times earlier? Tell me as many words from the list as you can remember in any order.

Time Started ____

Please record each word correctly recalled. Total score equals number of words recalled.

____

____

____

Total number of words recalled accurately: ____ or ____ of 10

6

STEP 6: DECISION

Domain	Date & time of assessment:		
Symptom number Child report (of 21) Parent report (of 21)			
Symptom severity score Child report (of 63) Parent report (of 63)			
Immediate memory	of 15 of 30	of 15 of 30	of 15 of 30
Concentration (of 6)			
Neuro exam	Normal Abnormal	Normal Abnormal	Normal Abnormal
Balance errors (5-9 y/o of 20) (10-12 y/o of 30)			
Delayed Recall	of 5 of 10	of 5 of 10	of 5 of 10

Date and time of injury: ____________

If the athlete is known to you prior to their injury, are they different from their usual self?

☐ **Yes** ☐ **No** ☐ **Unsure** ☐ **Not Applicable**

(If different, describe why in the clinical notes section)

Concussion Diagnosed?

☐ **Yes** ☐ **No** ☐ **Unsure** ☐ **Not Applicable**

If re-testing, has the athlete improved?

☐ **Yes** ☐ **No** ☐ **Unsure** ☐ **Not Applicable**

I am a physician or licensed healthcare professional and I have personally administered or supervised the administration of this Child SCAT5.

Signature: ____________

Name: ____________

Title: ____________

Registration number (if applicable): ____________

Date: ____________

SCORING ON THE CHILD SCAT5 SHOULD NOT BE USED AS A STAND-ALONE METHOD TO DIAGNOSE CONCUSSION, MEASURE RECOVERY OR MAKE DECISIONS ABOUT AN ATHLETE'S READINESS TO RETURN TO COMPETITION AFTER CONCUSSION.

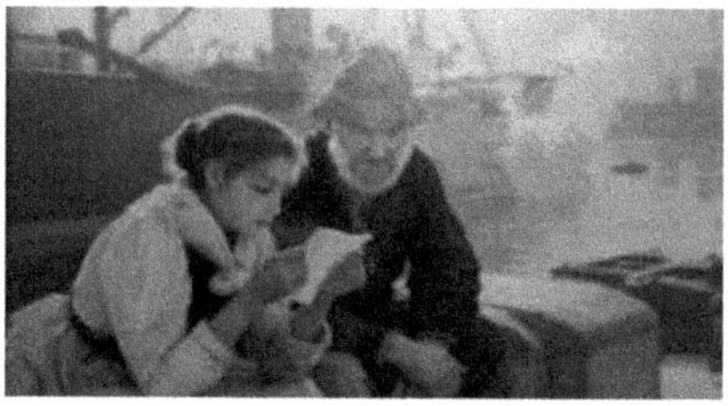

For the Neurological Screen (page 5), if the child cannot read, ask him/her to describe what they see in this picture.

Name:__________

DOB:__________

Address:__________

ID number:__________

Examiner:__________

Date:__________

CLINICAL NOTES:

Concussion injury advice for the child and parents/carergivers

(To be given to the person monitoring the concussed child)

This child has had an injury to the head and needs to be carefully watched for the next 24 hours by a responsible adult.

If you notice any change in behavior, vomiting, dizziness, worsening headache, double vision or excessive drowsiness, please call an ambulance to take the child to hospital immediately.

Other important points:

Following concussion, the child should rest for at least 24 hours.

- The child should not use a computer, internet or play video games if these activities make symptoms worse.
- The child should not be given any medications, including pain killers, unless prescribed by a medical doctor.
- The child should not go back to school until symptoms are improving.
- The child should not go back to sport or play until a doctor gives permission.

Clinic phone number:__________

Patient's name:__________

Date / time of injury:__________

Date / time of medical review:__________

Healthcare Provider:__________

Contact details or stamp

INSTRUCTIONS

Words in *Italics* throughout the Child SCAT5 are the instructions given to the athlete by the clinician

Symptom Scale

In situations where the symptom scale is being completed after exercise, it should still be done in a resting state, at least 10 minutes post exercise.

At Baseline	On the day of injury	On all subsequent days
• The child is to complete the Child Report, according to how he/ she feels today, and • The parent/carer is to complete the Parent Report according to how the child has been over the previous week.	• The child is to complete the Child Report, according to how he/ she feels now. • If the parent is present, and has had time to assess the child on the day of injury, the parent completes the Parent Report according to how the child appears now.	• The child is to complete the Child Report, according to how he/ she feels today, and • The parent/carer is to complete the Parent Report according to how the child has been over the previous 24 hours.

For Total number of symptoms, maximum possible is 21

For Symptom severity score, add all scores in table, maximum possible is 21 x 3 = 63

Standardized Assessment of Concussion Child Version (SAC-C)

Immediate Memory

Choose one of the 5-word lists. Then perform 3 trials of immediate memory using this list.

Complete all 3 trials regardless of score on previous trials.

"I am going to test your memory. I will read you a list of words and when I am done, repeat back as many words as you can remember, in any order." The words must be read at a rate of one word per second.

OPTION: The literature suggests that the Immediate Memory has a notable ceiling effect when a 5-word list is used. (In younger children, use the 5-word list). In settings where this ceiling is prominent the examiner may wish to make the task more difficult by incorporating two 5-word groups for a total of 10 words per trial. In this case the maximum score per trial is 10 with a total trial maximum of 30.

Trials 2 & 3 MUST be completed regardless of score on trial 1 & 2.

Trials 2 & 3: *"I am going to repeat the same list again. Repeat back as many words as you can remember in any order, even if you said the word before."*

Score 1 pt. for each correct response. Total score equals sum across all 3 trials. Do NOT inform the athlete that delayed recall will be tested.

Concentration

Digits backward

Choose one column only, from List A, B, C, D, E or F, and administer those digits as follows:

"I am going to read you some numbers and when I am done, you say them back to me backwards, in reverse order of how I read them to you. For example, if I say 7-1, you would say 1-7."

If correct, circle "Y" for correct and go to next string length. If incorrect, circle "N" for the first string length and read trial 2 in the same string length. One point possible for each string length. Stop after incorrect on both trials (2 N's) in a string length. The digits should be read at the rate of one per second.

Days of the week in reverse order

"Now tell me the days of the week in reverse order. Start with Sunday and go backward. So you'll say Sunday, Saturday ... Go ahead"

1 pt. for entire sequence correct

Delayed Recall

The delayed recall should be performed after at least 5 minutes have elapsed since the end of the Immediate Recall section.

"Do you remember that list of words I read a few times earlier? Tell me as many words from the list as you can remember in any order."

Circle each word correctly recalled. Total score equals number of words recalled.

Neurological Screen

Reading

The child is asked to read a paragraph of text from the instructions in the Child SCAT5. For children who can not read, they are asked to describe what they see in a photograph or picture, such as that on page 6 of the Child SCAT5.

Modified Balance Error Scoring System (mBESS)[5] testing

These instructions are to be read by the person administering the Child SCAT5, and each balance task should be demonstrated to the child. The child should then be asked to copy what the examiner demonstrated.

Each of 20-second trial/stance is scored by counting the number of errors. The This balance testing is based on a modified version of the Balance Error Scoring System (BESS)[5].

A stopwatch or watch with a second hand is required for this testing.

"I am now going to test your balance. Please take your shoes off, roll up your pants above your ankle (if applicable), and remove any ankle taping (if applicable). This test will consist of two different parts."

OPTION: For further assessment, the same 3 stances can be performed on a surface of medium density foam (e.g., approximately 50cm x 40cm x 6cm).

(a) Double leg stance:

The first stance is standing with the feet together with hands on hips and with eyes closed. The child should try to maintain stability in that position for 20 seconds. You should inform the child that you will be counting the number of times the child moves out of this position. You should start timing when the child is set and the eyes are closed.

(b) Tandem stance:

Instruct or show the child how to stand heel-to-toe with the non-dominant foot in the back. Weight should be evenly distributed across both feet. Again, the child should try to maintain stability for 20 seconds with hands on hips and eyes closed. You should inform the child that you will be counting the number of times the child moves out of this position. If the child stumbles out of this position, instruct him/her to open the eyes and return to the start position and continue balancing. You should start timing when the child is set and the eyes are closed.

(c) Single leg stance (10-12 year olds only):

"If you were to kick a ball, which foot would you use? [This will be the dominant foot] *Now stand on your other foot. You should bend your other leg and hold it up (show the child). Again, try to stay in that position for 20 seconds with your hands on your hips and your eyes closed. I will be counting the number of times you move out of this position. If you move out of this position, open your eyes and return to the start position and keep balancing. I will start timing when you are set and have closed your eyes."*

Balance testing – types of errors

1. Hands lifted off iliac crest
2. Opening eyes
3. Step, stumble, or fall
4. Moving hip into >30 degrees abduction
5. Lifting forefoot or heel
6. Remaining out of test position > 5 sec

Each of the 20-second trials is scored by counting the errors, or deviations from the proper stance, accumulated by the child. The examiner will begin counting errors only after the child has assumed the proper start position. The modified BESS is calculated by adding one error point for each error during the 20-second tests. The maximum total number of errors for any single condition is 10. If a child commits multiple errors simultaneously, only one error is recorded but the child should quickly return to the testing position, and counting should resume once subject is set. Children who are unable to maintain the testing procedure for a minimum of five seconds at the start are assigned the highest possible score, ten, for that testing condition.

Tandem Gait

Instruction for the examiner - Demonstrate the following to the child:

The child is instructed to stand with their feet together behind a starting line (the test is best done with footwear removed). Then, they walk in a forward direction as quickly and as accurately as possible along a 38mm wide (sports tape), 3 metre line with an alternate foot heel-to-toe gait ensuring that they approximate their heel and toe on each step. Once they cross the end of the 3m line, they turn 180 degrees and return to the starting point using the same gait. Children fail the test if they step off the line, have a separation between their heel and toe, or if they touch or grab the examiner or an object.

Finger to Nose

The tester should demonstrate it to the child.

"I am going to test your coordination now. Please sit comfortably on the chair with your eyes open and your arm (either right or left) outstretched (shoulder flexed to 90 degrees and elbow and fingers extended). When I give a start signal, I would like you to perform five successive finger to nose repetitions using your index finger to touch the tip of the nose as quickly and as accurately as possible."

Scoring: 5 correct repetitions in < 4 seconds = 1

Note for testers: Children fail the test if they do not touch their nose, do not fully extend their elbow or do not perform five repetitions.

References

1. McCrory et al. Consensus Statement On Concussion In Sport – The 5th International Conference On Concussion In Sport Held In Berlin, October 2016. British Journal of Sports Medicine 2017 (available at www.bjsm.bmj.com)
2. Jennett, B., Bond, M. Assessment of outcome after severe brain damage: a practical scale. Lancet 1975; i: 480-484
3. Ayr, L.K., Yeates, K.O., Taylor, H.G., Brown, M. Dimensions of postconcussive symptoms in children with mild traumatic brain injuries. Journal of the International Neuropsychological Society. 2009; 15:19–30
4. McCrea M. Standardized mental status testing of acute concussion. Clinical Journal of Sports Medicine. 2001; 11: 176-181
5. Guskiewicz KM. Assessment of postural stability following sport-related concussion. Current Sports Medicine Reports. 2003; 2: 24-30

CONCUSSION INFORMATION

If you think you or a teammate has a concussion, tell your coach/trainer/ parent right away so that you can be taken out of the game. You or your teammate should be seen by a doctor as soon as possible. YOU OR YOUR TEAMMATE SHOULD NOT GO BACK TO PLAY/SPORT THAT DAY.

Signs to watch for

Problems can happen over the first 24-48 hours. You or your teammate should not be left alone and must go to a hospital right away if any of the following happens:

- New headache, or headache gets worse
- Neck pain that gets worse
- Becomes sleepy/ drowsy or can't be woken up
- Cannot recognise people or places
- Feeling sick to your stomach or vomiting
- Acting weird/strange, seems/feels confused, or is irritable
- Has any seizures (arms and/or legs jerk uncontrollably)
- Has weakness, numbness or tingling (arms, legs or face)
- Is unsteady walking or standing
- Talking is slurred
- Cannot understand what someone is saying or directions

Consult your physician or licensed healthcare professional after a suspected concussion. Remember, it is better to be safe.

Graduated Return to Sport Strategy

After a concussion, the child should rest physically and mentally for a few days to allow symptoms to get better. In most cases, after a few days of rest, they can gradually increase their daily activity level as long as symptoms don't get worse. Once they are able to do their usual daily activities without symptoms, the child should gradually increase exercise in steps, guided by the healthcare professional (see below).

The athlete should not return to play/sport the day of injury.

NOTE: An initial period of a few days of both cognitive ("thinking") and physical rest is recommended before beginning the Return to Sport progression.

Exercise step	Functional exercise at each step	Goal of each step
1. Symptom-limited activity	Daily activities that do not provoke symptoms.	Gradual reintroduction of work/school activities.
2. Light aerobic exercise	Walking or stationary cycling at slow to medium pace. No resistance training.	Increase heart rate.
3. Sport-specific exercise	Running or skating drills. No head impact activities.	Add movement.
4. Non-contact training drills	Harder training drills, e.g., passing drills. May start progressive resistance training.	Exercise, coordination, and increased thinking.
5. Full contact practice	Following medical clearance, participate in normal training activities.	Restore confidence and assess functional skills by coaching staff.
6. Return to play/sport	Normal game play.	

There should be at least 24 hours (or longer) for each step of the progression. If any symptoms worsen while exercising, the athlete should go back to the previous step. Resistance training should be added only in the later stages (Stage 3 or 4 at the earliest). The athlete should not return to sport until the concussion symptoms have gone, they have successfully returned to full school/learning activities, and the healthcare professional has given the child written permission to return to sport.

If the child has symptoms for more than a month, they should ask to be referred to a healthcare professional who is an expert in the management of concussion.

Graduated Return to School Strategy

Concussion may affect the ability to learn at school. The child may need to miss a few days of school after a concussion, but the child's doctor should help them get back to school after a few days. When going back to school, some children may need to go back gradually and may need to have some changes made to their schedule so that concussion symptoms don't get a lot worse. If a particular activity makes symptoms a lot worse, then the child should stop that activity and rest until symptoms get better. To make sure that the child can get back to school without problems, it is important that the health care provider, parents/caregivers and teachers talk to each other so that everyone knows what the plan is for the child to go back to school.

Note: If mental activity does not cause any symptoms, the child may be able to return to school part-time without doing school activities at home first.

Mental Activity	Activity at each step	Goal of each step
1. Daily activities that do not give the child symptoms	Typical activities that the child does during the day as long as they do not increase symptoms (e.g. reading, texting, screen time). Start with 5-15 minutes at a time and gradually build up.	Gradual return to typical activities.
2. School activities	Homework, reading or other cognitive activities outside of the classroom.	Increase tolerance to cognitive work.
3. Return to school part-time	Gradual introduction of schoolwork. May need to start with a partial school day or with increased breaks during the day.	Increase academic activities.
4. Return to school full-time	Gradually progress school activities until a full day can be tolerated.	Return to full academic activities and catch up on missed work.

If the child continues to have symptoms with mental activity, some other things that can be done to help with return to school may include:

- Starting school later, only going for half days, or going only to certain classes
- More time to finish assignments/tests
- Quiet room to finish assignments/tests
- Not going to noisy areas like the cafeteria, assembly halls, sporting events, music class, shop class, etc.
- Taking lots of breaks during class, homework, tests
- No more than one exam/day
- Shorter assignments
- Repetition/memory cues
- Use of a student helper/tutor
- Reassurance from teachers that the child will be supported while getting better

The child should not go back to sports until they are back to school/ learning, without symptoms getting significantly worse and no longer needing any changes to their schedule.

References

1. McCrory P, Meeuwisse W, Duorak J, Aubry M, et al. Consensus statement on concussion in sport—the 5th international conference on concussion in sport held in Berlin, October 2016. Br J Sports Med. 2017;51:838–47. https://doi.org/10.1136/bjsports-2017-097699.
2. Bryan MA, Rowhani-Rahbar A, Comstock RD, et al. Sports-and recreation-related concussions in U.S. youth. Pediatrics. 2016;138(1):e20154635.
3. Hoofman JM, Dick R, Agel J. Epidemiology of collegiate injuries for 15 sports: summary and recommendations for injury prevention initiatives. J Athl Train. 2007;42:311–9.
4. Lincoln AE, Hinton RX, Almquist JL, et al. Head, face, and eye injuries in scholastic and collegiate lacrosse: a 4-year prospective study. Am J Sports Med. 2007;35:207–15.
5. Lincoln AE, Caswell SV, Almquist JL, Dunn RE, Norris JB, Hinton RY. Trends in concussion incidence in high school sports: a prospective 11-year study. Am J Sports Med. 2011;39(5):958–63.
6. Harmon KG, Drezner J, Gammons M, Guskiewicz K, et al. American medical society for sports medicine position statement: concussion in sport. Clin J Sport Med. 2013;23:1–18.
7. Langlios JA, Rutland-Brown W, Wald MM. The epidemiology and impact of traumatic brain injury: a brief overview. J Head Trauma Rehabil. 2006;21:375–8.
8. Bompadre V, Jinguji T, Yanez N, et al. Washington State's Lystedt law in concussion documentation in Seattle public high schools. J Athl Train. 2014;49(4):486–92.
9. Gessel L, Fields S, Collins C, et al. Concussions among U.S. high school and college athletes. J Ath Train. 2007;42(4):495–503.
10. Powell J, Barber-Foss KD. Traumatic brain injury in high school athletes. JAMA. 1999;282(10):58–63.
11. Barkhoudarian G, Hovda DA, Giza CC. The molecular pathophysiology of concussive brain injury. Clin Sports Med. 2011;30:33–48, vii–iii.
12. Prins ML, Hales A, Reger M, et al. Repeat traumatic brain injury in the juvenile rat is associated with increased axonal injury and cognitive impairments. Dev Neurosci. 2010;32:510–8.
13. Shrey DW, Griesbach GS, cc G. The pathophysiology of concussion in youth. Phys Med Rehabil Clin N Am. 2011;22:577–602, vii.
14. McCrory P, Meeuwisse W, Johnson K, et al. Consensus statement on concussion in sport. 3rd international conference on concussion in sport held in Zurich. November 2008. Br J Sports Med. 2009;43(suppl 1):i76–90.
15. Vagnozzi R, Tavazzi B, Signoretti S, et al. Temporal window of metabolic brain vulnerability to concussion: mitochondrial-related impairment—part i. Neurosurgery. 2007;61:379–88; discussion 388.
16. Esposito G, VanHorn JD, Weinberger DR, et al. Gender differences in cerebral blood flow as a function of cognitive state with pet. J Nucl Med. 1996;37:559–64.
17. Loughi L, Saatman KE, Fujimoto S, et al. Temporal window of vulnerability to repetitive experimental concussive brain injury. Neurosurgery. 2005;56:364–74; discussion 374.
18. Tavazzi B, Vagnozzi R, Signoretti S, et al. Temporal window of metabolic brain vulnerability to concussions: oxidative and nitrosative stresses—part ii. Neurosurgery. 2007;61:390–5; discussion 395–396.
19. Vagnozzi R, Signoretti S, Tavazzi B, et al. Temporal window of metabolic brain vulnerability to concussion: a pilot (1h-magnetic resonance spectroscopic study in concussed patients—part iii). Neurosurgery. 2008;62:1286–95; discussion 1295–1286.
20. Vagnozzi R, Signoretti S, Cristofori L, et al. Assessment of metabolic brain damage and recovery following mild traumatic brain injury: a multicentre, proton magnetic resonance spectroscopic study in concussed patients. Brain. 2010;133:3232–42.
21. Guskiewicz K, Waver N, Padua D, et al. Epidemiology of concussion in collegiate and high school football players. Am J Sports Med. 2000;28(5):643–50.
22. Meehan W, d'Hemecourt P, Comstock D, et al. High school concussions in the 2008–2009 academic year: mechanism, symptoms and management. Am J Sports Med. 2010;38(12):2405–9.

23. Herring SA, Cantu RC, Guskiewicz K, Putunkian M, Kibler WB, et al. Concussion (mild traumatic brain injury) and the team physician: a consensus statement—2011 update. Med Sci Sports Exerc. 2011;43(12):2412–22.
24. Echemendia RJ, Meeuwisse W, McCrory P, et al. The sport concussion assessment tool 5th edition (SCAT5). Br J Sports Med. 2017;51:848–50. https://doi.org/10.1136/bjsports-2017-097506.
25. Patricios J, Makdissi M. Fifth shades of grey: concussion complexities and constructive conclusions. Br J Sports Med. 2015;49(8):492–3. https://doi.org/10.1136/bjsports-2014-094284.
26. Coppel D. Use of neuropsychological evaluation. Phys Med Rehabil Clin N Am. 2011;22:653–64.
27. Iverson G. Evidence-based neuropsychological assessment in sport-related concussion. In: Webbe F, editor. The handbook of sport neuropsychology; 2011. p. 131–54.
28. McCrea M, Powell M. The concussion clinic: a practical, evidence-based model for assessment and management of sport-related concussion. J Clin Sport Psychol. 2012;6:275–92.
29. Resch J, McCrea M, Cullum C. Computerized neurocognitive testing in the management of sport-related concussion: an update. Neuropsychol Rev. 2013;23(4):335–49.
30. Thomas D, Apps J, Hoffman R, McCrea M, Hammeke T. Benefits of strict rest after acute concussion: a randomized controlled trial. Pediatrics. 2015;135(2):213–23.
31. Halstead M, McAvoy K, Devore C, Carl R, Lee M, Logan K. Return to learning after concussion. Pediatrics. 2013;132(5):948–57.
32. Concannon L. Effects of legislation on sports-related concussion. Phys Med Rehabil Clin N Am. 2016;27(2):513–27.
33. Silverberg N, Iverson G. Etiology of the post-concussion syndrome: physiogenesis and psychogenesis revisited. NeuroRehabilitation. 2011;29:317–29.
34. Cantu R, Green A. Second-impact syndrome and a small subdural hematoma: an uncommon catastrophic result of repetitive head injury with characteristic imaging appearance. J Neurotrauma. 2010;27(9):1557–64.
35. Kors E, Terwindt G, Vermeulen F, et al. Delayed cerebral edema and fatal coma after minor trauma: the role of the CACNA1C calcium channel subunit gene and relationship with familial hemiplegic migraine. Ann Neurol. 2001;49:753–60.
36. McCrory P. Does second impact syndrome exist? Clin J Sport Med. 2001;11:144–9.
37. McCrory P, Davis G, Makdissi M. Second impact syndrome or cerebral swelling after sporting head injury. Curr Sports Med Rep. 2012;11:21–3.
38. Iverson G, Gioia G. Returning to school following sport-related concussion. Phys Med Rehabil Clin N Am. 2016;27(2):429–36.
39. Committee on Sports-Related Concussions in Youth. Institute of Medicine National Research Council. Sports-related concussions in youth: improving the science, changing the culture. Washington DC: National Academies Press; 2013.
40. Meehan W, Mannix R, Zafone R, Pascual-Leone A. Chronic traumatic encephalopathy and athletes. Neurology. 2015;85:1–8.
41. Chrisman S, Schiff M, Chung S, Herring S, Rivara F. Implementation of concussion legislation and extent of concussion education for athletes, parents and coaches in Washington state. Am J Sports Med. 2014;42(5):1190–6.
42. Emery C, Kang J, Shrier I, Goulet C, et al. Risk of injury associated with body checking experience among youth hockey players. CMAJ. 2011;183(11):1249.
43. Kerr Z, Yeargin S, Valovich-McLeod T, Nittoli V, et al. Comprehensive coach education and practice contact restriction guidelines result in lower injury rates in youth American football. Orthop J Sports Med. 2015;3(7):1.

Chapter 21
Neurosurgery for Meningiomas

Michael W. Parsons, Paramita Das, and Pablo Recinos

Introduction

Meningiomas are the most common primary brain tumor in adults, accounting for 37% of all such masses, with an annual incidence of about 27,000 new cases currently [1]. The vast majority of these tumors (>80%) are classified as Grade I tumors, meaning that they do not infiltrate brain tissue or metastasize and are considered "mostly benign" [2]. However, these tumors can produce a variety of neurologic symptoms, including seizures and focal neurologic signs that relate to the brain regions most proximal to the tumor [3]. Cognitive symptoms are not uncommon in this population [4, 5]. The decision to resect meningiomas depends on many factors, including tumor location, rate of growth, size, and the patient's surgical risk factors. Neurologic and/or cognitive symptoms caused by the tumor are important factors in surgical decision-making. It is not uncommon that these symptoms are subtle and difficult to assess in a basic neurosurgical physical examination, or Mini-Mental State Examination may not be sensitive to the relevant symptoms [6]. Neuropsychological evaluation can be a helpful adjunct for neurosurgeons in their preoperative decision-making as well as postoperative evaluation to determine postoperatively whether resection of the tumor resolved the patient's symptoms. In this chapter, we present three cases with varying clinical presentations that illustrate the collaborative role of neuropsychology and neurosurgery in the care of these patients.

Case 1: Grade I Meningioma in the Context of Medical Comorbidities
Ms. A is a 73-year-old, right-handed female who presented to the neurosurgeon to consult for imaging findings. Relevant background factors include the fact that she

M. W. Parsons (✉)
Massachusetts General Hospital, Boston, Massachusetts, USA
e-mail: mwparsons@mgh.harvard.edu

P. Das · P. Recinos
Cleveland Clinic, Cleveland, Ohio, USA

K. M. Sanders (ed.), *Physician's Field Guide to Neuropsychology*,
https://doi.org/10.1007/978-1-4939-8722-1_21

had a medical history significant for left vertebral artery occlusion in the remote past, hypertension, hyperlipidemia, osteopenia, and kidney stones. She had completed high school education and had worked in a variety of clerical jobs before she retired several years ago. She was single, living alone, and had some support from a friend who accompanied her to the appointment. At the time of her initial presentation to the brain tumor service, her primary care doctor had recently retired and her care was transferred to a new primary care physician (PCP). As a part of her transition, her new PCP inquired about a report in her medical history of a vertebral artery occlusion, which the patient did not remember having. She was referred to a neurologist to evaluate this history, and during this workup an MRI was obtained that showed a 2.8 × 2.1 × 3.7 cm medial right temporal mass arising from the medial aspect of the greater wing of the sphenoid (Fig. 21.1).

Neuropsychological Evaluations

Evaluation 1: The patient was initially seen for a brief neuropsychological evaluation. Despite the fact that she herself was denying any cognitive symptoms, several worrisome details emerged during the neuropsychological interview. For instance, she reported the time that she had decided to stop taking her antihypertensive

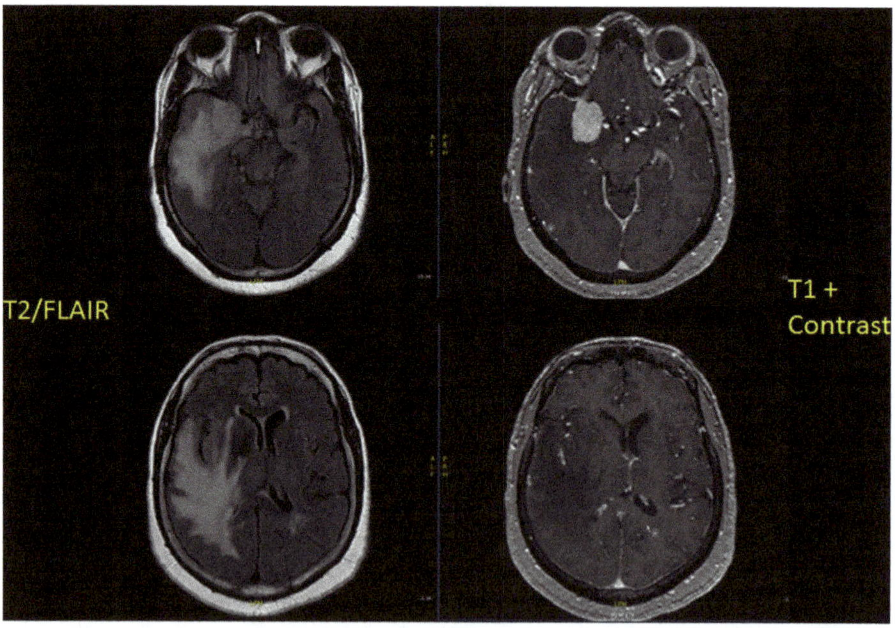

Fig. 21.1 Brain MRI at the time of presentation for Ms. A (Case 1). Note the contrast-enhancing mass lesion arising from the dural surface and impinging on the right medial temporal lobe. Fluid-attenuated inversion recovery (FLAIR) sequences show extensive edema extending into the right temporal and frontal lobes as well as subcortical areas

medications because she "did not trust them." Further discussion revealed that she was uncertain about what medications she should be taking. She stated that she believed she was fine without these medications because she had lived with hypertension since age 17 and "never had any problems." When tested in the clinic, her BP was found to be 192/116 mmHg. Hospital admission was recommended but she declined.

The initial brief neuropsychological evaluation demonstrated reductions from her expected baseline level of function on tests of visuospatial abilities and retrieval-based memory that were felt to be consistent with nondominant hemisphere dysfunction secondary to the right temporal mass/edema. We suspected that Ms. A's confusion could be attributed to the significant edema noted on neuroimaging, and we strongly encouraged her to adhere to her medication regimen to better assist with treatment planning.

Evaluation 2: The patient was stabilized on her medication, and the brain mass was followed with serial imaging for 1 year. The mass lesion appeared essentially unchanged, and she had persistent widespread edema throughout the right temporal and frontal lobes and subcortical structures. A repeat brief neuropsychological examination was conducted. At that time, she continued to live independently and denied any difficulties with activities of daily living. She was compliant with medications, and her blood pressure readings were normal (132/89 mmHg). Re-evaluation showed slight improvements in verbal memory retention and visuospatial abilities but continued demonstrating retrieval-based memory problems with mildly impaired visuospatial memory. The second battery was more extensive and demonstrated impairments in aspects of executive functioning, such as impaired problem solving and evidence of perseveration. Her improved performance was felt to reflect her medication adherence and relatively controlled hypertension. Nonetheless, there were residual cognitive impairments consistent with the right temporal mass and the surrounding edema.

Neurosurgeon's Perspective

Meningioma was the highest on the differential diagnoses when the patient presented to the clinic. This is due to its homogenous contrast enhancement and the fact that it appeared to be an extra-axial lesion. However, we discussed the potential of other pathologies, which could present this way. These included metastatic disease, lymphoma, malignant meningioma, or hemangiopericytoma. Some of these diagnoses require more urgent intervention. Surgery was discussed as a way to remove the mass causing the edema and for diagnosis. With her memory problems, she was also unable to fully adhere to her home medication schedule, and these issues would have to be addressed prior to surgery. Poorly controlled perioperative hypertension is a risk factor for intracranial hemorrhage after craniotomy [7]. We discussed observation, radiation therapy, or surgery with the patient and decided on a short 1–2-month course of observation, while management of her medical problems was optimized and neuropsychological evaluation was completed. The goal of the neuropsychological evaluation was to educate the patient appropriately on cognitive expectations after resection. The risks of the surgery were discussed with the patient, including subtotal resection, stroke (due to the proximity of the tumor to the middle cerebral artery), infection, or lack of improvement in cognitive symptoms. Neuropsychological assessment was also important to ensure that she had the capacity to understand these risks and make an informed decision about the surgery.

Ultimately, the patient underwent a right pterional craniotomy with orbitotomy for resection of the tumor. It was found to involve the dura of the cavernous sinus and was adherent to the internal carotid artery and middle cerebral artery. Simpson grade refers to the extent of resection, and for this patient it conferred that the intradural tumor was removed; however, the dural attachment was unable to be coagulated or resected. Her pathology returned as WHO Grade I meningioma, and she was followed closely with imaging to evaluate for recurrence. The neuropsychological evaluation played an important role in ensuring that she had adequate support to comply with medication schedules and improve control of her hypertension.

Neuropsychologist's Perspective

This case illustrates several of the typical features of meningioma. Specifically, it was discovered incidentally, was felt to be asymptomatic by the patient, and found to be producing cognitive symptoms upon evaluation. The neuropsychologist in this case played a role in understanding the potential for a relationship between cognitive and behavioral features related to the lesion and her overall health. Specifically, the extensive right hemisphere edema seen in this patient resulted in deficits on visuospatial function and executive function tests. These cognitive features were initially exacerbated by possible hypertensive encephalopathy, which appeared to have resolved by the time she presented for re-evaluation. Furthermore, the right hemisphere lesion may have been contributing to symptoms of reduced insight and judgment, including elements of anosognosia [8]. These features are commonly associated with right hemisphere lesions but may not be familiar to medical colleagues in the multidisciplinary neuro-oncology team. It is important for the neuropsychologist to point out the subtle ways in which idiosyncratic features of the patient's presentation may in fact be symptoms of the meningioma.

Key Point

The neuropsychologist's role in evaluating brain tumor patients includes not only measuring cognitive function or dysfunction but also assessing behavior, mood, and psychosocial issues that may be related to brain tumor surgery and outcome.

Part 2: Grade II and III Meningiomas

Although the majority of meningiomas are considered mostly benign, a significant minority of these tumors have more aggressive characteristics, with 15–20% being given a Grade II (atypical) designation and 1–2% a Grade III (malignant) diagnosis [2]. The classification as Grade II or III reflects a number of histopathological features that correlate with a more aggressive behavior and greater likelihood of brain invasion. A complete discussion of the diagnostic criteria is beyond the scope of this chapter, and the reader is referred to the neuropathological reference texts for more details [2]. For the purposes of discussion, it is necessary to understand that meningioma grade is an important predictor of the risk for tumor recurrence and correlates with a higher risk for neurologic symptoms and premature death. Even with gross total resection, Grade II meningiomas have a 5-year recurrence rate of 50% and Grade III tumors have a 5-year recurrence rate closer to 70–80% [3].

Because of their more aggressive growth characteristics, surgery is necessary for higher-grade meningiomas and is the cornerstone of treatment. Radiation therapy is considered standard of care treatment after resection for these meningiomas, though debate regarding the specific timing and method of delivery of treatment continues and there is little in the way of formal outcome data [9]. Chemotherapy agents are not routinely considered standard of care, though in recent years, the discovery of specific mutations has increased enthusiasm for the possibility of targeted therapies [10, 11]. Furthermore, Grade II and III meningiomas are more likely to induce extensive edema in the surrounding parenchyma than Grade I tumors [12], which may increase the likelihood of neurologic and cognitive symptoms.

Case 2: Atypical Meningioma of the Orbital Groove

Mr. B is a 52-year-old, right-handed, working attorney who had experienced some sporadic episodes of forgetfulness over the past 6 months, which led to a neurologic evaluation. His family reported that he lost his sense of smell and taste 2 years prior. He had also become increasingly irritable, lost interest in his usual activities, and had other personality changes. Brain imaging revealed a contrast-enhancing mass lesion arising from the cribriform plate, measuring about 3 × 4 × 5 cm, with substantial mass effect and edema in the frontal lobes bilaterally (see Fig. 21.2). The patient explained that there had been a couple of incidents of forgetting over the past 6 months that had raised concern. Even with reminders, he had only vague recollection. Other than these specific episodes, the patient reported that he had not noticed much in the way of significant cognitive change. The evaluation showed very subtle cognitive influence of tumor and edema on memory encoding and verbal fluency. Recommendations were for cognitive follow-up postoperatively.

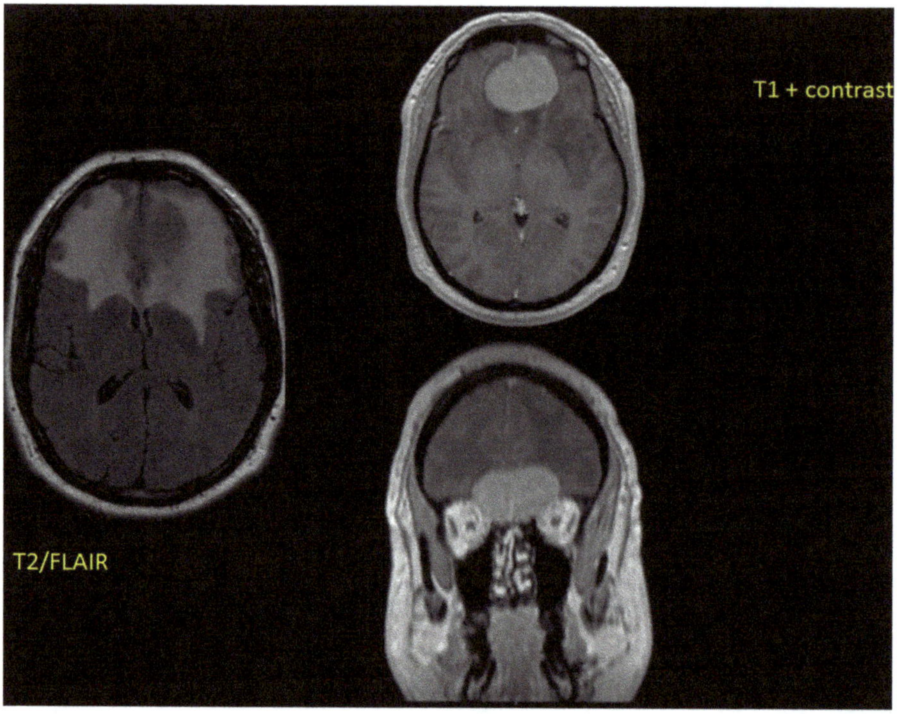

Fig. 21.2 Brain MRI prior to surgery for Mr. B (Case 2). The orbital groove meningioma shows homogeneous contrast enhancement with extensive bifrontal edema, most visible on FLAIR imaging

Neuropsychology Follow-Up

The patient felt that he improved after surgery relative to his preoperative baseline. The postoperative evaluation showed improved performance on memory tests and improved efficiency in executive functions compared with his preoperative evaluation. After undergoing radiation treatment and a 1-month period of recovery, the patient described his mood as "great." He had been active in his personal life and working full time with no problems. At that point, neuropsychological re-evaluation revealed normal cognitive performance. He had a slight weakness on his verbal memory test performance, though his performance on this assessment was significantly better than his initial presurgical evaluation. There was no evidence of generalized cognitive deficit or of any decline in performance over time.

Neurosurgeon's Perspective

Although options of observation or radiation therapy were discussed, surgery was the recommended treatment due to the patient's tumor-related cerebral edema. Although malignant meningiomas can have more edema than benign tumors, surgeons are not aware of the diagnosis until after final pathology, and therefore decisions in the clinic are not based off that knowledge. In all tumors that are believed to be meningiomas, the goal is total resection, if that can be achieved safely. Due to the imaging findings, the patient was started on a course of oral Decadron to help decrease cerebral edema. Due to the location, a bicoronal-transbasal approach was taken to prevent frontal lobe retraction. The procedure went smoothly and a Simpson Grade I resection was achieved. The patient was able to discharge home in a few days. The pathology returned as WHO Grade II. The patient completed radiation therapy to the resection cavity (54 Grey in 30 fx). He noticed minimal side effects during treatment other than experiencing some dryness of the eyes. He had some fatigue toward the end of radiation therapy, but this resolved within a week of completing treatment. He continues to have persistent loss of the sense of smell and taste.

In this case, the neuropsychological evaluation was originally requested due to the high level of cognitive functioning required by the patient's profession. Although the patient himself did not report any cognitive symptoms, the evaluation was able to demonstrate some weaknesses in functioning that appeared to be related to tumor/edema. This hypothesis was confirmed when the patient's postoperative neuropsychological evaluation showed improvement. In this case, the neuropsychological evaluation played a role in surgical planning and patient outcome.

Neuropsychologist's Perspective

This case illustrates the value of sensitive neuropsychological evaluation in the care of meningioma patients. In the brain tumor clinic, physicians quantify "performance status" using the Karnofsky Performance Scale [13]. This simple scale that classifies the level of functioning has been shown to be useful in cancer outcomes research for many decades, but it fails to capture a great deal of variance in cognitive function that falls within the "normal" range. Despite a substantial cognitive decline from his very high level of premorbid functioning, this patient was performing adequately in his cognitively demanding occupation and managing all complex activities of daily living. An individual who is expected to function at a high level of cognitive capability for their profession may continue to appear grossly normal during a standard medical office visit or neurologic exam. In these cases, neuropsychological evaluation illustrates the cognitive deficits that may be very relevant to professional work, even though they may not be apparent to the treatment team or the patient, and might be mistaken for more common changes (e.g., aging, stress, fatigue) by their family.

Part 3: Dual Diagnoses

As noted previously, meningioma is a relatively common diagnosis in older adults, with an incidence of 27–40 per 100,000 individuals between ages 65 and 85 years [1]. Because the incidence of other neurologic disorders also increases with age (e.g.,

Key Point
Grade II and III meningiomas account for 15–20% of all meningiomas and require postsurgical treatment and follow-up. They are more likely to recur, are accompanied by increased cerebral edema, and are more likely to induce cognitive deficits that may require long-term care.

Alzheimer's disease and other dementias, stroke), it is not uncommon to discover meningiomas in patients who may also be experiencing another neurologic disease. In these patients, determining whether or not the meningioma is causing cognitive deficits may be an important factor in deciding whether or not to proceed with surgery. The following case illustrates the complexities of this differentiation process.

Case 3: Meningioma and Dementia due to Multiple Sclerosis
Mr. C is a 63-year-old, right-handed man with a history of multiple sclerosis (MS). He had undergone a neuropsychological evaluation several years prior to the development of a brain mass to assess cognitive problems related to his MS diagnosis. That evaluation had shown significantly slowed processing speed, diminished visuospatial reasoning, and verbal memory impairment. These were considered to be cognitive symptoms related to his MS diagnosis.

The patient was lost to follow-up for about 4 years. When he underwent routine brain imaging for multiple sclerosis in 2015, the new study showed an extra-axial mass along the floor of the anterior cranial fossa in the orbital groove that had homogeneous and avid enhancement and minimal reaction in the surrounding brain, which was not evident on the prior study in 2011 (Fig. 21.3). There were also extensive stable multiple intracranial white matter lesions compatible with multiple sclerosis.

The patient was referred for a neuropsychological re-evaluation at that point. The goal of the evaluation was to determine whether or not there were cognitive or behavioral changes that would be attributable to the brain tumor. The implication would be that surgical resection could have the potential to improve his functioning if that were the case. Although the patient denied that he had noticed any significant cognitive problems or behavior change, his family members had noticed a subtle change in the patient's way of interacting with others over the past few years. Specifically, she described him as having a tendency to make jokes over and over again which, while not necessarily inappropriate or disinhibited, were repetitive and annoying. She stated that she did not see him as having significant decline in his cognitive functions, though she stated that he had long-standing cognitive problems related to MS, and that the family members had assisted him with complex activities of daily living (driving, medication management, finances) for several years.

Neuropsychological evaluation revealed impairment in multiple cognitive domains. Language functions were notably below expectation on tests of verbal fluency, reading, and confrontation naming. Visuospatial perceptual tasks also appeared to be below average, with some evidence of distortion and poor planning on visual designs. On tests of memory, the patient showed a retrieval-based impairment with intrusive and perseverative errors. Information processing speed was severely

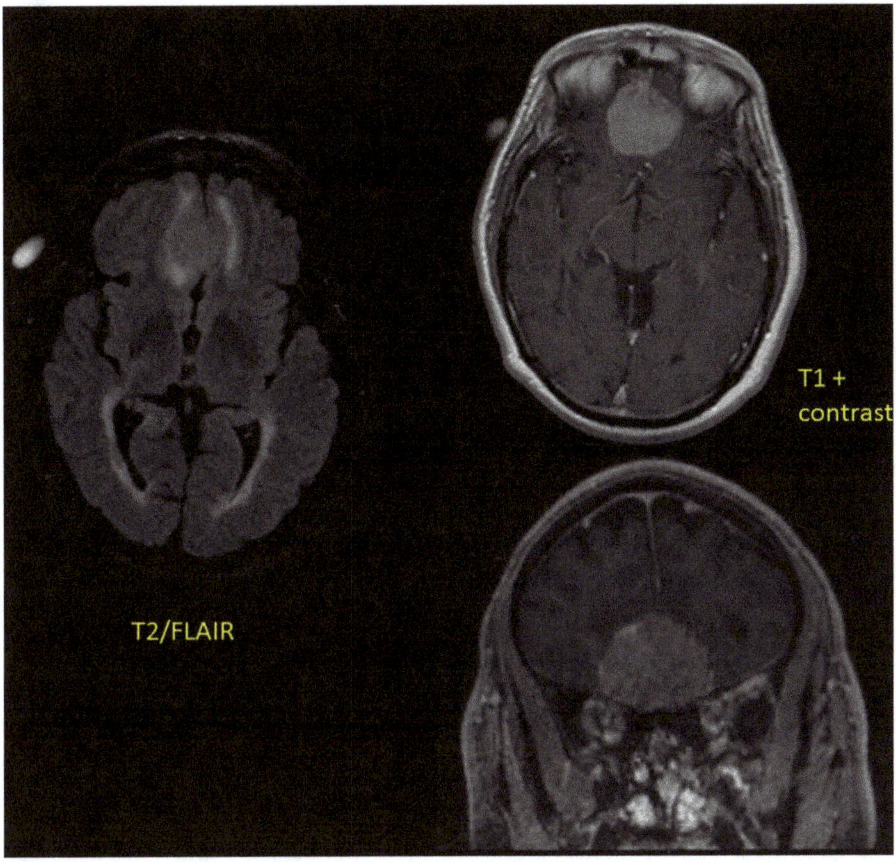

Fig. 21.3 Brain MRI prior to surgery for Mr. C (Case 3). Orbitofrontal meningioma has minimal surrounding edema. FLAIR imaging shows periventricular hyperintensity due to demyelination from multiple sclerosis

slowed. Perhaps his most severe impairment was seen on tests of executive function, on which he was essentially unable to engage in complex problem solving, cognitive set shifting, or conceptual/judgment decisions. In addition, there was evidence of executive function impairment across the battery in terms of his tendency to perseverate from one task to another.

Neuropsychologist's Perspective

The evaluation showed evidence of global impairment with a predominance of executive dysfunction. The test performance showed some variability compared with the prior evaluation, but no obvious or significant decline. Of note, because his prior evaluation was already so impaired, it may have been difficult to detect cognitive decline from his very low baseline level of functioning. Overall, the evaluation suggested that frontal lobe dysfunction was playing a large role in his behavioral presentation. Although it was considered likely that his long-standing history of multiple sclerosis was contributing significantly to these problems, it was also felt to be probable that some proportion of his executive dysfunction was related to the orbitofrontal meningioma and its compression of overlaying frontal cortex. In particular, the behavioral changes described by his family could be due in part to dysfunction in these brain regions.

Key Point
In some cases of meningioma, particularly those involving compression of the orbitofrontal cortex, changes in personality and behavior may be more significant than cognitive symptoms. Although such changes are difficult to quantify with objective neuropsychological tests, a comprehensive evaluation may be able to capture these changes and demonstrate the impact of those on the patient and their caregivers.

Neurosurgeon's Perspective

This case differs from the prior case, although both are meningiomas in similar locations. This patient has no edema surrounding his meningioma, and on presentation it was unclear if there was any effect of this mass on his cognitive function. Also the minimal edema is often a sign that it is a very slow-growing tumor. In a patient that may have frontal lobe dysfunction unrelated to mass effect, it is critical to avoid frontal lobe retraction. Any further injury to the frontal lobes may exacerbate decline in function rather than improve it after surgery. This is one of the risks which was discussed with the patient and his family. Also because the frontal sinus is invaded during the intranasal approach, cerebrospinal fluid leak can be a risk after this procedure. This is prevented by obliterating the frontal sinus during the closure of the procedure. The patient underwent a bilateral orbitofrontal/transbasal craniotomy. He had a Simpson Grade II resection. His meningioma returned WHO Grade II in pathology.

This clinical scenario shows that the absence of edema does not reliably rule out higher-grade pathology. This patient is being monitored on follow-up imaging to watch if there is any further growth of meningioma. If found radiation would be considered. In this case, the neuropsychological evaluation assisted in the surgical process by guiding expectations for cognitive outcome after surgery. It was important that they understand that the surgery would not help his neurocognitive deficits that were attributable to MS but may address other risks associated with meningioma.

Follow-Up

The patient was seen for neuropsychological follow-up 3 months after resection. He had been staying at a rehabilitation center and nursing facility since the surgical procedure and was soon going home with family support. The patient felt that there has been no problem with his cognitive function as he had felt prior to surgery. The family members noticed some improvement in functioning, particularly with an increase in his spontaneity, his sense of humor, and his social interactions. He had been participating in some rehabilitative activities and had been actively engaged in those activities. He was more spontaneous about his self-care and showed interest in social interactions with others at the nursing facility. They also felt his processing speed had improved somewhat relative to preoperative function, though it remained an area of difficulty.

The evaluation revealed an essentially stable pattern of significant cognitive impairment, but there were signs of improvement in his behavioral interactions. Although his test scores were consistently impaired, he did not show the level of cross-task perseveration in the postoperative battery that had been seen prior to surgery, suggesting qualitatively improved executive function. Given the recency of his resection and the complicated postoperative course, the fact that he was showing a stable cognitive profile and some possible behavioral improvements is a very positive sign. Nonetheless, he continued to have very significant cognitive impairment, consistent with a diagnosis of MS-related dementia.

Summary and Review

Given the many factors the neurosurgeon must consider when deciding whether or not surgery is indicated for a particular patient, cognitive issues may seem to be a minor issue. However, as the cases above illustrate, the cognitive issues encountered by patients with meningioma are often critical factors that relate to the decision to pursue surgery and to the patient's quality of life after treatment. A strong working relationship with neuropsychology can provide critical input into the decision-making process. Below, we present a brief review of the literature regarding cognitive issues in meningioma before concluding with a description of the multidisciplinary model we recommend for meningioma management.

Cognitive Symptoms in Meningioma

Although case reports of cognitive and behavioral symptoms of meningioma have been present for many years [14, 15], more systematic group studies of the issue have added to our understanding in the past two decades. In a series of studies of patients preparing for surgical resection of meningiomas, Tucha and colleagues demonstrated that cognitive deficits are common in these individuals. Using a formal neuropsychological battery, they initially demonstrated that older adults with meningioma were more likely to have cognitive deficits than a matched control group [16]. A follow-up study with a sample of patients with frontal lobe meningiomas, also compared to a matched group of healthy controls, demonstrated impairments on tests of executive function, attention, and memory [17]. Interestingly, these studies were initially conceived to determine whether or not neurosurgery resulted in cognitive detriments to the patients and, in fact, demonstrated significant cognitive improvements. These findings have been replicated in studies using brief cognitive screening tests, such as the Mini-Mental State Examination [18] and the modification known as the 3MS [19]. Very few studies have reported on incidence of cognitive impairment in meningioma. The exception is a computerized cognitive testing study, in which 69% of patients were reported to have a below normal score in at least one cognitive domain [20], which improved to 47% after surgery.

These findings have clearly demonstrated that meningiomas can cause cognitive deficits. However, it is important to keep in mind that a large proportion of meningiomas are asymptomatic and do not need treatment. Recently, Butts et al. examined the neuropsychological performance of patients who were incidentally found to have meningiomas on imaging they completed for a large-scale study of healthy aging in the population [4]. They found that 2% of patients had meningiomas in this healthy elderly sample (mean age of 77), most of which were small (<3 cm). The rate of diagnosis of mild cognitive impairment was no greater in patients with meningiomas than it was in a matched control group. Furthermore, performance on cognitive testing was similar between the two groups. Thus, it appears that asymptomatic meningiomas are not likely to cause cognitive impairment, even when measured with a sensitive neuropsychological test battery. In the subset of patients who come to clinical attention, either because they have experienced a symptom or their brain imaging has more concerning features (e.g., parenchymal edema), the risk of cognitive impairment is likely higher. It is for these patients that formal neuropsychological evaluation may provide important clinical information.

Integration of Neuropsychology and Neurosurgery in the Care of Patients with Meningioma

Because meningioma patients in general have excellent prognosis for overall survival, the relevance of their cognitive function is perhaps even more significant than in those with malignant brain tumors. Of course, surgical intervention and radiation for meningioma (when necessary) create additional risk for cognitive impairment. In patients selected by neurosurgery as good candidates for resection, the risks of surgery may need to be balanced against the presence of tumor-related cognitive symptoms. Therefore, preoperative assessment of cognition via a neuropsychological evaluation is recommended for our patients when cognitive symptoms are an issue in the decision-making process.

For suspected benign meningiomas, the role of neuropsychology is to determine whether or not cognitive symptoms are present and whether they are attributable to the tumor. The role of the neurosurgeon is to make a recommendation regarding treatment that balances the risks of surgery against the potential for cognitive benefit. For patients with malignant meningiomas, neuropsychology may also play a role in determining risk for cognitive deficits from subsequent treatments (e.g., radiation) and assisting in care management of the patient during and after such treatment.

Because meningioma is a common diagnosis, it may not be possible for all meningioma patients to complete formal neuropsychological evaluations. We recommend that patients be triaged for neuropsychological evaluation using a simple decision-making process. Refer patient for evaluation when:

- The patient, family, or physician observes a cognitive problem or raises a significant cognitive concern.
- The appearance of the tumor on imaging, by virtue of size (e.g., >3 cm), location (frontal lobes, left hemisphere), or surrounding edema, suggests that cognitive symptoms may be present.

Those patients then complete brief neuropsychological evaluation that includes an interview with the neuropsychologist, a core set of cognitive assessment tests, and potentially additional tests, depending on the specific symptoms that are of concern. The report should include the likely relationship of any neurocognitive symptoms to the tumor and the neuropsychologist's opinion about the potential for improvement in functioning as a result of surgery, if possible.

Postoperatively, the patient is re-evaluated after a 1–3-month recovery period. At that point in time, the patient and the surgeon can receive information about cognitive outcome from surgery. As has been noted in the literature, a substantial proportion of patients with meningioma who have cognitive deficits at baseline may continue to have cognitive issues postoperatively [5]. For those patients, additional cognitive treatment may then be recommended, and the specific findings from the evaluation may be relevant to cognitive rehabilitation therapists or physicians prescribing cognitive-enhancing medication. Other issues, such as recommendations for supportive services, documentation of deficits for the purpose of educational or occupational disability, and determination of decision-making capacity, may also be addressed at that time.

Chapter Review Questions

1. In addition to assessing cognition, neuropsychological evaluations also provide important information on which other factor(s) in patient outcome from meningioma surgery:
   A. Emotion, personality, and behavior change symptoms related to tumor.
   B. Psychosocial issues such as support available and caregiver burden that may play a role in the outcome.
   C. Insight into cognitive deficits.
   D. All of the above.
2. Grade II and III meningiomas:
   A. Are more common than benign meningiomas and less likely to induce cognitive symptoms.
   B. Are less common than benign meningiomas and more likely to induce cognitive symptoms.

   C. Require surgery as the cornerstone of treatment.
   D. B and C.

3. Useful criteria for deciding which meningioma patients may benefit from neuropsychological evaluation include all of the following, except:
   A. History of head injury.
   B. Family report of cognitive symptoms.
   C. Patient complaint of cognitive symptoms.
   D. Tumor location.

References

1. Ostrom QT, Gittleman H, Xu J, Kromer C, Wolinsky Y, Kruchko C, et al. CBTRUS statistical report: primary brain and other central nervous system tumors diagnosed in the United States in 2009–2013. Neuro Oncol. 2016;18(suppl_5):v1–v75.
2. Perry A, Brat D. Practical surgical neuropathology: a diagnostic approach. Philadelphia, PA: Churchill Livingstone Elsevier; 2010.
3. Daras M, Kaley TJ. Benign brain tumors and tumors associated with phakomatoses. Continuum (Minneap Minn). 2015;21(2 Neuro-oncology):397–414.
4. Butts AM, Weigand S, Brown PD, Petersen RC, Jack CR Jr, Machulda MM, et al. Neurocognition in individuals with incidentally-identified meningioma. J Neurooncol. 2017;134(1):125–32.
5. Meskal I, Gehring K, Rutten GJ, Sitskoorn MM. Cognitive functioning in meningioma patients: a systematic review. J Neurooncol. 2016;128(2):195–205.
6. Meyers CA, Wefel JS. The use of the mini-mental state examination to assess cognitive functioning in cancer trials: no ifs, ands, buts, or sensitivity. J Clin Oncol. 2003;21(19):3557–8.
7. Basali A, Mascha EJ, Kalfas I, Schubert A. Relation between perioperative hypertension and intracranial hemorrhage after craniotomy. Anesthesiology. 2000;93(1):48–54.
8. Adair J, Schwartz RL, Barrett AM. In: Heilman KM, Valenstein E, editors. Clinical neuropsychology. 4th ed. New York, NY: Oxford University Press; 2003. p. 185–214.
9. Walcott BP, Nahed BV, Brastianos PK, Loeffler JS. Radiation treatment for WHO Grade II and III meningiomas. Front Oncol. 2013;3:227.
10. Brastianos PK, Horowitz PM, Santagata S, Jones RT, McKenna A, Getz G, et al. Genomic sequencing of meningiomas identifies oncogenic SMO and AKT1 mutations. Nat Genet. 2013;45(3):285–9.
11. Brastianos PK, Carter SL, Santagata S, Cahill DP, Taylor-Weiner A, Jones RT, et al. Genomic characterization of brain metastases reveals branched evolution and potential therapeutic targets. Cancer Discov. 2015;5(11):1164–77.
12. Verheggen R, Finkenstaedt M, Bockermann V, Markakis E. Atypical and malignant meningiomas: evaluation of different radiological criteria based on CT and MRI. Acta Neurochir Suppl. 1996;65:66–9.
13. Karnofsky DA, Abelmann WH, Craver LF, Burchenal JH. The use of the nitrogen mustards in the palliative treatment of carcinoma—with particular reference to bronchogenic carcinoma. Cancer. 1948;1(4):634–56.
14. Avery TL. Seven cases of frontal tumour with psychiatric presentation. Br J Psychiatry. 1971;119(548):19–23.
15. Hunter R, Blackwood W, Bull J. Three cases of frontal meningiomas presenting psychiatrically. Br Med J. 1968;3(5609):9–16.

16. Tucha O, Smely C, Lange KW. Effects of surgery on cognitive functioning of elderly patients with intracranial meningioma. Br J Neurosurg. 2001;15(2):184–8.
17. Tucha O, Smely C, Preier M, Becker G, Paul GM, Lange KW. Preoperative and postoperative cognitive functioning in patients with frontal meningiomas. J Neurosurg. 2003;98(1):21–31.
18. Koizumi H, Ideguchi M, Iwanaga H, Shirao S, Sadahiro H, Oka F, et al. Cognitive dysfunction might be improved in association with recovered neuronal viability after intracranial meningioma resection. Brain Res. 2014;1574:50–9.
19. Yoshii Y, Tominaga D, Sugimoto K, Tsuchida Y, Hyodo A, Yonaha H, et al. Cognitive function of patients with brain tumor in pre- and postoperative stage. Surg Neurol. 2008;69(1):51–61; discussion 61.
20. Meskal I, Gehring K, van der Linden SD, Rutten GJ, Sitskoorn MM. Cognitive improvement in meningioma patients after surgery: clinical relevance of computerized testing. J Neurooncol. 2014;121(3):617–25.

Chapter 22
Adult Epilepsy

Erica M. Brandling-Bennett and David G. Vossler

Introduction

Epilepsy is one of the most common neurological diseases, with a worldwide prevalence of approximately 0.8% [1]. Epilepsies are defined as disorders in which individuals experience recurrent seizures along with alterations of their behavior [2]. They can arise from a variety of etiologies, such as structural brain malformations, genetic or metabolic abnormalities, birth anoxia, cerebrovascular insults, central nervous system infections, brain tumors, or moderate to severe brain injury. Most patients with epilepsy begin having seizures in childhood or adolescence, although accurate diagnosis can take years. Epilepsy can also begin at any point during adulthood, including older adulthood. In fact, the largest cohort of patients who experience unprovoked or idiopathic seizures is over the age of 60 years [3]. Regardless of a patient's age, a number of factors related to epilepsy, such as the underlying pathophysiology of seizures, age of onset, seizure type, seizure frequency, injury to the brain—either prior to the seizures or as a result of the seizures—and antiepileptic medication regimen, can all have an impact on both the transient and permanent aspects of intellectual and neurocognitive functioning. Given the heterogeneity of epilepsy, it is not surprising that patients with epilepsy can have vastly different levels of intellectual and neurocognitive functioning. Additionally, epilepsy impacts a number of other aspects of patients' lives, including psychosocial and emotional factors, all of which can further impact daily neurocognitive functioning and subjective feelings of neurocognitive health and overall wellbeing.

It is well beyond the scope of this chapter to try to characterize the intellectual, neurocognitive, psychosocial, and emotional functioning associated with all the different seizure types and epilepsy syndromes. Neuropsychological evaluations can, and often should, be used in patients with a variety of epilepsy syndromes in order

E. M. Brandling-Bennett (✉) · D. G. Vossler
UW Medicine—Valley Medical Center Neuroscience Institute, Renton, WA, USA

K. M. Sanders (ed.), *Physician's Field Guide to Neuropsychology*,
https://doi.org/10.1007/978-1-4939-8722-1_22

to assess their neurocognitive strengths and weaknesses so as to aid in understanding their level of functioning and in informing, planning, and evaluating various interventions and treatment plans. This chapter will briefly outline how comprehensive neuropsychological evaluations are generally used in assessing any and all patients with epilepsy. The main focus of the chapter is to provide a more comprehensive review of how neuropsychological evaluations are used in the pre- and post-surgical management of patients with epilepsy, most commonly in patients with medically intractable mesial temporal lobe epilepsy. Other common etiologies of epilepsy for which patients can undergo neurosurgical removal of an epileptic focus include tumors and post-traumatic epilepsy.

Neurological and Neuropsychological Management of Patients with Epilepsy

Neurologist's Perspective

The clinical management of patients with epilepsy is complex. While general neurologists can, and do, manage a number of patients with epilepsy, many patients are referred to fellowship-trained epileptologists, who are neurologists with specialized training in the treatment of patients with epilepsy. Epileptologists have specific training in medication management of patients with complex epilepsy syndromes or medically intractable epilepsy. Additionally, they have training in electroencephalography (EEG).

Adults and children with epilepsy are typically referred to epileptologists by general neurologists or primary care providers when seizures have been inadequately treated with antiepileptic drugs (AEDs). In the United States, epileptologists predominantly work at organized epilepsy centers. The time at which patients are referred varies, but over the last 15 years, we have consistently had patients referred earlier in their course than in the past after failure of one to three AEDs.

Patients with medically intractable seizures usually undergo scalp video-EEG monitoring to determine the types of seizures and the types of epilepsies they suffer from. Approximately one third are found to have psychogenic nonepileptic seizures. The remainder is found to have either focal-onset seizures or generalized-onset seizures. Of those with focal seizures, some may be candidates for focal neurosurgical resection.

Patients with medically intractable seizures with focal epilepsy who have either a lesion on brain MRI scan concordant with video-EEG monitoring or a normal brain MRI scan may be candidates for surgery. In both instances, the next step in the presurgical evaluation process is comprehensive neuropsychological testing. Such testing serves multiple purposes in the presurgical evaluation. One important purpose of neuropsychological testing in presurgical epilepsy patients is to identify areas of weakness in cognitive domains known to be subserved by certain brain areas. Identification of such weaknesses is important in providing another objective measure to localize the epileptogenic areas for surgical planning. If video-EEG monitoring, brain MRI scans, neuropsychological testing, and other techniques (e.g., PET scans, MEG, functional MRI) identify one concordant focus, in general the seizure reduction after surgery is good. When some presurgical findings, especially brain MRI scans, are normal, neuropsychological testing can play an even more important role in the localization of the focus. However, when EEG and MRI scans provide strongly lateralizing information, neuropsychological findings often add little additional information [4, 5]. Another possibly more important role of neuropsychological testing is to warn the epilepsy team about the risks of causing a permanent cognitive deficit if a neurosurgical resection is performed. The best example of this is the presurgical assessment of memory and language abilities in a patient who is being considered for a neurosurgical intervention to treat dominant lobe temporal lobe epilepsy, either with a standard anteromesial temporal resection or the newer technique, laser ablation of the hippocampus. In those cases, there is a risk to some aspects of language, particularly naming, as well as verbal memory functioning.

Key Point

Neuropsychological assessment of patients with epilepsy has become a critical portion of their neurological treatment. The National Association of Epilepsy Centers (NAEC) recommends that clinical neuropsychologists, particularly those who are fellowship trained in the assessment and treatment of patients with epilepsy, be part of a certified center, most notably Level 3 and Level 4 epilepsy specialty centers at which patients can be evaluated for and treated with neurosurgical interventions [6].

Key Point

Even in situations where patients with epilepsy are not being assessed for a neurosurgical intervention, a neuropsychological evaluation can be a valuable part of their clinical care. A significant portion of patients with epilepsy are disabled, at least in part due to the neurocognitive sequelae of experiencing seizures and the negative cognitive side effects caused by their AED regimen. Other causes for disability can be the underlying pathophysiology of their seizures or comorbid intellectual developmental disability, which frequently occurs in patients with epilepsy. Neuropsychological evaluations can provide essential information about a patient's neurocognitive functioning in order to assess their ability to perform in school or at work.

Neuropsychologist's Perspective

Findings from neuropsychological evaluations can be used to tailor accommodations and provisions that will allow patients with epilepsy to be as successful as possible, given their neurocognitive strengths and weaknesses. Perhaps more importantly, clinical neuropsychologists are trained in the comprehensive assessment and identification of psychosocial and psychological factors that can also have a significant impact on a patient's overall wellbeing.

Prevalence rates of depression in patients with epilepsy have been estimated between 20% and 60%, and depression certainly occurs at much higher rates than that in the general population [7, 8]. Anxiety is the second most common comorbid psychiatric disorder in patients with epilepsy, with prevalence rates estimated between 11% and 40% [8–10]. Additionally, countless studies have demonstrated that a variety of other psychiatric conditions and personality disorders occur in significantly higher rates among patients with epilepsy compared with the general population. Furthermore, some studies have also suggested a bidirectional relationship between psychiatric disorders and epilepsy [11]. It is critical that primary care physicians, neurologists, and neurosurgeons take into consideration the psychiatric health of patients with epilepsy. Comprehensive neuropsychological evaluations of patients with epilepsy should thoroughly assess various aspects of a patient's psychiatric wellbeing, because the relationship between epilepsy and psychiatric disorders is clearly significant and has a notable impact on both current patient functioning and long-term wellbeing.

Key Point
When conducting neuropsychological evaluations of patients with epilepsy, neuropsychologists need to be knowledgeable about the neuroanatomy that may be involved in the patient's seizures, including neuroanatomical correlates of performance on certain neuropsychological measures, as well as limitations of the neuroanatomical and ecological validity of neuropsychological measures.

There are certainly times when a patient's neurocognitive profile can clarify the location of an epileptogenic focus [12] or can clarify whether an elderly patient is suffering from dementia in addition to their seizure disorder [13]. However, there are also times when neuropsychological evaluations do not provide any lateralizing or localizing information about a patient's seizures [5]. Neuropsychologists also need to be informed about the potential neurocognitive side effects of the various AEDs that patients are taking. For example, it has been well established that topiramate and zonisamide cause a decline in verbal memory and verbal fluency in a subset of patients with epilepsy [14, 15]. Overall, it is critical that neuropsychologists are able to integrate all aspects of a patient's neurological, neurocognitive, psychiatric, and psychosocial profile to best understand how their overall quality of life may or may not be impacted by their epilepsy. Often, the clinical neuropsychologist is the practitioner on the epilepsy treatment team who integrates all those factors for the patient and for the entire treatment team in order to provide the most comprehensive overview of a patient's overall functioning.

Arguably one of the more valuable uses of neuropsychological evaluations in patients with epilepsy is in tracking their cognition over time. It has been demonstrated that patients with seizures that persist, despite treatment with AEDs and/or surgery, experience a significant decline in their cognitive abilities, particularly their memory abilities over time [16–18]. For neurologists, understanding the neurocognitive and psychiatric toll of repeated seizures can help them better care for their patients. For patients and their families, there can be a great deal of valuable information to be gained from understanding the neurocognitive impact of repeated seizures over many years, as it can help inform personal, occupation, and medical planning.

Neuropsychological Evaluation of Patients Being Considered for Neurosurgical Intervention to Treat Their Medically Intractable Seizures

Mesial Temporal Lobe Epilepsy

It has been estimated that focal-onset seizures make up about 60% and generalized-onset seizures comprise about 40% of seizure types in adults (and the reverse in children). By far, the most common focal epilepsy type is temporal lobe epilepsy. Two-thirds of temporal lobe epilepsies have an epileptogenic focus in mesial temporal areas, commonly involving the hippocampus, and the remaining third having an epileptogenic focus in lateral temporal lobe areas [19–23]. For the most part, temporal lobe epilepsy is not commonly associated with developmental delay or intellectual impairment [24]. However, cognitive and intellectual functioning in patients with temporal lobe epilepsy varies from individual to individual, with the occurrence of a series of generalized tonic-clonic (GTC) convulsive seizures or status epilepticus presenting the greatest risk factors for memory impairment (i.e., amnestic syndromes) and/or deficits in other areas of cognition, most commonly language deficits and executive dysfunction [25]. Furthermore, it has been demonstrated that patients with chronic, uncontrolled, intractable temporal lobe epilepsy often experience a significant decline in their overall intellectual abilities after about 30 years of uncontrolled seizure activity, although those findings are also mediated by a number of other factors, including the frequency and severity of the patient's seizures and whether or not they have experienced episodes of status epilepticus, as well as their premorbid cognitive and intellectual functioning [26]. Additionally, it has been demonstrated that some portion of patients with temporal lobe epilepsy have premorbid neurocognitive or intellectual weaknesses, presumably because cerebral infections (such as meningitis or encephalitis), lesions, malformations, areas of epileptogenesis, and seizures all interfere with brain development, which can have a global impact on neurocognitive development. This impact in development can lead to a decrease in overall intellectual functioning or a decline in specific neurocognitive abilities [24].

Many types of epilepsy can be relatively effectively treated and controlled with AEDs. However, there is a subset of patients with epilepsy whose seizures do not respond to AEDs, even if multiple AEDs are taken at once. The most common etiology for medically intractable seizures is temporal lobe epilepsy [27]. So, not only do temporal lobe epilepsies make up a significant proportion of diagnosed epilepsy they can also pose the most challenging treatment cases for epileptologists. Patients are considered to have medically intractable epilepsy when they have tried two different AEDs, but those have failed to result in sufficient seizure freedom or have caused the patient intolerable side effects. At that point, neurosurgical resection of anteromesial temporal structures should be considered.

A hallmark prospective randomized trial showed that once a patient has been determined to have medically intractable mesial temporal lobe epilepsy with mesial temporal sclerosis, then anteromesial temporal resection in conjunction with continued treatment with antiepileptic medication results in significantly greater rates of seizure freedom for at least 2 years, probably longer, compared with continued trials of multiple AEDs [28]. In other words, once a patient with medically intractable seizures has failed two or more AEDs, they should undergo a workup to determine if they are a candidate for neurosurgical resection to treat their seizures, as that is going to provide patients with the greatest opportunity for seizure freedom and potential for improvement in their quality of life. The workup for neurosurgical resection of anteromesial temporal structures as a treatment for medically intractable epilepsy is thorough and involves an extensive neurological evaluation, consultation with a neurosurgeon, and a comprehensive neuropsychological evaluation. The neurological evaluation includes inpatient video-EEG monitoring, along with neuroimaging studies, which can include a brain MRI as well as brain PET, MEG, and SPECT studies, and potentially even fMRI, if possible. If, after the comprehensive workup, a patient is still considered to be a potential candidate for neurosurgical treatment of their seizures, they often undergo a Wada test. Finally, many patients undergo intracranial EEG monitoring to further evaluate the nature and localization of their seizures.

Neuropsychological evaluations of patients who are being considered for a neurosurgical resection to treat their medically intractable temporal lobe epilepsy must be comprehensive, with a particular focus on both verbal and visual memory abilities. There are a number of goals involved in a presurgical neuropsychological evaluation including, but not limited to, establishing a baseline assessment of the patient's presurgical neurocognitive and emotional functioning, potentially supporting the lateralization and localization of an epileptogenic focus, predicting neurocognitive and emotional risks involved in the patient undergoing a neurosurgical resection, and providing recommendations for presurgical and postsurgical cognitive interventions that might minimize the neurocognitive risks involved in a neurosurgical intervention.

The literature has provided mixed findings on whether or not patients with mesial temporal lobe epilepsy show material-specific (i.e., verbal versus visual) memory deficits. The general consensus still holds that patients with dominant mesial temporal lobe epilepsy usually show deficits or impairments in verbal memory abilities [29, 30]. Thus, it is felt that weaknesses in dominant mesial temporal lobe functioning can be assessed using multi-trial verbal learning and memory tests, such as the California Verbal Learning Test-II (CVLT-II), Hopkins Verbal Learning Test (HVLT), or the Wechsler Memory Scale (WMS-IV) Verbal Paired Associates subtest [31]. In contrast, visual memory tests are less reliably linked to nondominant temporal lobe functioning [32, 33]. However, it is still important that both verbal and visual memory functioning be assessed in patients being considered for both dominant and nondominant mesial temporal lobe resections, as there is good evidence that findings from neuropsychological testing can support other findings from electrophysiological and neuroimaging findings about a possible seizure focus [34]. It is equally important that the neuropsychologist conducting the evaluation be well informed that there are a number of factors, most notably chronic duration of and frequency of seizures as well as known medication side effects, which can confound the predictive validity of neuropsychological measures.

Following a comprehensive neuropsychological evaluation, most patients who are still considered candidates for neurosurgical resection to treat their medically intractable epilepsy undergo an invasive intracarotid sodium amobarbital procedure, commonly called a Wada test. The purpose of the Wada test is to determine language lateralization and to assess the functioning of the nonoperative mesial temporal lobe [35, 36]. Ultimately, the goal is to assure that the nonoperative mesial temporal lobe is functioning well enough to support memory functioning once the contralateral, operative mesial temporal lobe is resected so as to avoid postsurgical amnesia [37, 38].

Over the past 20 years, more epilepsy centers have begun replacing the Wada test, which is an invasive procedure, with functional MRI (fMRI), which is a noninvasive procedure. Although there are limitations to the use of fMRI, the most obvious one being cost and access to the technique, the future possibilities are incredibly promising. It has now been well established that fMRI can be used to determine lateralization and localization of language with greater sensitivity and specificity than the Wada test [39–41]. Less reliably, fMRI has also been shown to determine lateralization of memory abilities [42, 43]. Additionally, fMRI has shown to be useful in postsurgical outcomes for seizure freedom [44], preservation of naming abilities [45, 46], and minimal decline in memory abilities [47, 48].

Importantly, in the comprehensive presurgical evaluation of patients who are being considered for a neurosurgical unilateral resection of one of their mesial temporal lobes to treat their medically intractable epilepsy, there is a great deal of clinical information that needs to be gathered and considered. The contribution of the neuropsychological evaluation not only provides information about the epileptic focus and possible seizure freedom after surgery but also provides important information about a patient's cognitive and psychological concerns both before and after surgery.

Key Point
The findings from the neuropsychological evaluation, Wada test, and fMRI can help identify an epileptic focus for neurosurgical resection; predict epileptic, cognitive, and psychological surgical outcomes; and inform postsurgical treatment plans.

Case Study

Left Mesial Temporal Lobe Epilepsy: The Following Case Report Outlines the Presurgical Workup of a Patient Who Was Diagnosed with Left (Dominant) Mesial Temporal Lobe Epilepsy

A.D. was a 28-year-old, right-handed, Caucasian female who reportedly had her first seizure, a generalized tonic-clonic (GTC) seizure, when she was 3 years old, shortly after having hit the left side of her head on a coffee table. After that, she reportedly started taking phenobarbital but only took that for a few months before discontinuing all medications. She was then seizure free until the age of 18 years, when she had another GTC seizure. In hindsight, A.D. said she remembers having very small, brief "episodes" starting around the age of 11 years, but she did not know what they were at the time. Since the age of 18 years, she had been experiencing recurrent seizures. She reportedly had three seizure types: a focal seizure without loss of consciousness, which frequently progressed to a focal seizure with loss of consciousness, which then rarely progressed to a tonic-clonic seizure.

From the age of 18 years until 28 years, A.D. underwent a number of neurological studies. When she was 24 years old, she reportedly had inpatient video scalp EEG monitoring at a major surgical epilepsy center, during which she had 22 subjective episodes as well as 2 episodes of word-finding difficulty without associated ictal EEG discharges. She then underwent repeat inpatient video-EEG monitoring at another hospital when she was 27 years old, during which she had 17 episodes, most of which were focal seizures with loss of consciousness, all of which were localized over the left temporal or left frontotemporal areas. An MRI of her brain showed left mesiotemporal hippocampal sclerosis.

Over the 10 years from the onset of her seizures until she underwent a neuropsychological evaluation, she reportedly tried six different AEDs. Despite trying those AEDs, alone and in combination, she continued to experience seizures. Thus, it was determined that she had medically intractable epilepsy. At the time of the neuropsychological evaluation, she was taking levetiracetam 1500 mg twice a day, lacosamide 200 mg twice a day, and clonazepam 1 mg once a day. However, she was still experiencing 1–3 focal seizures without loss of consciousness per day and 1–3 focal seizures with loss of consciousness per week. She had suffered approximately 5–8 GTC seizures in her life.

Cognitive Complaints: Regarding her cognition at the time of the neuropsychological evaluation, A.D. indicated that her memory was "poor." She said she often could not remember what her parents asked her to do, so she often did not accomplish what they asked her to do during the day. She said it was helpful to have a to-do list. She said she wrote notes for herself on her wrist, which she said was not a good system for her because she lost reminders when she washed them off. She also said she had been trying to use the calendar in her cell phone, but often set reminders for the wrong times. She said she often relied on her parents to help her remember important appointments and events. Her mother commented that A.D.'s father was her primary caretaker. A.D. endorsed frequent word-finding difficulties, hesitancy in her speech, and difficulty with mumbling. She denied visuospatial difficulties. Her mother said that A.D. was very disorganized, poor at planning activities, and often failed to follow through with her goals.

Neuropsychological Test Results: The neuropsychological evaluation documented average to high average functioning across all domains of cognition, including good attention, concentration, speed of cognitive processing, verbal working memory, language abilities, visuospatial skills, verbal and visual learning and memory, and executive abilities. See Table 22.1 for a comprehensive overview of her neuropsychological evaluation results. The most pertinent findings from the current evaluation were as follows:

- Given her academic and vocational history, as well as her current single-word reading ability, her premorbid level of cognitive functioning was estimated to be average (ACS TOPF = 97, 42nd %ile).
- Average overall intellectual functioning (WAIS-IV FSIQ = 103, 58th %ile). Her overall verbal abilities were high average (WAIS-IV VCI = 114, 82nd %ile) and her visuoperceptual reasoning abilities were average (WAIS-IV PRI = 102, 55th %ile). Overall, A.D.'s level of general cognitive functioning was at the high end of the average range and thus was generally commensurate with or exceeded expectation.
- Average speed of information processing (WAIS-IV PSI = 97, 42nd %ile). A.D. performed in the average to high average range across several timed tasks administered throughout the evaluation. Overall, her speed of cognitive processing was commensurate with expectation across a variety of cognitive domains.
- Average verbal working memory abilities (WAIS-IV WMI = 92, 30th %ile). Consistent with her good speed of cognitive processing, A.D. was able to hold simple information in working memory for a short period of time and manipulated it successfully, as she repeated five digits forward, recalled four digits backward, and sequenced six digits into numerical order, performing in the average range overall. She also performed in the average range on a more complex task of solving mental arithmetic problems. Overall, her verbal working memory ability was commensurate with expectation.
- Adequate brief and sustained attention. A.D. performed several visuomotor scanning tasks in the average range. Additionally, she was able to sustain her attention over the lengthy evaluation without taking many breaks. Overall, her attention was good throughout the evaluation.

Table 22.1 Neuropsychological evaluation data summary sheet

General intellectual function	**Raw score**	**Scaled score**	**%ile**	**Description**
ACS: Test of premorbid functioning	38	SS = 97	42	Average
WAIS-IV (standard norming)				
Verbal comprehension subtests				
Similarities	29	12	75	High average
Vocabulary	43	12	75	High average
Information	20	14	91	Superior
Comprehension	24	10	50	Average
Perceptual reasoning subtests				
Block design	52	11	63	Average
Matrix reasoning	18	9	37	Average
Visual puzzles	18	11	63	Average
Working memory subtests				
Digit span	26	9	37	Average
Arithmetic	11	8	25	Average
Processing speed subtests				
Symbol search	37	11	63	Average
Coding	62	8	25	Average
Index scores				
Full-scale IQ	105	SS = 103	58	Average
Verbal comprehension index	38	SS = 114	82	High average
Perceptual reasoning index	31	SS = 102	55	Average
Working memory index	17	SS = 92	30	Average
Processing speed index	19	SS = 97	42	Average
General ability index	69	SS = 108	70	Average
Academic abilities	**Raw score**	**Std score**	**%ile**	**Description**
WRAT-4				
Word reading (grade Eq = 12.7)	61	101	53	Average
Sentence comprehension (grade Eq = 12.9)	47	102	55	Average
Reading composite	203	101	53	Average
Spelling (grade Eq = 12.1)	43	96	39	Average
Math computation (grade Eq > 12.9)	43	101	53	Average
WJ-III word attack (grade Eq = 12.9)	29	100	50	Average
Attention and concentration	**Raw score**	**Scaled score**	**%ile**	**Description**
WAIS-IV				
Digit span	26	9	37	Average
Forward span	5			Cum% = 97.00
Backward span	4			Cum% = 83.50

(continued)

Table 22.1 (continued)

Sequencing span	6			Cum% = 72.50
Arithmetic	11	8	25	Average
Symbol search	37	11	63	Average
Coding	62	8	25	Average
D-KEFS				
Trails: Visual scanning	20″	10	50	Average
Errors	0			
Trails: Number sequencing	24″	12	75	High average
Errors	0			
Trails: Letter sequencing	27″	11	63	Average
Errors	0			
Speech and language	**Raw score**	**Scaled score**	**%ile**	**Description**
WAIS-IV				
Vocabulary	43	12	75	High average
Similarities	29	12	75	High average
D-KEFS				
Verbal fluency: Letter	36	10	50	Average
Verbal fluency: Category	40	11	63	Average
CW interfere: Color naming	27″	10	50	Average
Errors/self-corrections	0/1			
CW interfere: Word reading	23″	9	37	Average
Errors/self-corrections	0/0			
Boston naming test	54,0,4	$z = -0.65$	25	Average
Language screening	24/24			WNL
WRAT-4				
Word reading (grade Eq = 12.7)	61	SS = 101	53	Average
Sentence comprehension (grade Eq = 12.9)	47	SS = 102	55	Average
Reading composite	203	SS = 101	53	Average
WJ-III word attack (grade Eq = 12.9)	29	SS = 100	50	Average
Visuospatial skills	**Raw score**	**Scaled score**	**%ile**	**Description**
WAIS-IV				
Block design	52	11	63	Average
Visual puzzles	18	11	63	Average
Rey-O complex figure copy	36		>16	Average
Verbal memory	**Raw score**	**Z score**	**%ile**	**Description**
WMS-IV				
Logical memory I (17, 20)	37	ss = 14	91	Superior
Logical memory II (15, 16)	31	ss = 13	84	High average

(continued)

Table 22.1 (continued)

Logical memory recognition (14, 14)	28/30			Cum% > 75
Verbal paired assocs I (12, 13, 14, 14)	53	ss = 16	98	Very superior
Verbal paired associates II	13	ss = 12	75	High average
Verbal paired associates recognition	40/40			Cum% > 75
Auditory memory index	55	SS = 123	94	Superior
CVLT-II Total = (9, 15, 15, 15, 15)	69	$T = 68$	96	Superior
List A trial 1	9	1.0	84	High average
Trial 2	15	2.0	98	Very superior
Trial 3	15	1.5	93	Superior
Trial 4	15	1.0	84	High average
Trial 5	15	0.5	69	Average
List B	10	1.5	93	Superior
List A short delay free recall	15	1.0	84	High average
List A short delay cued recall	14	0.5	69	Average
List A long delay free recall	15	1.0	84	High average
List A long delay cued recall	14	0.5	69	Average
Recognition hits	15/16	−0.5	31	Average
Recognition false positives	0/32	(−0.5)	69	Average
Recognition discriminability	3.7	0.5	69	Average
Forced choice recognition	16/16			Cum% = 100
Visual memory	**Raw score**	**T score**	**%ile**	**Description**
WMS-IV				
Visual reproduction I recall	39	ss = 10	50	Average
Visual reproduction II recall	39	ss = 13	84	High average
Visual reproduction II recognition	7/7			Cum% > 75
BVMT-R Total = (7, 10, 12)	29	53	64	Average
Trial 1	7	50	50	Average
Trial 2	10	52	58	Average
Trial 3	12	60	84	High average
Delay	12	61	86	High average
Percent retention	100%		>16	Average
Recognition	6, 0fp		>16	Average
Rey-O complex figure				
3′ immediate recall	23.5	49	46	Average
30′ delayed recall	22.5	46	34	Average
Recognition	22/24	53	62	Average
Whole figure recognition	Yes			
Executive functions	**Raw score**	**Scaled score**	**%ile**	**Description**
WAIS-IV				

(continued)

Table 22.1 (continued)

Similarities	29	12	75	High average
Comprehension	24	10	50	Average
Matrix reasoning	18	9	37	Average
D-KEFS				
Trails: Visual scanning	20″	10	50	Average
Errors	0			
Trails: Number sequencing	24″	12	75	High average
Errors	0			
Trails: Letter sequencing	27″	11	63	Average
Errors	0			
Trails: Letter-number switching	72″	10	50	Average
Errors	1			
Trails: Motor speed	15″	13	84	High average
Verbal fluency: Letter	36	10	50	Average
Verbal fluency: Category	40	11	63	Average
Verbal fluency: Switching	13	9	37	Average
Verbal fluency: Switching accuracy	12	10	50	Average
Design fluency: Filled	13	13	84	High average
Design fluency: Empty	12	11	63	Average
Design fluency: Switching	10	12	75	High average
CW interfere: CW inhibition	51″	10	50	Average
Errors/self-corrections	0/2			
CW interfere: CW Inhib/switching	53″	11	63	Average
Errors/self-corrections	0/0			
WCST - # of trials administered	71			
# categories completed	6		>16	Average
Trials to first category	11		>16	Average
Errors	8	SS = 119	90	High average
Perseverative responses	4	SS > 145	>99	Very superior
Perseverative errors	4	SS > 145	>99	Very superior
Failure to maintain set	0		>16	Average
Learning to learn	0.00		>16	Average
Effort measures	**Raw score**		**%ile**	**Description**
ACS				
Word choice test	50		Cum% > 25	Valid
WAIS-IV digit span reliable digits	9		Cum% > 25	Valid
TOMM trial 1	50/50			Valid
CVLT-II forced choice	16/16		Cum% = 100	Valid
Mood/personality	**Raw score**	**T score**		**Rating**

(continued)

Table 22.1 (continued)

BDI-II	0			None
BAI	8			Mild
MMPI-2-RF				
VRIN-r	4	53		WNL
TRIN-r	9	65F		Clinically significant
F-r	4	61		WNL
Fp-r	1	51		WNL
Fs	5	83		Clinically significant
FBS-r	16	77		Clinically significant
L-r	3	52		WNL
K-r	8	52		WNL
Internalizing dysfunction	15	57		WNL
Thought dysfunction	3	57		WNL
Externalizing dysfunction	2	40		WNL
Demoralization	6	54		WNL
Somatic complaints	9	65		Clinically significant
Low positive emotions	6	58		WNL
Cynicism	5	47		WNL
Antisocial behavior	2	43		WNL
Ideas of persecution	0	43		WNL
Dysfunctional negative emotions	9	55		WNL
Aberrant experiences	5	63		WNL
Hypomanic activation	8	43		WNL

Note: "Descriptions" are qualitative descriptors derived from the quantitative percentile (%ile) data according to the following transformations: *impaired, ≤2nd %ile; borderline, 3rd to 8th %iles; low average, 9th to 24th %iles; average, 25th to 74th %iles; high average, 75th to 89th %iles; superior, 90th to 97th %iles; very superior, ≥98th %ile*

- On a brief screen of academic performance, A.D. demonstrated average phonemic processing abilities, single-word reading abilities, reading comprehension, and spelling abilities and at a greater than 12th grade level. Her performance on a mathematical computation task was also average and at a greater than 12th grade level. Overall, her performances on tests of academic achievement indicated that all of her academic abilities were commensurate with expectation and there was no evidence of a specific learning disability.
- Average language abilities. Specifically, A.D.'s expressive vocabulary, verbal abstract reasoning ability, and verbal social reasoning ability were all average to high average. Similarly, her confrontation naming was average. As stated earlier,

her phonemic processing abilities, her single-word reading abilities, and her reading comprehension abilities were average. Her phonemic and semantic fluencies were both average. Overall, her language abilities were average and thus were indicative of good dominant hemisphere functioning.

- High average performances across verbal learning and memory tasks. A.D.'s performance on an immediate verbal learning and memory measure was superior when information was presented in a context (short stories). After a 30-minute delay, she retained 84% of the information she had originally encoded, performing in the high average range. Her recognition for that contextual information was at least high average. On a measure of her ability to learn and recall word pairs, she performed in the very superior range, as she was able to learn 14 out of 14 word pairs after only 3 learning trials. After a 30-minute delay, she recalled 13 of the word pairs she was initially able to learn (93% retention), which was a high average performance. Her recognition for the word pairs was perfect. When memorization of a supra span word list was required, she demonstrated good initial encoding as she learned 15 out of 16 words after only 2 learning trials and maintained that performance over 5 learning trials. She recalled 15 words after both a short and a long delay (100% retention), which were both high average performances. Her recognition of the word list was average. Overall, A.D. demonstrated strong learning, encoding, retention, free recall, and recognition of verbal information, all of which is indicative of good functioning of dominant mesial temporal structures.
- Average simple and complex visuospatial processing and visuoperception. Specifically, she performed in the average range when asked to manipulate blocks to match a visual model and in the average range when asked to solve visually presented puzzles. Additionally, her reproduction of a complex figure was very good, as she was able to perceive the gestalt of the figure and then accurately organized the individual components of the figure. Overall, A.D. demonstrated good simple and complex visuoperceptual abilities, all of which is indicative of good nondominant hemisphere functioning.
- Average performances across visual learning and memory tasks. On a measure of simple visual memory, she performed in the average range immediately, and then in the high average range after a long delay as she retained 100% of the simple visual information she had initially encoded. Her recognition for that simple visual information was at least high average. Her learning of a six-item array of figures was average. After a delay, she recalled 100% of the visual information, which was a high average performance. Her recognition of the six items was perfect. On a more complex visual memory measure, she performed in the average range after both a short and a long delay. Her recognition of parts of the figure was also average, and she was able to correctly pick the figure out of a six-item array. Overall, A.D. demonstrated strong learning, encoding, retention, free recall, and recognition of visual information, all of which is indicative of good functioning of nondominant mesial temporal structures.

- Good performances on executive functioning tasks. She demonstrated high average verbal abstract reasoning as well as average verbal social reasoning and visual abstract reasoning. As mentioned before, her speed of cognitive processing and her verbal working memory abilities were average. Her performance was average when she was required to switch sets on a visuospatial sequencing task. Consistent with her average phonemic and semantic fluencies, her verbal fluency set shifting was also average. Her visual fluency and visual fluency set shifting was average to high average. Her ability to inhibit a prepotent verbal response was average. Additionally, on a task in which she had to use novel problem solving and hypothesis testing, she was able to easily identify all three sorting parameters for the cards and was able to easily sort the cards at an average level. Overall, A.D. demonstrated good performances across all tasks of executive functioning, including good switching, set shifting, inhibition, and novel problem solving.
- No endorsed symptoms of depression on a self-report measure of depression.
- Mild endorsed symptoms of anxiety on a self-report measure of anxiety. She indicated that she felt unsteady, nervous, and scared; had difficulty relaxing; and had a fear of losing control.
- Valid results on the MMPI-2-RF (VRIN-r = 53, TRIN-r = 65F, F-r = 61, FBS = 77, L-r = 52, K-r = 52). The following Restructured Clinical Scale was elevated: Somatic Complaints (65). Her pattern of responses was generally consistent with someone who was experiencing a number of vague neurological complaints, including headaches and fatigue, all to a significant degree. Her responses were best attributable to her seizure disorder rather than an inappropriate somatisizing of depression or anxiety. However, given that she was struggling with a variety of health concerns, it was possible that in the future she might become depressed or anxious if she felt that her health problems were overwhelming her and taking over her life.

Wada Test Results: A.D. then underwent a Wada test as part of her presurgical evaluation. The results of that procedure showed that she had left hemisphere dominance for all aspects of language. She demonstrated good episodic memory (83% recall) after a left hemisphere injection. However, she demonstrated only moderate episodic memory (50% recall) after a right hemisphere injection. The neuropsychological evaluation had suggested that A.D.'s verbal and visual memory abilities were both average and high average, which was suggestive of adequate functioning of the mesial temporal structures bilaterally. The findings from the Wada test suggested that both left and right mesial temporal structures were both encoding information, with right mesial temporal structures more functional than left mesial temporal structures. Given that A.D. was left hemisphere dominant for language, it was felt to be likely that left mesial temporal structures subserved verbal learning and memory abilities. In contrast, right mesial temporal structures likely subserved visual learning and memory abilities and were functioning at a higher level than left mesial temporal structures.

Summary and Impressions: The results of the neuropsychological evaluation indicated that A.D. was demonstrating globally good cognition, with particular strengths in her verbal and visual learning and memory abilities. Her cognitive profile indicated good bilateral mesial temporal functioning. Despite experiencing ongoing seizures for at least 10 years, probably longer, A.D. was demonstrating average to high average cognitive functioning across all domains of cognition, and there was no evidence that she is experiencing any current decline, dysfunction, or impairment in any aspect of her cognition. From the perspective of potential postsurgical cognitive deficits, the neuropsychological evaluation raised concerns about at least some decline in verbal memory abilities after she underwent a neurosurgical resection to treat her medically refractory seizures. The Wada test determined that she was left hemisphere dominant for language. Additionally, it showed that right mesial temporal structures were more functional than left mesial temporal structures. It was concluded that if left mesial temporal structures were resected, right mesial temporal structures should have been able to support memory functioning postsurgically. A.D. was told she might experience a decline (as can often happen in patients who undergo a dominant mesial temporal lobe resection) in her verbal memory abilities postsurgically, but she may be able to compensate for that decline with appropriate cognitive rehabilitation therapy aimed at providing her with strategies for improving verbal memory by using verbal memory aids, such as digital reminder systems and note taking. Additionally, A.D. was told that she might not notice a decline in her verbal memory abilities postsurgically if she had fewer or no seizures, as it is often ictal activity that negatively impacts subjective memory complaints. Finally, she was demonstrating little depression or other psychiatric concerns, which was also felt to be a positive indicator of a probable good outcome in her undergoing the surgical intervention to treat her medically refractory seizures.

Collaborative Process: Through the entire extensive presurgical workup, which includes the initial neurological consultation, initial EEG, antiepileptic medication trials, video-EEG monitoring, brain MRI scan, and other neuroimaging workups, comprehensive neuropsychological evaluation, neurosurgical consultation, Wada test, and final neurological and neuropsychological feedback to the patient, there is a collaborative method that involves a whole treatment team made up of the epileptologist, the neurosurgeon, and the neuropsychologist, as well as electrophysiology technicians, nurses, and other clinic and hospital support staff.

Outcome: A.D. underwent a standard left anterior temporal resection. She has now been seizure free for 3 years. She moved across the country and now lives independently and has a full-time job. She is able to drive herself independently and without difficulty. However, she has subjective complaints about memory difficulties and trouble with mental organization, which are consistent with the types of cognitive difficulties she was warned about based on the findings from the presurgical neuropsychological evaluation and the Wada test results. She has been advised to undergo another neuropsychological evaluation to determine the exact nature and extent of her current neurocognitive difficulties. Unfortunately, she has not yet undergone a postsurgical neuropsychological evaluation.

Chapter Review Questions

1. Why is it important to recommend that patients with epilepsy who have cognitive complaints undergo a comprehensive neuropsychological evaluation as opposed to undergoing just a quick mental status examination? Should only patients with medically intractable epilepsy be referred for neuropsychological evaluations? Explain.
2. Why is it important that neurologists and neuropsychologists assess and be aware of psychiatric comorbidities in patients with epilepsy?
3. What is the role of the neuropsychologist in the presurgical workup and treatment of patients with epilepsy who are being considered for a neurosurgical resection to treat their medically intractable epilepsy? How does the neuropsychologist complement the entire surgical epilepsy treatment team?
4. What are some of the cognitive concerns that may arise in patients with epilepsy who are experiencing frequent seizures? What are some of the cognitive concerns involved in undergoing a neurosurgical resection to treat medically intractable epilepsy?

References

1. England MJ, Liverman CT, Schultz AM, Strawbridge LM, editors. Epilepsy across the spectrum: promoting health and understanding. Washington, DC: The National Academics Press; 2012.
2. Engel J Jr, Pedley TA. Introduction: what is epilepsy? In: Engel J, Pedley T, editors. Epilepsy: a comprehensive textbook. Philadelphia, PA: Lippincott, Williams, & Wilkins; 2008. p. 1–7.
3. Hauser, WA, Annegers, JF, and Kurland, LT. Incidence of epilepsy and unprovoked seizures in Rochester, Minnesota: 1935–1984. Epilepsia. 1993; 34(3): 453–468.
4. Akanuma N, Alarcon G, Lum F, Kissani N, Koutroumanidis M, Adachi N, Binnie CD, Poley CE, Morris RG. Lateralising value of neuropsychological protocols for presurgical assessment of temporal lobe epilepsy. Epilepsia. 2003;44(3):408–18.
5. Swanson SJ. Neuropsychological testing is of limited value for predicting the epileptogenic zone. In: Silbergeld JMD, editor. Controversies in epilepsy surgery. New York, NY: Marcel Dekker Inc.; 2006. p. 214–20.
6. National Association of Epilepsy Centers (NAEC). Guidelines for essential services, personnel, and facilities in specialized epilepsy centers. Minneapolis, MN: NAEC; 2010.
7. Kessler RC, Berglund P, Demler O, Jin R, Merikangas KR, Walters EE. Lifetime prevalence and age-of-onset distributions of DSM-IV disorders in the National Comorbidity Survey Replication. Arch Gen Psychiatry. 2005;62(6):593–602.
8. Scott AJ, Sharpe L, Hunt C, Gandy M. Anxiety and depressive disorders in people with epilepsy: a meta-analysis. Epilepsia. 2017;58(6):973–82.
9. Kobau R, Gilliam F, Thurman DJ. Prevalence of self-reported epilepsy or seizure disorder and its associations with self-reported depression and anxiety: results from the 2004 HealthStyles Survey. Epilepsia. 2006;47(11):1915–21.
10. Wittchen HU, Kessler RC, Beesdo K, Krause P, Hofler M, Hoyer J. Generalized anxiety and depression in primary care: prevalence, recognition, and management. J Clin Psychiatry. 2002;63(Suppl 8):24–34.

11. Hesdorffer DC, Hauser WA, Olafsson E, Ludvigsson P, Kjartansson O. Depression and suicide attempt as risk factors for incident unprovoked seizures. Ann Neurol. 2006;59(1):35–41.
12. Loring DW, Strauss E, Hermann BP, Barr WB, Perrine K, Trenerry MR, Chelune G, Westerveld M, Lee GP, Meador KJ, Bowden SC. Differential neuropsychological test sensitivity to left temporal lobe epilepsy. J Int Neuropsychol Soc. 2008;14:394–400.
13. Helmstaedter C, Elger CE. Chronic temporal lobe epilepsy: a neurodevelopmental or progressively dementing disease? Brain. 2009;132. (Pt. 10:2822–30.
14. Brunbech L, Sabers A. Effect of antiepileptic drugs on cognitive function in individuals with epilepsy: a comparative review of newer versus older agents. Drugs. 2002;62(4):593–604.
15. Sommer BR, Mitchell EL, Wroolie TE. Topiramate: effects on cognition in patients with epilepsy, migraine headache and obesity. Ther Adv Neurol Disord. 2013;6(4):211–27.
16. Helmstaedter C, Kurthen M, Lux S, Reuber M, Elger CE. Chronic epilepsy and cognition: a longitudinal study in temporal lobe epilepsy. Ann Neurol. 2003;54(4):425–32.
17. Hermann BP, Seidenberg M, Dow C, Jones J, Rutecki P, Bhattacharya A, Bell B. Cognitive prognosis in chronic temporal lobe epilepsy. Ann Neurol. 2006;60(1):80–7.
18. Seidenberg M, Pulsipher DT, Hermann B. Cognitive progression in epilepsy. Neuropsychol Rev. 2007;17(4):445–54.
19. Crawford PM. Epidemiology of intractable focal epilepsy. In: Oxbury JM, Polkey CE, Duchowny M, editors. Intractable focal epilepsy. London: WB Saunders; 2000. p. 25–40.
20. Hauser WA, Annegers JF, Kurland LT. The prevalence of epilepsy in Rochester, Minnesota: 1940–1980. Epilepsia. 1991;32(4):429–45.
21. Panayiotopoulos CP. A clinical guide to epileptic syndromes and their treatment. Oxfordshire: Bladon Medical Publishing; 2002.
22. Vossler DG, Rostad SW, Haltiner AM, Davis B, Powell TW, Bell AJ, Kraemer DL. Increased ictal discharge frequency and neocortex gliosis in lateral temporal lobe epilepsy. J Clin Neurophysiol. 2012;29(5):449–57.
23. Wiebe S. Epidemiology of temporal lobe epilepsy. Can J Neurol Sci. 2000;27(Suppl 1):S6–S10.
24. Sauerwein HC, Gallagher A, Lassonde M. Neuropsychological deficits in children with temporal lobe epilepsy. In: Arzimanoglou A, Aldenkamp A, Cross H, Lassonde M, Moshé S, Schmitz B, editors. Cognitive dysfunction in children with temporal lobe epilepsy. Paris: John Libbey Eurotext; 2005. p. 1–12.
25. Lee TM, Yip JT, Jones-Gotman M. Memory deficits after resection from left or right anterior temporal lobe in humans: a meta-analytic review. Epilepsia. 2002;43(3):283–91.
26. Jokeit H, Ebner A. Effects of chronic epilepsy on intellectual functions. Prog Brain Res. 2002;135:455–63.
27. Engel J Jr. Etiology as a risk factor for medically refractory epilepsy: a case for early surgical intervention. Neurology. 1998;51(5):1243–4.
28. Engel J Jr, McDermott M, Wiebe S, Langfitt J, Stern J, Dewar S, Sperling M, Gardiner I, Erba G, Fried I, Jacobs M, Vinters H, Mintzer S, Kieburtz K, the ERSET Study Group. Early surgical therapy for drug-resistant temporal lobe epilepsy: a randomized trial. JAMA. 2012;307(9):922–30.
29. Loring DW, Lee GP, Martin RC, Meador KJ. Material-specific learning in patients with partial complex seizures of temporal lobe origin: convergent validation of memory constructs. J Epilepsy. 1988;1:53–9.
30. McDonald CR, Bauer RM, Grande L, Gilmore R, Roper S. The role of the frontal lobes in memory: evidence from unilateral frontal resections for relief of intractable epilepsy. Arch Clin Neuropsychol. 2001;16:571–85.
31. Jones-Gotman M, Zatorre RJ, Olivier A, Andermann F, Cendes F, Staunton H. Learning and retention of words and designs following excision from medial or lateral temporal-lobe structures. Neuropsychologia. 1997;35:963–73.
32. Barr WB, Chelune GJ, Hermann BP, Loring DW, Perrine K, Strauss E, Trenerry MR, Westerveld M. The use of figural reproduction tests as measures of nonverbal memory in epilepsy surgery candidates. J Int Neuropsychol Soc. 1997;3(5):435–43.

33. Pigott S, Milner B. Memory for different aspects of complex visual scenes after unilateral temporal- or frontal-lobe resection. Neuropsychologica. 1993;31:1–15.
34. Holmes MD, Miles AN, Dodrill CB, Ojemann GA, Wilensky AJ. Identifying potential surgical candidates in patients with evidence of bitemporal epilepsy. Epilepsia. 2003;44:1075–9.
35. Chelune GJ. Hippocampal adequacy versus functional reserve: predicting memory functions following temporal lobectomy. Arch Clin Neuropsychol. 1995;10:413–32.
36. Wada J. A new method for the determination of the side of cerebral speech dominance. A preliminary report of the intra-carotid injection of sodium amytal in man. Igaku Seibutsugaki. 1949;14:221–2.
37. Loring DW, Meador KJ, Lee GP, King DW. Amobarbital effects and lateralized brain function: the Wada test. New York: Springer-Verlag; 1992.
38. Milner B, Branch C, Rasmussen T. Study of short-term memory after intracarotid injection of sodium amytal. Trans Am Neurol Assoc. 1962;87:224–6.
39. Bookheimer S. Pre-surgical language mapping with functional magnetic resonance imaging. Neuropsychol Rev. 2007;17(2):145–55.
40. Janecek JK, Swanson SJ, Sabsevitz DS, Hammeke TA, Raghavan M, E Rozman M, Binder JR. Language lateralization by fMRI and Wada testing in 229 patients with epilepsy: rates and predictors of discordance. Epilepsia. 2013;54(2):314–22.
41. Swanson SJ, Sabsevitz DS, Hammeke TA, Binder JR. Functional magnetic resonance imaging of language in epilepsy. Neuropsychol Rev. 2007;17(4):491–504.
42. Binder JR, Swanson SJ, Sabsevitz DS, Hammeke TA, Raghavan M, Mueller M. A comparison of two fMRI methods for predicting verbal memory decline after left temporal lobectomy: language lateralization versus hippocampal activation asymmetry. Epilepsia. 2010;51(4):618–26.
43. Vannest J, Szaflarksi JP, Privitera MD, Schefft BK, Holland SK. Medial temporal fMRI activation reflects memory lateralization and memory performance in patients with epilepsy. Epilepsy Behav. 2008;12(3):410–8.
44. Killgore WD, Glosser G, Casasanto DJ, French JA, Alsop DC, Detre JA. Functional MRI and the Wada test provide complementary information for predicting post-operative seizure control. Seizure. 1999;8(8):450–5.
45. Janecek JK, Swanson SJ, Sabsevitz DS, Hammeke TA, Raghavan M, Mueller W, Binder JR. Naming outcome prediction in patients with discordant Wada and fMRI language lateralization. Epilepsy Behav. 2013;27(2):399–403.
46. Sabsevitz DS, Swanson SJ, Hammeke TA, Spanaki MV, Possing ET, Morris GL 3rd, Mueller WM, Binder JR. Use of preoperative functional neuroimaging to predict language deficits from epilepsy surgery. Neurology. 2003;60(11):1788–92.
47. Binder JR, Sabsevitz DS, Swanson SJ, Hammeke TA, Raghavan M, Mueller WM. Use of preoperative functional MRI to predict verbal memory decline after temporal lobe epilepsy surgery. Epilepsia. 2008;49(8):1377–94.
48. Labudda K, Mertens M, Aengenendt J, Ebner A, Woermann FG. Presurgical language fMRI activation correlates with postsurgical verbal memory decline in left-sided temporal lobe epilepsy. Epilepsy Res. 2010;92(2–3):258–61.

Chapter 23
Multiple Sclerosis

Kevin N. Alschuler and Annette Wundes

Multiple sclerosis (MS) is a chronic and progressive disease of the central nervous system. Over 45% of individuals with multiple sclerosis experience cognitive deficits [1, 2]. Just as with most symptoms of MS, cognitive problems are variable in presence, severity, and impact. It is generally understood that individuals with MS primarily present with cognitive problems in areas of complex attention, learning/acquisition of new information, speed of information processing, and executive functioning; however, there is variability in presentation between individuals and with relation to MS disease course [3]. While patients may voice concerns that they are experiencing dementias such as Alzheimer's disease, there is no evidence to support that these dementias are more common in individuals with MS. (See Box 23.1 for summary and [1, 2, 4] for comprehensive reviews.)

Given that MS-related cognitive changes tend to have gradual onset and progress over time and that other symptoms are also often changing simultaneously, it is often difficult for both patients and providers to recognize that cognitive changes have occurred. Studies of self-reported cognitive dysfunction have suggested that self-report is not particularly well correlated with objective measures of cognitive functioning and may, in fact, be better correlated with factors such as depression [5]. As with many symptoms of MS (or any chronic disease), cognitive complaints are most frequently brought to the attention of the physician or psychologist due to the perceived interference of symptoms on activities and quality of life. Common referrals emerge in the setting of difficulty at work or school or changes that have interfered with family relationships.

K. N. Alschuler (✉) · A. Wundes
Department of Neurology, University of Washington School of Medicine, UW Medicine Multiple Sclerosis Center, Seattle, WA, USA

Department of Rehabilitation Medicine, University of Washington School of Medicine, UW Medicine Multiple Sclerosis Center, Seattle, WA, USA
e-mail: kalschul@uw.edu

K. M. Sanders (ed.), *Physician's Field Guide to Neuropsychology*,
https://doi.org/10.1007/978-1-4939-8722-1_23

Box 23.1: Key Info of Cognitive Impairment in MS

- Seen in 40% to >60% of MS patients.
- Most common cause of employment disability.
- Key impairments are short-term memory, processing speed, multitasking, and attention, whereas dementia is extremely rare.
- No correlation with physical disability.
- Can occur early in the disease process.

Table 23.1 Comparison of assessment methods

	BICAMS	MACFIMS	Comprehensive assessment
Functioning across cognitive domains	Very limited assessment (processing speed and learning memory only)	Limited assessment specifically targeted at common domains affected by MS (processing speed/working memory, learning and memory, executive function, visual-spatial processing, word retrieval)	Complete assessment of cognitive domains that fully assesses cognitive functioning
Assessments of intelligence and/or academic achievement	None	None	Yes
Personality assessment	None	None	Yes

In recent years, cognitive evaluation for individuals with MS has transitioned toward a graduated approach. A working group of MS-focused neuropsychologists developed a brief screening battery (<15 minutes), as well as a 90-minute evaluation. The screening—Brief International Cognitive Assessment for MS (BICAMS)—is designed to be administered in medical clinics by trained staff to identify the presence of cognitive concerns in the areas of processing speed and learning memory [6]. The 90-minute evaluation—Modified Assessment for Cognitive Functioning in MS (MACFIMS) [7]—is a concise but relatively comprehensive evaluation of processing speed/working memory, learning and memory, executive function, visual-spatial processing, and word retrieval. Finally, the most comprehensive means for assessing cognitive changes is through a comprehensive neuropsychological evaluation (NSE), which is often a half- to full-day thorough evaluation of cognitive functioning. The comprehensive evaluation extends beyond the MACFIMS by more comprehensively evaluating functioning across each cognitive domain, while also incorporating intelligence, academic achievement, and/or personality assessments [4] (Table 23.1).

Case Summary

Background and history. Peter, a 30-year-old married man, presented to our center in early spring 2013 for evaluation of possible central nervous system (CNS) demyelinating disease. At the time of his initial assessment, he worked full time as an administrative coordinator and was pursuing an online degree in information technology. His past medical history included sleep apnea (using continuous positive airway pressure) and childhood asthma. His family history was negative for MS and neurological or autoimmune disease apart from remote family member with lupus disease.

Circumstances leading to MS diagnosis. In January 2014, out of good health and without preceding fever, infection, trauma, vaccination, or toxin exposure, the patient started to have sunburn-like sensations (in winter) in his abdominal area, and within a 2-week timeframe developed neurological symptoms consisting of sunburn-like sensations from the rib cage downward, bladder retention, erectile dysfunction, weakness in both legs with ability to ambulate only a few steps at a time, fatigue, and left eye blurry vision associated with pain with eye movements. Though his presentation is classical for transverse myelitis (TM) and optic neuritis (ON), those symptoms were not initially recognized by local providers.

The patient was referred to a local neurologist for further diagnostic workup around 6–8 weeks from initial onset, at which time his symptoms had spontaneously improved but not yet fully resolved. A spine MRI demonstrated several cervical and thoracic spine lesions, some with acute inflammation, as illustrated by contrast enhancement. This triggered a brain MRI where several lesions in localization and distribution consistent with MS were noted with overall low lesion load though one subcentimeter enhancing lesion. Evaluation of cerebrospinal fluid (CSF) ruled out an acute infection, and CSF markers for MS (OCB, IgG index) were normal. Blood work for mimics of MS was non-yielding. Clinical, MRI, and laboratory parameters were not suggestive of neuromyelitis optica.

Engagement with MS specialist. The patient was referred from a community neurology provider for a second opinion with presumed newly diagnosed relapsing-remitting MS and MS management. His condition was confirmed to be definite relapsing-remitting MS per McDonald 2010 criteria [8]. On neurological exam, his visual acuity was 20/20 without red desaturation in either eye. Trace weakness in left thumb-index finger opposition, a wide-based gait with instability on tandem gait, and inability to walk fast/jog were noted; otherwise, strength, coordination, sensation, and reflexes were without impairment at that time, which was 3 months after initial onset of symptoms. As residual gait impairment interfered with daily activities and work, and a recent MRI demonstrated ongoing acute disease activity, a 3-day course of intravenous 1000 mg solu-methylprednisolone was initiated, which is the standard treatment for an acute MS relapse. The patient was also started on baclofen for painful spasms interfering with sleep. His symptoms subsequently improved.

Approximately 6 weeks later, the patient developed recurrence of some prior symptoms, as well as new-onset blurry vision without pain upon eye movements in his contralateral eye, dizziness, sunburn-like sensation in areas previously not affected, difficulties with urination, and cognitive complaints. Repeat MRIs were pleasingly stable and without signs of acute worsening. He was given another 3-day course of intravenous 1000 mg solu-methylprednisolone for a clinical relapse, and his symptoms resolved back to baseline. The patient was consulted regarding the benefit of disease-modifying therapy to reduce the risk of future relapse, MRI disease activity, and progression of disability over time. After careful consideration of various treatment options, the patient was started on a newer oral agent requiring twice daily administration.

On this agent for more than 1 year, he had no further clinical relapse, MRI progression, or new findings on neurological exam. He endorsed subjective leg weakness at times, but he was physically active and could walk for 1 mile without a break. Other baseline symptoms included mild imbalance (described as drifting to the side at times and having to concentrate on walking), a certain level of fatigue, and difficulties maintaining an erection. He no longer used baclofen as spasms resolved. Upon specific questioning regarding possible cognitive difficulties during a routine follow-up visit, the patient acknowledged a mild concern for memory impairment. He also reported that his thinking seems slower to him, that it takes longer to capture information and to draw conclusions, and he finds himself staring at the computer more often. At the same time, he recently successfully completed his online information technology degree and started a position switching from administration to the information technology field and denied any cognitive difficulties interfering with his work performance. The provider discussed not only the possibility of neurocognitive impairments in the setting of MS but also how other confounders, such as increased demands in a new position, stressors related to trying to have a baby, adjustment to his new MS diagnosis, MS symptoms like fatigue, and other medical conditions (e.g., sleep apnea), may contribute. Availability of different neurocognitive testing modalities was discussed. The patient was interested in further assessment through our rehabilitation psychology provider.

Cognitive Evaluation

The patient was seen on the referral of the neurologist to assess whether his cognitive concerns were a reflection of cognitive deficits, the impact of fatigue on cognition, the demands of a new occupation, or the combination of multiple factors. Given that the patient did not have concerns at this time about his work performance, the purpose of the referral was primarily for information, so as to better understand the patient's cognitive functioning, identify targets for intervention, and collect quasi-baseline data that could be used in the future to better understand whether the patient's cognitive functioning was changing.

The first step of the cognitive evaluation was to conduct a standard clinical interview. The patient reported that he had the primary concern of a declined ability to acquire new information, which emerged within the past 6 months. He reported that this was most bothersome in the context of reading, such that he frequently had to reread information. He reported that he was pursuing a new line of work and that this rereading was bothersome in the setting of his retraining. Upon further evaluation, the patient also endorsed decreased processing speed and diminished ability to multitask. He otherwise had no concerns about his cognitive functioning or about the possibility that his cognitive functioning was negatively impacting his performance in work, school, or home life.

Following the clinical interview, a number of factors were considered to determine the most appropriate method of evaluation. A primary deciding factor was that the patient's and referring provider's goal for the assessment was to obtain a clearer understanding of the patient's level of cognitive functioning, so as to be able to characterize the extent of the concerns, as well as to differentiate symptoms as cognitive functioning in nature versus manifestations of fatigue or workplace stress. In most cases, including this one, these questions can be sufficiently answered with the 90-minute MACFIMS. In the context of this patient, if the goals were academic or work accommodations, or the possibility of needing to pursue disability, a comprehensive NPE would have been prescribed to ensure that sufficient information was available to satisfy the educator, employer, or government. We ultimately settled on the MACFIMS-type battery as the most appropriate assessment method. It is the philosophy of our clinic to tailor assessments to the patient's needs; therefore, the final cognitive assessment battery was a modification of the MACFIMS, utilizing measures of attention, verbal fluency, verbal learning and memory, visual learning and memory, processing speed, working memory, and executive functioning. The evaluation was conducted and the patient returned to learn of the results and recommendations.

The first area of interest was whether weaknesses were indeed present. Ultimately, three primary areas of weakness were identified: a portion of verbal memory, processing speed, and verbal fluency. Regarding *verbal memory*, consistent with the patient's presenting concern, there was evidence of difficulty with acquisition of novel information. The verbal memory test thoroughly examines the process of memory and revealed two related weaknesses: First, the patient's performance suggested difficulty with the storage of learned information, such that the patient performed at lower-than-expected levels on the initial learning trials of the test. Second, the patient made a significant number of errors on a recognition subtest, which asks patients to identify the presence of words from the "target" (learned) list from among a list that also includes words that were on a "distractor" list and words that were not on any list. The patient's errors were primarily the endorsement of distractor list words as being from the target list, suggesting he was recognizing he had heard the information previously, but was unable to benefit from an organization of information that allowed him to determine which list the words were from. On a positive note—and consistent with most individuals with MS—the patient performed at expected levels in terms of retention, suggesting that while he may have had difficulty learning the information, he did not have difficulty retaining the pieces he did learn. Regarding *processing speed* and consistent with the patient's self-report, he performed worse than expected on tests of processing speed, particularly on tests that were written (vs. verbal). Finally, surprisingly to the patient, his lowest performance was on tests of *verbal fluency*, with scores <10th percentile (1st percentile for category fluency). This was an important finding, as the patient is quite strong verbally in conversation and would not have been an obvious candidate for such low scores on this portion of the evaluation if assessed on interview alone.

The second area of interest was whether the weaknesses were indicative of MS-related cognitive changes. Indeed, the patient's presentation was consistent with MS-related cognitive changes in many ways, particularly for an individual with a relatively new diagnosis. Consistent with MS, the patient showed weaknesses in common MS-related domains, such as the acquisition of information, processing speed, and verbal fluency. Consistent with a new diagnosis of MS, the magnitude of the weaknesses was subtle, but there were early signs of interference on functioning. At the same time, there were valid reasons to consider other potential causal factors. For example, it was not unreasonable to expect that the patient's symptoms—subjectively or objectively—would become more pronounced when fatigued. Additionally, given the patient's difficulty with learning new information, it was not surprising that the symptoms were most noticeable in the context of his retraining in a new occupation.

Recommendations

The decision to refer this patient for a cognitive evaluation was beneficial for a number of reasons:

First, findings for this patient importantly highlight that cognitive difficulties in MS can be difficult to detect. They are independent from any physical disability. Additionally, they may easily either go unnoticed or be underestimated when a patient presents with strong verbal skills and a number of other symptoms that dominate focus in the medical appointment. Additionally, this case highlights that cognitive impairments can occur despite a low lesion load on brain MRI and may be already present in the early stages of MS. Even at this stage, cognitive impairments may cause significant disruptions and functional impairments for people with MS in interpersonal relationships or at work.

Second, the test results contributed to a better understanding of the patient's cognitive complaints and impacted medical decision-making. The assessment revealed an unanticipated severity of weaknesses, as well as weaknesses in unexpected domains (e.g., verbal fluency), despite reports of good work performance and no obvious cognitive impairments notable to the neurologist or psychologist during interview.

Third, the assessment results alerted both the provider and the patient to the presence of this concern and highlighted the need to monitor his cognitive functioning over time. The current evaluation will serve as a useful "baseline" when assessing for interval change in the future.

Fourth, monitoring cognitive functioning provides the neurologist another avenue for monitoring MS disease activity, in addition to regular clinic visits, neurological exams, and repeat MRIs. Given the presence of cognitive changes, the neurologist may be more inclined to consider escalating disease-modifying therapies (DMT), as optimal control of MS disease activity by appropriate DMT is considered a critical element in preventing progression of neurocognitive impairments due to MS. However, these results do not suggest the use of agents like cholinesterase inhibitors (e.g., donepezil (Aricept®) and memantine (Namenda®)) used in dementia due to Alzheimer's disease as such agents were found to be ineffective in MS and have been associated with worsening of MS symptoms in clinical trials.

Fifth, the results of the cognitive evaluation may serve as another reason for the neurologist to encourage the patient and other treating physicians to optimize medical management of comorbidities, such as sleep disorder, possible mood disorder, and MS symptoms (e.g., MS-related fatigue, neuropathic pain, and spasticity) due to their potential negative impact on cognitive functioning. Fatigue, in particular, is a challenging element of MS and often requires both non-pharmaceutical and pharmaceutical management. Optimal lifestyle choices, such as regular exercise, good sleep hygiene, a healthy diet, and weight management, are critical elements of medical management. Depending on the level of MS fatigue, stimulating agents such as modafinil (Provigil®), armodafinil (Nuvigil®), and methylphenidate-related agents (Ritalin and others®)—FDA-approved for sleep apnea or attention deficit hyperactivity disorder—may be considered for off-label use.

Sixth, and finally, rehabilitation therapies may be recommended. In the current patient's case, a referral was initiated to a speech-language pathologist with expertise in cognitive rehabilitation. The purpose of such a referral is to provide the patient with an opportunity to learn new strategies that improve functioning by compensating for areas of weakness [4]. Additionally, a referral to vocational counseling was initiated so that the patient would have assistance, if needed, in workplace or academic accommodations. While not necessary in this case, additional services are sometimes considered, including a referral to rehabilitation psychology for coping with the impact of symptoms on functioning and quality of life.

Box 23.2: Case #2: Another Example of Clinical Presentation, Neurocognitive Evaluation, and Implications for Patient Management in a Young Female with MS

A 25-year-old female with early relapsing-remitting MS diagnosed after a single, self-limiting episode of numbness/tingling with intermittent dizziness and imbalance, some mild MRI progression over time, and CSF findings consistent with MS. Only mild lesion load on brain MRI and normal neurological exam.

- Failed MCAT four times and patient felt, at least in more recent attempts, that anxiety did not play a role in her test performance.
- Referral to full NPE to assess for otherwise not obvious difficulties with cognition.
- NPE result: Bright individual with well-preserved ability in most cognitive functioning areas but mild to moderate difficulties in areas of attention, memory, abstract reasoning, and aspects of executive functioning. Also fatigue is a significant symptom and when increased could be expected to further erode quality and consistency of cognitive abilities. No emotional stress affecting testing.
- Implications: NPE results were incorporated in working with patient on career development and triggered a referral to speech therapy to work on compensatory strategies to enhance attentional focus on daily tasks and to optimize her ability to rapidly develop well-organized approaches to complex tasks.

MCAT Medical College Admission Test, *NPE* neuropsychological evaluation.

Chapter Review Questions

1. Which neuropsychological domains are most commonly affected in MS?
   A. Intelligence.
   B. Aspects of short-term memory.
   C. Processing speed.
   D. Visual-spatial skills.
   E. A and C.
   F. B and C.
   G. All of the above.

2. Cognitive impairment in MS:
   A. Correlates with age at MS diagnosis.
   B. Correlates with baseline intellectual capacities.
   C. Is seen only in patients with advanced physical disability.
   D. Is seen only in patients with prolonged disease duration of disease.
   E. A and B.
   F. All of the above.
   G. None of the above.

3. Cognitive impairment presents in:
   A. <5% of patients with MS.
   B. 5–20% of patients with MS.
   C. 40–70% of patients with MS.
   D. 80–90% of patients with MS.

4. The BICAMS (Brief International Cognitive Assessment of MS) is a validated neurocognitive screening for patients with MS and tests for the following components:
   A. Verbal fluency.
   B. Assessment of academic achievements.
   C. Processing speed.
   D. Learning memory.
   E. A and C.
   F. C and D.
   G. A, C, and D.
   H. All of the above.

References

1. Chiaravalloti ND, DeLuca J. Cognitive impairment in multiple sclerosis. Lancet Neurol. 2008;7(12):1139–51.
2. DeLuca J, Nocentini U. Neuropsychological, medical and rehabilitative management of persons with multiple sclerosis. NeuroRehabilitation. 2011;29(3):197–219.
3. Benedict RH, Cookfair D, Gavett R, et al. Validity of the minimal assessment of cognitive function in multiple sclerosis (MACFIMS). J Int Neuropsychol Soc. 2006;12(4):549–58.
4. Pepping M, Brunings J, Goldberg M. Cognition, cognitive dysfunction, and cognitive rehabilitation in multiple sclerosis. Phys Med Rehabil Clin N Am. 2013;24(4):663–72.
5. O'Brien A, Gaudino-Goering E, Shawaryn M, Komaroff E, Moore NB, DeLuca J. Relationship of the Multiple Sclerosis Neuropsychological Questionnaire (MSNQ) to functional, emotional, and neuropsychological outcomes. Arch Clin Neuropsychol. 2007;22(8):933–48.
6. Langdon DW, Amato MP, Boringa J, et al. Recommendations for a Brief International Cognitive Assessment for Multiple Sclerosis (BICAMS). Mult Scler. 2012;18(6):891–8.
7. Benedict RH, Fischer JS, Archibald CJ, et al. Minimal neuropsychological assessment of MS patients: a consensus approach. Clin Neuropsychol. 2002;16(3):381–97.
8. Polman CH, Reingold SC, Banwell B, et al. Diagnostic criteria for multiple sclerosis: 2010 revisions to the McDonald criteria. Ann Neurol. 2011;69(2):292–302.

Chapter 24
Schizophrenia Case Study: Residual Thought Disorder versus Emerging Dementia

Bernice A. Marcopulos and Robert Gardella

Introduction

This is a case of an older adult with a long history of a schizophrenia-spectrum disorder, who presented with exacerbation of psychotic symptoms, aggression, and cognitive concerns. The patient and his psychiatrist wondered about the source of the cognitive deficits and how this would affect his treatment options and prognosis. In addition to a long-standing serious mental illness, this patient had a number of possible medical conditions associated with cognitive decline and was also taking medications that affect cognition.

Key Question

1. Is this man's cognitive symptom the result of a residual thought disorder associated with schizophrenia-spectrum illness or is a dementia emerging?

This case study highlights the difficulties inherent in evaluating cognitive complaints in the presence of multiple risk factors for cognitive impairment. The interprofessional collaboration between the psychiatrist and neuropsychologist was

B. A. Marcopulos (✉)
Department of Graduate Psychology, James Madison University, Harrisonburg, VA, USA

Department of Psychiatry and Neurobehavioral Sciences, University of Virginia Health Sciences Center, Charlottesville, VA, USA
e-mail: marcopba@jmu.edu

R. Gardella
Department of Psychiatry and Neurobehavioral Sciences, University of Virginia Health Sciences Center, Charlottesville, VA, USA

Western State Hospital, Staunton, VA, USA

K. M. Sanders (ed.), *Physician's Field Guide to Neuropsychology*,
https://doi.org/10.1007/978-1-4939-8722-1_24

critical in differentiating the cognitive deficits in schizophrenia-spectrum illness from deficits heralding the onset of a progressive dementia such as Alzheimer's disease. Neuropsychological assessment assisted the psychiatrist and the patient in understanding the nature and etiology of his cognitive concerns and selecting the best treatment options.

Key Point: Cognitive Deficits in Major Mental Illness
Schizophrenia is a serious and chronic mental illness with a typical onset in early adulthood [1]. It is thought to be a neurodevelopmental disorder with both genetic and environmental influences. Perceptual alterations (hallucinations), delusions, disorganized behavior and thoughts, and disturbances in mood wax and wane over the course of the lifetime. These symptoms cause impairment in daily functioning, negatively impacting social relationships and academic and occupational success. Antipsychotic medications are usually prescribed to address the symptoms of psychosis and to help maintain stability. Neuropsychological deficits are seen in the majority of individuals with schizophrenia-spectrum illness, most often in verbal learning and memory [2–4], with much variability among patients in terms of nature and severity. These cognitive deficits have a strong negative impact on adaptive functioning and predict outcome better than hallucinations and delusions [5, 6]. Amelioration of cognitive deficits is a focus of treatment, and new drugs are being developed to enhance cognition [7].

Key Point: Aging and Schizophrenia
The prevalence of schizophrenia in older adults is lower than younger adults due to reduced life expectancy [8, 9]. Older adults do develop new-onset psychotic symptoms as they age, usually due to medical disorders [10]. Persons who age with schizophrenia may become more stable over time [11, 12].

Several reviews, including a quantitative meta-analysis [13, 14] on cognitive aging and schizophrenia, concluded that there is little evidence to suggest that persons with schizophrenia will show a greater decline in cognitive functioning as they age compared to peers without schizophrenia. Although some studies have suggested that older adults with schizophrenia do not have a higher risk of developing dementia, several recent population-based cohort studies showed increased risk [15, 16]. Because schizophrenia is associated with cognitive deficits, such as memory dysfunction, detecting cognitive change associated with impending dementia may be challenging. The associated cognitive symptoms of schizophrenia can be quite significant, and in older adults may mimic dementia, which makes differential diagnoses very difficult. Neuropsychological testing can be very helpful in discerning whether the cognitive symptoms are due to thought disorder or signify the onset of a progressive dementia.

Referral

Mr. R is a 62-year-old married white male with a history of schizoaffective disorder, substance use disorder, and a learning disability. He has type 2 diabetes with peripheral neuropathy, history of gastroesophageal reflux disease, history of hypertension, and history of coronary artery disease (CAD) with placement of right coronary artery stent and hernia repair. He had recently been verbally and physically aggressive toward his family and reported experiencing auditory hallucinations. This prompted him to seek a consultation with his psychiatrist.

Psychiatric Findings

Mr. R reported auditory hallucinations and chronic mood instability. He indicated that he had previously done well in the past on a combination of fluphenazine and risperidone. He is currently prescribed only fluphenazine 40 mg/day (but recently at a dose higher than his prior dose of 15 mg b.i.d.) along with benztropine to prevent extrapyramidal symptoms. He was hesitant to stop benztropine because he was concerned that he would experience stiffness in his arms and tremors.

He was diagnosed with schizophrenia in his early 20s and has had at least 20 hospitalizations. He has a history of polysubstance dependence, including crack cocaine, marijuana, opiates, hallucinogens, and stimulants. He stopped substances approximately 20 years ago. He graduated from the 12th grade and has done some odd jobs such as working for a moving company but is not currently employed. He has been married twice, currently to a woman in her 70s who is not in good health. He has a son by his first wife but they have rarely spoken and he is not a source of support. He suspects that his mother had some type of mental illness but was not diagnosed, and she developed Alzheimer's dementia in her 60s. Mr. R's vital signs are normal, including blood pressure of 109/77 and heart rate of 89. His body mass index is 22; O_2 saturation is 90% on room air. There were no signs of acute medical or neurological problems on physical exam except mild peripheral neuropathy of the distal lower extremities. EKG was normal. Laboratory studies (including comprehensive metabolic profile, TSH, CBC, B-12, folate, RPR, and HIV) were all normal except for an elevated fasting blood sugar of 171 and HgA1c of 7.5 (prompting his primary care physician to adjust his diabetic medications), and vitamin D was 24.1 (supplement ordered).

Key Point: Anticholinergic Drugs and Cognition and Psychotropic Drugs and Cognition

The brain neurotransmitter acetylcholine plays an important role in attention and memory [17]. A reduction of cholinergic neurons projecting from the nucleus basalis of Meynert to the frontal lobes is implicated in the memory loss of Alzheimer's disease [18]. Many medications have anticholinergic properties and have the potential to reduce attention and memory, particularly in older adults [19]. Antipsychotic medications, as well as medication to control the extrapyramidal side effects of antipsychotic medications, have potent anticholinergic properties. These medications can exacerbate the attention, learning, and memory difficulties already apparent in schizophrenia [20, 21]. For instance, Mitzenberg, Poole, Benton, and Vinoradov [22] found that routine doses of medications with anticholinergic properties significantly exacerbate the attention and memory deficits in patients with schizophrenia.

Mental Status Exam

Mr. R presents as a white male older than his stated age. He is calm, cooperative, and appropriately groomed. He demonstrates good eye contact, and there is no evidence of abnormal involuntary movements, tremor, or akathesia. His speech is of normal tone and latency rate but of quiet volume. He describes his mood as "tired" and his affect is euthymic. He denies current perceptual disturbances but he acknowledges recent breakthrough auditory hallucinations. He felt that the higher dose of fluphenazine he has taken over the last 4 weeks has not been beneficial in reducing the auditory hallucinations. Thought processes are logical and goal oriented. He does complain of some difficulty with his memory and has difficulty incorporating new information on interview. For example, he had difficulty processing the discussion about medications and asked that the details be repeated several times. Thought content is reality based without current evidence of paranoia or grandiose ideas.

Initial impression: A 62-year-old man with a history of schizoaffective disorder and current presentation of residual psychosis and some cognitive impairment (including memory), which may be indicative of emerging dementia. He has some difficulty sleeping, but otherwise does not have substantial mood-related symptoms on presentation. Although he has a past history of substance use, there is no current evidence of an active substance component, withdrawal, or intoxication. He does have diabetes with some peripheral neuropathy.

Despite his residual symptoms, Mr. R was able to give competent informed consent for treatment and was interested in aggressive treatment to resolve auditory hallucinations as a priority and also addressing his memory deficit, if possible. Among the various treatment options discussed, he initially requested to augment fluphenazine with risperidone as this had been previously effective. He was aware of the metabolic, anticholinergic, and psychomotor movement risks of his choice.

Key Point: Cognitive Effects of Metabolic Syndrome

Stone and Keshavan [23] reviewed the literature on medical conditions in schizophrenia and found that they had a higher prevalence of medical disorders known to affect cognition. Persons with schizophrenia are more likely to develop "metabolic syndrome." "Metabolic syndrome" is a term used to describe a cluster of abnormalities including abnormal glucose and/or insulin metabolism, abdominal obesity, dyslipidemia, and cardiovascular disease [24–26]. These diseases have a deleterious effect on cognitive functioning and increase risk of dementia [27, 28]. Careful monitoring and treatment of the conditions constituting metabolic syndrome can prevent exacerbation of cognitive affects.

Risperidone was initiated at 2 mg q.h.s. and then increased to 3 mg per day, but he experienced some dizziness, so risperidone was decreased to 2 mg. Following this experience, he was interested in other medication options which might be better tolerated. He previously had a trial of aripiprazole but was concerned that it may not be covered by his insurance. His pharmacy indicated that he would be able to get it at this point for low co-pay, so he agreed to switch from fluphenazine, risperidone, and benztropine to aripiprazole. He was also interested in converting to a long-acting intramuscular form to address concern that he might forget to take doses. Oral aripiprazole was converted to long-acting injection. Fluphenazine, risperidone and benztropine were discontinued in an effort to reduce anticholinergic load, which could worsen cognition, especially given his concern about memory. Despite these medication changes yielding remission of auditory hallucination, improved subjective mood, and resolution of aggression, he continued to report "memory problems" and demonstrated persistent difficulty incorporating new information and remembering information during follow-up appointments. *In an effort to clarify if he had emerging symptoms of dementia, the psychiatrist sought neuropsychological testing.*

Differential Diagnosis

This gentleman has multiple risk factors for cognitive impairment: chronic schizophrenia, history of polysubstance abuse, diabetes, hypertension, and family history of Alzheimer's. Neuropsychological assessment added additional information that was helpful to the physician making a differential diagnosis and devising appropriate treatment. Specifically, neuropsychological assessment revealed patterns of cognitive performance that were associated with either his long-standing psychotic illness or could indicate a new problem, such as degenerative dementia.

Neuropsychological Evaluation

Mr. R had a number of neuromedical issues that are likely to impact cognition. The neuropsychologist was faced with the difficulty of characterizing current cognitive impairments in a complex and long-standing history of serious mental illness (schizophrenia-spectrum), drug use, as well as a history of learning disabilities. His history of verbal-based learning disabilities was expected to result in relative weaknesses on some verbal measures, something to be considered when interpreting his cognitive test profile. Hypertension and diabetes are associated with cognitive impairment and increased risk of cerebrovascular disease [27, 28]. Mr. R complained of memory impairment, and his psychiatrist noted some difficulties in memory registration during his exam. There was a family history of Alzheimer's disease. The neuropsychologist needed to carefully select a test battery that would validly clarify this very complex clinical picture [29].

Test Results. Mr. R presented to the test sessions as alert and oriented to person and location. He was mostly oriented to time but mis-stated the date by 1 day. Conversational speech was normal although he spoke rapidly at times. His answers to interview questions were generally logical and goal-directed with some tangential statements that could have represented confabulations or misunderstandings. He described memory problems over the past 3 years and non-specific communication problems. Mr. R became quite nervous during tests, especially memory measures. Due to his anxiety, the tests were carried out over several days. Scores on measures of performance validity (Test of Memory Malingering, Dot Counting) were within normal, except for one session which were thought to reflect his high level of distress that day. Tests administered included a test of premorbid functioning, a mood questionnaire (Beck Depression Inventory, 2nd edition), language tests (Boston Naming Test, 2nd edition, Controlled Oral Word Association), motor tests (finger tapping, grooved pegboard), a cognitive screening instrument (Repeatable Battery for Assessment of Neuropsychological Status), and problem-solving (Tower of London), visuomotor (Trail Making Test), intellectual (WAIS-IV), and academic (Wide Range Achievement Test) tests (Table 24.1).

Key Point: The Importance of Determining Test Validity

Accurate interpretation of neuropsychological test results, as well as all psychological testing, is predicated on the assumption that the patient exerted full effort on the tests to demonstrate their typical cognitive capacity or personality features and psychiatric symptoms. Patients may approach the test with attitudes that may threaten test validity. They may be concerned about how the test results will be used to make decisions about their care or be concerned about legal repercussions. They may also not comprehend the purpose of testing and not try their best. As a result, neuropsychologists have developed a number of specific tests and procedures designed to detect "response bias," that is, whether the patient might be underperforming or perhaps exaggerating their deficits [30]. Modern neuropsychological practice guidelines strongly recommend that test batteries include procedures for assessing response bias and "effort" [31, 32].

Table 24.1 Neuropsychological test data

Test	Standard score (percentile)	Interpretation
WAIS-IV		
Verbal comprehension	85 (16)	Low average
Similarities	9 (37)	
Vocabulary	7 (16)	
Information	6 (9)	
Perceptual reasoning	84 (14)	Low average
Block design	6 (9)	
Matrix reasoning	7 (16)	
Visual puzzles	9 (37)	
Working memory	74 (4)	Borderline
Digit span	6 (9)	
Arithmetic	5 (5)	
Processing speed	71 (3)	Borderline
Symbol search	4 (2)	
Coding	5 (5)	
Full scale IQ	75 (5)	Borderline
General ability	82 (12)	Low average
Dot Counting		Normal
Test of Memory Malingering		Normal
Boston Naming 53 (raw)	$T = 42$ (21)	Below average
Controlled Oral Word Association		
Phonemic	$T = 26$	Mild impaired
Semantic	$T = 43$	Below average
Finger tapping		
Right hand	$T = 37$ (10)	Mild impaired
Left hand	$T = 29$ (1)	Mod impaired
Grooved pegboard		
Right hand	$T = 23$ (<1)	Mod impaired
Left hand	$T = 28$ (1)	Mod impaired
RBANS total	54 (1)	Extremely low
TOL		
Total correct	88 (21)	Low average
Trail Making Test		
TMT A	$T = 36$	Mild impaired
TMT B	$T = 31$	Mod impaired
WRAT 4		
Reading composite	73 (32)	Borderline
Beck Depression Inventory	30 (raw)	Severely depressed

Results: Mr. R's premorbid intellectual abilities were estimated to be average. Current borderline performance on intelligence measures was lower than premorbid estimates, primarily due to low working memory and processing speed. His verbal and visual skills, although lower than premorbid estimates, were low average. His reading ability was borderline, which was consistent with his report of learning difficulties as a child. Performance on a brief measure of cognitive functioning (Repeatable Battery for the Assessment of Neuropsychological Status [RBANS]) was extremely low overall, again with extremely low attention as well as extremely low learning and recall. Language and visual skills were generally intact. Basic attention was average to borderline, and he demonstrated slowed processing speed overall. Motor speed and dexterity were also generally impaired. Executive functions were broadly intact when speed was not taken into account. His performance on memory testing was well below average, but he was able to retain some of the verbal information he initially learned. His self-reported depression symptoms were rated as severe on the Beck Depression Inventory.

The neuropsychological report concluded that he demonstrated overall cognitive performance that was slightly lower than premorbid expectations. The most significant difficulties included motor and processing speed and learning and recall of information, although he was able to retain some initially learned information. Other neuropsychological functions were generally consistent with his low average to borderline general functioning. The interpretation of his test results indicated inefficiencies in cognitive speed and learning, which were most likely related to long-standing symptoms of schizoaffective disorder, chronic polysubstance use, and his poorly controlled medical comorbidities, including diabetes and hypertension. *In conclusion, Mr. R's current cognitive functioning was more closely consistent with serious mental illness substance use and medical comorbidities rather than a profile that would be suggestive of Alzheimer's dementia.*

Mr. R's cognitive strengths and weaknesses, as shown on formal testing, provided important information about his adaptive functioning and evidence against a diagnosis of Alzheimer's disease. He was able to retain some memory information, which would not be expected if his deficits were due to Alzheimer's disease.

Key Point: Efficacy of Neuropsychological Testing in Detecting Dementia

Neuropsychological assessment plays a key role in detecting cognitive changes associated with Alzheimer's disease and other dementias [33]. Deficits in episodic memory (i.e., recalling an event) can differentiate Alzheimer's disease from normal cognitive aging. Neuropsychological tests can also distinguish among types of dementia [34]. Although it is more difficult to delineate these deficits in patients with a long history of serious mental illness, a pattern of rapid forgetting and ineffectiveness of cues characterizes abnormal memory in geropsychiatric patients [35].

Collaboration Considerations and Questions from Referral through Feedback

What does neuropsychology contribute to the case, and how does the information gleaned from the assessment complement the psychiatric evaluation? Why was a neuropsychological evaluation important in this diagnostic work-up of chronic schizophrenia?

The results of neuropsychological evaluation reassured this patient and his psychiatrist that the cognitive difficulties he was experiencing were most likely related to his long-standing mental and physical health issues, rather than emerging dementia. He was interested in further improving his mood stability and cognition, so his psychiatrist offered N-acetylcysteine, lamotrigine, and melatonin to augment aripiprazole. They are metabolically safe and could *potentially* improve his cognition, promote mood stability, and reduce residual thought disorder symptoms [36, 37]. In addition to normalizing the sleep/wake cycle, melatonin has been reported to potentially reduce the risk of appetite increase/metabolic problem context of treatment with atypical antipsychotic and has even been noted to improve Positive and Negative Syndrome Scale (PANSS) scores in a study [38]. Following psychiatric consultation, his medication regimen included melatonin 6 mg q.h.s., metformin 1000 mg b.i.d., N-acetylcysteine 600 mg b.i.d., ASA 81 mg enteric-coated QAM, atorvastatin 10 mg q.h.s., cholecalciferol vitamin D3 50,000 units PO q. week, DSS 100 mg q.h.s., glipizide 10 mg ER QAM, glargine insulin 20 units subcutaneous q.h.s., lamotrigine 25 mg b.i.d., and aripiprazole long-acting injection 400 mg IM Q4 weeks. It was recommended that lamotrigine be further titrated up to a goal of 100–400 mg per day in split doses as tolerated and effective.

Key Issues

1. Patients with schizophrenia-spectrum disorder frequently have cognitive impairment. In an older adult, this cognitive impairment may mimic dementia.
2. Neuropsychological testing reveals a unique pattern of strengths and weaknesses that can help differentiate the cognitive deficits seen in schizophrenia from the deficits seen in dementia. It is common to have impairment in schizophrenia, but the extent and nature is unique to each individual.
3. Medication effects on cognition are an important consideration in patient education on risks and benefits of a particular drug regimen.

Chapter Review Questions

1. How does thought disorder differ from the cognitive changes seen in early dementia?
2. What is the relative risk of Alzheimer's disease in persons with schizophrenia?
3. What is the mechanism for cognitive impairment with anticholinergics?

References

1. American Psychiatric Association. Diagnostic and statistical manual of mental disorders. 5th ed. Arlington, VA: American Psychiatric Association; 2013.
2. Heinrichs RW, Zakzanis KK. Neurocognitive deficit in schizophrenia: a quantitative review of the evidence. Neuropsychology. 1998;12(3):426–45.
3. Mesholam-Gately RI, Giuliano AJ, Goff KP, Faraone SV, Seidman LJ. Neurocognition in first-episode schizophrenia: a meta-analytic review. Neuropsychology. 2009;23(3):315.
4. Owoso A, Carter CS, Gold JM, MacDonald AW, Ragland JD, Silverstein SM, Strauss ME, Barch DM. Cognition in schizophrenia and schizo-affective disorder: impairments that are more similar than different. Psychol Med. 2013;43(12):2535–45.
5. Bowie CR, Harvey PD. Cognitive deficits and functional outcome in schizophrenia. Neuropsychiatr Dis Treat. 2006;2(4):531.
6. Green MF. What are the functional consequences of neurocognitive deficits in schizophrenia? Am J Psychiatry. 1996;153:321–30.
7. Keefe RSE, Harvey PD. Cognitive impairment in schizophrenia. In: Novel antischizophrenia treatments. Berlin, Heidelberg: Springer; 2012. p. 11–37.
8. Copeland JR, Dewey ME, Scott A, Gilmore C, Larkin BA, Cleave N, et al. Schizophrenia and delusional disorder in older age: community prevalence, incidence, comorbidity, and outcome. Schizophr Bull. 1998;24(1):153.
9. Hjorthøj C, Stürup AE, McGrath J, Nordentoft M. SA57. Life expectancy and years of potential life lost in schizophrenia: a systematic review and meta-analysis. Schizophr Bull. 2017;43(Suppl 1):S133–4.
10. Östling S, Skoog I. Psychotic symptoms and paranoid ideation in a nondemented population–based sample of the very old. Arch Gen Psychiatry. 2002;59(1):53–9.
11. McGlashan TH. A selective review of recent North American long-term followup studies of schizophrenia. Schizophr Bull. 1988;14(4):515.
12. Thara R. Twenty-year course of schizophrenia: the Madras longitudinal study. Can J Psychiatry. 2004;49:564–9.
13. Depp CA, Loughran C, Palmer BW. Neuropsychological considerations in older adults with schizophrenia. In: Marcopulos BA, Kurtz M, editors. Clinical neuropsychological foundations of schizophrenia. New York: Psychology Press; 2012. p. 141–58.
14. Irani F, Kalkstein S, Moberg EA, Moberg PJ. Neuropsychological performance in older patients with schizophrenia: a meta-analysis of cross-sectional and longitudinal studies. Schizophr Bull. 2011;37(6):1318–26.
15. Ribe AR, Laursen TM, Charles M, Katon W, Fenger-Grøn M, Davydow D, Chwastiak L, Cerimele JM, Vestergaard M. Long-term risk of dementia in persons with schizophrenia: a Danish population-based cohort study. JAMA Psychiatry. 2015;72(11):1095–101.
16. Köhler S, Allardyce J, Verhey FR, McKeith IG, Matthews F, Brayne C, Savva GM. Cognitive decline and dementia risk in older adults with psychotic symptoms: a prospective cohort study. Am J Geriatr Psychiatry. 2013;21(2):119–28.

17. Sarter M, Bruno JP. Cognitive functions of cortical acetylcholine: toward a unifying hypothesis. Brain Res Rev. 1997;23(1):28–46.
18. Vallés AS, Borroni MV, Barrantes FJ. Targeting brain α7 nicotinic acetylcholine receptors in Alzheimer's disease: rationale and current status. CNS Drugs. 2014;28(11):975–87.
19. Fox C, Richardson K, Maidment ID, Savva GM, Matthews FE, Smithard D, et al. Anticholinergic medication use and cognitive impairment in the older population: the medical research council cognitive function and ageing study. J Am Geriatr Soc. 2011;59(8):1477–83.
20. Strauss ME, Reynolds KS, Jayaram G, Tune LE. Effects of anticholinergic medication on memory in schizophrenia. Schizophr Res. 1990;3(2):127–9.
21. Tracy JI, Monaco C, Giovannetti T, Abraham G, Josiassen RC. Anticholinergicity and cognitive processing in chronic schizophrenia. Biol Psychol. 2001;56(1):1–22.
22. Minzenberg MJ, Poole JH, Benton C, Vinogradov S. Association of anticholinergic load with impairment of complex attention and memory in schizophrenia. Am J Psychiatry. 2014;161(1):116–24.
23. Stone W, Keshavan M. Medical co-morbidity in schizophrenia. In: Marcopulos BA, Kurtz M, editors. Clinical neuropsychological foundations of schizophrenia. New York: Psychology Press; 2012. p. 159–80.
24. Holt R, Peveler R, Byrne C. Schizophrenia, the metabolic syndrome and diabetes. Diabetic Med. 2004;21(6):515–23.
25. Newcomer JW. Metabolic syndrome and mental illness. Am J Manag Care. 2007;13(7 Suppl):S170–7.
26. Reaven GM. Banting lecture 1988. Role of insulin resistance in human disease. Diabetes. 1988;37(12):1595–607.
27. Muller M, van Raamt F, Visseren FL, Kalmijn S, Geerlings MI, Mali WP, et al. Metabolic syndrome and cognition in patients with manifest atherosclerotic disease: the SMART study. Neuroepidemiology. 2010;34(2):83–9.
28. Dickinson D, Gold JM, Dickerson FB, Medoff D, Dixon LB. Evidence of exacerbated cognitive deficits in schizophrenia patients with comorbid diabetes. Psychosomatics. 2008;49(2):123–31.
29. Lezak MD, Howieson DB, Bigler ED, Tranel D. Neuropsychological assessment. New York: Oxford University Press; 2012.
30. Boone KB. Assessment of feigned cognitive impairment: a neuropsychological perspective. New York, NY: Guilford Press; 2007.
31. Bush SS, Ruff RM, Tröster AI, Barth JT, Koffler SP, Pliskin NH, et al. Symptom validity assessment: practice issues and medical necessity: NAN Policy & Planning Committee. Arch Clin Neuropsychol. 2005;20(4):419–26.
32. Heilbronner RL, Sweet JJ, Morgan JE, Larrabee GJ, Millis SR. American Academy of Clinical Neuropsychology consensus conference statement on the neuropsychological assessment of effort, response bias, and malingering. Clin Neuropsychol. 2009;23(7):1093–129.
33. Bondi MW, Jak AJ, Delano-Wood L, Jacobson MW, Delis DC, Salmon DP. Neuropsychological contributions to the early identification of Alzheimer's disease. Neuropsychol Rev. 2008;18(1):73–90.
34. Karantzoulis S, Galvin JE. Distinguishing Alzheimer's disease from other major forms of dementia. Expert Rev Neurother. 2011;11(11):1579–91.
35. Marcopulos BA, Gripshover DL, Broshek DK, McLain CA, McLain RH. Neuropsychological assessment of psychogeriatric patients with limited education. Clin Neuropsychol. 1999;13(2):147–56.
36. Berk M, Malhi GS, Gray LJ, Dean OM. The promise of N-acetylcysteine in neuropsychiatry. Trends Pharmacol Sci. 2013;34(3):167–77.
37. Zoccali R, Muscatello M, Bruno A, Cambria R, Mico U, Spina E, et al. The effect of lamotrigine augmentation of clozapine in a sample of treatment-resistant schizophrenic patients: a double-blind, placebo-controlled study. Schizophr Res. 2007;93(1):109–16.
38. Modabbernia A, Heidari P, Soleimani R, Sobhani A, Roshan ZA, Taslimi S, et al. Melatonin for prevention of metabolic side-effects of olanzapine in patients with first-episode schizophrenia: randomized double-blind placebo-controlled study. J Psychiatr Res. 2014;53:133–40.

Chapter 25
Neuroimaging and Neuropsychology

Erin D. Bigler

Neuroimaging has revolutionized all of the clinical neurosciences because of the exquisite manner in which the living brain can now be visualized [1, 2]. But it is more than just neuroanatomy; contemporary neuroimaging permits mapping of structure with function, as well as some aspects of brain metabolism. The fact that the 1979 Nobel Prize in Physiology or Medicine involved computed tomography (CT) and the 2003 prize was for magnetic resonance imaging (MRI) is a testament of the contribution that these imaging techniques have made to medicine and neuroscience.

Although neuropsychology is the discipline that utilizes psychometric technique to assess the behavioral and cognitive effects of neurological and neuropsychiatric disorder [3], the integration of neuroimaging findings with neuropsychology, both structural and functional, is rapidly emerging [4, 5]. In fact these advancements lead Kelly and Castellanos [6] to indicate the importance that neuroimaging adds to "… the neuropsychologist's toolbox for evaluating the sequelae of brain insult (p. 63. e-print)."

This chapter will give an overview of the general principles of neuroimaging that are relevant to neuropsychological assessment as well as to various medical disciplines. The interface of what the psychologist may interpret about brain-behavior relations using neuroimaging enhances medical decision making using the same information. Given the commonness of CT and MRI, for most patients with some type of neurological and/or neuropsychiatric disorder, some form of neuroimaging will have been performed. This chapter uses several cases to highlight how neuropsychologists utilize neuroimaging findings.

E. D. Bigler (✉)
Department of Psychology, Brigham Young University, Provo, UT, USA

Neuroscience Center, Brigham Young University, Provo, UT, USA

Magnetic Resonance Imaging Research Facility, Brigham Young University, Provo, UT, USA

Department of Psychiatry, University of Utah, Salt Lake City, UT, USA
e-mail: erin_bigler@byu.edu

K. M. Sanders (ed.), *Physician's Field Guide to Neuropsychology*,
https://doi.org/10.1007/978-1-4939-8722-1_25

CT and MRI Comparisons

The neuroimaging review by Wilde et al. [7] provides a more thorough overview of neuroimaging principles than what can be covered in this chapter. Figure 25.1 provides a brief synopsis of CT and MRI comparisons using the standard, conventional clinical imaging methods. CT derives the tomographic image by detecting the passage of X-ray beams through tissue at different orientations allowing computer reconstruction of a two-dimensional section of the tissue (see Fig. 25.1). The image reflects tissue density where the bone is bright white, water [cerebral spinal fluid (CSF)] or air is dark, gray matter is light gray, and white matter is darker gray.

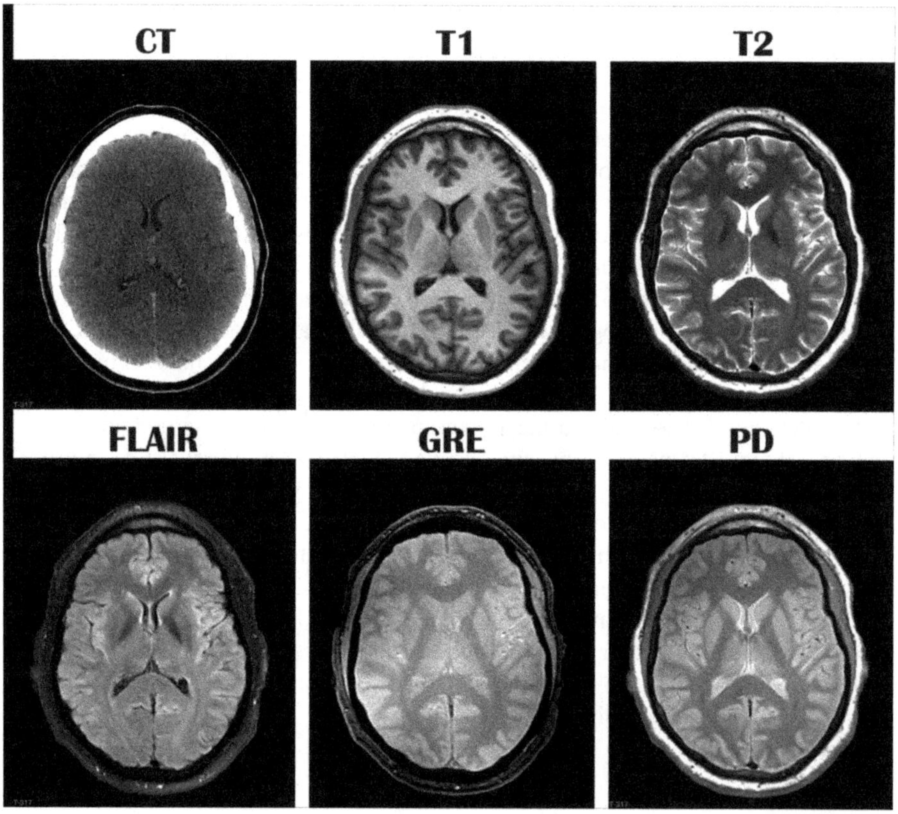

Fig. 25.1 The images are all from the same individual and all performed at approximately the same level in a 45-year-old male control with no abnormalities. *CT* computed tomography, *T1* T1-weighted anatomical MRI with distinct white-gray matter boundaries, *T2* T2-weighted MRI where the hyperintense (white) signal indicates CSF or higher water content, *FLAIR* fluid-attenuated inversion recovery MRI sequence that is best in detecting abnormal white matter, *GRE* gradient-recalled echo that is particularly sensitive to blood by-products like hemosiderin but what is referred to as susceptibility-weighted imaging (SWI) shows even better detection for hemorrhage and associated findings, and *PD* proton density-weighted MRI also good at detecting pathology

Although CT contrast agents may be given and the procedure is modified for blood perfusion and radiotracer uptake studies such as that done with positron-emission or single-photon emission computed tomography, the basic image is the same.

With MRI, there is considerably greater range of imaging sequences designed to detect different aspects of neuropathology (see Fig. 25.1). With magnetic resonance (MR), different imaging sequences reflect differences in tissue types and pathologies. As shown in Fig. 25.1, there are several standard, conventional MR sequences. Each sequence depends on differences in the excitation pulses of strong magnetic fields separated by a repetition time. This is why each is referred to as a "pulse sequence" associated with an acronym, as listed in Fig. 25.1. Within each pulse sequence, the image findings are described in terms of signal intensity in the detection of the radiofrequency wave. The T1 sequence is often referred to as the anatomical sequence and provides an overall view of the brain, where gray matter is dark gray, white matter is light gray to white, and CSF is dark. T2 highlights CSF, and because differences in water content often characterize pathological changes, the T2 sequence is better at detecting pathological changes. The fluid-attenuated inversion recovery (FLAIR) sequence is particularly sensitive in detecting white matter pathology and the gradient-recalled echo (GRE) at detecting blood by-products (i.e., hemosiderin) as is the susceptibility-weighted imaging (SWI) sequence (not shown in Fig. 25.1). Diffusion tensor imaging (DTI) is an additional method for examining white matter integrity of the brain. Magnetic resonance spectroscopy permits quantification of certain aspects of metabolism.

Clinical Integration of Neuroimaging and Neuropsychology

Figure 25.2 presents the MRI findings in a 31-year-old with multiple sclerosis (MS). Cognitively, neuropsychological testing demonstrated generally intact functioning except for reduced speed of processing, a common finding in MS. Emotionally, though, anxiety-mediated problems were prominent, with frequent panic-anxiety attacks. Figure 25.2 shows the classic pattern of white matter hyperintensities on the FLAIR and T2 sequences typical of MS, and the fact that several of the abnormalities involved corpus callosum and deep white matter tracts represents a consistent finding with motor slowing and diminished processing speed.

However, the largest signal abnormality was actually in the right temporal lobe, within the temporal stem, as shown in Fig. 25.3. Using the T1 anatomical image to slice through that region, it is readily visualized that these white matter regions are adjacent to the hippocampus and amygdala. In that these are prominent regions involved in emotional control and regulation, some of the emotional dysregulation in this patient is likely related to pathology at this level of the temporal lobe.

By knowing functional neuroanatomy, the knowledge of how common neuropsychological symptoms/problems map on to neural function permits the integration of neuroimaging findings with those from neuropsychological testing and consultation. Some MS lesions may not be producing a detectable neuropsychological

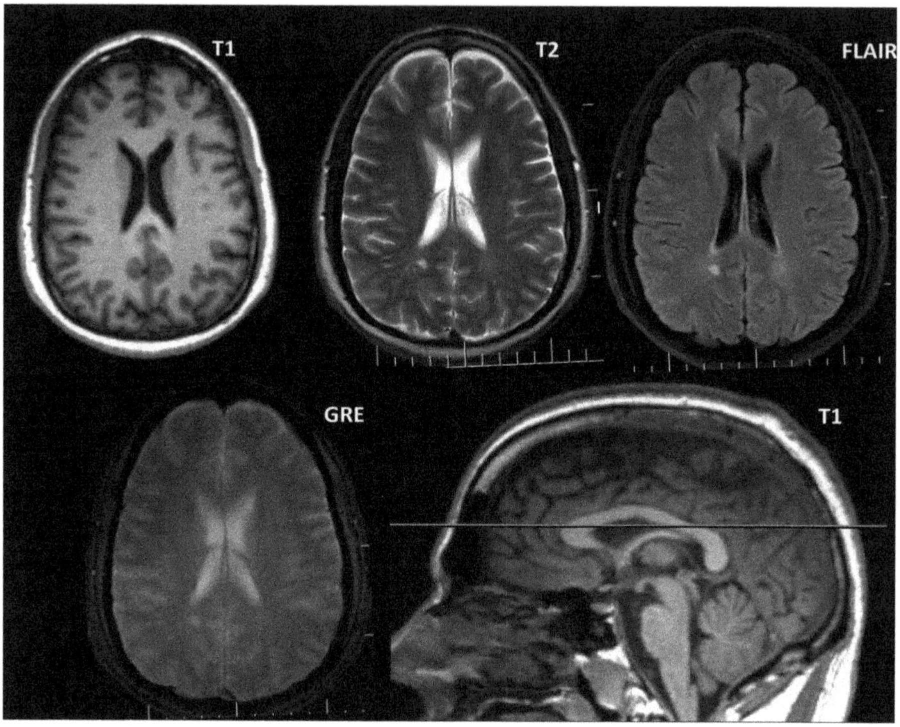

Fig. 25.2 These MRI studies are from a 31-year-old male with MS. Note the hyperintense signal abnormality in both the T2 and FLAIR images, characteristic of MS. Also note on the FLAIR sequence the subtle yet hyperintense signal in the posterior periventricular area and the outer extent of the forceps major. Also note that the T1 and GRE sequences are not very sensitive in detecting the MS pathology. The sagittal T1 image in the lower right depicts the plane at which the horizontal sections were taken

impairment, hence performing a comprehensive neuropsychological examination is important.

While the images in Figs. 25.2 and 25.3 distinctly identify areas of white matter abnormality, because of issues related to resiliency and plasticity, the precise location of MS lesions is not necessarily predictive of the type and level of cognitive impairment [8, 9]. Accordingly, while neuroimaging findings are critical in establishing the MS diagnosis, the neuropsychological examination defines the cognitive, emotional, and neurobehavioral deficits that may accompany the disorder. Furthermore, because MS pathology may change, particularly in relapse and remitting MS, the neuropsychological studies provide an ongoing reference for the level of function and potential treatment programming. The collaboration between physician and psychologist, as in this case, provides a more comprehensive and thorough assessment along with better understanding of the medical and cognitive-emotional issues in a patient with MS.

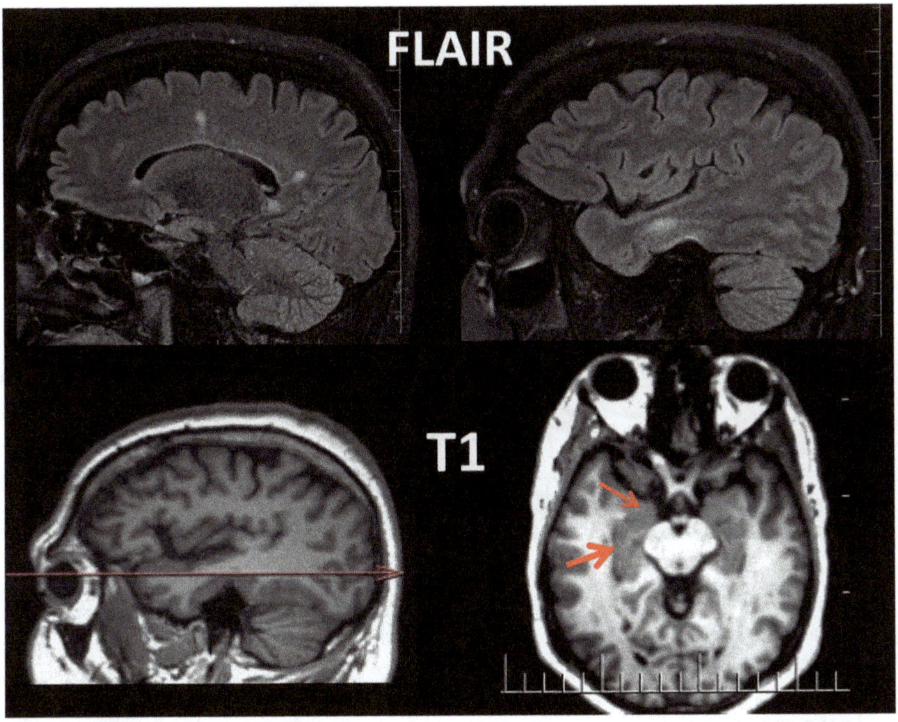

Fig. 25.3 Sagittal FLAIR images at the level of the outer margins of the corpus callosum and beginning of the corona radiata (left) through the temporal stem of the temporal lobe (right). The anatomical sagittal T1 at the bottom left shows the plane for the axial cut, and the bottom right depicts the location of the hyperintense signal in the temporal lobe adjacent to the hippocampus (bottom arrow) and amygdala (top arrow)

Key Point
The neuropsychological test findings demonstrate the relative importance of the lesion on behavior and cognition.

Tracking Pathology over Time

Figure 25.4 shows the day-of-injury (DOI) CT scan from a patient with severe traumatic brain injury (TBI). It shows a distinct but small petechial hemorrhage. This is an obvious abnormality, but CT is less sensitive in detecting small hemorrhage associated with TBI where MRI techniques, especially the GRE and SWI sequences, are superior. Additionally, MRI findings, several weeks to months post-injury, better relate to the neuropsychological outcome.

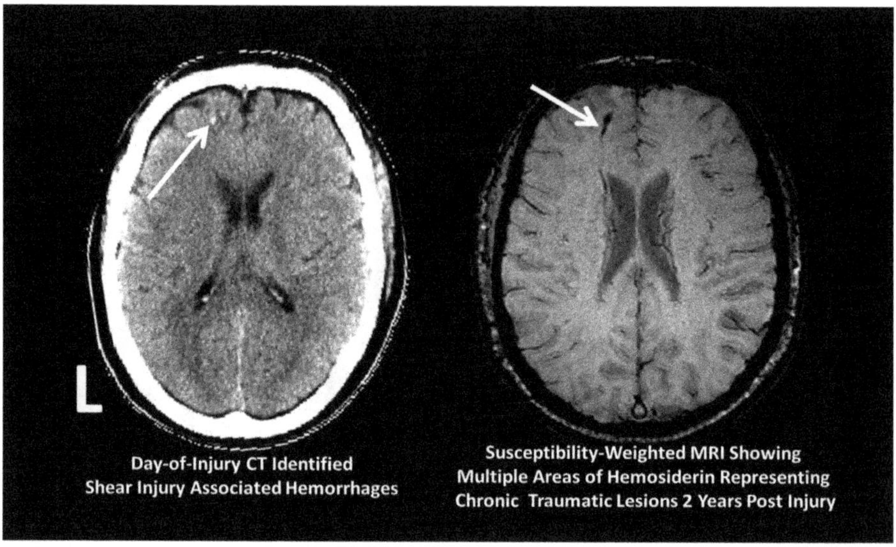

Fig. 25.4 (Left) Day-of-injury (DOI) CT with a solitary petechial hemorrhage in the frontal lobe. (Right) Contrast susceptibility-weighted imaging (SWI) shows that the hemorrhagic lesion was larger than that detected by the CT. Because the images in Fig. 25.5 are presented in 3-D, these axial images show left on the viewer's left

In the subacute timeframe, this patient had some of the typical cognitive impairments in memory and executive functioning commonly experienced in those who have sustained a severe TBI, but the DOI CT scan had only shown a small solitary frontal hemorrhage, so the treating physicians were optimistic about the outcome. However, a very prominent deficit in motivation and drive emerged post-discharge from rehabilitation even though cognitive ability improved. As this patient was followed neuropsychologically which documented that cognitive function had in large part returned to baseline, one explanation for the clinical presentation of poor motivation would be a frontal lobe-type disorder that affected drive and motivation more than cognitive ability. Furthermore, there was a need to determine whether this was post-injury depression or something more specific to the residual brain damage from the TBI.

Accordingly, in this patient when follow-up MR imaging was performed, as shown in Fig. 25.5, a rather dramatic evidence for larger and multiple hemorrhagic lesions were found throughout the frontal lobes, beyond what would have been predicted by the DOI CT. This type of hemorrhagic lesion formation reflects underlying shear injury to the brain and is a biomarker for diffuse axonal injury (DAI). Furthermore, when a DTI sequence was applied, which permits the demonstration of aggregate white matter tracts in the brain, it was apparent that significant white matter damage had occurred throughout the anterior projections of the corpus callosum, disengaging both frontal lobes from optimal level of connectivity. Taken together, this trauma-related pathology was much more extensive, as demonstrated

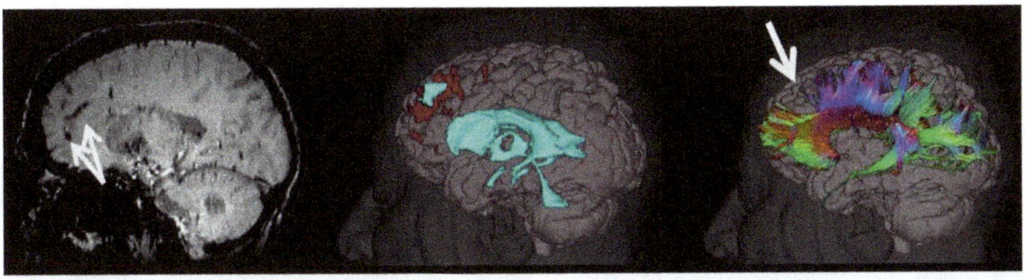

Fig. 25.5 (Left) Sagittal SWI shows the true extensiveness of the hemorrhagic lesions (white arrows) and when plotted on 3-D images. (Middle) 3-D rendered lateral view where red depicts all of the locations where hemosiderin was detected. Aquamarine outlines the ventricle and a pocket of CSF that developed around where the shear lesions occurred. (Right) DTI of the corpus callosum where the color map shows the directionality of the projecting fiber tracts. Green indicates more lateral projection, blue more vertical, and warm (red-orange) reflecting side-to-side or laterally projecting fibers. The white arrow points to a major loss of projecting tracts

on MRI, than what would have been predicted if only the DOI CT scan had been performed. Furthermore, this type of brain pathology was consistent with the type of frontal lobe disorder that the patient exhibited.

In this patient, the synergism between using neuropsychological assessment findings to monitor the recovery of cognitive function simultaneously with documenting the emergence of a frontal lobe behavioral disorder, with neuroimaging confirmation, demonstrates how useful these assessment modalities may be. In other words, imaging or neuropsychological testing would not have answered the clinical question; however, the confluence of the two assessment modalities comprehensively addressed the diagnostic question. Furthermore, because outwardly this patient had recovered physical function and did not appear impaired, having the objective neuroimaging information to show the spouse, family, and treatment team assisted all in understanding the frontal lobe disorder.

Figure 25.6 compares the DOI neuroimaging with follow-up and shows the initial CT scan from a patient who unfortunately had an aneurysm involving the internal carotid artery on the right at the point it branches into the middle cerebral artery (MCA). When it ruptured a massive infarction along the distribution of the MCA ensued, as shown in the figure. Post-injury encephalomalacic and porencephalic cystic changes dominated the entire right hemisphere, and there had been a secondary infarction involving the left frontal area. Neuropsychologically, she exhibited a dense left hemiplegia, complete left hemianopia, and left-side visual neglect. She had a prominent expressive aphasia but remarkably some spared receptive abilities. Nonetheless, given the extensiveness of damage, minimal expectation for improvement or even recommendations for cognitive therapies seemed indicated other than to maintain the level of function.

This case provides another example of the interface between neuroimaging and neuropsychology because neuroimaging provides a physical example of the damaged brain that the neuropsychologist may use in providing feedback to the family as well as the treatment team. The obliteration of the left hemisphere in this

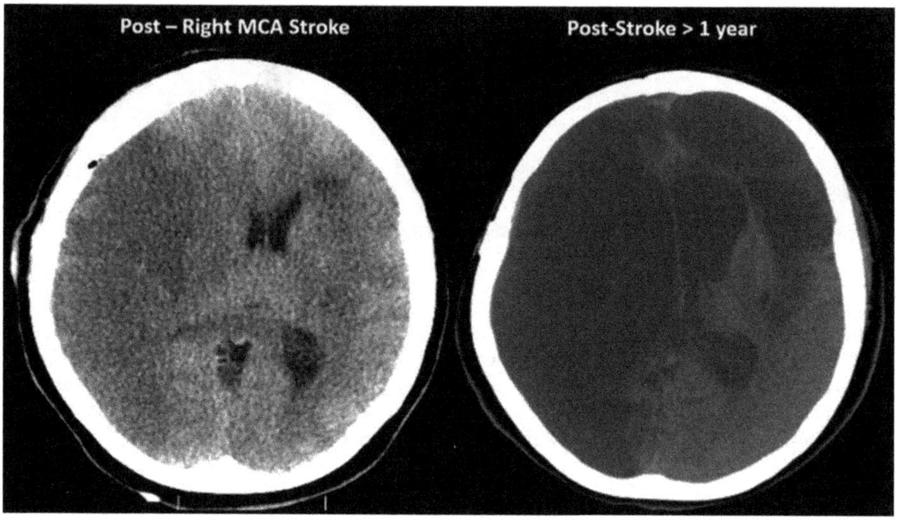

Fig. 25.6 (Left) This patient experienced a rupture of a carotid artery aneurysm leading to a right middle cerebral artery (MCA) stroke. The CT on the left was performed at about 48 h post-incident and depicts the generalized infarction along the distribution of the entire right MCA with extensive brain edema and midline shift. (Right) More than 1 year post-injury, extensive regions of cystic formation as a consequence of the infarction along with a large secondary left frontal infarction, likely a result of the massive cerebral edema that occurred

case combined with the massive frontotemporal damage to the right simply meant minimal survivable cortical tissue, limiting the possibility for shifting recovery to less damaged cortical regions. Furthermore, most of the behavior observed was reflective of subcortical, cerebellar, and brainstem functions. Using the objective findings from the neuroimaging studies provided the opportunity to explain the profound neuropsychological impairments to the family.

Key Point
Neuroimaging provides objective visual information for physicians and neuropsychologists to explain test findings and diagnostic conclusions to patients and families.

Quantitative Neuroimaging

There is a simple but elegant fact about gross brain anatomy, as imaged by MRI. White matter, gray matter, and CSF have distinct signal intensity differences and typically clear boundaries, wherein an image voxel can be defined as representing all or mostly one tissue type. By first "segmenting" the brain MRI into white matter-, gray matter-, or CSF-defined regions, the image can be then "classified" according to traditional anatomic designation. These methods are now automated

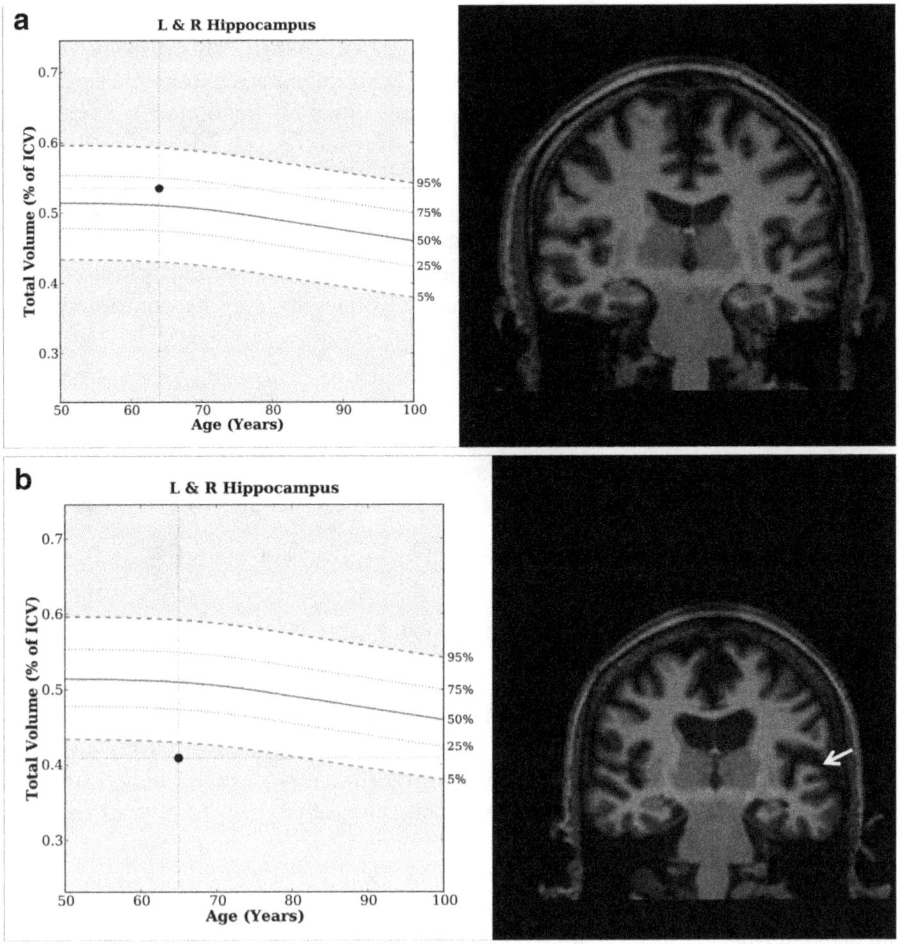

Fig. 25.7 (**a**) The author's quantitative imaging based on segmented and classified MRI. The colorized region-of-interest map of a coronal section shows the hippocampus highlighted in yellow with the age plot showing above-average volume, adjusted for brain volume. (**b**) For comparison, this patient has significant deficits in memory and executive functioning and likely a dementing illness. Note that the hippocampal volume is distinctly below the 5th percentile, and as can be seen the white arrow points to a prominent Sylvian fissure, indicative of temporal lobe atrophy, and the hippocampus is visibly smaller than what is observed in (**b**)

and may be completed with minimal time [10]. For example, the image shown in Fig. 25.7 is the classified coronal image of a 64-year-old (this is in fact the author when he was that age compared to a similarly aged patient with memory and cognitive deficits). Furthermore, by acquiring the image in 3-D with known slice thickness and no gap between slices, determination of region of interest (ROI) volume may be obtained for any region. Part of successful aging relates to the rate of normal apoptosis and development of atrophic changes with age. The hippocampus is critical in that process, and Fig. 25.7a shows that in comparison with those 64 years of age, the author's hippocampal volume is above average. This also provides a baseline, and by combining memory testing with quantitative imaging, cognitive functioning may be tracked over time in conjunction with anatomical changes. For example, the patient shown in Fig. 25.7b has neuropsychological findings of impaired cognitive ability and likely has a dementing illness. As shown in the figure, this patient who was of a similar age to the author has hippocampal volume dramatically below what would be age-typical. This approach provides an excellent demonstration of the interface between neuroimaging and neuropsychology and how both neuropsychological testing and neuroimaging may be contrasted with age-mediated differences.

Key Point
Quantitative neuroimaging permits identification of regions of interest to assess their anatomical integrity in relation to neurocognitive and neurobehavioral functioning.

Functional Neuroimaging

Within MRI technology is the capability of measuring changes in blood flow by detecting differences in the blood oxygen level-dependent (BOLD) contrast. Because neuronal activation is coupled with differences in blood flow, using the BOLD signal to detect differences in magnetization of oxygen-rich versus oxygen-poor regions actually reflects differences in underlying neuronal activation. Using sophisticated image analysis tools to detect the most prominent BOLD signal differences in the brain, the areas of greatest activation coincide with brain regions most involved during a neuropsychological task when the neurocognitive probe is modified for test administration within the scanner. By having an individual perform cognitive tasks in the scanner, activation plots may be derived which show the greatest likelihood of which brain regions are involved in a particular function. An example is given in Fig. 25.8 showing areas of activation involving the commonly used neuropsychological measurement referred to as the Trail Making Test (TMT, [11]). The TMT taps both speed of sequential processing and executive planning where the patient has to string together using a pencil to "connect the dots" in sequence (see Fig. 25.8). The faster one performs the task, the better, and to perform the task most efficiently requires planning and integration [12]. Using the BOLD technique and adapting the TMT to be able to perform in the scanner allow the plotting of the primary regions of activation associated with performing the task, as shown in Fig. 25.7. From what is depicted in Fig. 25.7 in this right-handed individual, it is quite straightforward to visualize the pathways and ROIs involved in this task. The visual-spatial component obviously dominates, especially involving the right occipitoparietal region but also the left frontal areas involved in primary motor cortex of the right body side with motor activation extending into premotor areas involved in

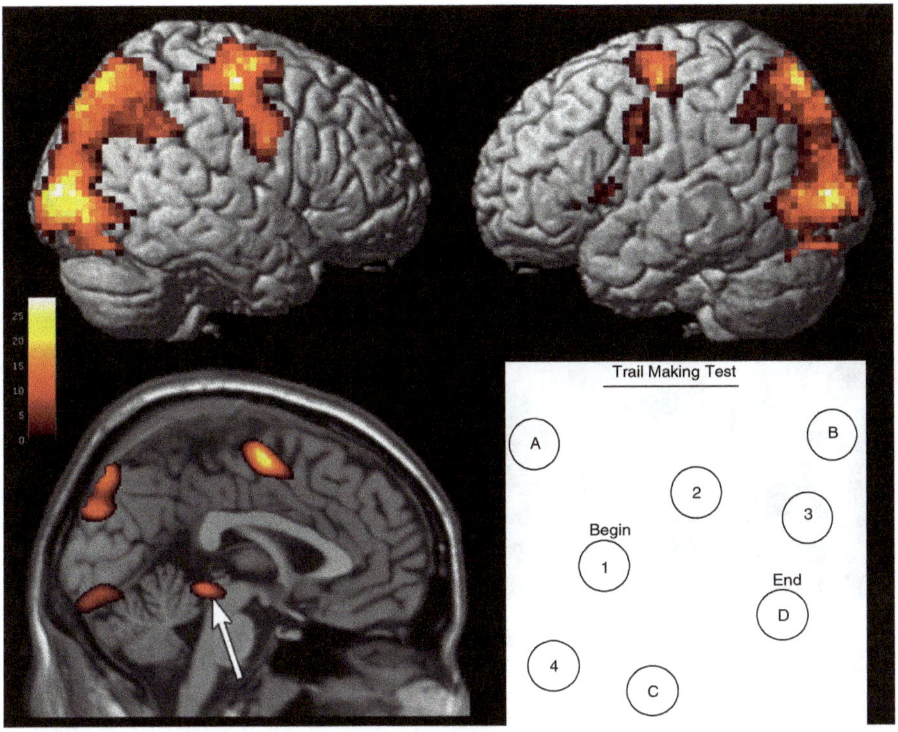

Fig. 25.8 Functional MRI where the BOLD signal of main activation during performance of the Trail Making Test is plotted. A protype example of the Trail Making Test is shown in the lower right. Arrow points to activation at the level of the superior colliculus

motor planning. The bilateral activation patterns would require interhemispheric pathways across the corpus callosum, and the posterior activations to connect with frontal would also engage the superior longitudinal fasciculus. The arrow in Fig. 25.8 points to the superior colliculus of the midbrain, likely mediating eye-tracking movements necessary to perform the task. From these kinds of images, inferences can be made about underlying tracts that would need to be intact to perform TMT which could then be investigated with other imaging modalities like DTI and what is referred to as resting state functional connectivity mapping [13].

Although technically a structural imaging technique, DTI also permits answering questions about functional integrity. The image shown in Fig. 25.9 depicts the postsurgical resection of a large astrocytoma that was in the inferior posterior temporal-occipital lobe region. Neuropsychologically, the patient had left-side hemianopia without neglect, but with visual memory defects as visual retention of information tends to be most affected with right hemisphere damage in those who are right handed, which was the case with this individual. The neuropsychological question was whether it would be better to try compensatory training for visual memory by turning visual tasks into more verbally mediated ones or a more direct approach of retraining visual memory. As can be seen in the imaging, the residual damage was extensive as reflected in the T2 axial image, but the DTI distinctly

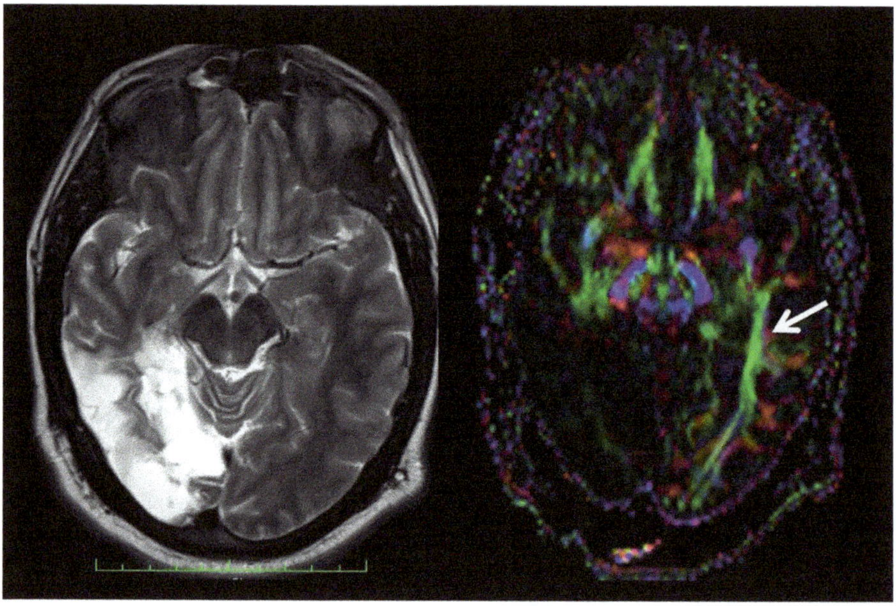

Fig. 25.9 (Left) Axial T2 MRI post-resection for an astrocytoma involving much of the right posterior temporal-occipital region. (Right) DTI at a similar axial section demonstrates the absence of any viable white matter connections of the right hemisphere. The arrow points to an intact occipitotemporal fasciculus. Scans in a radiological perspective, with left on the viewer's right

shows no viable white matter pathways that would likely need to be present if direct visual retraining were to be attempted. Indeed, the verbal compensatory method facilitated this individual's return to college, with eventual graduation.

The case in Fig. 25.9 and the fact that this individual had compensated well, given the size of the post-tumor resection and residual damage, provides another example of the beneficial relation between the information that comes from medicine and neuropsychology. One look at Fig. 25.9 and the amount of structural damage is obvious and would be expected to produce devastating cognitive impairments. However, neuropsychological testing and consultation was able to guide and direct cognitive and rehabilitative therapies resulting in the patient's return to college. Furthermore, using the neuropsychological and neuroimaging information, accommodations were achieved that permitted this individual to complete a college education. Other than the patient's residual visual field defect, other intact regions were able to take over function. Without neuropsychological input, the neuroimaging findings could have been overinterpreted in terms of the residual functional deficits.

Key Point

Neuropsychological consultation and assessment help define the neurobehavioral and neurocognitive consequences of brain abnormalities observed in neuroimaging studies.

The Future

In this author's opinion, much of the neuropsychological assessment will be integrated with neuroimaging over the next decade. With rapid automated neuroimaging methods providing volumetric and morphometric information about critical brain regions, understanding the relation between volume and morphology derived from neuroimaging with neuropsychological test findings will only improve over the next decade (see [4]). Algorithms will be developed that incorporate multiple neuropsychological, neuroimaging, and other relevant medical variables into predictive modeling related to diagnosis and outcome. Furthermore, with advances in functional neuroimaging, neurocognitive probes will become refined in their ability to identify critical brain regions that participate in certain functions, as well as improve techniques to investigate networks and their functioning in terms of neuropsychological test performance.

Chapter Review Questions

1. Given the type and location of certain pathologies, as shown in neuroimaging studies, the neuropsychological examination may assist in defining the:
   A. Relation between emotional findings and brain pathology.
   B. Relation between neurobehavioral functioning and brain pathology.
   C. Relation between neurocognitive functioning and brain pathology.
   D. All of the above.
2. The future of the neuroimaging-neuropsychology interface will see the development of:
   A. Quantitative neuroimaging providing normative data about brain structural integrity.
   B. Algorithms that integrate neuropsychological test findings with quantitative neuroimaging.
   C. Direct cognitive testing from functional neuroimaging probes.
   D. All of the above.

References

1. Bigler ED. Neuroimaging biomarkers in mild traumatic brain injury (mTBI). Neuropsychol Rev. 2013;23(3):169–209. https://doi.org/10.1007/s11065-013-9237-2.
2. Kloppel S, Abdulkadir A, Jack CR Jr, Koutsouleris N, Mourao-Miranda J, Vemuri P. Diagnostic neuroimaging across diseases. [Review]. NeuroImage. 2012;61(2):457–63. https://doi.org/10.1016/j.neuroimage.2011.11.002.
3. Lezak MD, Howieson DB, Bigler ED, Tranel D. Neuropsychological assessment. 5th ed. New York: Oxford; 2012.

4. Bilder RM. Neuropsychology 3.0: evidence-based science and practice. [Historical Article Research Support, N.I.H., Extramural Research Support, Non-U.S. Gov't Review]. J Int Neuropsychol Soc. 2011;17(1):7–13. https://doi.org/10.1017/S1355617710001396.
5. Chanraud S, Zahr N, Sullivan EV, Pfefferbaum A. MR diffusion tensor imaging: a window into white matter integrity of the working brain. [Research Support, N.I.H., Extramural Review. Neuropsychol Rev. 2010;20(2):209–25. https://doi.org/10.1007/s11065-010-9129-7.
6. Kelly C, Castellanos FX. Strengthening connections: functional connectivity and brain plasticity. Neuropsychol Rev. 2014;24(1):63–76. https://doi.org/10.1007/s11065-014-9252-y.
7. Wilde EA, Hunter JV, Bigler ED. A primer of neuroimaging analysis in neurorehabilitation outcome research. [Review]. NeuroRehabilitation. 2012;31(3):227–42. https://doi.org/10.3233/NRE-2012-0793.
8. Chiaravalloti ND, Genova HM, DeLuca J. Cognitive rehabilitation in multiple sclerosis: the role of plasticity. [Review]. Front Neurol. 2015;6:67. https://doi.org/10.3389/fneur.2015.00067.
9. DeLuca GC, Yates RL, Beale H, Morrow SA. Cognitive impairment in multiple sclerosis: clinical, radiologic and pathologic insights. [Research Support, Non-U.S. Gov't]. Brain Pathol. 2015;25(1):79–98. https://doi.org/10.1111/bpa.12220.
10. Bigler ED, Abildskov TJ, Wilde EA, McCauley SR, Li X, Merkley TL, et al. Diffuse damage in pediatric traumatic brain injury: a comparison of automated versus operator-controlled quantification methods. [Comparative Study Research Support, N.I.H., Extramural]. NeuroImage. 2010;50(3):1017–26. https://doi.org/10.1016/j.neuroimage.2010.01.003.
11. Reitan RM. The relation of the trail making test to organic brain damage. J Consult Psychol. 1955;19(5):393–4.
12. Allen MD, Fong AK. Clinical application of standardized cognitive assessment using fMRI. I. Matrix reasoning. Behav Neurol. 2008;20(3):127–40. https://doi.org/10.3233/BEN-2008-0223.
13. Nielsen JA, Zielinski BA, Fletcher PT, Alexander AL, Lange N, Bigler ED, et al. Abnormal lateralization of functional connectivity between language and default mode regions in autism. Mol Autism. 2014;5(1):8. https://doi.org/10.1186/2040-2392-5-8.

Chapter 26
Traumatic Brain Injury Rehabilitation Case Study

Samantha L. Backhaus and Ana Durand-Sanchez

Case Example: Rehabilitation of Traumatic Brain Injury (Physician's Field Guide)

Neuropsychological testing and treatment—the importance of assessment of cognition and mood and the importance of collaboration to help achieve positive outcome goals.

Introduction

This is a case example of traumatic brain injury (TBI) using neuropsychological (NP) and neurological evaluations and follow-ups to assist the patient in helping her reach her long-term rehabilitation goals. The largest obstacles to achieving success included the patient's defensiveness and psychological reactions to her situation, fatigue, and higher-level cognitive challenges, which were detected on neuropsychological assessment.

S. L. Backhaus (✉)
Department of Physical Medicine and Rehabilitation, Rehabilitation Hospital of Indiana—Indiana University, Indianapolis, IN, USA
e-mail: samantha.backhaus@rhin.com

A. Durand-Sanchez
Department of Physical Medicine and Rehabilitation, Indiana University School of Medicine, Indianapolis, IN, USA

K. M. Sanders (ed.), *Physician's Field Guide to Neuropsychology*,
https://doi.org/10.1007/978-1-4939-8722-1_26

Key Questions

1. What are the benefits of conducting a neuropsychological examination, and how can this data be used to help the physiatrist manage the overall care?
2. How can the neuropsychologist and the physiatrist collaborate effectively to help the patient reach her neurorehabilitation goals?

This case study helps to demonstrate the value of NP testing in the treatment of TBI, as well as the value of establishing a strong collaborative relationship between the neuropsychologist and the physiatrist specializing in brain injury rehabilitation.

Key Point
A traumatic brain injury (TBI) is an injury to the brain that generally results from an impact or blow to the head. Closed head injuries can be caused by motor vehicle accident (causing acceleration/deceleration of the brain) falls, violent assaults, electrocution, and blast injuries occurring in military situations. Open head injuries can be caused by penetrations to the brain tissue from moving objects, open head wounds, and gunshot wounds [1]. The consequences of TBI can be devastating for the patient and can affect the individual from a holistic standpoint. Specifically, TBI most often causes challenges to cognitive, emotional, behavioral, and physical functions. Long-term cognitive effects on patients typically include but are not limited to deficits in learning and memory, attention, processing speed, and higher-level executive functions. Neurobehavioral consequences can include lack of initiation, emotional lability, aggression, agitation, lack of awareness, behavioral rigidity, and impulsivity. Emotional difficulties are also common and include depression, anxiety, apathy, frustration, and suicidality. Medical and health-related consequences can occur, including changes in sexual functioning, sleep, and metabolic and endocrine abnormalities [2–4]. Together, these challenges can affect one's ability to return to important aspects of life, including participation in vocational, social, marital, relational, financial, and other community-related tasks. Unfortunately, research findings suggest that individuals who experience moderate-to-severe TBI are likely to experience these problems over long periods of time post-injury [5].

Referral Question

Patient: 27-year-old female
Education: Associate degree
Occupation: Registered nurse (RN)

The patient is a 27-year-old female who suffered traumatic brain injury (TBI) in a work-related incident (to be described in further detail below) and was referred for a neuropsychological examination to determine her neurocognitive status as well as obtain appropriate treatment recommendations. The patient's overall care was managed and directed by her workman's compensation case worker to assist her in receiving evaluations and recommended treatments.

Medical Treatments and Concerns

To briefly review, the patient suffered a motor vehicle accident (MVA) while at work. According to medical records, she sustained multiple head injuries including skull fracture, contusion of the anterior frontal lobe and right central lobe, subarachnoid contusion, fractures of the left occipital bone, pneumocephalus of the left middle cranial fossa, and right frontal parietal intracranial hemorrhage requiring emergent right craniectomy and decompression. Her initial Glasgow Coma Scale (GCS) was 3 (lowest score possible), and she was lifelined to a local level 1 trauma center where she was emergently treated and received neurosurgery. Her hospitalization was complicated by recurrent high intracranial pressure. Once she was stabilized at the acute hospital, she was transferred to an inpatient brain injury rehabilitation hospital to obtain comprehensive brain injury care. Following her discharge from the inpatient rehabilitation hospital, she was transferred to another transitional rehabilitation hospital to focus on receiving specialized neurobehavioral therapies, as many of her challenges centered around her neurocognitive and neurobehavioral disruptions, including episodes of agitation, impaired awareness of deficits, akathisia, impaired attention and memory, as well as sleep–wake cycle dysregulation and abnormality of gait. Following completion of rehabilitation treatment at the transitional facility, she returned home to temporarily live with her parents, who could provide supervision. She was referred to the current physiatrist to manage ongoing outpatient neurorehabilitation care, as well as to a local brain injury comprehensive outpatient neurorehabilitation center where she was primarily followed by the neuropsychologist. The neuropsychologist and physiatrist continued to closely collaborate to help manage her overall rehabilitation care and help achieve goals.

Such goals included the following:

- Return to making independent decisions.
- Able to be alone and requiring no supervision.
- Return to independent living with minimal assistance.
- Return to driving with minimal assistance.
- Return to working as a RN with minimal accommodations or assistance.
- Maintain and monitor overall neurobehavioral status and mood as to achieve optimal psychological health and well-being.

Based on a patient's symptoms, the physician must attempt to clarify the best management approach. At times, workup of possible underlying problems will be needed. Other times, the management will be targeted toward the relief of symptoms, assuming that acute or potentially threatening issues have been addressed or ruled out. Ensuring comorbidities are assessed and managed is important in order to keep them from worsening TBI-related symptoms and from acting as confounding variables or impediments to the recovery process.

Physical Concerns

Fatigue is a common symptom after TBI. It can occur in up to 70% of individuals early after injury and has a prevalence of 44% [6, 7]. While it often improves over time, not all patients return to their pre-injury baseline. In this case, the patient struggled with moderate fatigue in the first 6 months after her injury, which kept her from being active for more than a few hours a day and forced her to take naps and to use energy "budgeting" strategies to accomplish her most important goals on a given day. After her discharge from post-acute rehabilitation, she was weaned off antipsychotics to avoid their sedative effects. Various formulations and schedules (frequencies) of methylphenidate were used to help her get through the better part of the day with the use of only a 30–45-minute nap. Later on, she returned to work and continued to struggle with cognitive fatigue that she described as "hitting a wall" as early as 1 p.m. on most days. Her pituitary function (TSH, FT4, and cortisol) was assessed, and no abnormalities were found, so we continued to ensure adequate management of mood, sleep, and energy conservation strategies, along with adjustment of neurostimulants. Finally, over a year after her injury, she was able to stay alert and focused until the late afternoon or early evening without taking a nap on the days that she worked. Almost 2 years after her injury, she continued to struggle with cognitive fatigue. Although her fatigue is less frequent, she continues to experience less cognitive and emotional efficiency later in the day. She continues to practice energy conservation strategies by doing more challenging tasks in the day, taking power naps earlier in the day, and ensuring that she gets adequate sleep at night.

Headaches are among the top complaints of post-TBI patients. In a prospective study, the cumulative incidence was 91% over 1 year [8]. Given the traumatic, often high-speed mechanisms of injury involved in TBI, it is important to assess the type of headache, taking into consideration the frequent musculoskeletal changes present in this population. These are often present along with other types of headaches (e.g., cervicogenic or tension type), and at times the only etiology may be cervicogenic head pain. Important considerations include the development of hydrocephalus in patients with a history of intracranial bleeds or that of subclinical seizures [9]. In this case fortunately, the patient did not report suffering with any post-traumatic headaches.

Visual deficits are another frequent complaint in this population [10]. Unfortunately, the patient's symptoms are often dismissed after normal reading chart and fundoscopic examination. However, the most common etiology of visual deficits in this population is related to abnormal activity or incoordination of the muscles that drive eye movements or to the brain's inability to superimpose or decode acquired images accurately. It is important to remember that these deficits can and often do impact the patient's headache symptoms and are at times the only trigger of pain and fatigue with visual tasks including phone, computer work, reading, and writing. In this case, the patient was found to have vague visual deficits early on and was referred to a neurooptometrist, who is an optometrist that subspecializes in the visual ailments of people with neurologic conditions. Given the tremendous impact visual deficits can have in daily function and quality of life, the specialized clinical and diagnostic tests required to determine these deficits, and the importance of obtaining an appropriate visual rehabilitation plan, it is strongly recommended that patients with TBI be referred specifically to a neurooptometrist, even if they have already seen an ophthalmologist for other concerns. The patient's visual challenges gradually improved over time and were not noted to impact her functionality in any way.

Dyssomnias have been reported in up to 70% of TBI patients [11]. These can be quite difficult to treat and should not be ignored, as sleep–wake cycle disturbances can drive other physical, cognitive, and emotional challenges suffered in this population. Dyssomnias may be TBI-related sleep–wake cycle dysregulation, related to fatigue, pain, decreased level of activity and exercise, premorbid or acute obstructive sleep apnea (OSA), medication side effects, anxiety and/or depression [12], or poor sleep hygiene habits. This patient was seen by a sleep specialist due to sleep impersistence despite various single and combination medication regimens for sleep. A trial of morning-only short-acting neurostimulants was attempted, to ensure that her sleep would not be affected by taking a stimulant later in the day. However, the trial was unsuccessful due to her significant afternoon fatigue, but she did respond well to a different formulation of methylphenidate (combination of 30% IR and 70% ER) every morning, as well as treatment with trazodone 150 mg at bedtime and stricter sleep hygiene.

Endocrine abnormalities, in particular pituitary dysfunction, are more prevalent when skull base fractures are present, especially in the area of the pituitary sella. Symptoms may vary from persistent fatigue, decreased libido, and unexplained weight gain or loss to abnormal serum electrolytes (e.g., sodium levels), abnormal sleep pattern, decreased overall energy level, depression, constipation, and dry skin. When hypopituitarism or other abnormal hypothalamic–pituitary function is suspected, in part due to symptoms that fail to improve or have no other clear explanation, a hormone screening panel can be obtained. In this case, approximately 6 months after the injury, the patient complained of excessive night sweats that had started after her accident. That paired with persistent, moderate-to-severe fatigue and depression triggered an endocrine consult. She was diagnosed with post-TBI hypothalamic–pituitary dysfunction, but no treatment was instituted due to concern about the significant side effects of the medications indicated for hyperhidrosis. The patient's symptoms resolved months later without medications.

Emotional Concerns

Mood impairments may include one or a combination of the following: depression, anxiety, irritability, anger, aggression, oppositional behavior, and panic attacks. Depression is among the most common consequences [13]. Major depressive disorder is the most frequently diagnosed psychiatric illness following traumatic brain injury [14]. Reports of frequency of depression in patients with TBI have ranged from 42% to 77% [15–17], with differential findings being related to variability in the assessment methodology. Depression is common in patients with both mild and moderate-to-severe TBI, with it being greater in the former [18]. The rates of depression are high in the first year following a brain injury, and the risk for developing depression is elevated at any time after injury [19]. The presence of depression can negatively affect a person's ability to benefit from their rehabilitation by increasing feelings of fatigue and attenuating motivation and overall cognitive functioning [20]. Several studies have found associations between depression and reduced functional outcome in individuals with TBI [21, 22]. Depression is also found to be related to increased functional disability, decreased participation in activities of daily living, increased stress, decreased potential for employment, increased divorce rate, increased burden of caregiving, difficulties in sexual functioning, and overall reduced quality of life [23].

Once again, the approach should include the clarification of their etiology (premorbid, acute, or preexisting but exaggerated by TBI) and interactions between symptoms (e.g., depression worsening fatigue or cognitive deficits worsening irritability Trexler, Ph.D. and frustration); it should not be assumed that a symptom is related to the TBI only, until proven otherwise. In this case, the patient struggled with a history of depression that was exacerbated by her functional deficits related to her injury. Early on, she also had difficulty trusting providers and allowing people to participate in her care, especially when it came to medication management. Due to her impaired awareness of her higher-level cognitive deficits, she had difficulty accepting feedback from practitioners and caregivers, and that caused further emotional stress for her and delayed her progress, affecting her overall rehabilitation outcome. This patient eventually developed a major depressive disorder, as well as anxiety disorder. Given the frequent presence of single and multiple mood disturbances in TBI patients, the physiatrist's knowledge on treatment of mood is paramount. Without such management, physicians are unlikely to be able to provide an optimal milieu for the rehabilitation of their patients. Furthermore, there are an insufficient number of psychiatrists in the United States, and access is increasingly limited by insurance restrictions and physicians' level of comfort in treating someone with a history of TBI. These factors will often require that a physiatrist initiate treatment efforts to maximize patient's benefit from a neurorehabilitation program. However, when patients fail to improve with trials of antidepressants despite allowing for adequate time and dosage, a psychiatric evaluation should be requested and at times diligently pursued. Optimal treatment for the mood disturbances should include the combination of psychopharmacological treatments and psychotherapy by someone who understands rehabilitation and trauma challenges. In this case, the physiatrist and neuropsychologist consulted together to provide this treatment for this patient who continued to take an SSRI along with a neurostimulant and also underwent careful surveillance of thyroid function due to history of hypothyroidism.

Cognitive Concerns

The management of cognitive deficits demands that aspects like sleep, mood, fatigue, and endocrine status be taken into consideration. Cognitive deficits are often magnified or complicated by some or all of these factors, and treating one alone would not render best results for the patient. Two methods often used to manage cognitive challenges are through neuropsychological testing and use of medications. Neuropsychological testing is a powerful diagnostic and management tool in neurorehabilitation. While physicians should always be thorough in the neurologic and psychiatric evaluation of their patients, office visits are not designed to provide in-depth information about specific subsets of cognitive functions. There are times when it might be more appropriate to obtain brief mental status examination such as a Folstein Mini Mental Status Examination (MMSE) or a Montreal Cognitive Assessment (MoCA) and times when it may not be as appropriate. Although caution should be exercised when commenting on an individual's degree or pattern of cognitive impairment based solely on their performance on the total MoCA and its subscores, some findings suggest that the MoCA is useful as an easily tolerated "first pass" to give a sense of the most likely stage and profile of an individual's cognitive deficits. If it is consistent with the suspected diagnosis, treatment and prognosis might reasonably be given when further testing is not available, but if the suggested pattern is unanticipated and in keeping with an alternate diagnosis, further detailed neuropsychological testing and investigation should be sought if available. Thus, more than a screening tool, the MoCA can serve as an indicator of the need for further neuropsychological assessment, or serve as a fair proxy, when more detailed standard testing is unavailable or impractical [24]. Additionally, the MoCA demonstrated more differences in cognitive profile between TIA, stroke, and memory research subjects without major cognitive impairment than the MMSE. The MoCA showed between-group differences even in those with normal MMSE and would thus appear to be a useful brief tool to assess cognition in those with MCI, particularly where the ceiling effect of the MMSE is problematic [25]. Full neuropsychological testing may be beneficial prior to sending a patient back to work, school, or being able to participate in independent home living tasks (driving, financial affairs, etc.), so that information regarding cognitive and emotional strengths and weaknesses can be obtained. A detailed description of their deficits and recommendations/accommodations for managing them would help. This may allow physicians and therapists to better tailor a rehabilitation plan to serve that particular patient's needs. This not only provides a more efficient allocation of effort, time, and financial resources but allows for the establishment of a baseline and the monitoring of the patient over time with neuropsychological follow-up and repeat assessments when needed.

It is also important to keep in mind that one medication may at times be used to address more than one issue (e.g., SSRI's for attention motor deficits and mood elevation [26]; methylphenidate for attention and fatigue; or amantadine, to address attention, irritability, and akathisia) when present at a given time. Other interventions like therapy, family education, and environmental modifications should always accompany pharmacologic treatment efforts in order to maximize the benefits of the latter and the permanence of healing and functional gains.

Treatment Needs

From a medical and neurological standpoint, the major treatment needs of this patient seemed to revolve around managing her fatigue, higher-cognitive dysfunctions (which she was unaware of), and increasingly negative psychological reactions to circumstances. This patient responded best to the use of a combination of amantadine and methylphenidate for cognitive inefficiencies and irritability. Several doses and formulations were trialed prior to finding the combination that allowed her to stay focused during the day and feel less fatigued, without feeling anxious or jittery. Amantadine and an SSRI were used to help control irritability, and the SSRI was also meant to target her chronic depression, which had been well controlled but was exacerbated by the accident.

Neuropsychological Testing

The patient was eventually discharged from the transition rehabilitation hospital, as noted above, and was then sent to an outpatient brain injury rehabilitation facility (closer to where she lives) as part of her continuum of brain injury rehabilitation care for neuropsychological examination and evaluation of outpatient therapies. She was referred for testing by the treating physiatrist, who specializes in brain injury rehabilitation. Her overall care was managed by her workman's compensation case manager. As part of the evaluation and admission process to this rehabilitation program, she participated in a neuropsychological examination approximately 3 months following her initial injury. During the first 2 h of this evaluation process, the patient and her parents participated in a clinical interview with the neuropsychologist to obtain initial psychosocial data as well as information about her current complaints and functioning.

During this interview, she was able to state when the accident happened but could not recall any details regarding the accident. She told the neuropsychologist that her last memory before the accident was the night before and she could not remember anything on the day of the accident, demonstrating a period of retrograde amnesia nearly 21–24 h prior to the accident. Her first memory after the accident is of waking up at the local inpatient rehabilitation facility. She was able to state some details that were told to her about the accident. She was also able to state that she is aware of where some of the brain injuries were. Based on her neuropathological injuries and period of retrograde amnesia for details regarding the accident, the severity of her TBI was judged to be a moderate-to-severe injury.

The patient ambulated independently. She reported that she was functioning well physically. She reported experiencing some headaches but believes that they have improved and may be related to premenstrual symptoms. She complained of some problems with fatigue, which she believed were improving a bit however. Cognitively, she noted some forgetfulness and difficulty multitasking, but felt these were improving as well. She also reported she does have some anger and frustration that is different for her; however, she denied issues with depression. Overall, she reported coping well. Clinically, she seemed to be quite aware of some of her challenges, and her behavior was entirely appropriate and actually quite pleasant. The things that she was concerned about seemed to be natural given her current circumstances. Interestingly, it was not until at about 6–9 months following her injury did issues with mood disturbance really start to arise.

The patient reported that her goals were to improve her fine motor skills, memory, ability to multitask, and vision with the overall goals of returning to work, living independently, and driving. However, she knew she had to remain seizure-free until February 2014 before she can be assessed for driving.

Rationale to neuropsychological testing: Following her clinical interview with the neuropsychologist, the patient participated in 4–5 h of neuropsychological testing that was prescribed by the neuropsychologist. Assessment of cognitive and psychological functions provides data to properly plan and effectively implement neurorehabilitation procedures and therapies [27]. The use of neuropsychological assessment data has grown in its contributions in determining appropriate patient care and treatment [17]. According to the authors, adequate and logical planning of rehabilitative needs usually depend on an understanding of the person's strengths and weaknesses, psychological changes, and adjustment to the injury and the impact of these alterations on their experiences and on their behavior. Neuropsychological assessment data is often used to answer questions regarding ability to engage in self-care activities [28], ability to drive and make roadside decisions [29], return to work, supervision level needed, independence in decision-making, or overall functional outcome [30], the need for other types of interventions (e.g., psychological assessment, neuro-opthalmology assessments, etc.) and services (e.g., Office of Vocational Rehabilitation), and information that cannot merely be obtained by simple mental status examination in a physician's office.

Specifically, neuropsychological data can provide cogent information regarding cognitive and neurobehavioral status following a traumatic brain injury [31]. Currently, neuropsychology involvement in the treatment of individuals with neuropathological conditions plays an important role [32]. The knowledge and data derived from neuropsychological techniques can provide important information regarding effective behavioral interventions for those with neuropathological conditions [33]. Specifically,

> Sensitive, broad-gauged, and accurate neuropsychological assessment is necessary for determining the most appropriate treatment for each rehabilitation candidate with brain dysfunction (p. 9)
>
> —Lezak [17]

Approach and selection of neuropsychological test battery: In general, completing an intensive neuropsychological examination typically does not occur during the acute and early post-acute stages since the patients may continue to be confused, delirious, unable to complete the testing, or be minimally responsive. Thus, comprehensive neuropsychological testing typically gets undertaken after the patient clears from post-traumatic confusion, is able to complete such a battery, and is used for planning and rehabilitation purposes and/or at specific time points from the injury [17]. At this point, the patient would have been approximately 3 months post-injury. She was fully oriented, out of post-traumatic confusion, had completed both inpatient and post-acute neurorehabilitation programs, and was entering into the next phase of her rehabilitation, outpatient neurorehabilitation.

Specific approaches to neuropsychological assessment have been developed that emphasize the strategies or processes that patients utilize when performing multifactorial, complex cognitive functions. There are several approaches to selecting which battery of tests would be most appropriate for the client. For a most extensive review, the author recommends a review of Lezak [17] and Parker [34]. In general, Parker [34] contends that there is no one-size-fits-all approach to selecting the proper test battery. Based on several of the aforementioned authors cited directly above, factors that influence the selection procedure should include knowledge regarding the clinical population being tested and expected deficits from this population, attempted use of up-to-date procedures, well-validated assessment tools with robust psychometric properties, appropriately normed tools, as well as assessment procedures sensitive to detecting impairments based on the injury. Neuropsychologists can utilize a fixed battery approach (using the same tests each time in the same order) or a flexible approach (one that is more patient-centered and is guided by the hypotheses formulated by the neuropsychologist after reviewing information about the patient) [35].

The approach utilized by this clinician entails using a core fixed battery, with tests added or eliminated based upon the individual patient's characteristics, abilities, referral question, and needs. This utilizes a fixed–flexible approach, which is often used by neuropsychologists in the assessment of brain injury. The current test battery consisted of measures of estimation of prior level of intellectual functions (to establish an estimation of where the person should be functioning on some cognitive measures), estimations of current intelligence, neurocognitive functions that may influence other cognitive functions and affect functions in therapy (language, visual spatial functions, and sensory/motor abilities), as well as functions often affected by this particular injury (attention, learning and memory, visuomotor processing speed, executive functions, and emotional functions).

As such, this test battery consisted of measures of estimated intelligence, sensory/motor functions, attention, learning and memory, visual spatial abilities, executive functions, language skills, and emotional functions. Such tests included sensory perceptual examination (tactile, visual), finger-tapping test, Boston naming test, animal naming, FAS, Judgment of Line Orientation, Continuous Performance Test, Brief Test of Attention, California Verbal Learning Test-2, Rey/Taylor Complex Figure, Wechsler Memory Scale-IV (Logical Memory 1 and 2), Trail Making Test, Stroop Color and Word Interference Test, Wisconsin Card Sorting Test, Zoo Map Test, Wechsler Adult Intelligence Scale-3 (WAIS-3) short form, Wechsler Test of

Adult Reading (WTAR), Beck Depression Inventory-2 (BDI-2), Frontal Systems Behavior Executive Scale (FrSBe), and Personality Assessment Inventory (PAI).

Observations made during the testing process: During test administration, it is standard practice for the technician to observe and document any behaviors, speech patterns, thinking processes, attention and alertness levels, emotional reactions, neurobehavioral disturbances, and additional verbal responses that may influence the test results. Of course, if everything is "normal," then such notes should also be made. During the test administration, the patient was alert and oriented. Her grooming was good and eye contact was excellent. She displayed fluent and spontaneous speech, although she did have some mild misspeaking of words and would sometimes stumble on her words. There was also some mild paraphasias and dysnomia noted in the conversation. The patient spontaneously reported to the technician that she had previously been diagnosed with dyslexia but not until college. She did have some naming difficulty and some naming errors that seemed to be related to semantic paraphasias. However, she sometimes self-corrected. Comprehension of directions seemed intact. Thought processes were generally goal directed and logical, although every once in a while she was mildly tangential. She was also somewhat distractible and impulsive. Psychomotor behavior was noted to be normal. Hearing was good. Vision seemed okay for testing, although she reported some double vision when she gets fatigued. She was not always aware when she was struggling with test items, but for the most part, she did have some appropriate reaction when she was aware that she struggled. Her mood was normal and she was always very pleasant. She put forth adequate effort on testing and remained cooperative. For these reasons, the present test results were considered to be a valid reflection of her neuropsychological functioning, and test results were interpreted.

Neuropsychological Test Results

Intelligence: Psychometric estimation of her prior level of intellectual functioning, as assessed by word reading test (WTAR Demographic Predicted FSIQ = 103), fell within the average range. Fund of general knowledge, also thought to reflect premorbid intelligence, fell within the average range. Although these are only estimates, it is likely that her prior level of intellectual functioning likely fell around the average range of functions.

She completed subtests of the WAIS-3 to provide estimates of her current level of intellectual functioning. Only several of the tests were selected to obtain an estimation of intellectual functions due to time constraints. Based on test results, her estimated Full Scale IQ fell within the low average range. Verbal abilities were slightly better than nonverbal abilities, with verbal abilities falling in the average range and nonverbal falling in the low average range. It was thought that based on estimation of prior level of intellectual functions, these scores may reflect a mild deflation in intellectual functions and that she likely had not yet returned to baseline functions (Tables 26.1 and 26.2).

Table 26.1 Summary of WAIS-3 Index standard scores

Index	Standard score	Descriptor
Working memory	95	Average
Processing speed	88	Low average
Full Scale IQ	88; 21st percentile	Low average
Verbal IQ	92	Average
Performance IQ	84	Low average

Table 26.2 Performances on measures of attention

Index	Scores	Descriptor
Working memory index	95 standard score	Average
Processing speed index	88 standard score	Low average
Brief auditory attention span	9 scaled score	Average
Auditory verbal working memory	10 scaled score	Average
Graphomotor processing speed	6 scaled score	Low average
Selective attention	25–75th percentile	Average
Basic visuomotor processing speed	$T = 49$; 47th percentile	Average
Vigilance and sustained attention	4 atypical measures	Impaired

Attention: Overall, patient's performances ranged from low average to average in comparison to normative expectations, with sustained attention being a weakness for her. Specifically, she displayed average performances on test of brief auditory attention span, auditory verbal working memory, selective attention, and visuomotor processing speed. In contrast, processing speed index on the WAIS-3 fell within the low average range. Sustained attention and vigilance on a computerized test were just impaired (Table 26.2).

Memory: The patient's test performances on tests of encoding, consolidation, and retrieval for verbal information generally fell within functional limits. However, she did demonstrate a mildly reduced rate of learning as well as recall for information that required complex organizational ability, suggesting some inefficiencies in short-term memory. Ability to recall visual information was slightly weak in comparison to what would be expected for her.

Specifically, she displayed a low average to average learning curve on the word list learning test, recalling 13 out of 16 words when following five learning trials. Her recall for this information following a short delay was marginally deficient and improved to the low average range when following a long delay, suggesting she had the ability to consolidate verbal information, albeit slow. It also suggested that she may have benefitted from repetition and cueing of information. In contrast, when verbal information was placed within a context, she was able to recall a higher than average amount of information when following both short and long delays (84th percentiles). When asked to recall visual information, her performance fell at the 24th percentile when following both short and long delays, which is at the lowest end of the average range and again slightly weaker than expectations. It may be likely that her weaker performance here could have been affected by her poor visual organization of the information. Again, this information suggests that her memory, per se, is not affected. However, higher-level organizational abilities may be contributing to some inefficiency of recall (Table 26.3).

Table 26.3 Performances on memory tests

Index	Score	Descriptor
Word list learning	13/16 after 5 trials $T = 43$	Average
Short delay	8/16 raw	Marginally impaired
Long delay	11/16 raw	Low average
Recognition on word list	13/16 raw	Mildly low
Story memory short delay	13 scaled score; 84th percentile	High average
Story memory long delay	13 scaled score; 84th percentile	High average
Visual recall short delay	8 scaled score; 24th percentile	Average (low end)
Visual recall long delay	8 scaled score; 24th percentile	Average (low end)

Table 26.4 Performances on language tests

Index	Score	Descriptor
Prorated VIQ	92 standard score	Average
Confrontation naming	44/60 4th percentile	Mild-to-moderately impaired
Category fluency	$T = 50$	Average

Language functions: In conversation, expressive speech was fluent. She did not demonstrate any frank aphasic errors. Likewise, she was able to follow along in conversation, demonstrating functionally intact comprehension for basic communication. On formal assessment, the patient showed some variability in expressive language abilities. She seemed to demonstrate some challenges with confrontation naming, as her performance fell at the 4th percentile and was mild-to-moderately impaired. However, her performance was at the 50th percentile on a measure of semantic fluency. Likewise, prorated Verbal IQ fell within the average range. Auditory comprehension was not assessed due to time constraints. There was no indication during testing that this was a significant issue, so the speech therapist attempted to further assess if suspected issues arose in the future (Table 26.4).

Sensory motor functions: The patient did not show any suppressions on tests of bilateral simultaneous stimulation when measured in tactile and visual modalities. Thus, there was no evidence of a sensory inattention or neglect. She is right-hand dominant. Fine motor speed was bilaterally intact with no significant difference between her hands. Thus, fine motor speed was not thought to have affected her neuropsychological test performances on motor tasks. Fine motor coordination, however, was not affected and was left to the occupational therapist to evaluate.

Visual spatial functions: Visual spatial abilities were generally lower than average in comparison to a normative population, and seemed mildly weak at times. There was some slowness and mildly reduced visual organization of information. Specifically, on a shortened version of a judgment of line orientation task, she produced a superior performance. However, visual construction and praxis were mildly

Table 26.5 Performances on visual spatial tests

Index	Score	Descriptor
Prorated performance IQ	84 standard score	Low average
Judgment of line orientation	86th percentile	High average to superior
Visual construction	16th percentile	Low average
Visual spatial reasoning	6 scaled score	Low average

Table 26.6 Performances on measures of executive functions

Index	Score	Descriptor
Interference control and response inhibition	43 – T-score	Low average to average
Problem-solving and concept formation	6/6 categories	Within normal limits
Perseverative errors	43 – T-score	Within normal limits
Spatial planning and reasoning	2/4	Poor
Cognitive flexibility	42 – T-score	Low average
Rapid phonemic generative naming	41– T-score	Low average to marginal

weak. She experienced some difficulty obtaining the gestalt of the figure, and this did not seem to be due to any motor control issues. On a visual spatial reasoning and constructional praxis test, her performance was lower than average. Prorated performance IQ, measuring perceptual reasoning abilities, fell within the low average range (Table 26.5).

Executive functions: Executive abilities were at times weaker than expectations, as she demonstrated mild slowness when completing these types of tasks and reduced organizational ability when completing these tasks. Specifically, problem-solving ability, concept formation, and abstract reasoning performance fell within normal limits. She achieved six out of six categories and did not lose a set once. She was not significantly perseverative on this test either. Interference control was low average. Cognitive flexibility and visuomotor processing speed fell at the 21st percentile and was lower than average. This is likely to be relatively lower than expectations for her. Spatial reasoning and planning was mildly low, but not grossly impaired. Rapid phonemic generative naming fell at the 19th percentile, which is considered marginally impaired (Table 26.6).

Emotional functions: As emotional challenges are common following TBI, the patient was administered a depression-screening inventory, the BDI-2, as well as personality testing. The BDI-2 was chosen because it provides a little more clarity on specific items that are bothersome to the individual. In addition to its usefulness for detecting symptoms of depression, it can also be used to help guide specific clinical interventions, if necessary. Thus, it can provide some insight into specific deviations in mood and emotional functions, behavioral challenges, negative attributions, and physical/cognitive symptoms often similar to those seen directly from the TBI. The client completed all items on this measure and generated a score that fell within the mild range. Specifically, she endorsed mild symptoms of pessimism, feelings of failure, feelings of guilt, loss of confidence, self-criticism, agitation, indecisiveness, some feelings of worthlessness, loss of energy, sleeping less than usual, irritability, decreased appetite, disturbed concentration, and fatigue. Her pattern did not suggest the presence of a major depressive disorder, but it did suggest some possible adjustment issues with some depressive features, specifically entailing some negative attributions about herself and her current circumstances, disturbed mood (more irritability than sad mood), neurovegetative symptoms, and some cognitive issues. It did not include any anhedonia or severe emotional disturbance as the irritability she was endorsing appeared to be reportedly mild in nature.

She completed the Personality Assessment Inventory, which is a personality test that is often used to assess for emotional and specifically mood disturbances. Utilizing the framework of the Diagnostic and Statistical Manual-IV (DSM-IV), it provides more data concerning Axis I (mood) than for specific Axis II (personality) disorders. Review of validity indices revealed that she completed it in a manner that was valid. She did not attempt to endorse items in a primarily negative way, attempt to make herself look desirable, nor was she highly defensive. Her profile suggested that she may have some ongoing concerns about her physical functioning and disruptions in physical areas of life that may produce some stress and leave her feeling tense and worried. Thus, she may have some anxiety or fears surrounding her current situation. She may also have some significant symptoms related to a traumatic stressor. Finally, she may be a little bit leery of others and may be vigilant of others' intentions toward her, as her profile suggested some levels of paranoia. This profile was not surprising since she recently reported having gone through some negative experiences at her recent hospitalization and was outwardly voiding distrust of some her recent medical providers.

Neuropsychological conclusions: The results of the neuropsychological examination showed that the patient was actually doing fairly well from a neurocognitive standpoint given the severity of her injury. She seemed to be slightly below her normal expectations on tests of intellectual functions and as such had likely not returned to full baseline level of functions. However, she did demonstrate average level verbal intelligence, intact basic auditory attentional skills, intact verbal learning and memory for contextual information, superior visual perceptual functions, preserved semantic fluency, and intact executive functions. This was surprising given the severity of her TBI and neuropathological injuries.

In contrast, she primarily showed some decreased processing speed in comparison with what would be expected from her. It was thought that this could affect her higher-level attentional abilities and ability to multitask or divide her attention, problem-solving ability, and spatial reasoning, as slowness tended to impact those scores on testing rather than those specific cognitive abilities, per se. Likewise, she also showed some decreased confrontation naming and visual organizational abilities. She was likely to see mostly the details but may have a difficult time seeing the big picture. Some of these performances were consistent with what would be expected in TBI and, in particular, from right hemisphere injuries.

From an emotional standpoint, the patient did show some adjustment reactions that were more on depressiveness and irritability in nature, along with some tension and anxiety. Her affect was quite pleasant however and her demeanor is quite appropriate. She did not overtly demonstrate irritability, dysphoria, or anxious responses. Personality testing also revealed that she was experiencing some caution about others' intentions toward her. On measures of neurobehavioral functioning, she did not see herself as having a significant level of neurobehavioral dysfunction but did report some mild levels of impulsivity. This was corroborated by her family, who also completed a family rating form. They do see her as being a little bit more impulsive than she sees herself.

She was doing much better than what the records state of how she did during her inpatient stay as well as at the other rehabilitation center. She was coping very well given her circumstances and seemed to be quite appropriate, in spite of documented neurobehavioral and emotional disturbances during inpatient rehabilitation. However, majority of individuals who worked with her during her later inpatient stay and transitional rehabilitation stay documented eventual high levels of defensiveness and unwillingness to receive any feedback from others, as well as a tendency to put on a positive front with others. The neuropsychologist concluded that although she was doing better than expected from a neurocognitive standpoint, given the severity of her traumatic brain injury, she was likely to have some high-level cognitive challenges that may be difficult to detect in very simple tasks. Of note, neuropsychological test performances should not just be viewed as "normal" for just average scores. It is quite often that "average" scores may not always represent the person's prior level of functions. Individuals often do worse under stressful situations, when fatigued or in non-structured environments. Thus, the highly structured neuropsychological testing situation may not always provide adequate ecological validity in predicting how one might perform under real-life circumstances. It was thought that when placed in a work situation where there is a lot going on around her and there are a lot of expectations or high levels of stress, she may be likely to struggle but may not always see it. In addition, based on her prior psychological history, as well as reported emotional challenges during her inpatient admissions, it was believed that she could be at risk for experiencing psychological challenges further out if she is disappointed with her expectations for recovery. It was cautioned that given her defensiveness, and possible decreased levels of awareness, she may actually try to present herself much better than she was and this could place her at risk for experiencing challenges. In fact, as noted earlier, months later, she developed worsening of mood.

Based on her neuropsychological profile, it was recommended that the patient participate in a comprehensive brain injury day treatment program to help her achieve her outcome goals. This program consisted of individual sessions of speech therapy to address specific impairments in naming and verbal expression, attention and processing speed (some issues were found on the attention process training examination during speech therapy evaluations), and occupational therapy to address helping her return to complex activities of daily living as she had not returned to these tasks at the time of evaluation. It also consisted of group therapies guided by neuropsychological milieu. Such group therapies included (1) a cognitive skills group, consisting of psychoeducation in understanding deficits in attention, memory, and executive functions, group exercises to work on those cognitive skills, and opportunities to plan community outings; (2) a life skills group, aimed at teaching individuals to cook, plan, and execute various life skills tasks, and engage in community outings; and (3) a neuropsychology group, consisting of group sessions of psychoeducation and neuropsychological support within a small group setting. As part of this program, patients also participate in individual weekly sessions with the neuropsychologist with the aims of improving awareness and adjustment to injury, as well as helping to reinforce self-monitoring strategies. The day treatment program consists of no more than six to eight individuals, at any one time, who typically go through the program together to establish bonds and build rapport with the therapists. The focus on doing group interventions consists both of content and process approaches utilizing Yalom's group therapy factors. Members are expected to help improve each other's awareness as well as provide positive and constructive feedback. She would also be expected to follow up with the neuropsychologist in individual sessions once weekly to help improve awareness and mood and problem-solve ongoing challenges. It is estimated that she should participate in this program for a period of 12–16 weeks, with the main outcome goals being (1) return to work with modified independence, (2) return to driving, (3) return to living independently, (4) have positive adjustment to injury as evidenced by either neutral or positive well-being or lack of significant negative well-being, (5) require no supervision, (6) cook independently, (7) complete finances independently, (8) complete her own medication management independently, and (9) complete home management tasks independently.

The patient begrudgingly participated in the recommended treatments, noting all along that she was not like other TBI patients, she did not have problems at other patients, and she felt that she was being demeaned by staff. Although she participated, she was disengaged, and multiple times, she asked to discontinue treatment. Anytime she experienced neurocognitive challenges on therapy or community tasks, she provided a reasonable explanation as to why these challenges occurred. Thus, she was eventually discharged from treatment. However, by the end of treatment, the patient had accomplished the goals of not requiring any supervision, independent living with occasional assistance and check-ins (due to reported fatigue issues), and driving. She was able to cook and do medication management and finances independently with occasional check-ins but would sometimes make poor decisions with medication management. It was unclear whether this was due to brain injury or psychological responses to her injury, as she often noted that she is an intelligent nurse and knows how to manage her own medications. The neuropsychologist continued to follow her to help assess or manage any ongoing psychological or neurobehavioral difficulties. The neuropsychologist also worked in collaboration with the physiatrist to help manage challenges and assist with reaching her return to work goal, even until the present.

Collaboration Considerations and Questions

The patient had obviously made some improvements and was functioning at a much higher level at the time of her neuropsychological testing. Given that she had such difficulties with awareness, emotional functioning, and neurobehavioral functions, it would have been difficult to guess whether she would be functioning as well as she did 3 months post-injury. However, given the aforementioned challenges, she was also at risk for not being aware of when she was experiencing challenges. She also had not been placed in challenging situations that would require observation of these functions. Her family seemed to have somewhat of a "halo" effect given how they viewed her prior level of functions, as well as her current level of functions, as they repeatedly noted that they were "just thankful" that she survived such an injury and is with them now. They rarely contributed much information to the process and would become tearful when discussing her functioning, so thankful for her survival. Thus, it is likely that we were unable to obtain fully accurate information regarding her true level of functioning. Thus, in this case, it was important to obtain neuropsychological data, not only to demonstrate that she was, in fact, making significant neurological and neurocognitive gains but that she also had some deviations in higher-attentional functions (processing speed), decreased ability to see the big picture, and decreased planning/organizational ability that may be likely to affect her functionally in higher-demand situations. This would be especially important given that she had goals to return to working as a nurse.

Importantly, the patient was attempting to return to work as a nurse in a setting that was much more complex than her previous setting, and as such, much new learning would be required from her. This is something that is often recommended that be avoided to the best extent possible because it is best to try to send someone back to an environment that is familiar and overlearned to them. It is also important to note that she was reporting significant fatigue that was likely to affect her functioning even more in those situations and that she would not be able to return to work immediately due to these issues. As such, this information would be valuable in terms of knowing what she would and would not be able to do, as well as if she would require ongoing therapies. Additionally, it was valuable to note how she was functioning psychologically, if she was being defensive, and had any lack of awareness or any significant neurobehavioral challenges that would also affect her prognosis for recovery and subsequent recommendations for treatment.

The patient eventually returned to her hospital and attempted to reintegrate into the new department. The physiatrist and neuropsychologist collaborated with the workman's compensation case manager, her immediate supervisor, and the entire clinical team to assist her in gradually returning to work. Due to issues with reported fatigue and missing critical elements on the job, it took her too long to return full time to that position, so the position was lost. Both clinicians followed up with the team to provide recommendations regarding medications to increase attention and alertness, reduce fatigue, and address increasing anxiety and depression as awareness slowly emerged.

Recommendations

1. *Repeat neuropsychological testing*: At some point, workmen's compensation sent the patient for another neuropsychological examination with a different neuropsychologist to gather objective data. The results showed similar patterns of

strengths and weaknesses as the first evaluation, although with some improvements. This information was important to obtain to assure the patient and team that she was making improvements but was, in fact, still experiencing some cognitive challenges. Given the patient's continued high level of defensiveness, it was important for her to receive this feedback from someone objective so she could see that she needed to make some alterations and go for further treatments.

2. *Further functional assessment*: Following this examination, the patient was able to find a program that would test out her skills in medication administration since she lost her job. She went through the course and passed the testing. Once she was cleared, she was given permission by the treating physiatrist to be able to return to nursing again with ability to administer medications independently, in a noncomplex or demanding environment. Once she passed this testing, she was able to market herself to her hospital and apply for other types of nursing positions, as she discovered that the setting to which she attempted to return was too complex and contributing to significant fatigue.
3. *Medication alterations*: The physiatrist continued to alter medications to manage fatigue, sleep, and attention. She was eventually able to find the proper dosing schedule for such medications but still requires practicing energy conservation strategies.
4. *Neuropsychology follow-ups*: The patient also continues to work with the neuropsychologist to process awareness and psychological reactions to her current challenges, relationship issues caused by the TBI, and help develop a new sense of identity. In spite of her continued defensiveness at times, it appears that the according to the patient's family and workman's compensation case manager, the neuropsychologist and physiatrist are the only two healthcare professionals which she will confide in.

Key issues in this case would be:

- Managing fatigue
- Managing anxiety and depression:
  - Premorbid depression was well controlled with SSRIs, and their use was continued after TBI.
  - Methylphenidate was chosen to target fatigue, processing speed, and higher-level cognitive deficits and to support mood elevation (mild additive effect).
  - Neurorehabilitation therapies to address functional deficits that added to the patient's mood complaints.
  - Neuropsychology to improve anxiety, depression, and coping skills.
  - Trazodone to improve sleep and decrease anxiety and depression (mild additive effect due to low dose).
  - Referral to a psychiatrist was not completed due to patient doing well with her medical regimen and psychological therapy. Another consideration was her pre-TBI history of depression which complicates coverage for this treatment as part of the TBI case unless a clear relationship can be established. In the

patient's case, it appears there will likely always be a combination of premorbid psychological factors that may be exacerbated by the injury and more difficult to control. For basic psychopharmacological management then, either the PCP (depending on their expertise) or the physiatrist can continue lifelong treatment. Should the patient fail to thrive functionally with these interventions, a psychiatric evaluation would be indicated and pathophysiologic and situational considerations used to tie the worsening of depression to the current TBI.

- Providing a safe structure for disappointments and setbacks/failures

Chapter Review Questions

1. In this case, the diagnosis of TBI was already known. Given this information, how was it useful to obtain neuropsychological testing data, and how did this guide the treatment recommendations for the patient's outpatient treatment, particularly given that she appeared so "high-level" and obtained some "average" scores?
2. Why was it important to recommend that a more comprehensive neuropsychological test be given as opposed to providing a basic mental status examination for this patient? Are there times when administering mental status examinations can be useful?
3. Why was it important for the physiatrist to have some knowledge on treatment of mood disturbances, and when would it have been a good idea to refer out to a psychiatrist?
4. How does collaboration with a neuropsychologist help a physician better monitor a patient's cognitive progress and rehabilitation process? How does it help synergize the management of mood disturbances?

References

1. Lezak MD, Howieson DB, Bigler ED, Tranel D. Neuropsychological assessment. New York: Oxford University Press; 2012.
2. Brooks N, McKinlay W, Symington C, Beattie A, Campsie L. Return to work within the first seven years of severe head injury. Brain Injury. 1987;1(1):5–19.
3. Thomsen IV. Late outcome of very severe blunt head truma: a 10–15 year second follow-up. J Neurol Neurosurg Psychiatry. 1984;47:260–8.
4. Kolakowsky-Hayner SA, Miner KD, Kreutzer JS. Long-term life quality and family needs after traumatic brain injury. J Head Trauma Rehabil. 2001;16(4):374–85.
5. Ponsford JL, Olver JH, Curran C, Ng K. Prediction of employment status 2 years after traumatic brain injury. Brain Injury. 1995;9(1):11–20.

6. Borgaro SR, Baker J, Wethe JV, et al. Subjective reports of fatigue during early recovery from traumatic brain injury. J Head Trauma Rehabil. 2005;20:416–25.
7. Cantor JB, Bushnik T, Cicerone K, Dijkers MP, Gordon W, Hammond FM, Kolakowsky-Hayner SA, Lequerica A, Nguyen M, Spielman LA. Insomnia, fatigue, and sleepiness in the first 2 years after traumatic brain injury: a NIDRR TBI model system module study. J Head Trauma Rehabil. 2012;27(6):E1–14.
8. Lucas S, Hoffman JM, Bell KR, Dikmen S. A prospective study of prevalence and characterization of headache following mild traumatic brain injury. Cephalalgia. 2014;34(2):93–102.
9. Godbolt AK, Stenberg M, Jakobsson J, Kimmo S, Krakau K, Stalnacke FM, DeBoussard CN. Subacute complications during recovery from severe traumatic brain injury: frequency and associations with outcome. BMJ Open. 2015;5(4):e007208.
10. Barnett BP, Singman EL. Vision concerns after mild traumatic brain injury. Curr Treat Options Neurol. 2015;17(2):329.
11. Gardani M, Morfiri E, Thomson A, O-Neill B, McMillan T. Evaluation of sleep disorders in patients with severe traumatic brain injury during rehabilitation. Arch Phys Med Rehabil. 2015;15:418–9.
12. Ponsford JL, Sinclair KL. Sleep and fatigue following traumatic brain injury. Psychiatr Clin North Am. 2014;37(1):77–89.
13. Seel RT, Kreutzer JS, Rosenthal M, Hammond FM, Corrigan JD, Black K. Depression after traumatic brain injury: a national institute on disability and rehabilitation research model systems multicenter investigation. Arch Phys Med Rehabil. 2003;84:177–84.
14. Deb S, Lyons I, Koutzoukis C, Ali I, McCarthy G. Rate of psychiatric Illness 1 year after traumatic brain injury. Am J Psychiatry. 1999;156:374–8.
15. Kreutzer JS, Seel RT, Gourley E. The prevalence and symptom rates of depression after traumatic brain injury: a comprehensive examination. Brain Injury. 2005;15(7):563–76.
16. Varney NR, Martzke JS, Roberts RJ. Major depression in patients with closed head injury. Neuropsychology. 1987;1(1):7–9.
17. Lezak M. Relationship between personality disorders, social disturbances, and physical disability following traumatic brain injury. J Head Trauma Rehabil. 1987;2(1):57–69.
18. Dickmen SS, Bombardier CH, Machamer JE, Fann JR, Temkin NR. Natural history of depression in traumatic brain injury. Arch Phys Med Rehabil. 2004;85(9):1457–64.
19. Jorge RE, Robinson RG, Arndt SV, Starkstein SE, Forester AW, Geisler F. Depression following traumatic brain injury: a 1 year longitudinal study. J Affect Disord. 1993;27(4):233–43.
20. MacNiven E, Finlayson MA. The interplay between emotional and cognitive recovery after closed head injury. Brain Injury. 1993;7:241–6.
21. Malec JF, Moessner AM. Self-awareness, distress, and post-acute rehabilitation outcome. Rehabil Psychol. 2000;45:227–41.
22. Rosenthal M, Christensen BK, Ross TP. Depression following traumatic brain injury. Arch Phys Med Rehabil. 1998;79:90–103.
23. Cantor JB, Ashman TA, Schwartz ME, Gordon WA, Hibbard MR, Brown M, Spielman L, Charatz HJ, Cheng Z. The role of self-discrepancy theory in understanding post-traumatic brain injury affective disorders: a pilot study. J Head Trauma Rehabil. 2005;20(6):527–43.
24. Lam B, Middleton LE, Masellis M, Stuss DT, Harry RD, Kiss A, Black SE. Criterion and convergent validity of the Montreal cognitive assessment with screening and standardized neuropsychological testing. J Am Geriatr Soc. 2013;61(12):2181–5.
25. Pendlebury ST, Markwick A, deJager CA, Zombini G, Wilcock GK, Rothwell PM. Differences in cognitive profile between TIA, stroke and elderly memory research subjects: a comparison of the MMSE and MoCA. Cerebrovasc Dis. 2012;34(1):48–54.
26. Breceda EY, Dromerick AW. Motor rehabilitation in stroke and traumatic brain injury: stimulating and intense. Curr Opin Neurol. 2013;26(6):595–601.
27. Trexler L, Webb PM, Zappala G. In: Christensen AL, Uzzell Barbara P, editors. Strategic aspects of neuropsychological rehabilitation. As seen in brain injury and neuropsychological rehabilitation: international perspectives. Hillsdale, NJ: Lawrence Erlbaum Associates, Publishers; 1994.

28. Galski T, Ehle HT, McDonald MA, Mackevich J. Evaluating fitness to drive after cerebral injury: basic issues and recommendations for medical and legal communities. J Head Trauma Rehabil. 2000;15:895–908.
29. Dawson JD, Uc EY, Anderson SW, et al. Neuropsychological predictors of driving errors in older adults. J Am Geriatr Soc. 2009;58:1090–6.
30. Sigurdardottir S, Andelic N, Roe C, Schanke AK. Cognitive recovery and predictors of functional outcome 1 year after traumatic brain injury. J Int Neuropsychol Soc. 2009;33:202–10.
31. Wilde EA, Whiteneck GG, Bogner J, Bushnik T, Cifu DX, Dikmen S, French L, Giacino JT, Hart T, Malec JF, Millis SR, Novack TA, Sherer M, Tulsky DS, Vanderploeg RD, von Steinbuechel N. Recommendations for the use of common outcome measures in traumatic brain injury research. Arch Phys Med Rehabil. 2010;91:1650–60.
32. Vanderploeg RD, Collins RC, Sigford B, Date E, Schwab K, Warden D. Practical and theoretical considerations in designing rehabilitation trials: the DVBIC cognitive-didactic versus functional-experiential treatment study experience. J Head Trauma Rehabil. 2006;21:179–93.
33. Christensen AL, Uzzell BP. International handbook of neuropsychological rehabilitation. New York: Kluwer Academic/Plenum Press; 2000.
34. Parker RS. Traumatic Brain Injury and Neuropsychological Impairment: sensorimotor, cognitive, emotional, and adaptive problems of children and adults. New York: Springer-Verlag; 1990.
35. Mitrushina MN, Boone KB, D'Elia LF. Handbook of normative data for neuropsychological assessment. New York: Oxford University Press; 1999.

Chapter 27
Neuropsychological Assessment of Adult Attention Deficit/Hyperactivity Disorder

Margaret Lanca, Flannery Geier, and Lenna Finger

Introduction

Attention-deficit/hyperactivity disorder (AD/HD) is a developmental brain disorder that is marked by persistent inattention and/or hyperactivity/impulsivity that interferes with daily functioning. It is normal for everyone to have some distractibility and impulsivity, but for children and adults with this disorder, these symptoms are more pervasive and interfere with their ability to function at school, home, and work. Children and adults with this disorder can be forgetful in their daily activities, have difficulty concentrating or sustaining their attention on a task, struggle to sit still for longer periods of time, feel constantly restless or as if driven by a motor, or talk nonstop. A full description of the scope of these symptoms is outlined in the *Diagnostic and Statistical Manual of Mental Disorders* (DSM-5) [1]. AD/HD is a heterogeneous disorder with three subtypes: predominantly inattentive, predominantly hyperactive/impulsive, and combined subtype. The prevalence of AD/HD in childhood in the United States is estimated at 5% [1], and prospective longitudinal studies have demonstrated that AD/HD persists into adulthood with an estimated prevalence of approximately 3.3–5.3% [2], though estimates vary widely depending on the variables and methods used [3–6]. Although the exact cause of AD/HD is unknown, vast epidemiological, neuroscience, cognitive, genetic, and psychiatric research has described various aspects of the disorder [1, 2, 7, 8]. Despite this, the diagnosis of AD/HD remains tricky due to the high comorbidity and/or overlap of symptoms with other psychiatric, developmental,

M. Lanca (✉) · L. Finger
Harvard Medical School, Cambridge Health Alliance, Cambridge, MA, USA
e-mail: Margaret_Lanca@hms.harvard.edu

F. Geier
Harvard Medical Center/Cambridge Health Alliance, Cambridge, MA, USA

K. M. Sanders (ed.), *Physician's Field Guide to Neuropsychology*,
https://doi.org/10.1007/978-1-4939-8722-1_27

and medical disorders [9]. The following case highlights a typical case presented in a primary care clinic in which a neuropsychological evaluation was requested to assist with diagnostic clarity.

Referral

Patient: 21-year-old female
Education: high school degree
Occupation: bartender at a restaurant

Reason for Referral

Ana was struggling with inattention, disorganization, and forgetfulness in the context of ongoing anxiety and depression. She recently withdrew from her first semester at a community college because she felt overwhelmed by her course load and her grades were slipping. Ana's psychological distress appeared to be related to and exacerbated by her ongoing cognitive complaints. Neuropsychological testing was deemed helpful for diagnostic clarity, identification of cognitive strengths and weaknesses, and offering diagnostic clarification around current emotional and cognitive functioning.

Case Presentation

Ana described chronic problems with disorganization, procrastination, forgetfulness, and following through with tasks dating back to childhood in Argentina and persisting as an adult. She explained that she misplaces her parking stub at work almost every day and added that she tends to run back and forth from her house to her car in the morning to collect important items she inadvertently leaves behind. Overall, she is independent with activities of daily living and most instrumental activities of daily living but not without a great deal of effort. She described using multiple compensatory strategies to assist her with attention and organization in daily life. She maintains a desk calendar with sticky note reminders for her doctor appointments and financial obligations so that she is able to pay bills on time. However, she routinely forgets to take her medication as prescribed and estimated that she misses a dose three times per week on average. With household chores, she reported that she is "scatterbrained" but gets them done weekly as a way to help her mother around the house.

Ana's medical history was significant for asthma, which was diagnosed approximately 6 months ago after she experienced respiratory distress, for which she was being prescribed albuterol. She reported prior nightly marijuana use but stated she discontinued after she was diagnosed with asthma. She estimated 9–10 h of sleep per night but noted she feels better when she gets 11–12 h. Her family history is negative for AD/HD or learning disorders, though admittedly her family has never sought prior treatment.

In terms of psychiatric history, Ana reported a history of anxiety and episodic depression and had been witness to domestic violence between her parents as a child. She explained she always had a tendency to worry but that her anxiety and depressive symptoms peaked in high school. She described a second episode of depression 2 years prior in the context of academic and work demands. At that time, she quit her job and neglected her self-care, spent days in bed, and isolated from others. She had a first panic attack at that time and had approximately five panic attacks since then with the most recent occurring the week prior to her testing appointment. Her panic symptoms were characterized by increased heart rate, sweating, shaking, chest pain, dizziness, and tingling. These symptoms reportedly peaked within 6–7 minutes of onset. She recently began psychotherapy for anxiety and panic episodes. She was being treated with fluoxetine, 20 mg, which was prescribed 1 year prior only with modest benefit. She was previously tried on two different SSRIs (citalopram and sertraline) but with no benefit.

MD Perspective

Key Point

There is a high rate of overlap among AD/HD and mood disorders. The National Comorbidity Survey estimated that more than 80% of those who meet the DSM-4 criteria for AD/HD also met criteria for a mood disorder such as bipolar disorder or major depressive disorder [8].

As a primary care physician, it can be challenging to make a diagnosis of AD/HD, particularly in adulthood. AD/HD generally presents with symptoms of inattention and/or trouble with concentration. These symptoms, however, are common in other psychiatric disorders such as mood disorders. Therefore, making the right diagnosis can be complicated as there is so much overlap in symptomatology between AD/HD and mood disorders.

Ana presented initially with complaints of anxiety and had been a witness of domestic violence. It was unclear if the trouble with focus and concentration she was experiencing in school was related to a primary diagnosis of anxiety/depression or if she in fact had AD/HD or both.

In terms of medical history, she had a history of asthma, which sometimes can increase feelings of anxiety if asthma is poorly controlled. Her asthma was generally well controlled with albuterol and probably not a significant factor in her symptoms, but medical conditions should always be considered when evaluating a psychiatric disorder. In addition, she was a marijuana user, which also affects concentration, attention, and mood [10–12], and it was important to determine how much of a contributor her drug use was to the clinical picture.

Key Point

Research suggests that AD/HD is associated with elevated substance use disorders [13–15]. Childhood AD/HD has been related to an increased odds of lifetime marijuana use, and one meta-analysis indicated that children with AD/HD were nearly three times more likely to have reported ever having used marijuana than children without AD/HD [16].

Ana reported some difficulty in school in childhood but had not been diagnosed with AD/HD in childhood. There remains some debate about how often AD/HD persists in adulthood. One meta-analysis estimates that about 50% of individuals with AD/HD in childhood have AD/HD that persists into adulthood [17, 18], but findings vary widely. Therefore, a diagnosis of AD/HD in childhood alone (or a suspicion of this as with Ana) is not enough to make this diagnosis in adulthood. Moreover, learning disorders may also co-occur with AD/HD, and these may present as problems with attention and concentration [1, 19]. Thus, evaluation for learning disorders becomes an important piece of the assessment.

When presented with these potential AD/HD cases, it is critical to make the right diagnosis/diagnoses so that the proper treatment (nonpharmacological or pharmacological) can be prescribed to the patient. This is of particular importance in the diagnosis of AD/HD as there are many important treatment considerations that must be taken into account. While there are various treatments, AD/HD is commonly treated with amphetamines, which are medications that can be abused. Approximately 3–10% of college-age students abuse amphetamines as they improve cognitive function even in those without any psychiatric disorder [20]. Not only do amphetamines carry a risk of abuse, but there is also some evidence in animal studies that they may cause neurotoxicity [20]. These medications can also exacerbate symptoms of anxiety, insomnia, and mania in patients with these conditions [20]. For these reasons, prescribing amphetamines cannot be taken lightly, and it is important to have a comprehensive understanding of the clinical picture before prescribing such medications.

In cases like Ana's, when there are multiple complicating factors, neuropsychological testing and assessment is critically important to decipher the relative contribution of the multiple psychiatric, developmental, and medical conditions to the clinical picture of possible AD/HD. Neuropsychological testing helps to tease out if the problems with concentration and attention are primarily related to an anxiety or mood disorder, a learning disorder, a substance use disorder, AD/HD, or a combination of these. Not only is neuropsychological evaluation a crucial part of the diagnostic process, it also provides guidance to patients for nonpharmacological interventions to manage the symptoms. These interventions can be as important, if not more, as pharmacological interventions and have the benefit of less risk. The assessment of the neuropsychologist aids in determining any accommodations in the school setting that can promote student success. Neuropsychological testing provides valuable information to help guide patients and providers on the most appropriate treatments/interventions to maximize the AD/HD patient's ability to function at the highest level possible.

Key Point
An important element of a neuropsychological evaluation is the guidance provided to patients and their families for nonpharmacological interventions (behavioral management, cognitive remediation, academic accommodations) to manage the symptoms. These interventions can be as important, if not more important, as pharmacological interventions and have the benefit of less risk.

Referring to Neuropsychology

Despite a clear-cut history of attention difficulties since childhood, Ana also expressed learning difficulties as well as depression and anxiety beginning in childhood. Neuropsychological assessment was indicated to differentiate among AD/HD, a learning disorder, and depression and anxiety. It was also requested to help develop a treatment plan for Ana to improve her level of functioning at school and home.

The Role of Neuropsychology

Questions to be addressed by a neuropsychological assessment are as follows: Does this patient meet the criteria for AD/HD? What are her cognitive abilities? Are there any other comorbid psychiatric disorders or learning disorders?

Key Point
AD/HD and learning disorders can co-occur in a significant minority of children with each disorder, and comorbidity has been estimated to be 45% [19]. Individuals with specific learning disorder may appear inattentive due to frustration, low interest, or limited abilities [1]. According to the DSM-5, learning disorders reflect specific deficits with learning academic skills, while AD/HD poses a challenge in realizing academic abilities.

Neuropsychological Testing

Neuropsychological Perspective of Adult AD/HD

AD/HD is diagnostically challenging, particularly in adults. Because AD/HD is a neurodevelopmental disorder that first presents in childhood with symptom onset before age 12 [1], diagnosis in adulthood requires a thorough developmental history that integrates childhood and adult symptom profiles. A significant challenge in diagnosing adult AD/HD involves obtaining accurate accounts of AD/HD symptoms throughout the life span. Self-report of childhood symptoms in adulthood may be unreliable as a function of time [21]. Additionally, collateral information documenting childhood symptoms (e.g., school records, informant reports) may not be as readily available or accessible for adults [21].

Key Point

Because AD/HD is currently classified as a childhood-onset disorder, a thorough developmental history is essential for diagnostic clarification. Through interview and testing, patients are asked to describe their behaviors during childhood across contexts (at home, school, etc.) and fill out questionnaires describing current and historical symptoms, and when possible collateral information is gathered from caregivers and school transcripts.

Questions that may aid inquiry of childhood symptoms:

- What kind of student were you in elementary school?
- How did your kindergarten or first grade teachers describe you?
- Did you ever repeat a grade?
- Were you ever in a specialized classroom or did you work with a teacher's aid?
- Did you get sent to the principal's office? How often and for what?

Another challenge with diagnosis is the high level of comorbid psychiatric disorders with AD/HD. Approximately 50% of children and adults with AD/HD have a co-occurring psychiatric disorder [8, 22]. Nearly one-quarter of children have a co-occurring behavior disorder (e.g., conduct disorder or oppositional defiant disorder), and in adults, they commonly have co-occurring depression (38.3%), anxiety (47.1%), substance use disorders (15.2%), and impulse control disorders (19.6%; [8]). These psychiatric disorders can also cause attention and executive impairment. Medical conditions such as asthma, allergies, anemia, hypoglycemia, thyroid disorders, toxic exposure, vitamin deficiencies, and hearing or visual impairments can also disrupt attention [23]. Importantly, sleep disorders are also common among individuals with AD/HD [24] and well known to impair cognition, particularly attention, learning, and memory.

Key Point

Research has also shown evidence of a bidirectional relationship between AD/HD and sleep disturbances [25]. Sleep problems were part of the initial diagnostic criteria for AD/HD in DSM-3 [26]. The most common sleep disorder associated with AD/HD is initial insomnia or difficulty falling asleep [27]. For individuals with AD/HD, sleep problems may be intensified by anxiety and depression [28]. Introducing sleep hygiene strategies can be critical to improving concentration and treating AD/HD.

Thus, these co-occurring disorders can mask, mimic, or exacerbate AD/HD symptoms, thereby increasing the complexity of diagnosis and specialized knowledge of provider training. Therefore, it is not surprising that even though cognitive difficulties associated with AD/HD are often first reported in primary care settings [29], many adult primary care providers (48%) are uncomfortable diagnosing adult AD/HD [30, 31]. Consequently, they are more likely to defer to a specialist to assess AD/HD when compared to other disorders [32].

The Psychiatric Interview

A thorough history and establishment of presence of clinically significant AD/HD symptoms is the primary method of diagnosis, although neuropsychological testing can be used to support the diagnosis, rule in or out other causes, and develop a treatment plan that includes individualized cognitive remediation and/or indications for academic accommodations. Therefore, a detailed clinical interview was conducted with Ana, and school records were obtained for collateral input.

During the clinical interview, Ana acknowledged behavioral difficulties beginning in elementary school in Argentina. She recalled behavioral problems that resulted in her getting in trouble at school and at home (e.g., having constant problems completing her homework and disobedience). She was required to attend summer school in third and fourth grade and needed a tutor for homework help. Her difficulties persisted after she immigrated to the United States with her family in the fifth grade (10 years old). She was initially in ESL classes and then mainstreamed in middle school. She noted that learning English was easy. She reportedly earned Bs and Cs through middle school but would frequently stay after school for extra support. In high school, her grades were variable (As to Ds), though she mostly earned Bs and Cs. She reported that she began skipping classes and did not complete her assignments, in part because of disorganization and procrastination. Her teachers encouraged her to meet minimum requirements so that she could graduate. She graduated high school on time with a low GPA. Ana linked significant declines in her academic performance with the onset of anxiety and depression; this timeline was corroborated by a review of her academic transcripts from high school. However, her struggles in more theory-oriented, writing classes raised the question of a possible undetected learning disorder, especially in the context of second-language learning. After taking off 1 year after high school, she enrolled at a local community college where she struggled academically and emotionally and withdrew during her second semester. At home, she was having difficulty keeping up with her chores and appointments.

Adult AD/HD is marked by ongoing symptoms of inattention, impulsivity, and/or hyperactivity, which significantly impair functioning across multiple settings, such as at home, school, or work; with friends or relatives; or in other activities. These symptoms may be exacerbated by external demands [30]. Therefore, it was critical to evaluate current functional impairment across domains in Ana's life. Based on presenting concerns, it was apparent that she was experiencing significant functional impairment at school and in her home life (e.g., medication noncompliance, difficulty keeping appointments). Notably, Ana denied major functional impairment at work though she trained herself to use multiple compensatory strategies (e.g., writing down all orders) in her job as a bartender. As a child, she struggled academically, notably even in Argentina, before immigrating and prior to onset of depression and anxiety. Taken together, this symptom history and review of her transcripts and the AD/HD questionnaires completed (see below) were consistent with AD/HD, combined type. The neuropsychological testing was further helpful in delineating the types of cognitive difficulties, performance validity, and assessing for a learning disorder.

Approach and Selection of Neuropsychological Test Battery

Neuropsychological tests are modestly reliable in diagnosing adults with AD/HD, though the absence of impairment on testing does not rule out behavioral impairment in daily functioning [33]. This is due, in part, to the significant symptom variability in adults with AD/HD [24]. However, adults with AD/HD have demonstrated difficulties on neuropsychological tests of activation (e.g., organization, prioritization, task initiation), attention (e.g., focused, sustained, and/or divided attention), alertness (e.g., regulating alertness, sustaining effort, processing speed), memory (e.g., working memory, recall), and/or action (e.g., monitoring and regulating self-action) [30].

While AD/HD has been consistently characterized by impaired executive functioning (planning, inhibitory control, organization), cognitive deficits are found on both executive and nonexecutive tasks, including verbal fluency, inhibition, set shifting, response consistency, word reading, and color naming [34]. In fact, at least some degree of impairment has been evidenced across all cognitive domains [35] when comparing adults with and without AD/HD. Though effect sizes vary by test, some of the most robust findings signal the utility of measuring complex and sustained attention, verbal memory, and abstract verbal problem-solving that involves working memory [36].

In Ana's case, issues of bilingualism were also of consideration, especially in evaluating a learning disability. Patients who have English as a second language and/or are from a different culture have been shown to underperform on cognitive tests that are normed on English-speaking Americans [37]. Although there is significant research in the areas of acquisition of second language and impact of bilingual education on learning, there is scant research on how to evaluate the presence of a learning disability in a patient with English as a second language [33]. This is related to the fact that proficiency in a second language varies greatly as a function of age of acquisition and degree and years of exposure to the second language, to name a few variables. In Ana's case, she began to learn English at the age of 10 and completed more years of education in English than Spanish, making her a fluent conversational bilingual. She remarked that she considered English to be her current dominant language. Testing was therefore conducted in English. Academic testing in English was conducted to determine her level of proficiency in English and assist with a diagnosis of a learning disorder. It should be noted that because of the sequential nature of second-language learning (Ana learned Spanish first and then English), some performance variability of academic testing and neuropsychological testing was expected (Note: a thorough review of the effects of second language on neuropsychological testing is beyond the scope of this chapter; see [33, 38]).

As mentioned above, potential for secondary gain (e.g., academic accommodations, stimulant abuse) can result in symptom exaggeration or even fabrication. Sullivan et al. [39] found that 47% of college students evaluated for AD/HD did not pass performance validity tests (i.e., Word Memory Test), which are designed to detect a patient's level of effort and performance consistency. In another study, individuals feigning or exaggerating symptoms of AD/HD completed self-report questionnaires and neurocognitive testing in a manner that was difficult to distinguish from patients with AD/HD [40]. Self-report questionnaires are especially easy to feign; Jachimowicz and Geiselman [41] showed that 75–90% of college students successfully feigned AD/HD symptoms when directed to do so. As a result, performance validity tests are routinely administered in neuropsychological evaluations to ensure consistent effort throughout testing.

In order to assess Ana's current cognitive and emotional functioning, tests were selected:

- *Intelligence and premorbid functioning*: Wechsler Adult Intelligence Scale—Fourth Edition (WAIS-IV), Test of Premorbid Functioning from Advanced Clinical Solutions
- *Attention*: Digit Span from WAIS-IV; Conners' Continuous Performance Test—Third Edition
- *Executive functioning*: Trail Making Test, Verbal Fluency, and Color-Word Interference Test from the Delis-Kaplan Executive Functioning System

- *Memory*: California Verbal Memory Test—Second Edition; Logical Memory subtest from the Wechsler Memory Scale—Fourth Edition; Brief Visuospatial Memory Test—Revised
- *Visual-spatial abilities*: Rey-Osterrieth complex figure test
- *Performance validity*: Test of Memory Malingering, Advanced Clinical Solutions—Word Choice; Reliable Digit Span: Rey 15-Item
- *Academic achievement*: select subtests of Woodcock-Johnson Fourth Edition Tests of Achievement; Nelson-Denny Reading Test
- *Behavioral functioning*: Behavior Rating Inventory of Executive Function; *Barkley Adult ADHD Rating Scale-IV*
- *Mood functioning*: Beck Depression Inventory—Second Edition; Adult Manifest Anxiety Scale, Adult Version; Panic and Agoraphobia Scale; Panic Attack Questionnaire

Neuropsychological Domains and Test Findings (See Table 27.1)

Performance validity: Ana showed sufficient task engagement and performance consistency on neuropsychological testing for the results to be a valid representation of her current cognitive functioning.

Table 27.1 Neuropsychological test results

	Standard/scaled score	Percentile
Wechsler Adult Intelligence Scale—Fourth Edition		
Verbal Comprehension Index	80	9
Perceptual Reasoning Index	98	45
Working Memory Index	105	63
Processing Speed Index	94	34
Vocabulary	6	9
Similarities	5	5
Information	8	25
Block design	8	25
Matrix reason	11	63
Visual puzzles	10	50
Digit span	12	75
Arithmetic	10	50
Coding	10	50
Symbol search	8	25
Advanced Clinical Solutions		
Test of Premorbid Functioning	96	39
Conners' Continuous Performance Test Third Edition		
d'	48	42
Omissions	58	79

(continued)

Table 27.1 (continued)

	Standard/scaled score	Percentile
Commissions	37	10
Perseverations	59	82
Hit RT	90	>99
Hit RT SD error	75	99
Variability	60	84
Hit RT Block Chg	42	21
Hit RT ISI Chg	85	>99
Delis-Kaplan Executive Function System: Trail Making Test		
Visual scanning	9	37
Number sequencing	9	37
Letter sequencing	13	84
Number-letter sequencing	12	75
Number-letter sequencing errors	12	75
Delis-Kaplan Executive Function System: Verbal Fluency		
Letters	9	37
Category	11	63
Switching accuracy	16	98
Set-loss errors	13	84
Repetitions	8	25
Delis-Kaplan Executive Function System: Color-Word Interference		
Colors	7	16
Words	9	37
Inhibition	11	63
Switching	12	75
Inhibition errors	12	75
Switching errors	12	75
California Verbal Learning Test—Second Edition		
List A total (trials 1–5)	68	96
List A short-delay free recall	1	84
List A short-delay cued recall	1	84
List A long-delay free recall	1.5	93
List A long-delay cued recall	1	84
Wechsler Memory Scale—Fourth Edition		
Logical memory immediate recall	11	63
Logical memory delayed recall	10	50
Brief Visuospatial Memory Test—Revised		
Total recall (trials 1–3)	67	96
Delayed recall	59	82
Cued recall	–	>16
Rey-Osterrieth complex figure test		
Copy	–	11–16

(continued)

Table 27.1 (continued)

	Standard/scaled score	Percentile
Woodcock-Johnson Tests of Achievement—Fourth Edition		
Letter-word identification	97	42
Applied problems	116	85
Spelling	95	37
Passage comprehension	93	32
Calculation	99	47
Writing samples	109	73
Word attack	99	47
Oral reading	92	31
Sentence reading fluency	108	69
Math facts fluency	106	66
Sentence writing fluency	99	47
Nelson-Denny Reading Test		
Comprehension	206	49
Reading rate	188	28
Behavior Rating Inventory of Executive Function (BRIEF)		
Inhibition	80	>99
Shifting	73	99
Emotional control	78	>99
Self-monitoring	80	>99
Initiation	79	>99
Working memory	86	>99
Planning/organizing	89	>99
Task monitoring	72	99
Adult Manifest Anxiety Scale		
Worry	60	84
Physiological worry	71	98
Test	77	>99
Social concern/stress	62	88
Total anxiety	71	98
Raw		
Beck Depression Inventory	23	Significant
Barkley Adult ADHD Rating Scale		
Childhood inattention	5	Significant
Childhood hyperactivity	8	Significant
Current inattention	8	Significant
Current hyperactivity	9	Significant
Test of Memory Malingering		
Initial presentation	50	Pass
Second presentation	50	Pass
Advanced Clinical Solutions		
Word choice	50	Base rate: >25%

Premorbid Functioning and IQ. Ana performed within the average range on a measure of word reading, which is used to estimate baseline cognitive abilities. There is a strong association between word reading and IQ, and this relationship is relatively stable and uninfluenced by brain pathology [42].

Consistent with premorbid estimates, Ana obtained an overall IQ score in the low average to average range. For specific index scores, she earned average scores on indices of perceptual reasoning, processing speed, and working memory. She performed in the low average range on the Verbal Comprehension Index. Within this domain of verbal intelligence, she performed in the average to borderline range on subtests. Though she demonstrated average abilities with regard to crystallized information or school-based knowledge (information), she struggled more on a measure of verbal reasoning (similarities was borderline), and her vocabulary knowledge was low average. Even though she was fluently bilingual, Ana did not acquire English until she was approximately 10 years old, which likely affected her vocabulary knowledge. Overall, Ana's pattern of intellectual performances was intact across domains. She did not demonstrate significant deficits in areas of processing speed or basic attention that are sometimes observed in individuals with attention disorders.

Academic Achievement. Across measures of academic skills, Ana performed consistently in the average range compared to her grade-related American peers on tests of spelling, writing, reading, and mathematics. Significant disparity among academic skills is expected in individuals with learning difficulties as well as observed impairment in target areas. Given her performance on these tests, there was no evidence of a learning disorder. Moreover, these academic scores reflected well-developed skills in reading and writing in English, even with her later-onset bilingual status.

Attention and Executive Functioning. Ana's basic auditory attention (repeating numbers) and complex working memory (repeating numbers in backward order) were in the high average and superior range, respectively. In contrast, Ana's performance on measures of sustained visual attention was impaired, signaling difficulties with inattentiveness and vigilance. Further, self-report forms indicated concerns for both inattention and hyperactivity. Ana's performances on various executive functioning measures ranged from average to superior and did not suggest significant problems with mental flexibility, impulsivity, or inhibitory control. In contrast, Ana endorsed significant levels of executive dysfunction on a self-report measure (see Behavioral functioning section).

While Ana performed largely within the expected range across measures of attention and executive functioning, an isolated area of weakness was noted when tasks challenged her ability to sustain and focus her attentional resources. Qualitatively, Ana's observed impulsivity and distractibility during testing were consistent with the type of challenges often associated with AD/HD.

Memory and Learning. No deficits were noted across measures of verbal and visual memory. Ana's learning and retention of unstructured verbal information (word list), structured verbal information (stories), and visual information (figures) were consistently strong with performances ranging from average to superior.

Visual Spatial Functioning: Ana's performance was low average when copying a complex geometric figure. Notably, she struggled to copy this figure in an organized and efficient fashion, suggestive of poor visual organization abilities.

Behavioral Functioning: On an executive function scale, Ana reported very significant challenges with all aspects of executive functioning. Specifically, she reported difficulty with initiation of tasks, working memory, planning and organization, task monitoring (e.g., making errors on tasks), and self-monitoring of behaviors. On an AD/HD self-report scale, she endorsed symptoms of both inattention and hyperactivity that met criteria for AD/HD both in childhood and in the past 6 months that met criteria for AD/HD combined type, reinforcing the diagnosis from the interview.

Mood Functioning: Ana rated her symptoms on anxiety and depression on broad-based rating scales. The results of self-report measures revealed clinically significant levels of anxiety and depression, including indecisiveness, agitation, irritability, disrupted sleep, pervasive worrying, test anxiety, as well as somatic and cognitive symptoms. These findings are consistent with Ana's clinical interview description: ongoing anxiety, depression symptoms, and the recent emergence of panic attacks. On the Panic Attack Questionnaire, she reported five panic attacks in the past year, with the last one being the prior week, lasting 6–7 minutes. Both anxiety and depression commonly co-occur with AD/HD. The pattern and severity of her reported symptoms were consistent with generalized anxiety disorder, panic disorder, and major depressive disorder (moderate, recurrent).

Diagnoses

F90.0 Attention-deficit/hyperactivity disorder (AD/HD), combined presentation
F33.1 Major depressive disorder, recurrent, moderate
F41.1 Generalized anxiety disorder
F41.0 Panic disorder

Collaborative Discussion

AD/HD in adults is a significantly impairing disorder that affects virtually every sphere of daily functioning (i.e., education, occupation, relationships, financial management) [2, 43]. One study at the University of Massachusetts showed that the areas most affected by AD/HD were education (worse in the hyperactive subtype), followed by home responsibilities and occupational functioning, and then, to a lesser extent, relationships and social activities [2]. Adults with AD/HD have elevated risk for tobacco and drug use, antisocial behavior, and sleep problems [44]. Adults with hyperactive subtype especially are at higher risk for injury, have higher rates of nonsurgical hospitalizations and poisonings, and have lower rates of consistent exercising. Research has also revealed that these individuals have a greater risk of coronary heart disease [2, 45]. Therefore, neuropsychologists target not only acute symptoms of attention but also larger psychosocial disturbances. The following recommendations were made to Ana by the neuropsychologist (and primary care physician for some of the recommendations) in a feedback session.

1. *Psychopharmacological Treatment for AD/HD*: Psychostimulant medication is the most effective pharmacologic treatment for adults with AD/HD with response rates ranging from 25% to 78% [46, 47]. The factors predicting the wide response rate include stimulant dosage levels, presence of co-occurring mood disorders, and the various methods of measuring response rates.

   In the current case, Ana had suffered recent panic attacks, so even though prescription of a stimulant medication was recommended, the potential for increased panic attacks needed to be taken into consideration. The primary care physician directed Ana continue to take fluoxetine, 20 mg, for depression and panic in addition to the psychostimulant.
2. *Psychotherapy*: Given Ana's ongoing symptoms of anxiety and depression, she was encouraged to continue in psychotherapy to treat these conditions. Psychotherapy would help her feel better emotionally, but as her mood and anxiety improved, her attention was predicted to improve as well [48].
3. *Sleep Hygiene*: It was recommended that Ana follow up with prescription for continuous positive airway pressure. Sleep helps replenish memory and maintain optimal cognitive functioning, as well as enhancing overall well-being [49]. Therefore, it was important for Ana to develop reliable sleep hygiene as a self-care habit. She was educated on sleep hygiene at neuropsychology feedback (provided with a sleep hygiene handout as well) and was encouraged to make behavioral changes to improve the quality and duration of her sleep.
4. *Substance Use*: Ana was encouraged to continue to abstain from marijuana use. Ongoing use can negatively impact attention, processing speed, as well as anxiety and depressive symptoms [10–12, 50].
5. *Exercise*: Research shows that regular aerobic exercise helps improve attention by activating the part of the brain that controls focus, concentration, organization, and planning [51, 52]. Ana was encouraged to engage in aerobic exercise.
6. *Self-Care*: Maintaining physical and cognitive health through consistent self-care including a well-balanced diet, adequate regular sleep where possible, and regular physical activity (if not medically contraindicated) was strongly recommended. These behaviors are also well known to reduce mood and attention symptoms [49, 53, 54]. Ana was advised to focus on the holistic nature of treatment, emphasizing her self-care and lowering stress.

7. *AD/HD Coaching*: Ana was recommended to work with an AD/HD coach to develop specific compensatory strategies for her school or workplace and home life.

Academic

1. *Academic Accommodations*

   Accommodations, especially testing accommodations, have become increasingly prevalent, in part from an effort to provide persons with disabilities the ability to demonstrate their skills and compete fairly with nondisabled persons. However, there is not always a consistent metric of application of accommodations provided to individuals with disabilities, and greater research-based practice is needed to determine which accommodations are helpful and improve functional/academic outcomes [55]. Accommodations can be recommended for both work and educational settings. Academic accommodations, specifically, can be classified into several domains [56]: (1) setting accommodations which includes taking a test in a separate location from other students, (2) presentation accommodations for test instructions or test questions using a different communication medium (e.g., audio versus written), (3) scheduling accommodations such as taking a test at a different time of the day, (4) timing accommodations such as being provided with addition time or additional break, and (5) response accommodations such as responding to test items using alternative means (e.g., a scribe) (Table 27.1).

   There is not much formal research outcome efficacy of test accommodations for AD/HD, though evaluators typically make recommendations based on the patient's/student's cognitive symptom profile. Based upon Ana's diagnosis of AD/HD, her symptom and cognitive profile, the following academic accommodations were recommended:

   (a) Taking extra breaks during in-class exams and tests as well as standardized tests
   (b) Testing in a separate classroom, which offers a distraction-free environment
   (c) Permission to stand in the back of academic lectures or classes as needed to minimize fidgetiness
   (d) Permission to take notes standing up during academic lectures or classes as needed

2. *Study/Homework Strategies*

   Ana was also provided with cognitive strategies to assist with studying and homework based on her neurocognitive profile:

   (a) She was instructed to take frequent, short breaks while studying. Breaks typically need only be 1 or 2 minutes in duration. Noting when attention begins to diminish will help determine the optimal time for a break.

(b) Break down assignments into smaller steps or chunks.
(c) Schedule regular, consistent homework/study time into your day with firm start and end times.
(d) Use active, engaging study strategies such as note-taking or highlighting main points while reading, using electronic media (audio books, books on iPad), joining a study group, or explaining concepts to peers.

Chapter Review Questions

1. True/False: Because many individuals present for the first time with complaints of inattention and disorganization in adulthood, the DSM-5 recognizes AD/HD may have an adult onset.
2. True/False: There are three subtypes of AD/HD.
3. True/False: AD/HD causes sleep disturbance.
4. True/False: AD/HD is associated with elevated rates of substance abuse including marijuana use.
5. Which is the primary method of diagnosing AD/HD symptoms in adults?
   A. Neuropsychological testing.
   B. Review of academic transcripts.
   C. Clinical interview.
   D. Self-report measures.
6. Which of the following treatments are recommended for individuals diagnosed with AD/HD?
   A. Stimulant medications.
   B. Physical exercise.
   C. Sleep hygiene.
   D. All of the above.

References

1. American Psychiatric Association. Diagnostic and statistical manual of mental disorders. 5th ed. Washington, DC: APA; 2013.
2. Barkley RA, Murphy KR, Fischer M. AD/HD in adults: what the science says. New York: Guilford Press; 2008.
3. Antshel KM, Barkley R. Overview and historical background of attention deficit hyperactivity disorder. In: Evans SW, Hoza B, editors. Treating attention deficit hyperactivity disorder: assessment and intervention in developmental context. Kingston: Civic Research Institute; 2011. p. 1–30.

4. Lara C, Fayyad J, de Graaf R, Kessler RC, Aguilar-Gaxiola S, Angermeyer M, Demytteneare K, de Girolamo G, Haro JM, Jin R, Karam EG, Lépine JP, Mora ME, Ormel J, Posada-Villa J, Sampson N. Childhood predictors of adult attention-deficit/hyperactivity disorder: results from the World Health Organization World Mental Health Survey Initiative. Biol Psychiatry. 2009;65(1):46–54.
5. Biederman J, Petty CR, Clarke A, Lomedico A, Faraone SV. Predictors of persistent ADHD: an 11-year follow-up study. J Psychiatr Res. 2011;45(2):150–5.
6. Mannuzza S, Castellanos FX, Roizen ER, Hutchison JA, Lashua EC, Klein RG. Impact of the impairment criterion in the diagnosis of adult ADHD: 33-year follow-up study of boys with ADHD. J Atten Disord. 2011;15:122–9.
7. Biederman J, Newcorn J, Sprich S. Comorbidity of attention deficit hyperactivity disorder with conduct, depressive, anxiety, and other disorders. Am J Psychiatr. 1991;148(5):564–77.
8. Kessler RC, Alder RC, Barkley R, Biederman J, Conners CK, Demler O, Zaslavsky AM. The prevalence and correlates of adult AD/HD in the Unites States: results from the National Comorbidity Survey Replication. Am J Psychiatr. 2006;163:716–23.
9. Newcorn JH, Weiss M, Stein MA. The complexity of AD/HD: diagnosis and treatment of the adult patient with comorbidities. CNS Spectr. 2007;12(8S):1–16.
10. Crean RD, Crane NA, Mason BJ. An evidence-based review of acute and long-term effects of cannabis use on executive cognitive functions. J Addict Med. 2011;5(1):1–8.
11. Pope HG, Yurgelun-Todd D. The residual cognitive effects of heavy marijuana use in college students. J Am Med Assoc. 1996;275(7):521–7.
12. Tapert SF, Schweinsburg AD, Brown SA. The influence of marijuana use on neurocognitive functioning in adolescents. Curr Drug Abuse Rev. 2008;1(1):99–111.
13. Clure C, Brady KT, Saladin ME, Johnson D, Waid R, Rittenbury M. Attention deficit/hyperactivity disorder and substance use: symptoms pattern and drug choice. Am J Drug Alcohol Abuse. 1999;25:441–8.
14. Katusic SK, Barbaresi WJ, Colligan RC, Weaver AL, Leibson CL, Jacobsen SJ. Psychostimulant treatment and risk for substance abuse among young adults with a history of attention-deficit/hyperactivity disorder: a population-based, birth cohort study. J Child Adolesc Psychopharmacol. 2005;15:764–76.
15. Whalen CK, Jamner LD, Henker B, Delfino RJ, Lozano JM. The ADHD spectrum and everyday life: experience sampling of adolescent moods, activities, smoking, and drinking. Child Dev. 2002;73(1):209–27.
16. Lee SS, Humphreys KL, Flory K, Liu R, Glass K. Prospective association of childhood attention-deficit/hyperactivity disorder (ADHD) and substance use and abuse/dependence: a meta-analytic review. Clin Psychol Rev. 2011;31(3):328–41.
17. Biederman J, Faraone S, Mick E. Age dependent decline of ADHD symptoms revisited: impact of remission definition and symptom subtype. Am J Psychiatr. 2000;157:816–7.
18. Mick E, Faraone SV, Biederman J, Spencer T. The course and outcome of ADHD. Primary Psychiatry. 2004;11(7):42–8.
19. Dupaul GJ, Gormley MJ, Laracy SD. Comorbidity of LD and ADHD: implications of DSM-5 for Assessment and Treatment. J Learn Disabil. 2012;46(1):43–51.
20. Vergne D, Whitham E, Barroilhet S, Fradkin Y, Ghaemi S. Adult ADHD and amphetamines: a new paradigm. Neuropsychiatry. 2011;1(6):591–8.
21. Murphy KR, Alder LA. Assessing attention-deficit/hyperactivity disorder in adults: focus on rating scales. J Clin Psychiatry. 2004;65:12–7.
22. Biederman J, Faraone SV, Spencer T, Wilens T, Norman D, Lapey KA, et al. Patterns of psychiatric comorbidity, cognition, and psychosocial functioning in adults with attention deficit hyperactivity disorder. Am J Psychiatr. 1993;150:1792–8.
23. Monastra VJ. Medical conditions that mimic AD/HD. In: Unlocking the potential of patients with AD/HD: a model for clinical practice. Washington, DC: American Psychological Association; 2008. p. 49–66.
24. Wasserstein J. Diagnostic Issues for adolescents and adults with AD/HD. J Clin Psychol. 2005;61(5):535–47.

25. Owens JA. The AD/HD and sleep conundrum: a Review. J Dev Behav Pediatr. 2005;26: 312–22.
26. American Psychiatric Association. Diagnostic and statistical manual of mental disorders: DSM-III. Washington, DC: Author; 1980.
27. Barkley RA, McMurray MB, Edelbrock CS, Robbins K. Side effects of methylphenidate in children with attention deficit hyperactivity disorder: a systemic, placebo-controlled evaluation. Pediatrics. 1990;86:184–92.
28. Mayes SD, Calhoun SL, Bixler EO, Vgontzas AN, Mahr F, Hillwig-Garcia J, et al. ADHD subtypes and comorbid anxiety, depression, and oppositional-defiant disorder: differences in sleep problems. J Pediatr Psychol. 2008;34(3):328–37.
29. Montano B. Diagnosis and treatment of AD/HD in primary care. J Clin Psychiatry. 2004;65:18–21.
30. Brown TE. ADD/AD/HD and impaired executive function in clinical practice. Curr Psychiatry Rep. 2008;10:407–11.
31. Weiss MD, Weiss JR. A guide to the treatment of adults with ADHD. J Clin Psychiatry. 2004;65(Suppl 3):27–37.
32. Adler L, Shaw D, Sitt D, Maya E, Morrill MI. Issues in the diagnosis and treatment of adult AD/HD by primary care physicians. Prim Psychiatry. 2009;16(5):57–63.
33. Mapou R. Adult learning disabilities and ADHD: research informed assessment. New York: Oxford University Press; 2009.
34. Boonstra AM, Oosterlaan J, Seargeant JA, Buitelaar JK. Executive functioning in adult AD/HD: a meta-analytic review. Psychol Med. 2005;35:1097–108.
35. Hervey AS, Epstein JN, Curry JF. Neuropsychology of adults with attention-deficit/hyperactivity disorder: a meta-analytic review. Neuropsychology. 2004;18(3):485–503.
36. Schoechlin C, Engel R. Neuropsychological performance in adult attention-deficit hyperactivity disorder: meta-analysis of empirical data. Arch Clin Neuropsychol. 2005;20(6): 727–44.
37. Fortuny LA i, Mullaney HA. Neuropsychology with Spanish speakers: language use and proficiency issues for test development. J Clin Exp Neuropsychol. 1997;19(4):615–22.
38. Robillard R. Neuropsychological considerations in bilingual assessment: the underlying basis of language disability. In: Clinton A, editor. Assessing bilingual children in context: an integrated approach. Washington DC: APA; 2014.
39. Sullivan BK, May K, Galbally L. Symptom exaggeration by college adults in attention-deficit hyperactivity disorder and learning disorder assessments. Appl Neuropsychol. 2007;14(3):189–207.
40. Marshall PS, Hoelzle JB, Heyerdahl D, Nelson NW. The impact of failing to identify suspect effort in patients undergoing adult attention-deficit/hyperactivity disorder (AD/HD) assessment. Psychol Assess. 2016;28:1290–302.
41. Jachimowicz G, Geiselman RE. Compariosn of ease of falsification of attention deficit disorder diagnosis using standard behavioral rating scales. Cogn Sci Online. 2004;2:6–20.
42. Miller E. Some basic principles of neuropsychological assessment. In: Crawford JR, Parker DM, McKinlay WW, editors. A handbook of neuropsychological assessment. Hove: Lawrence Erlbaum; 1994. p. 7–20.
43. Halmony A, Frasmer OB, Gillberg C, Haavik J. Occupational outcome in adult AD/HD: impact of symptom profile, comorbid psychiatric problems, and treatment: a cross-section study of 414 clinically diagnosed adult AD/HD patients. J Atten Disord. 2009;13:175–87.
44. Barkley RA, Fischer M, Smallish L, Fletcher K. Young adult outcome of hyperactive children: adaptive functioning in major life activities. J Am Acad Child Adolesc Psychiatry. 2006;45(2):192–202.
45. Nigg JT. Attention-deficit/hyperactivity disorder and adverse health outcomes. Clin Psychol Rev. 2013;33:215–28.
46. Dotson WW. Pharmacotherapy of adult AD/HD. J Clin Psychol. 2005;61:589–606.

47. Goksory PK, Nottestad JA. The burden of untreated AD/HD among adults: the role of stimulant medication. Addict Behav. 2008;33:342–6.
48. Ramsay JR. Current status of cognitive-behavioral therapy as a psychosocial treatment for adult attention-deficit/hyperactivity disorder. Curr Psychiatry Rep. 2007;9:427–33.
49. Blunden S, Milte C, Sinn N. Diet and sleep in children with ADHD: preliminary data in Australian children. J Child Health Care. 2011;15(1):14–24.
50. Wilens TE. Impact of AD/HD and its treatment on substance abuse in adults. J Clin Psychiatry. 2004;65:38–45.
51. Gapin JI, Labban JD, Etnier JL. The effects of physical activity on attention deficit hyperactivity disorder symptoms: the evidence. Prev Med. 2011;52:S70–4.
52. Pontifex MB, Saliba BJ, Raine LB, Picchietti DL, Hillman CH. Exercise improves behavioral, neurocognitive, and scholastic performance in children with ADHD. J Pediatr. 2013; 162(3):543–51.
53. Lopresti AL, Hood SD, Drummond PD. A review of lifestyle factors that contribute to important pathways associated with major depression: diet, sleep and exercise. J Affect Disord. 2013;148(1):12–27.
54. Stein D, Pat-Horenczyk R, Blank S, Dagan Y, Barak Y. Sleep disturbances in adolescents with symptoms of attention-deficit/hyperactivity disorder. J Learn Disabil. 2002;35(3):268–75.
55. Lovett BJ, Lewandowski LJ. Testing accommodations for students with disabilities: research-based practice. Washington DC: APA; 2015.
56. Thurlow ML, Elliott JL, Ysseldyke JE. Testing students with disabilities: practical strategies for complying with district and state requirements. 2nd ed. Thousand Oaks: Corwin Press; 2003.

Part III
Related Issues in Collaboration: Specialties and Essential Considerations

Chapter 28
Neuropsychology in the Twenty-First Century: The Rise of Multicultural Assessments

Margaret Lanca and Emily K. Wilner

Racial, cultural, and linguistic diversity in the United States is growing exponentially. Between 2000 and 2010, the US population grew 9.7%, and the majority of this growth comprised individuals who identify as nonwhite or Hispanic/Latino [1]. There was a 43% increase in the US Latino population from 2000 to 2010, which represents more than half of the total population growth [1]. As of 2012 the US immigrant population consisted of 40.7 million people, which represented a 31.2% increase from 2000 [2]. In 2010 about 21% of individuals 5 years and older reported speaking a language other than English at home, which represented a 158.2% increase since 1980 [3]. Of these individuals, 15% reported speaking English "not well," and 7% spoke English "not at all" [3]. These statistics reflect the changing landscape of the US demographic population, which inevitably will alter the field of clinical neuropsychology.

Whereas multicultural neuropsychological assessment was once considered a subspecialty, it is quickly migrating toward center stage. Consequently, neuropsychologists have been integrating culturally informed neuropsychological assessments into their practice to better serve the vast array of multicultural patients. At minimum, culturally informed assessments incorporate (1) greater sensitivity to the psychological factors that affect evaluation of multicultural populations, (2) understanding of the ways in which culture impacts the testing environment, (3)

M. Lanca (✉) E. K. Wilner
Harvard Medical School, Cambridge Health Alliance, Cambridge, MA, USA
e-mail: Margaret_Lanca@hms.harvard.edu

K. M. Sanders (ed.), *Physician's Field Guide to Neuropsychology*,
https://doi.org/10.1007/978-1-4939-8722-1_28

multicultural assessment tools and evaluation techniques, and (4) knowledge of how to work with interpreters, if necessary. These will be discussed in this chapter.

Key Point
Multicultural assessments are culturally informed assessment techniques that incorporate:

- Sensitivity to psychological factors affecting multicultural groups
- Understanding of how culture impacts testing
- Use of multicultural assessment tools
- Knowledge of how to work with interpreters

Cultural Factors in Neuropsychological Testing

The terms *race*, *ethnicity*, and *diversity* are often bantered in medical settings sometimes without much thought to the specificity of each term. *Culture* is a more comprehensive term, which refers to sets of customs and ways of life belonging to a particular group [4]. This chapter will use the terms *culture* and *multiculturalism* to refer to the diverse range of experiences patients of various races, ethnicities, nationalities, religions, linguistic groups, and other backgrounds bring to the neuropsychological assessment process.

Cultural factors are well known to play a role in multiple aspects of medical care. This includes vast differences in symptom expression and coping mechanisms across cultures, as well as the decision to report symptoms to a professional and which symptoms to discuss [5]. Cultural factors may also dictate the level of stigma attached to a disorder as well as beliefs about the characteristics of the individual who is diagnosed with a particular disorder [5]. This is especially true for psychiatric disorders that are often significantly stigmatized cross-culturally. In many cultures physical symptoms are more acceptable than psychiatric symptoms. Therefore, a neuropsychologist discussing behavioral symptoms of a neurologic disorder may choose to discuss them in the context of the medical condition as opposed to labeling them as a psychiatric symptom [6]. Such findings emphasize the importance of awareness and knowledge of the patient's cultural values and beliefs in order to establish a therapeutic alliance and protect against miscommunication due to cultural differences [7].

Attention to the role of culture and the need for culturally informed approaches to neuropsychological assessment continues to gain traction in the field of neuropsychology (e.g., [8, 9]). There is increasing awareness of many cultural variables embedded in assessment, which can impact the outcome of an evaluation (e.g., [4, 6, 10]). These include, for example, knowing how to work with patients from other cultures, especially those from collectivist cultures, who may be unfamiliar with the testing environment or the emphasis on a one-to-one relationship with an authority figure in an isolated environment. Neuropsychological measures also depend on specific test stimuli (e.g., blocks, pictures) that are culture specific and may not be equally familiar to individuals depending on their cultural background. Importantly, the validity of neuropsychological test data depends upon a patient's ability to put forth his/her best performance. This orientation and expectation are most familiar to individuals from cultures that value formal assessment and competition but may be completely novel and even uncomfortable for other patients. Similarly, performance on many cognitive tests depends on speed of task completion; however, perceptions and attitudes toward time and speed are culturally dependent. Furthermore, speed and quality of performance may be considered at odds with each other [4].

Literacy and education are major factors that influence cognition and are themselves related to culture (e.g., [10–15]). Research has shown that literacy influences both the functional and structural development of the brain (e.g., [16, 17]), as well as nearly all domains of cognition (for a review see [11]). These cognitive enhancements can be attributed to improvement in visual perception and logical reasoning (i.e., executive functioning), memory strategies, access to lexical storage, explicit phonological processing, and working memory. Thus, it is not a surprise that reading level, as assessed by a reading test, has been found to be a significant predictor of neuropsychological test performance [18]. While education has implications for literacy, years of education is not always a sufficient proxy for literacy given the variability in education quality, achievement expectations, and curricula internationally [11]. World illiteracy levels are shockingly high with UNESCO (2017) [19] reporting 14% of the adult world population to be illiterate with the greatest regions of illiteracy in Southern Asia (49%) and sub-Saharan Africa (27%). These findings have strong implications for neuropsychological testing, which often assume a certain level of literacy for the patient's age and raise possible confounds in the interpretation of test results if literacy and education are not accounted for. Therefore, the need to assess literacy as well as preliteracy skills (i.e., knowledge of numbers and letters) for patients with low education is of paramount importance prior to administering and interpreting neuropsychological measures [20].

Key Point

There are a wide range of cultural variables that can influence neuropsychological test performance. These include:

- Cultural orientation toward test-taking
- Cultural perceptions and attitudes toward time and speed
- Culture-specific test stimuli
- Literacy and educational attainment
- Language proficiency
- Acculturation level
- Bilingualism

Similarly, education and schooling have widespread implications for neuropsychological test performance as the quality, intensity, and scholastic curriculum of a patient's educational experience can impact neuropsychological assessment. Though focused on assessing cognitive domains (e.g., learning, memory, language, etc.), neuropsychological tests capture skills reinforced in school, and it is well-established that individuals with formal education perform better on cognitive testing than those without (e.g., [13, 15, 21]). For example, schooling helps develop strategies for recalling new information [11] and increases operational thinking. Thus, patients whose education in their home country is less intensive or formal (e.g., half-day schools), or predominated by cultural or religious curriculum, will have an experience that is different from mainstream North American education. Subsequently their performance on neuropsychological tests that were developed and normed on individuals raised in the United States will also be affected.

When patients immigrate to the United States from another country, their brain networks are inevitably altered as they incorporate a new culture, academic experience, and often a new language into their life. Level of acculturation (including language preference, level of English proficiency, first exposure to English, as well as years of residence and education in the United States) is an important consideration in multicultural neuropsychological testing. Not surprisingly, level of acculturation has been linked to neuropsychological test performance. As patients become more acculturated to the American culture, neuropsychological test performance increases, suggesting that familiarity with and approach toward test-taking may influence results obtained on neuropsychological measures, especially American-based measures [14]. For example, in their research, Boone et al. [10] found that the ability to identify drawings of common American objects was significantly related to the number of years of education in the United States, as well as the number of years in the United States and the age at which conversational English was learned. The ability to repeat numbers was also significantly associated with the age at which English was learned and years spent in the United States. Additionally, Razani et al. [14] found that monolingual English-speaking individuals performed better on tasks of information processing and attention than multicultural, English-speaking individuals. This finding cautions against the assumption that English-speaking American norms, even for nonverbal tests, are applicable to all English-speaking individuals.

For bilingual individuals, there are additional factors to consider. Bilinguals have been shown to outperform monolinguals in some areas of cognition but lag behind in other areas of cognition (as reviewed in [22]). Research has also shown that level of proficiency in both languages (i.e., *balanced* versus *unbalanced* bilinguals) can impact performance on neuropsychological tests, such as the Boston Naming Test (BNT) [23]. Unfortunately, the field of neuropsychology has not yet established clear-cut guidelines on how to best determine language(s) of assessment.

Specific Cultural Considerations in the Neuropsychological Evaluation

In general, there is a dearth of formalized guidelines for neuropsychological testing with multicultural populations [8]. The American Academy of Clinical Neuropsychology Practice Guidelines for Neuropsychological Assessment and Consultation [24] provided a general framework for multicultural testing. These guidelines discuss the influence of cultural factors in neuropsychological assessment process, including implications for test selection and interpretation, and the importance of education and training when administering tests and interpreting findings vis-a-vis a patient's cultural background. Others have also promoted tailored approaches and suggested guidelines for the assessment for specific cultural populations (e.g., [6]). The following sections will illustrate some considerations for assessing multicultural populations at each time point in the neuropsychological evaluation process.

Case Preparation

Knowledge about a patient's cultural background is crucial to all aspects of the neuropsychological evaluation. Gaining an understanding of the patient's culture *prior* to meeting the patient can assist in facilitating rapport and the therapeutic alliance. For example, in Latino cultures, there may be an emphasis on friendliness and warmth (*personalismo*) when interacting with healthcare providers or clinicians [25]. This may manifest in nonverbal communication such as physical contact (handshakes, hugs) and interactions at a closer distance. A lack of *personalismo* on the part of the clinician can affect the nature and extent of personal information a patient is inclined to share during the evaluation, as well as preclude the development of rapport and alliance.

While there is great variability in customs and traditions within cultural groups, awareness of broader group characteristics can also be helpful in interpreting behavior that might be unfamiliar to the clinician [6]. For example, Wong and Fujii discuss how emphasis on the family unit in Asian cultures may help explain an adult child's reluctance to place an elderly parent with dementia in an assisted living center or nursing home. Respect for elders is another prominent value in Chinese culture, which in the context of a neuropsychological evaluation, may preclude family members from openly reporting or discussing concerning symptoms or behaviors of a parent unless specifically asked in a sensitive manner [6].

In addition to understanding cultural values and normative behaviors, learning about the social and economic conditions, immigration trends, and education system of a patient's home country is also recommended [6]. This information can be obtained through reading, professional consultation, and education/training.

Key Point
Cultural considerations in case preparation include gaining awareness and understanding of cultural values, customs, and normative behaviors. Knowledge about socioeconomic conditions, immigration patterns, and education in the patient's country or culture of origin is also recommended.

Conducting the Interview

Given the aforementioned variability within cultural groups, it is of paramount importance to assess the extent to which cultural factors play a role in the patient's day-to-day life. In addition to standard inquiries regarding symptoms, as well as medical, developmental, and psychosocial history during the clinical interview, it can be useful to ask questions that shed light on the patient's symptoms and development in the context of his/her culture of origin. As discussed by Takushi and Uomoto [26], this may include inquiries about cultural expectations regarding the behavior or abilities for individuals the patient's age, the patient's or family's beliefs regarding those expectations, and the supports or resources available to individuals experiencing these types of challenges or symptoms.

In neuropsychological assessment as well as many other medical disciplines, it is also crucial to evaluate acculturation level [6]. Inquiries about a patient's immigration history, including reasons for immigration, recency of immigration, and experience entering and integrating into the host culture, can provide useful information about a patient's degree of acculturation [26], immigration trauma, and level of psychosocial stressors. Questions regarding frequency and extent of English use in social, leisure, educational, and work environments can also shed light on acculturation level as majority language use is the primary predictor of acculturation [27].

Key Point
The clinical interview can provide an opportunity to evaluate the extent to which cultural factors play a role in the patient's daily life. This may include inquiries about immigration history, English language use, and education.

Another important area of neuropsychological assessment is premorbid functioning [6]. Premorbid functioning refers to a patient's baseline cognitive and functional abilities. Given the influence of culture on cognition and behavior, coupled with limitations in the use of existing measures (i.e., a reading test) for estimating premorbid abilities in multicultural populations, inquiry regarding educational and occupational history is often useful, particularly for immigrants. In addition to learning about the patient's schooling and work history prior to immigration as well as his/her current employment or academic functioning (as applicable), it may be useful to ask about the educational and work history of the parents, the typical level of educational and occupational achievement in the patient's native country, and how this compares with that of the patient and other members in his/her family [6].

Key Point
The term *premorbid functioning* refers to a patient's baseline cognitive and functional abilities. In multicultural populations, tests assessing premorbid abilities such as a reading test may not be valid. Baseline abilities may be better estimated via inquiry into the patient's schooling and work history and comparing this with cultural expectations of educational and occupational achievement in the home country.

For patients whose native language is not English, the interview is also an opportunity to evaluate the level of English proficiency for the purpose of test selection and decisions regarding the language in which to conduct the evaluation. As recommended by Wong and Fujii [6], this may include administration of brief measures of reading comprehension or vocabulary, such as the Auditory Comprehension subtest of the Boston Diagnostic Aphasia Examination [28] or items of the Peabody Picture Vocabulary Test (PPVT) (most recent version PPVT-4; [29]). Questions about a patient's familiarity with and use of English, including age of first exposure, type and length of formal education or instruction in English, and use of English (vs. other languages) in daily life, are also helpful in determining the language of assessment.

Test Selection

Many core neuropsychological tests and measures are sensitive to cultural/linguistic factors. Not surprisingly, these include verbally based tasks or measures assessing language such as object naming (Boston Naming Test; [30]), verbal fluency [31], and verbal learning and memory (California Verbal Learning Test; [32]). What might be more surprising is that nonverbally mediated tasks can also be impacted by culture. For example, nonverbal measures assessing visuoconstruction/planning and organization (Rey-Osterrieth Complex Figure Test; [33]) have been shown to be culturally skewed (as reviewed in [10]). Consequently, neuropsychologists need to be mindful that translations of tests developed and normed on US populations can threaten the validity of these measures in all aspects of validity criterion (i.e., item, method, and construct; [34]). To address these threats in a multicultural assessment, neuropsychologists sometimes adopt nontraditional assessment techniques such as employing assessment strategies that do not require a standardized normative approach, including direct observation, charting of behavioral changes over time, criterion-referenced testing, direct comparisons with a group of demographically similar peers, or comparison with demographically similar groups in published research studies [35].

Key Point
Both verbal *and* nonverbal neuropsychological tests are sensitive to cultural influences.

Common neuropsychological measures have been translated into other languages (e.g., Wechsler Adult Intelligence Scale-Fourth Edition (WAIS-IV) [36] in over 20 languages, Montréal Cognitive Assessment (MoCA) [37] in 30 languages); however, it remains important to consider issues of construct validity when using translated measures (i.e., test content does not necessarily have the same familiarity, significance, or meaning in other languages/cultures). For example, the most challenging item on the Boston Naming Test [30], an abacus, may be easily named by an older Asian patient [6]. Adaptation of tests for use with other cultural/linguistic groups (i.e., Boston Naming Test, Ponton-Satz version; [38]) has attempted to address issues of cross-cultural validity. However, it is also important to note that the availability of translated/adapted tests/batteries varies widely depending on the cultural group (i.e., there are more options for Spanish speakers than most other languages).

Key Point
Translations of tests into other languages do not mean that the test has retained its construct validity. In other words, translation does not guarantee the same familiarity or significance of test items from one language to another.

The development of normative data for specific cultural groups has strongly improved interpretation of neuropsychological test performance across cultures. These norms include large databases such as Mayo's Older African Americans Normative Studies (MOAANS), which provides norms for African American individuals over the age of 55 on commonly administered neuropsychological tests [39], and the Spanish Multicenter Normative Studies (NEURONORMA), which provides norms for Spanish-speaking individuals over 49 years of age for tests on attention, language, visuo-perceptual abilities, constructional tasks, memory, and executive function [40]. Normative data for commonly used measures (e.g., verbal fluency, Trail Making Test) are also available for various linguistic groups, including Spanish-, Portuguese-, and Chinese-speaking individuals [41–43]. Additionally, there are neuropsychological test batteries that have been developed for and normed on specific cultural and linguistic groups, including the *Evaluación Neuropsicológica Breve en Español* (NEUROPSI; [44]) for monolingual Spanish speakers.

Recently there has been a movement toward the development of measures with cross-cultural validity, often referred to "culture-fair" tests [45]. Examples of these measures include the Test of Nonverbal Intelligence, Fourth Edition (TONI-4) [46], a language-free measure of cognition; the MOCA Test Basic [47], a cognitive screening tool for illiterate or minimally educated patients (less than 5 years); or Color Trails Test (CTT) [48], a graphomotor test of visual scanning, complex attention, information sequencing, and mental flexibility analogous to Trail Making Test, which replaced letters with colors. These types of tests hold promise for the field because they reduce the necessity for multiple normative data sets across culture and language. They also uniquely pinpoint elements of cognition that are universal and emphasize *etic* perspectives of cognition and minimize *emic* differences [49].

Key Point
While no test is entirely culture-free, several "culture-fair" tests (measures with cross-cultural validity) have been developed. Common culture-fair tests include:

- TONI-4
- MOCA Test Basic
- Color Trails Test

Test Interpretation

The core of a neuropsychological evaluation rests in test interpretation, conclusions, and delivery of feedback to patients. Test interpretation and resulting conclusions go beyond the test scores and rely on a trained neuropsychologist with knowledge of current published literature in the field. A neuropsychologist is required to interpret the test findings in the context of a patient's history and symptoms, direct observation of the patient, levels or patterns of test performance associated with specific clinical presentations, and the current knowledge regarding the neurological, psychiatric psychosocial, and cultural influences on test performance and daily functioning. This interpretation is individualized and does not follow a "cookbook" approach [24]. In a multicultural setting, the test scores must also be interpreted within the cultural framework. Test interpretation may be constrained by numerous factors such as test translation, inadequate normative data for the patient's language and ethnicity, unfamiliarity with the patient's culture and language, and/or the use of interpreters. The cumulative result of these constraints can range from mild considerations to invalidation of the test findings depending on the range and type of constraints. It is crucial that the neuropsychologist states these limitations in his/her report. Sometimes, conclusions may be limited to functional descriptions of test findings and/or a recommendation for repeated testing to track cognition over time.

Key Point
Interpretation of test data in multicultural populations may be affected by many factors, including:

- Test translation
- Lack of normative data
- Lack of familiarity with patient's culture or language
- Use of interpreters

Medical Interpreters

A growing reality for many neuropsychologists across the country is the inclusion of medical interpreters in their practice given the discrepancy between the rising number of multicultural patients and lack of multilingual neuropsychologists. The American Psychological Association (APA) Ethics Code recognizes the impact of cultural factors in assessment with culturally diverse populations. The Code instructs psychologists to conduct assessments in the patient's preferred language as appropriate to the purpose of the assessment and to use measures that have been established for use with the cultural group being tested [50]. Under the ideal conditions, a bilingual/bicultural neuropsychologist is available to conduct testing in the patient's preferred language with measures that have been designed and validated for use with that population. While this may be more feasible for some languages and populations (e.g., Spanish-speaking patients), in many instances it is not possible to refer to a bilingual/bicultural neuropsychologist or access language- or culture-specific tests despite an increasing need for neuropsychological assessments for multicultural populations [8]. As a result, neuropsychologists are frequently being asked to assess patients whose cultural and linguistic backgrounds are not native English-speaking from North America and for whom tests and measures have not yet been developed.

Although working with medical interpreters is not ideal for neuropsychological assessment for many of the reasons already discussed in this chapter, learning how to work effectively with medical interpreters is an increasingly crucial aspect of clinical practice. At the outset, employing medical interpreters who are trained as professionals and subscribe to national standards of practice (i.e., [51]) is of paramount importance. Choosing a family member or friend to interpret can introduce conflict of interest, lack of confidentiality, and destabilization of family systems. Medical interpreters are typically with college education and a facility with both languages that is important in a medical setting. A trained interpreter knows how to build rapport with both the patient and the medical provider and understands the patient's culture to convey cultural biases in the evaluation. It is also important that the neuropsychologist understands the interpreter's biases, especially in the areas of socioeconomic status, gender, and more subtle language issues (e.g., dialect) [52], which can affect rapport with the patient and possibly negatively impact the evaluation.

Key Point

Effective work with medical interpreters includes:

- Building rapport between all three parities (patient, interpreter, medical provider)
- Education of HIPAA privacy rules applicable to interpreters
- Explaining the rationale for using an interpreter to the patient
- Asking for permission from patient to use an interpreter

Obviously working with interpreters places certain pressures and constraints on the neuropsychological evaluation, but there are ways in which the examiner can minimize these pressures, improve test validity, and minimize bias. Ideally, a neuropsychologist can select an entire test battery designed and normed for a given culture and administer it with the assistance of a medical interpreter. Neuropsychologists who frequently evaluate patients with the same medical interpreter may have the opportunity to train that interpreter to function largely as a psychometrician who administers the tests normed and developed for that language/culture. In less ideal but equally viable situations, the neuropsychologist can select some measures normed for the patient's language and use other tests that are translated using formal translation procedures; an interpreter can then assist in administering these measures. Since test administration is a more formalized process than conversation, interpreters are further trained by neuropsychologists to minimize bias by translating test instructions as concisely as possible (e.g., not elaborating on instructions), and not providing coaching/clarification without examiner consent.

An equally critical aspect of working with medical interpreters is knowing how to facilitate a positive triadic relationship. Bolton [53] writes that the use of interpreters can act as a barrier for communication, especially when the provider is deemed as an "out-group." The neuropsychologist must therefore look for the "hidden patient," his or her needs, motives, and intentions, which can easily be obscured through translation. Occasionally, patients are reluctant to have a medical interpreter. They may believe that their English is sufficient and are not aware of cultural/linguistic test norms or the level of language fluency required to complete some neuropsychological tests (e.g., measures that are used to assess language). Other times, the cultural community is small, and the interpreter may be known to the patient. Education of HIPAA privacy rules may need to be explained to the patient as extending to medical interpreters. In some cases, patients may have taken a psychological distance to their home country, especially in situations where patients were oppressed, traumatized, or abused in their homeland, and may not want contact with another member of their country. Thus, obtaining permission from patients and explaining the rationale for using an interpreter should not be overlooked. Even when patients are amenable to interpreters, the presence of a third person can alter the examiner-patient relationship. Thus, evaluations with interpreters can be improved when neuropsychologists educate medical interpreters about the neuropsychological testing process, are aware of potential biases that can arise, are knowledgeable of multicultural test availability and normative data sets for different cultural groups, and know how to interpret findings within a cultural context.

Conclusions

In tandem with the growing racial, ethnic, and linguistic diversity within the United States, neuropsychologists are increasingly evaluating diverse patient populations, which has led to the development of culturally informed neuropsychological assessments. Cultural factors are well known to play a role in multiple aspects of medical care, including disclosure and expression of symptoms, attitudes toward illness, and coping mechanisms.

Within the field of neuropsychology, there has been growing attention to and appreciation of the ways in which cultural factors permeate each step of the neuropsychological assessment process. This includes consideration of cultural variables embedded in neuropsychological measures and the testing environment as well as attention to the impact of a variety of factors such as literacy, education, acculturation, and language proficiency on cognition and test performance. Despite the relative dearth of formalized guidelines for neuropsychological testing with multicultural populations, current approaches propose a set of practices aimed at promoting greater understanding of the patient's cultural background to facilitate rapport as well as guide test selection, interpretation, and the use of medical interpreters. The ability to make these determinations rests on understanding the cultural values and customs prior to the initial meeting and inquiring about aspects of a patient's history and cultural background that may not be part of a standard interview (e.g., immigration story, acculturation level). Familiarity with existing multicultural neuropsychological measures and normative data is also crucial to conducting culturally informed assessments. At present, the availability of multicultural tests, normative data, and neuropsychologists proficient in the patient's native language and/or culture is far behind the demand. This highlights the importance of developing and promoting more multicultural tests, as well as continuing to improve all aspects of culturally informed assessments and increasing the linguistic and cultural diversity of neuropsychologists in the field.

Chapter Review Questions

1. All of the following are useful approaches when assessing a patient whose cultural background is different from one's own except:
   A. Memorizing the specifics of the culture's customs, values, and beliefs prior to meeting the patient.
   B. Familiarizing oneself with broader characteristics of the culture (e.g., cultural values, normative behaviors) through reading, professional consultation, etc.

   C. Assessing premorbid functioning by way of questions about a patient's educational and occupational history as opposed to using formal measures (e.g., reading test).
   D. Querying the patient/family about cultural expectations regarding educational and occupational attainment, functioning, etc.

2. You are asked to urgently assess a 75-year-old Bengali-speaking gentleman with limited education for possible dementia. Which of the following approaches and techniques would be best suited for this assessment?
   A. Assess memory functioning using nonverbal measures only.
   B. Use a medical interpreter to translate memory tests developed for US populations into Bengali.
   C. Administer "culture-fair" measures of memory functioning and supplement with nontraditional assessment techniques.
   D. Attempt to refer the case to a Bengali-speaking provider.

3. Which of the following are common reasons why a patient may be reluctant to use a medical interpreter?
   A. The patient may believe their level of English is sufficient.
   B. The patient may know or be acquaintances with the medical interpreter from interactions outside the medical setting (e.g., belong to the same church).
   C. The patient may not want contact with their native country for psychological reasons.
   D. All of the above.

References

1. U.S. Census Bureau. Overview of race and Hispanic origin: 2010 U.S. Census Briefs. 2011. http://www.census.gov/prod/cen2010/briefs/c2010br-02.pdf. Accessed 1 Aug 2015.
2. Center for American Progress Immigration Team. Facts on immigration today. 2014. https://cdn.americanprogress.org/wpcontent/uploads/2013/04/ImmigrationFact-brief-10.23.pdf. Accessed 1 Aug 2015.
3. Ryan C. Language use in the United States: 2011. American Community Survey Reports. 2013. https://www.census.gov/prod/2013pubs/acs-22.pdf. Accessed 1 Aug 2014.
4. Ardila A. Cultural values underlying psychometric cognitive testing. Neuropsychol Rev. 2005;15:185–95.
5. U.S. Department of Health and Human Services, Public Health Office, Office of the Surgeon General. Mental health: culture, race, and ethnicity—A supplement to mental health: a report of the surgeon general. 2001. http://mentalhealth.samhsa.gov/cre/toc.asp.
6. Wong TM, Fujii DE. Neuropsychological assessment of Asian Americans: demographic factors, cultural diversity, and practical guidelines. Appl Neuropsychol. 2004;11:23–36.
7. American Psychological Association. Guidelines on multicultural education, training, research, practice, and organizational change for psychologists. Am Psychol. 2003;58:377–402.
8. Mindt MR, Byrd D, Saez P, Manly J. Increasing culturally competent neuropsychological services for ethnic minority populations: a call to action. Clin Neuropsychol. 2010;24(3):429–53.
9. Romero HR, Lageman SK, Kamath V, Irani F, Sim A, Suarez P, Manly JJ, Attix DK. Challenges in the neuropsychologist assessment of ethnic minorities: Summit proceedings. Clin Neuropsychol. 2009;23:761–79.

10. Boone KB, Victor TL, Wen J, Razani J, Ponton M. The Association between neuropsychological scores, ethnicity, language, and acculturation variables in a large patient population. Arch Clin Neuropsychol. 2007;22:355–65.
11. Ardila A, Bertolucci PH, et al. Illiteracy: neuropsychology of cognition without reading. Arch Clin Neuropsychol. 2010;25:689–712.
12. Gonzalez da Silva C, Peterson KM, Faisca L, Ingvar M, Reis A. The effects of literacy and education on quantitative and qualitative aspects of semantic verbal fluency. J Clin Exp Neuropsychol. 2004;26:266–77.
13. Manly JJ, Jacobs DM, Sano M, Bell K, Merchant CA, Small SA, Stern Y. Effect of literacy on neuropsychological test performance in nondemented, education-matched elders. J Int Neuropsychol Soc. 1999;5:191–202.
14. Razani J, Burciaga J, Madore M, Wong J. Effects of acculturation on tests of attention and information processing in an ethnically diverse group. Arch Clin Neuropsychol. 2007;22:333–41.
15. Ostrosky-Solis F, Ardila A, Rosselli M, Lopez-Arango G, Uriel-Mendoza V. Neuropsychological test performance in illiterate subjects. Arch Clin Neuropsychol. 1998;13(7):645–60.
16. Castro-Caldas A. Relationship between functional brain organization and education. In: Uzzell BP, Ponton MO, Ardila A, editors. International handbook of cross-cultural neuropsychology. Mahwah, NJ: Lawrence Erlbaum Associates; 2007.
17. Castro-Caldas A, Cavaleiro Miranda P, Carmo I, Reis A, Leote F, Ribeiro C, Ducla Soares E. Influence of learning to read and write on the morphology of the corpus callosum. Eur J Neurol. 1999;6(1):253–28.
18. Manly JJ, Byrd DA, Touradji P, Stern Y. Acculturation, reading level, and neuropsychological test performance among African American elders. Appl Neuropsychol. 2004;11(1):37–46.
19. UNESCO. Literacy rates continue to rise from one generation to the next. UIS Fact Sheet No. 45. 2017. http://uis.unesco.org/sites/default/files/documents/fs45 literacy-rates-continue-rise-generation-to-next-en-2017_0.pdf. Accessed 14 July 2018.
20. Wilner EK, Geier FM, Wershba R, Chow C, Lanca M Cross-cultural literacy screening in low-educated immigrants: a pilot study. Poster presented at the International Neuropsychological Society Annual Meeting. 2016.
21. Ardila A, Rosselli M. Neuropsychological assessment in illiterate: visuospatial and memory abilities. Brain Cogn. 1989;11:147–66.
22. Mindt MR, Arentoft A, Germano KK, D'Aquila E, Scheiner D, Pizzirusso M, Sandoval TC, Gollan TH. Neuropsychological, cognitive, and theoretical considerations for evaluation of bilingual individuals. Neuropsychol Rev. 2008;18(3):255–68.
23. Gollan T, Fennema-Notestine C, Montoya R, Jernigan T. The bilingual effect on Boston naming test performance. J Int Neuropsychol Soc. 2007;13:197–208.
24. American Academy of Clinical Neuropsychology. American Academy of Clinical Neuropsychology (AACN) practice guidelines for neuropsychological assessment and consultation. Clin Neuropsychol. 2007;21:2009–231.
25. Flores G. Culture and the patient-physician relationship: achieving cultural competency in health care. J Pediatr. 2000;136(1):14–23.
26. Takushi R, Uomoto JM. The clinical interview from a multicultural perspective. In: Suzuki LA, Ponterotto JG, Meller PJ, editors. Handbook of multicultural assessment. San Francisco, CA: Jossey Bass; 2001. p. 47–66.
27. Lanca M, Alksnis C, Roese N, Gardner RC. Effects of language choice on acculturation: a study of Portuguese immigrants in a multicultural setting. J Lang Soc Psychol. 1994;13:315–30.
28. Goodglass H, Kaplan E, Barresi B. Boston diagnostic aphasia examination. 3rd ed. Philadelphia, PA: Lippincott Williams & Wilkins; 2001.
29. Dunn LM, Dunn DM. Peabody picture vocabulary test, fourth edition (PPVT-4). Minneapolis, MN: Pearson; 2007.
30. Kaplan EF, Goodglass H, Weintraub S. The Boston naming test. 2nd ed. Philadelphia: Lea & Fibiger; 1983.
31. Benton AL, Hamsher K, Rey GL, Sivan AB. Multilingual aphasia examination. 3rd ed. Iowa City, IA: AJA Associates; 1994.

32. Delis DC, Kramer JH, Kaplan E, Ober BA. California verbal learning test. Second ed. Bloomington, MN: Pearson; 2000.
33. Meyers JE, Meyers KR. Rey complex figure test and recognition trial. Lutz, FL: Psychological Assessment Resources, Inc.; 1995.
34. Van de Vijver F, Hambleton RK. Translating tests. Eur Psychol. 1996;1(2):89–99.
35. Manly JJ. Advantages and disadvantages of separate norms for African Americans. Clin Neuropsychol. 2005;19:270–5.
36. Wechsler D. Wechsler adult intelligence scale. 4th ed. San Antonio, TX: Psychological Corporation; 2008.
37. Nasreddine Z, Phillips NA, Bedirian V, Charbonneau S, Whitehead V, Collin I, Cummings JL, Chertkow H. The Montreal Cognitive Assessment, MoCA: a brief screening tool for mild cognitive impairment. J Am Geriatr Soc. 2005;53(4):695–9.
38. Ponton MO, Satz P, Herrera L, Young R, Ortiz F, D'elia L, Namerow N. Modified Spanish version of the Boston naming test. Clin Neuropsychol. 1992;3(6):334.
39. Lucas JA, Ivnik RJ, Willis FB, Ferman TJ, Smith GE, Parfitt FC, Petersen RC, Graff-Radford NR. Mayo's Older African Americans normative studies: normative data for commonly used clinical neuropsychological measures. Clin Neuropsychol. 2005;19(2):162–83.
40. Peña-Casanova J, Blesa R, Aguilar M, Gramunt-Fombuena N, Gómez-Ansón B, Oliva R, Molinuevo JL, Robles A, Barquero MS, Antúnez C, Martínez-Parra C, Frank-García A, Fernández M, Alfonso V, Sol JM. Spanish Multicenter Normative Studies (NEURONORMA Project): methods and sample characteristics. Arch Clin Neuropsychol. 2009;24(4):307–19.
41. Cavaco S, Goncalves A, Pinto C, Almeida E, Gomes F, Moreira I, Fernandes J, Teixeira-Pinto A. Semantic fluency and phonemic fluency: regression-based norms for the Portuguese population. Arch Clin Neuropsychol. 2013;28:262–71.
42. Lu L, Bigler E. Normative data on trail making test for neurologically normal Chinese-speaking adults. Appl Neuropsychol. 2002;9:219–25.
43. Ponton MO, Satz P, Herrera L, Ortiz F, Urrutua C, Young R, et al. Normative data stratified by age and education for the Neuropsychological Screening Battery for Hispanics (NeSBHIS): initial report. J Int Neuropsychol Soc. 1996;2:96–104.
44. Ostrosky-Solis F, Ardila A, Rosselli M. NEUROPSI Evaluación Neuropsicológica Breve en Español. D.F. Mexico: Publingenio, S.A. de C.V.; 1997.
45. Gasquoine PG. Race-norming of neuropsychological tests. Neuropsychol Rev. 2009;19:250–62.
46. Brown L, Sherbenou RJ, Johnsen SK. Test of nonverbal intelligence, Fourth Edition (TONI-4). Austin, TX: Pro-ed; 2010.
47. Julayanont P, Tangwongchai S, Hemrungrojn S, Tunvirachaisakul C, Phanthumchinda K, Hongsawat J, Nasreddine ZS. The Montreal Cognitive Assessment—basic: a screening tool for mild cognitive impairment in illiterate and low-educated elderly adults. J Am Geriatr Soc. 2015;63(12):2130–5.
48. D'Elia LF, Satz P, Uchiyama CL, White T. Color trails test. Odessa, FL: Psychological Assessment Resources, Inc.; 1994.
49. Lonner WJ. The search for psychological universals. In: Triandis HC, Lambert WW, editors. Handbook of cross-cultural psychology: perspectives, vol. 1. Needham Heights, MA: Allyn & Bacon; 1980.
50. American Psychological Association. Ethnical principles of psychologists and code of conduct. Am Psychol. 2002;57:1060–73.
51. National Council on Interpreting in Health Care. National standards of practice for interpreters in health care. 2005. http://www.ncihc.org/assets/documents/publications/NCIHC%20National%20Standards%20of%20Practice.pdf.
52. Vasquez C, Javier R. The problem with interpreters: communicating with Spanish-speaking patients. Hosp Community Psychiatry. 1991;42(2):163–5.
53. Bolton J. The third presence: a psychiatrist's experience of working with non-English speaking patients and interpreters. Transcult Psychiatry. 2002;39:97–114.

Chapter 29
Forensic Challenges in Medical Settings for Physicians and Neuropsychologists

Bernice A. Marcopulos, Michael Welner, and Kristen T. Campbell

Physicians may encounter forensic issues when treating and evaluating their patients. The decisions made in the clinical care environment are used to guide treatment planning, social services, or hospital discharge disposition, but deliberations regarding civil capacity in treatment settings, such as informed consent to treatment and competency to refuse treatment and guardianship, are difficult for patients and their families. The physician may be the first to broach the need for a guardian for finances, after their patient suffered a stroke, traumatic brain injury (TBI), or other brain disease affecting cognition, putting them at potential risk for abuse or exploitation. A physician may also be the entry point for consideration of whether their patient is competent to sign a contract or to give sexual consent. Capacity issues such as these require relatively intact cognitive functioning, and physicians may enlist the help of a neuropsychologist to perform a more detailed assessment. Physicians and neuropsychologists can collaborate to ensure careful documentation of medical conditions and cognitive abilities affecting these treatment decisions and legal implications. Also, a patient may have committed a crime, and their medical status and cognitive functioning may be seen as relevant to their culpability. Physicians and neuropsychologists can work well together to address legal matters that arise during routine patient care or from attorney referrals once a matter becomes a legal dispute in civil or criminal court. This chapter will provide a brief overview of the various civil and criminal legal proceedings that patients

B. A. Marcopulos (✉)
Department of Graduate Psychology, James Madison University, Harrisonburg, VA, USA

Department of Psychiatry and Neurobehavioral Sciences, University of Virginia Health Sciences Center, Charlottesville, VA, USA
e-mail: marcopba@jmu.edu

M. Welner
The Forensic Panel, New York, NY, USA

K. T. Campbell
Department of Graduate Psychology, James Madison University, Harrisonburg, VA, USA

K. M. Sanders (ed.), *Physician's Field Guide to Neuropsychology*,
https://doi.org/10.1007/978-1-4939-8722-1_29

may face and how these legal matters can be addressed with collaboration between physicians and neuropsychologists. The literature on forensic issues in medical practice and psychology and neuropsychology is much too extensive to be adequately covered in this chapter. The reader is encouraged to consult with current texts and journal articles for a more in-depth discussion [1, 2].

When medical professionals become involved in a legal matter involving their patients, this greatly alters their care provider role. The court may ask the physician to be a "fact" witness or an "expert" witness. These are distinct roles. It is very important for medical professionals to be clear in their role with the courts. Physicians may be the source of a referral, and may be asked to testify in a proceeding involving a patient in their care, but have inherent conflicts as treaters and advocates for their patient that render them partial in the court context. If a physician or other medical professional is testifying on behalf of a patient one is currently treating, one is testifying as a fact witness. They are not an expert witness. An expert witness is retained by the court or attorneys to address a particular legal question, using one's experience, training, and knowledge of the science supporting one's medical specialty [3]. For instance, a pediatric neurologist could testify either to the facts surrounding their care of their 10-year-old patient who suffers from seizures (fact witness), or they could testify about the likely causes of seizures in children in a medical malpractice case where a medical procedure is blamed for causing seizures (expert witness). The expert must be unbiased and objective, while the treating physician would not be expected to be unbiased regarding their own patient.

Sometimes referrals come to physicians from attorneys asking for an evaluation to be billed under insurance, which would imply routine patient care. This often happens in mild traumatic brain injury (mTBI) cases. An example would be a person who hit their head after a fall in a store parking lot. The person did not seek medical care at the time of the accident but several months later consulted an attorney about suing the store. The attorney advised the person to obtain a medical evaluation to document a brain injury for the purposes of litigation. It would be improper to bill insurance for a legal case. Prior to accepting the referral, the medical professional may attempt to confirm that the referral is indeed to assist clinical diagnosis and treatment and not for litigation. However, when an attorney initiates the referral, careful consideration of the circumstances would make it clear that even if the referral is not immediately meant for forensic application, the medical professional may eventually be brought into court to testify about one's findings.

Within civil, employment, and criminal law, one finds a wide range of indications for neuropsychological testing and its integration with medical data or input from physicians. Because legal cases involve fact finding and a timeline geared toward gathering objective evidence, forensic examiners are expected to integrate available evidence into their analysis to a degree not expected in the clinical realm. For that reason, neuropsychological testing for litigation may be more extensive than that expected in the clinical realm.

Civil Cases

Civil Capacity

Civil competency and capacity are sometimes considered to be synonymous, but they actually refer to slightly different applications. Competency is a legal term used by the courts. It refers to an individual's ability to perform a specific function, such as executing a will or understanding court proceedings in a criminal trial. The term capacity is used in clinical contexts in which a medical professional will render an opinion about a patient's ability to make a decision about their medical care. Medical disorders that affect mental abilities may render a person incompetent from a legal perspective, or lacking capacity from a medical perspective, but one does not follow from the other [4]. For example, the fact that an examinee was recently diagnosed with dementia does not automatically mean that one lacks the capacity to write one's will or consent to medical treatment [5, 6].

Neuropsychologists administer tests in order to assess cognitive functioning of individuals with neurological disorders or serious mental illnesses and make recommendations about an individual's capacity to consent and make decisions [7, 8]. A patient with a developmental disability may lack the intellectual ability to weigh the risks and benefits of a complicated medical procedure. An aging adult with significant cognitive decline suggestive of dementia may have a questionable capacity to create a will or sign a legal contract and may be susceptible to undue influence by others who may not have the patient's welfare in mind [9, 10].

One concern regarding adults with cognitive impairment is their capacity to make medical decisions. There are four legal standards of consent: expressing choice, appreciation, reasoning, and understanding [11]. That is, in order to have the capacity to consent and make decisions, an individual should have the ability to reach a decision, appreciate a situation and its potential consequences, reason through potential outcomes, and understand information relevant to the situation [12]. Each of these standards should be assessed when considering if an adult with dementia has the capacity to make their own medical decisions [8, 13].

One particular challenge confronting the application of neuropsychological testing in the capacity arena is a lack of ecological validity. Capacity is task specific. Neuropsychological testing identifies deficits in a variety of cognitive functions on standardized, norm-referenced tests. The tests do not directly address a specific task needed for a particular capacity (e.g., consent to medical treatment, handle finances). The capacity needed for competency to invest may be very different from capacity to give informed consent for medical procedures. If testing demonstrates problems calculating, those deficiencies are empirically determined. But decisions regarding one's investments are based upon individual strategies and one's consideration about what is best for that person. Moreover, capacity may shift over time, and the timing of testing must be carefully cross-referenced to medical status, psychiatric status, and medications one is taking. The application of neuropsychological testing in decision-making necessitates extensive collateral history, forensic psychiatric assessment, and perhaps even neuroimaging to embed it in the facts of a legal case.

Case example: A 75-year-old investment client of a brokerage dies. His widow sues the brokerage firm, alleging that her husband traded during periods of incapacity. She presents evidence of his aggressive trading of his accounts and investments that failed. She also presents a neuropsychological evaluation showing that the examinee had dementia for approximately 2 years prior to his death. In response, the brokerage firm presents evidence that the investor was a brilliant businessman who actively led his businesses until only weeks before his death. He was making decisions, considering alternatives, and showing reasoning specific to these business concerns – even months after he had a Mini-Mental Status Exam of 16. Moreover, the aggressive investment strategy he maintained was no different from one he followed all of his life. His wife, in the weeks leading up to his death, was actively negotiating with him over her share in his trust, even as she knew of his dementia diagnosis. A neurological exam, including neuroimaging (PET), did not support a diagnosis of dementia. The examinee had numerous medical problems and a history of delirium when hospitalized for complications of some of those problems. In response, the wife presents evidence that the brokerage was making investment decisions during times in which the subject was hospitalized.

The above example illustrates how important it is for neuropsychological testing and medical evaluations to integrate in the backdrop of exactly what capacity is being tested and in a context that converges history relevant to what is being tested. In this case, investment correspondence, transaction records, trust documents, email chains, phone records, and even legal representation and direction to his staff were relevant. Timing is also important – the sequence of his acute medical problems, their instability, nature of treatment and recovery, and correlation with available documentation. Medical information from the physician and neuropsychological test data accurately interpreted by the neuropsychologist, along with a clear understanding of the legal issue being contested, can help resolve these capacity issues.

Perhaps the most established area of neuropsychological testing input is in personal injury civil litigation. Those involving mild TBI can be quite contentious. Mild TBI is an arena of great current debate, owing in part to concussion litigation in sports, with some parties asserting that even a mild injury can have lasting consequences. Neuropsychologists bring to bear an armamentarium of standardized tests to ascertain the functional ramifications of brain injury. Brain injury claims illustrate the integration of physician input, such as psychiatric assessment on confounding diagnoses, corroborating and contradictory history, neuropsychological testing data, and neuroimaging data.

Case example: A construction worker falls at a jobsite and later asserts a head injury. A neuropsychological evaluation reveals findings that would objectively support that claim. In response, the defendant jobsite provides evidence that the examinee was involved in a motor vehicle accident 3 years earlier in which he lost consciousness. Neuroimaging findings reveal a brain tumor.

Employment law applications of neuropsychological testing overlap and often with the above challenges. The Americans with Disabilities Act allows that for a person who can perform the essential functions of their duties, an employer must provide reasonable accommodations to that employee. Neuropsychological testing may be very informative about the nature of deficits. However, without a clear understanding about what it is that said employee does, and the range of expectations for that particular position, the relevance of neuropsychological testing data to questions of a person's abilities to perform essential functions is unclear. Here again, ecological validity matters. Moreover, since many positions attracting these legal disputes have interpersonal demands, psychiatric diagnostic evaluations that integrate understandings of conflicts and personality dynamics and patterns of interpersonal relatedness are necessary whether other issues are at play. Employment matters likewise illustrate the advantages of integrating neuropsychological testing with neuroimaging and psychiatric data, as litigation follows its course.

Consider the case of a litigation partner who is fired from his firm. He files a claim with workmen's compensation and with a disability policy, asserting that he can no longer work as an attorney because he had a stroke. The hospital record and neurology consultation recorded that such a stroke occurred. He is in psychiatric treatment for depression. Neuroimaging reflects markings consistent with a stroke. Neuropsychological testing demonstrates a variety of deficits. The examinee awarded his disability policy.

Several years later, the attorney becomes involved in litigation. It seems he resumed work at some point, worked in a firm for several months, and was then fired. He asserts that he was able to perform the essential functions of his duties and that his law firm did not accommodate his disability but could have. The employer presents his previous evaluation and records of his being awarded a benefit for disability. Neuropsychological testing, conducted again, demonstrates considerable improvement in a number of functional parameters. The psychiatrist who is deconstructing the dynamics of the workplace adapts these findings, along with a better understanding of his strengths and weaknesses, to a forensic investigation of his responsibilities and whether that profile of strengths and weaknesses would allow for his ability to perform his duties.

Criminal Cases

A collaboration between a neuropsychologist and a physician contribute to the resolution of many aspects of criminal proceedings and potentially add insight into the connections between the history, cognitive functioning, and illegal and sometimes unimaginable behavior of the individual. Forensic psychiatrists who are routinely involved in evaluations of this type may find the input and collaboration with the neuropsychologist to have a pivotal and complementary synergy in a number of areas across the life cycle of a criminal case. These areas include pretrial assessments of disputed confessions, trial competency challenges, criminal responsibility and diagnostic considerations for affirmative defenses (self-defense, battered person, extreme emotional disturbance insanity), detecting malingering, and pre-sentencing evaluations of mitigation, alternatives to incarceration, and possibility of intellectual disability.

Assessments can also be used to determine the mental state of the individual before the alleged crime, at the time of the offense and at the time of testing [14]. A unique quality that neuropsychological evaluations have over clinical interviews and medical tests is that they provide quantitative, standardized data about cognitive functioning and inferences about a person's behavior directly related to his or her cognitive capacities. Diagnostic standards for clinical and forensic assessment are identical. The expectations of diligence and adherence to scientific standards for the forensic setting are more intensely scrutinized; neuropsychologists and physicians qualified to testify are not only sufficiently trained but must also be presenting an analysis that is not only relevant and valid but reliable. That means such examination reflects the standards of practice and interpretation, rather than one's own idiosyncratic opinion.

Criteria were established for expert testimony as a result of the US Supreme Court decision in Daubert v. Merrell Dow Pharmaceuticals [15]. These are called Daubert criteria. Several guidelines have been proposed for meeting the criteria: use methods for gathering information that have been proven to be reliable and valid, base conclusions on scientific data, and be prepared and able to competently answer cross-examination inquiries that call into question the methods used to collect the information on which conclusions are based [16].

Disputed Confession

A suspect's confession may be the most meaningful evidence against him/her at trial. Therefore, there is great pressure on defense attorneys to suppress such confession from coming before a jury at trial or to blunt its impact if it does. Neuropsychological testing is helpful to inform an understanding of an examinee's cognitive abilities and how the dynamic between the officer and suspect leads to a self-incriminating statement or even a false confession. Forensic psychiatry relies upon neuropsychological testing to explore whether cognitive vulnerabilities exist. The assessment of suspect vulnerability is a pre-consideration of disputed confession claims in which physical coercion is not alleged to have taken place.

Competency to Stand Trial

Competency to stand trial, also known as adjudicative competence, is an important legal standard that resulted from the *Dusky v. United States* (1960) decision [17]. The resolution of competency is one more area in which neuropsychologists and psychiatrists complement each other well. To be deemed competent to stand trial, a defendant must demonstrate an ability to understand the nature of the charges one confronts, as well as the range of punitive outcomes. In addition, the defendant must be able to assist with his or her defense by working with a lawyer – either as an informant, to appraise potential witnesses, to identify evidence or sources that might be helpful, or to engage in discussion on overall trial approach and the defense to be adopted. Defendants must demonstrate knowledge of basic legal concepts, such as the roles of lawyers and judges, the nature of pleas, and the role of witnesses [18]. A defendant is at a severe disadvantage if unable to assist his lawyer with his defense. For this reason, the greater the gravity of the charges, the more sensitive the evaluation to ensure one is competent to stand trial, to plead, to represent one's self, or to receive sentencing.

Competency is often primarily a cognitive construct because a defendant must have the ability to reason through the legal proceedings and consider possible outcomes [19, 20]. To gain insight into how a defendant's cognitive functioning impacts his competency, a forensic psychiatrist working to restore a defendant's competency may refer the defendant for neuropsychological testing. There are five main ways neuropsychologists can assist in competency evaluations: (1) provide descriptions of the defendant's specific cognitive abilities, (2) present a plausible explanation for deficits in abilities related to competency, (3) examine the importance of the defendant's cognitive deficits in relation to his competency, (4) state an opinion about the defendant's competence, and (5) prescribe cognitive treatment and rehabilitation techniques to improve the defendant's likelihood of restoration [11]. Just because a defendant demonstrates significant deficits on testing and she/he has neuroimaging evidence for brain injury or disease, this does not automatically mean they are not competent to stand trial. This must be determined by examining the defendant on the legal standard using functional assessment. A defendant could be quite impaired on formal testing yet adequately display the requisite knowledge and ability to rationalize his case with his attorney.

Insanity, Diminished Capacity, and Criminal Responsibility

Insanity is strictly a legal, not clinical, concept. Laws differ by state, but most focus on being unable to distinguish right from wrong. Less frequently, the standards involve the inability to conform one's conduct and rarely, being unable to resist an impulse. Neuropsychological testing can also offer insight into a suspect's level of cognitive functioning at the time of the crime [21]. Because conditions fluctuate, and improve, and because psychotropic medication can affect cognition as well as reality perception, the challenge for courts and examiners is to conduct testing with time proximity to the instant offense, in order to capture the mental state as it was at the time of the crime. This is far easier to ensure when the issues at hand involve brain damage that was known to be present prior to the offense.

Testing may inform insanity defense standards that include the inability to conform conduct. Deficits in impulse control, emotional control, and other executive functions more directly relate to conduct questions. Inability to perceive right from wrong may be affected by psychiatric conditions that do not necessarily manifest in neuropsychological testing data (e.g., paranoid delusions). Alternatively, appreciation for wrong may also reflect values and other historical context. But like capacity and competency, the presence of a psychiatric or neurological diagnosis does not preclude a determination of insanity. This is a legal term, not a clinical diagnosis, and this is determined by the courts, not by healthcare providers [1].

Diminished capacity is likewise a consideration of decreased criminal responsibility as a result of emotional or cognitive limitation. Input from neuropsychological testing may be useful in demonstrating diminished capacity when the defendant otherwise does clearly demonstrate appreciation of wrong, and ability to conform one's conduct, as illustrated in this example.

The defendant was charged with theft and fraud in connection with taking thousands of dollars of heavy equipment that did not belong to him. An extensive historical background in the forensic psychiatric exam revealed him to be a successful contractor, knowledgeable about his work. He had peculiarities to his personality, such as volatility and poor boundaries. He was ashamed of what he had done, and while he denied an awareness of why, he – as many defendants – denied an awareness of his actions to both distance himself from the event and to mislead the interviewer. The forensic psychiatrist referred the examinee for neuropsychological testing. His medical history was notable for migraine headaches and chronic and related pain, for which he was addicted to opiates. Neuropsychological testing showed a variety of deficits not to be expected in a person of his responsibilities as a contractor. Neuroimaging, requested on the basis of the neuropsychological test findings, revealed brain lesions that were later demonstrated to be due to migraine stroke. The court took into account this mitigating information and sentenced the examinee to time served.

Malingering

Clinicians operate with the presumption of trust that patients are truthfully reporting symptoms for which they seek help. Because forensic cases involve litigants invested in the outcome of one's case, an examinee has inherent motivation to misrepresent history or to embellish or even fabricate symptoms (malinger). Malingering is defined as exaggerating or feigning illness or symptoms [22–25]. It is important to consider malingering in any forensic examination for which an interview is necessary [26]. The challenge of examination is that any invested litigant has greater motivation to manage impressions on the ability of an examiner to uncover elemental truth. Memory loss, psychosis, or the effects of head trauma could be a genuine issue; however, it is important to verify that these issues are true because of the potential benefits that an examinee could gain by malingering [25, 27].

Malingering is not typically considered in routine patient care, and the patient's self-report is accepted at face value. However, if a patient is involved in a legal matter, it can be suspected in the clinical interviews and observations conducted by physicians or psychologists, by the quantity and quality of inconsistent history. However, neuropsychological assessments provide much more information regarding inconsistency of claims, what symptoms are exaggerated, and to what extent they are fabricated [28]. Specifically, neuropsychologists have developed a number of standardized tests to evaluate the veracity of neuropsychological symptoms. These techniques are referred to as symptom validity and performance validity measures. The basis of these tests is to compare how a claimant or defendant's performance matches either patients who truly have the condition with those who do not but are feigning symptoms of the condition. That is, does the defendant's presentation of symptoms match any known diagnosis, or do they tend to endorse symptoms that are rare, extreme, or unlikely to occur together? If so, it is likely that the defendant is not actually experiencing those symptoms, and thus malingering is suspected [29]. The tests also could show if an examinee is putting in a reasonable amount of effort or engagement while taking the tests to ensure a valid reflection of their true cognitive abilities. A possibility of invalid test scores is indicated if the claimant or defendant scores below a certain cutoff point that designates suboptimal performance. That is, one is likely failing to put in effort in an attempt to perform poorly on the test, thus distorting one's true level of impairment [24].

Summary

Physicians may be asked to provide an opinion on legal matters affecting their patients. This chapter outlined several civil and criminal issues patients may face and described the collaborative relationship between physicians and neuropsychologists which is well-established in civil and criminal forensic settings. A variety of legal matters lend critical importance to the application of neuropsychological testing data. Neuropsychology as practiced in the forensic context has more specific indications, and relies on much greater access to historical context, and can contribute depth to a court's deliberation of the brain and how it relates to behavior. With greater attorney sophistication, collaboration between psychiatry and other physicians and neuropsychology, and neuroradiology and neuropsychology, allows for greater validity and reliability.

At the same time, courts may have unrealistic expectations of neuropsychological as well as medical testing. The ability of neuropsychological testing to address certain questions tempts courts and practitioners to extend interpretations to areas for which testing is not truly validated. The pressures of advocacy in an adversarial system push neuropsychologists and physicians to apply their evaluations to answer questions despite a lack of ecological validity. Courts in some instances may push physicians and neuropsychologists into testifying about areas beyond their own expertise or beyond the available science. Moreover, the arcane quality of medical and neuropsychological test data and statistical jargon could result in the presentation of data in biased ways, particularly in sensitive and high-profile cases.

Neuroimaging data in particular poses the same advantages and pitfalls of neuropsychological testing [30].

Interdisciplinary collaboration and even mutual oversight allow for judicious and ethical application of neuropsychological testing integrated with medical information to its true potential. Physicians and neuropsychologists continue to cultivate a collaboration borne of the seamless integration of contextually relevant history and the testing data that looks beyond what one may only appreciate at a surface level. Collaboration between physicians and neuropsychologists fortifies the integrity of forensic medicine by mutual checks and balances, ensuring the adherence to expertise, the limits of the science, and the interpretive limits of available history and data. Neuroimaging advances herald not only an emerging physician relationship with neuropsychological testing but also the responsibilities of disciplining new advances with the responsible and ecologically valid application of the technology to medicolegal questions. Again, the collaboration of professionals with mutual consideration of how we learn from each other assists courts in a mission to use science for justice and good.

Chapter Review Questions

1. True/False: Treating providers should not also serve as expert witnesses for their patients.
2. True/False: The Dusky standard refers to the mental status sufficient to refuse treatment.
3. True/False: Neuropsychological testing is critical to evaluate the nature and validity of cognitive complaints.
4. True/False: The term capacity is used in clinical contexts in which a medical professional will render an opinion about a patient's ability to make a decision about their medical care.
5. True/False: A patient can be diagnosed with dementia and still have the capacity to make medical decisions.
6. True/False: Insanity is a clinical concept, not a legal definition.

References

1. Melton GB, Petrila J, Poythress NG, Slobogin C, Lyons PM Jr, Otto RK. Psychological evaluations for the courts: a handbook for mental health professionals and lawyers. 3rd ed. New York, NY: Guilford Press; 2007.
2. Simon RI, Gold LH. Textbook of forensic psychiatry. Washington, DC: American Psychiatric Publishing; 2010.

3. Strasburger LH, Gutheil TG, Brodsky A. On wearing two hats: role conflict in serving as both psychotherapist and expert witness. Am J Psychiatry. 1997;154(4):448–56.
4. Ganzini L, Volicer L, Nelson WA, Fox E, Derse AR. Ten myths about decision-making capacity. J Am Med Dir Assoc. 2004;5(4):263–7.
5. American Bar Association and American Psychological Association Assessment of Capacity in Older Adults Project Working Group. Assessment of older adults with diminished capacity: a handbook for psychologists. Washington, DC: American Bar Association and American Psychological Association; 2008.
6. Morgan J, Marcopulos BA. Capacity evaluations in the elderly: neuropsychological perspectives. In: Ravdin LD, Katzen HL, editors. Clinical handbook of the neuropsychology of aging and dementia. New York: Springer Science; 2012.
7. Gurrera RJ, Moye J, Karel MJ, Azar AR, Armesto JC. Cognitive performance predicts treatment decisional abilities in mild to moderate dementia. Neurology. 2006;66:1367–72.
8. Demakis GJ. Civil capacities in clinical neuropsychology: research findings and practical applications. New York: Oxford University Press; 2012.
9. Shulman KI, Cohen CA, Hull I. Psychiatric issues in retrospective challenges of testamentary capacity. Int J Geriatr Psychiatry. 2005;20:63–9.
10. Shulman KI, Cohen CA, Kirsh FC, Hull IA, Champine JD. Assessment of testamentary capacity and vulnerability to undue influence. Am J Psychiatry. 2007;164:722–7.
11. Appelbaum PS. Assessment of patients competence to consent to treatment. N Engl J Med. 2006;357:1834–40.
12. Marson DC, Cody HA, Ingram KK, Harrell LE. Neuropsychological predictors of competency in Alzheimer's disease using a rational reasons legal standard. Arch Neurol. 1995;52:955–9.
13. Okonkwo OC, Griffith HR, Belue K, Lanza S, Zamrini EY, Harrell LE, Brockington JC, Clark D, Raman R, Marson DC. Cognitive models of medical decision-making capacity in patients with mild cognitive impairment. J Int Neuropsychol Soc. 2008;14:297–308.
14. Denney RL, Wynkoop TF. Clinical neuropsychology in the criminal forensic setting. J Head Trauma Rehabil. 2000;15(2):804–28.
15. Daubert v. Merrell Dow Pharmaceuticals, Inc., 509 U.S. 579, 113 S.Ct. 2795. 1993.
16. Krafka C, Dunn MA, Johnson MT, Cecil JS, Miletich D. Judge and attorney experiences, practices, and concerns regarding expert testimony in federal civil trials. Psychol Public Policy Law. 2002;8(3):309–32.
17. Dusky v. United States, 362 U.S. 402. 1960.
18. Grisso T. Evaluating competencies: forensic assessments and instruments. 2nd ed. New York: Springer Science; 2003.
19. Ryba NL, Zapf PA. The influence of psychiatric symptoms and cognitive abilities on competence-related abilities. Int J Forensic Ment Health. 2011;10:29–40. https://doi.org/10.1080/14999013.2010.550982.
20. White AJ, Meares S, Batchelor J. The role of cognition in fitness to stand trial: a systematic review. J Forens Psychiatry Psychol. 2014;25:77–99. https://doi.org/10.1080/14789949.2013.868916.
21. Yates KF, Denney RL. Neuropsychology in the assessment of mental state at time of offense. In: Denney RL, Sullivan JT, editors. Clinical neuropsychology in the criminal forensic setting. New York: Guilford; 2008.
22. Larrabee GJ. Detecting of malingering using atypical performance patterns on standard neuropsychological tests. Clin Neuropsychol. 2003;17(3):410–25.
23. Larrabee GJ. Performance validity and symptom validity in neuropsychological assessment. J Int Neuropsychol Soc. 2012;18:1–7.
24. Lees-Haley PR, Iverson GL, Lange RT, Allen LM III. Malingering in forensic neuropsychology: Daubert and the MMPI-2. J Forensic Neuropsychol. 2003;3(1-2):167–203.
25. Denney RL. Symptom validity testing of remote memory in a criminal forensic setting. Arch Clin Neuropsychol. 1996;11(7):589–603.

26. Bush SS, Ruff RM, Troster AI, Barth JT, Koffler SP, Pliskin NH, Reynolds CR, Silver CH. Symptom validity assessment: practice issues and medical necessity NAN Policy & Planning Committee. Arch Clin Neuropsychol. 2005;20:419–26. https://doi.org/10.1016/j.acn.2005.02.002.
27. Marcopulos BA, Hedgar L, Arredondo B. Dissociative amnesia or malingered amnesia? A case report. J Forensic Psychol Pract. 2016;16(2):106–17.
28. Boone KB. Clinical practice of forensic neuropsychology: an evidence-based approach. New York: Guildford Press; 2012.
29. van Oorsouw K, Merckelbach H. Detecting malingered memory problems in the civil and criminal arena. Legal Criminol Psych. 2010;15:97–114.
30. Meltzer CC, Sze G, Rommelfanger KS, Kinlaw K, Banja JD, Wolpe PR. Guidelines for the ethical use of neuroimages in medical testimony: report of a multidisciplinary consensus conference. AJNR Am J Neuroradiol. 2014;35(4):632–7.

Chapter 30
Neuropsychological Interventions for Individuals with Brain Injury

Samantha L. Backhaus and Summer L. Ibarra

Introduction

Acquired brain injury (ABI) and traumatic brain injury (TBI) are significant healthcare and psychosocial issues, necessitating appropriate treatment, education, and support. Approximately 1.5 million Americans sustain a traumatic brain injury [1]. Almost 10 million Americans are stroke survivors or are living with the challenges following a TBI [2–4]. Consequences of BI can be devastating for individuals with brain injury. Long-term effects of brain injury typically include effects on physical, cognitive, neurobehavioral, as well as personality and emotional functioning (see Table 30.1).

Specific emotional difficulties can include depression, anxiety, mania, frustration, and suicidality. Personality changes are also quite common after brain injury. One study showed that half of relatives of those with severe TBI reported personality changes at 3 months post-injury, and two-thirds reported changes at 6 and 12 months in a sample of 33 cases [5]. Emotional problems and personality changes post brain injury are often the focus of neuropsychological interventions due to the significant effect on the rehabilitation outcome. Depression is among the most common consequences [6] with major depressive disorder being the most frequently diagnosed psychiatric illness following TBI [7]. Reports of frequency of depression in patients with TBI have ranged from 24% [8] to 77% [6, 9–11]. Depression is common in patients with both mild and moderate-to-severe TBI, with some reports of it being greater in the former [12]. Depression is also common in individuals with

S. L. Backhaus
Department of Physical Medicine and Rehabilitation, Rehabilitation Hospital of Indiana, Indiana University, Indianapolis, IN, USA
e-mail: Samantha.backhaus@rhin.com

S. L. Ibarra (✉)
Rehabilitation Hospital of Indiana, Indianapolis, IN, USA
e-mail: Summer.ibarra@rhin.com

K. M. Sanders (ed.), *Physician's Field Guide to Neuropsychology*,
https://doi.org/10.1007/978-1-4939-8722-1_30

Table 30.1 Common consequences of a brain injury

Physical impairments
Balance and vestibular dysfunctions
Sensory dysfunctions (vision, hearing, taste, olfactory, tactile functions)
Speech and language impairments (articulatory disorders, dysphagia, swallowing)
Sensation or motor deficits in extremities affecting movement or ambulation
Headaches and pain disorders
Dizziness or vertigo
Endocrine or metabolic abnormalities
Fatigue
Sexual dysfunction
Sleep disturbances
Light and noise sensitivity
Cognitive impairments
Attention impairments (focused, selective, alternating, divided, sustained, processing speed)
Memory deficits (learning, verbal memory, visual retrieval)
Visual spatial and construction dyspraxia
Language disorders including dysnomia, paraphasias, or problems with comprehension
Executive dysfunctions (impairments in problem-solving, decision-making, inhibitory control, abstract reasoning and concept formation, planning, judgment, organization, mental flexibility, safety awareness)
Emotional problems
Mood disorders including depression, anxiety, mania
Irritability and anger dyscontrol
Aggression
Frustration intolerance
General changes in personality
Behavioral changes
Apathy and loss of initiation
Impulsivity and disinhibition of thoughts and actions
Social inappropriateness and inability to read or interpret social cues
Hyperverbosity or circumlocutious speech
Tangential thoughts

ABI, such as stroke, with rates ranging from 20% to 63% [13, 14]. The rates of depression tend to be high in the first year following a brain injury, but the risk for developing depression is elevated at any time after injury [1]. Some studies have shown that depression may be more likely to occur after the initial phases of recovery due to increased awareness and slowness of recovery at that stage [15]. Thus, it is important to evaluate for depression no matter the severity of the BI, as well as assess for depression for years following the actual injury.

As a result of these challenges, overall rehabilitation outcome is likely to be affected [13]. Significant problems can occur in vocational, marital, financial, academic, social, interpersonal, and physical functioning [16–19]. For example, individuals with brain injury can experience significant declines in their ability to return to work or be involved in productive activities [20]. Moreover, research findings suggest individuals who experience moderate-to-severe TBI are likely to experience these problems over long periods of time post-injury [21]. Recent evidence from the TBI Model Systems National Database suggests that it is more common for individuals to change in their functioning than to stabilize in persons with moderate-to-severe TBI [22]. As a matter of fact, a recent statement was made at the consensus conference stating, "Injury to the brain can evolve into a lifelong health condition termed chronic brain injury (CBI). CBI impairs the brain and other organ systems and may persist or progress over an individual's life span. CBI must be identified and proactively management as a lifelong condition to improve health, independent function and participation in society" [23].

Multifaceted Nature of Neuropsychological Interventions

Given the complexity of challenges following a brain injury and their detrimental effects on the person's overall outcome and functioning, it is important to address these issues early after the brain injury. Brain injury is a heterogeneous disorder that can require treatment throughout the course of recovery [24]. There are several types of treatment approaches available to help individuals adjust to and compensate for the challenges. Neuropsychological interventions typically include, but may not be limited to, a neuropsychological assessment to provide specific recommendations, neuropsychological therapies (individual, family, or group), cognitive remediation, and/or comprehensive neuropsychological rehabilitation. Neuropsychological interventions typically involve providing a specialized and individualized treatment program depending on the person's severity of injury and challenges following the injury, premorbid personality and psychosocial functioning, and current emotional and psychosocial functioning, support systems, as well as their specific rehabilitation goals [25, 26].

To illustrate, Lance Trexler ([25]; see Fig. 30.1) provides a conceptualization of a brain injury recovery model. He proposes that individuals have their own set of premorbid personality and psychosocial characteristics, including strengths and weaknesses, coping resources, and cognitive reserves. Then the point of injury occurs, causing a set of either transient or permanent sequelae caused by the injury. Individuals' rehabilitation outcome may be influenced by the severity of such challenges, potential remediation of these challenges, as well as ability to compensate for them. At some point in the person's recovery, they hopefully become aware of their deficits. Each person then has their own reaction to this awareness (based on factors including, but not limited to, severity of challenges from injury and cognitive limitations, current emotional functions, past coping strategies, and current psychosocial circumstances). This psychological reaction can either be healthy and natural (e.g., a person goes through a typical response of grieving and adjusting to the injury effects but works through challenges using a positive problem-solving orientation) or a catastrophic reaction (e.g., one in which they start to feel they are incapacitated by their challenges and do not have the coping resources to deal with

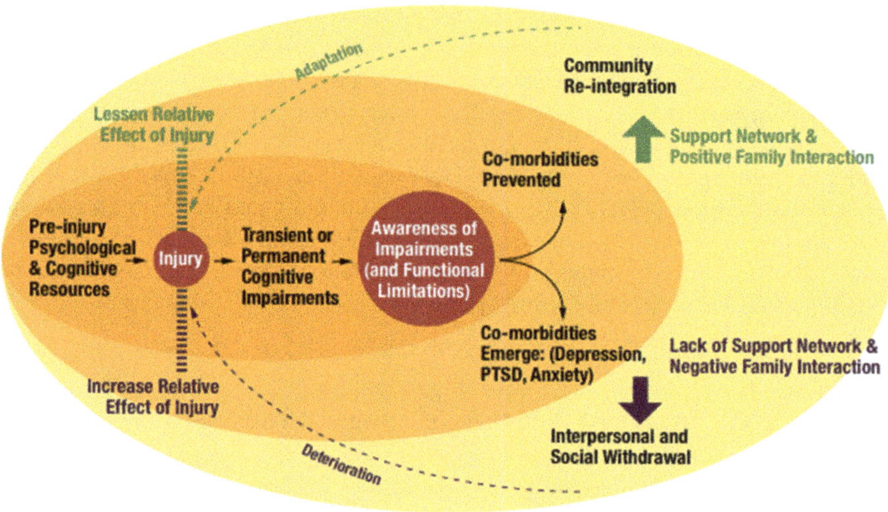

Fig. 30.1 Recovery model for brain injury. Taken with permission from Lance Trexler [25]

them). Trexler notes that this is a pivotal point in the recovery, leading to the possibility of comorbidities. He notes that in the ideal situation, these comorbidities are prevented by way of services that proactively assess and intervene accordingly. These psychological reactions can contribute to either a positive rehabilitation outcome if the responses are healthy or negative outcome if they are catastrophic. Another factor influencing rehabilitation outcome includes the presence of positive family/community support. If the individual has adequate and effective family, social, and/or community support, they are likely to have a better rehabilitation outcome. If they have a negative or limited support, this is likely to affect their overall rehabilitation outcome. Thus, the role of the neuropsychologist is to positively influence each area of functioning (cognitive functions, psychological reactions, family functioning) by providing appropriate neuropsychological interventions in order to help promote the most positive outcome for the individual with brain injury.

Neuropsychological Interventions

Neuropsychological Testing

Even if the individual does not have physical challenges, referral for neuropsychological examination can be valuable. This examination typically consists of a clinical interview with the patient and a significant other or caregiver, as well as a half to full day of neurocognitive and psychological assessments. Generally, neuropsychological testing should be able to provide information regarding cognitive strengths and weaknesses, as well as psychological status related to the injury and any premorbid personality or emotional issues that may affect present coping strategies. Testing will generally include assessment of estimates of intelligence, orientation and attention, learning and memory, language functions, visual-spatial abilities, executive functions such as mental flexibility and problem-solving, sensory and motor abilities, and emotional/personality functions. In a post-acute rehabilitation setting, however, the neuropsychologists are additionally called upon to discuss and provide insights regarding the level of disability caused by the brain injury, not just the impairments [27]. There is a greater focus on the person's ability to function within their specific environments. The purpose of the testing is to also generate the most appropriate treatment plan for the patient, whether in a brain injury rehabilitation setting or whether the referral comes from an outside physician. Recommendations can address, but are not limited to, (1) what kind of therapies may be helpful in rehabilitating or remediating deficits, (2) strategies for compensating functional daily challenges, (3) level of supervision needed, (4) level of independence in making decisions, (5) driving, (6) return to work or school, (7) ability to parent independently, (8) suggestions on improving mood, and (9) pharmacological recommendations for cognitive and psychological challenges. In particular, neuropsychological testing often plays an important role in providing psychological recommendations, as it can obtain a sample of behavior and coping strategies when faced with challenges. It provides some insight into level of awareness, as well as inappropriate or appropriate reactions. Often, individuals are unaware of their challenges and overestimate the extent to which they are truly functioning, presenting a positive picture for physicians and other clinicians who do not have the experience observing their true everyday functioning.

Neurorehabilitation

The purpose of rehabilitation is to help the individual achieve their maximum potential of functioning following a brain injury [28]. It is to help the person reintegrate into their roles, both professionally and personally. This can include restoration of functions or teaching compensatory strategies to adapt to the presence of cognitive and behavioral challenges. Unfortunately, this may not always be their exact previous level of functioning. The amount and comprehensiveness of neurorehabilitation required often depends on the person's rehabilitation needs and often requires involvement of a physician, cognitive therapies, and neuropsychological therapies for management of behaviors and mood. According to Trexler [29], brain injury rehabilitation continuum anticipates the biopsychosocial dimensions of brain injury, from mild to severe brain injury, with the goal of achieving the maximum optimal outcome, defined by productivity, participation in the family and community, functional independence, and quality of life (see Fig. 30.2).

Neurorehabilitation is best managed by a physician specializing in brain injury recovery, the physiatrist. The role of the physiatrist is to manage any physical (e.g.,

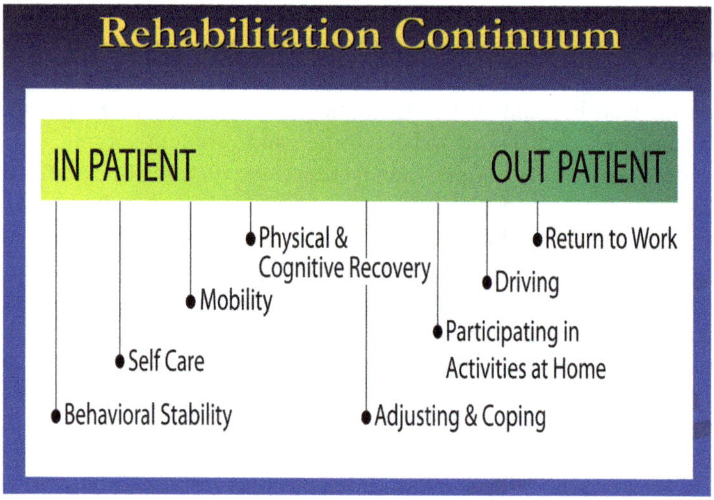

Fig. 30.2 Rehabilitation continuum of persons with brain injury. Taken with permission from Lance [29]

hemiparesis, spasticity, fatigue, visual problems, sleep disturbances, headaches, etc.), cognitive (attention or memory dysfunction), and/or emotional challenges from a medical or pharmacological standpoint. They are likely to make specific recommendations regarding medication management of some of these challenges, guide overall neurorehabilitation care or complications, make recommendations for pertinent therapies required, and provide recommendations regarding returning to previous level of activities. In a rehabilitation setting, the physiatrist often collaborates with the neuropsychologist to help manage these challenges. For the purposes of this chapter, we will defer on discussing specific psychiatric as well as pharmacological interventions for brain injury and focus more on neuropsychological aspects of brain injury interventions. However, for information on managing the medical and physiatric aspects of brain injury, the authors refer you seek out additional resources [30].

The rehabilitation of individuals with BI has moved away from the notion of a "cookie-cutter" approach to treatment, where everyone receives the same therapies based on diagnosis alone. According to Malec [31], there has been a movement to provide rehabilitation treatments as individualized to the person as possible, depending on the person's challenges, strengths, goals, psychological functioning, and psychosocial circumstances. If the individual only has "minor" or circumscribed limitations (e.g., mildly decreased short-term memory, relatively reduced processing speed, hemiparesis of an extremity, etc.), reasonable level of awareness, and impairments which are considered to be mild, then referral to a traditional outpatient therapy for speech, occupational, or physical therapy may be of benefit. In this context, the person would participate in therapy services at an "impairment" level. Such goals could include something like "improving memory functions to 85% of the time using external memory aids." In a traditional outpatient setting, the patient may end up in a single or multidisciplinary setting, with each therapist addressing separate challenges. There is very little coordination between therapists. Majority of individuals with brain injuries will likely fit into this category.

However, as is often the case in individuals with BI, patients can often present with several impairments, moderate-to-severe deficits, decreased insight, and neurobehavioral or emotional challenges and have goals of returning to home- or community-level activities (employment, school, home management, etc.). A common scenario may include someone with a TBI who is now experiencing deficits in short-term memory, attention, processing speed, word retrieval, and various executive functions. Neurobehavioral deficits are often present, such as decreased initiation or the converse, impulsivity, and disinhibition. They may be unaware of the extent to which these challenges are present and may believe they are capable of doing much more than what is recommended for them (e.g., driving). Their mood may be somewhat labile or even irritable. They may have some weakness on an extremity, balance issues, language disturbances, or even some visuospatial or vision deficits. This person has not been cleared for driving, returning to work, being left alone without any supervision, and may even be experiencing some challenges with home management. In this scenario, referral for a comprehensive neurorehabilitation or holistic day treatment program (DTP) is strongly recommended [31].

Holistic DTPs were founded by Yehuda Ben-Yishay [32] and were further elaborated by works of Prigatano [33]; Christensen et al. [34]; and Diller [28]. Essential elements of a DTP have been identified and defined. One of the foci of this type of program is to help the individual increase their level of self-awareness, which may require an intensity of services. This type of program focuses on the provision of group treatments promoting a therapeutic or neuropsychological milieu to enhance awareness, acceptance, and social pragmatics; psychotherapy to promote positive coping strategies and prevention of catastrophic reactions; cognitive retraining carried out in individual and group settings utilizing evidence-based approaches; supported work trials; family education and training, as well as emotional support if the family requires; and follow-up procedures. These programs can often last from 6 to 16 weeks on average. Staff is often transdisciplinary, meaning that each therapist is aware of the core principles and therapeutic techniques that should underlie the therapy from session to session, no matter which therapist is working with the client. For example, if disinhibition and impulsivity are neurobehavioral challenges that will affect overall outcome goals, then even the physical therapist who is working on dynamic gait balance should be utilizing strategies to address the impulsive behavior and promoting self-regulation (one of the ultimate goals of neurorehabilitation).

The effectiveness of holistic neuropsychologically oriented post-acute rehabilitation programs has been studied for years [24], but it can still be difficult to conduct adequate research such as prospective controlled trials [18]. Nevertheless, these types of programs have been found to be effective in increasing productivity when compared to controls. Sarajuuri et al. [24] found that 89% of the patients treated in their neurorehabilitation program were productive (defined as working, studying, or participating in volunteer activities) when compared to the 55% of the controls at follow-up. The authors concluded that comprehensive neuropsychologically oriented rehabilitation programs can improve psychosocial functioning with respect to obtaining productivity in a sample of moderate-to-severe TBI. Klonoff et al. [20] found that 73.9% of patients discharged from a milieu-based day treatment neurorehabilitation program were productive in a long-term outcome study of individuals with multiple brain injury types. Malec [35] evaluated the impact of a holistic day treatment program in individuals with acquired brain injury. Subjects consisted of 96 program graduates, with either a TBI (72%), stroke (19%), or other types of acquired brain injury (9%, e.g., anoxia), whose outcome data were analyzed after participating in a comprehensive day (holistic) outpatient brain injury rehabilitation program. Admission to the program required individuals with limited self-awareness of disabilities, cognitive deficits, poor social and communication skills, and limited emotional and coping resources, as well as decreased behavioral self-control. Examination of data revealed that graduates achieved significant improvements in specific treatment goals set, significant reductions in disability, and improvements as measured by the Mayo-Portland Adaptability Index—22 [36], including reduced physical disabilities, increased self-awareness and emotional self-regulation, as well as effective participation in interpersonal activities. These changes were also associated with significant improvements in social participation including living independently or unsupervised living, as well as employment status at the end of the program.

Cognitive Rehabilitation

If an individual with BI possesses cognitive or neuropsychological impairments affecting their everyday functioning, they may still benefit from cognitive therapies, regardless of whether it is in a traditional outpatient setting or DTP. Traditionally, these types of treatments are provided by speech and language pathologists, occupational therapists (OT), or neuropsychologists, depending on the type of cognitive or neuropsychological impairments demonstrated. The topic of cognitive rehabilitation has been of great interest for over a decade [37] and has come to be viewed as a standard component of medical and rehabilitative care following TBI or stroke [38]. However, it is a complex topic [39] and debatable in terms of which interventions are considered to be the most efficacious or would be recommended as practice standards or guidelines [40]. Due to this complexity, the National Institutes of Health (NIH), as well as other professional organizations in Europe and the United States, has been focused on providing some evidence-based practice guidelines to clinicians practicing cognitive therapies. In 1992, the Brain Injury-Interdisciplinary Special Interest Group (BI-ISIG) of the American Congress of Rehabilitation Medicine (ACRM) published practice guidelines for cognitive rehabilitation after stroke and TBI [41], although some of these guidelines have also received criticism as being based on expert opinion rather than on empirically driven [42].

Nevertheless, Cicerone et al. [43–45] have also published guidelines examining the most exhaustive reviews of the literature on cognitive treatments. Based on these reviews, the Cognitive Rehabilitation Manual [46] was published to provide specific guidelines and recommendations for practicing clinicians who conduct cognitive rehabilitation. This is the first type of specific treatment manual of its kind and was published by ACRM. Treatment strategies were graded based on the strength of the empirical evidence examined and found in the literature by the BI-ISIG task force. Level of recommendations falls into specific categories, including (1) practice standards, strategies which have shown "substantive evidence of effectiveness"; (2) practice guidelines, strategies which have shown "probable effectiveness"; and (3) practice options, strategies which have shown "possible effectiveness" but require further research evidence for stronger recommendations (see Table 30.2 for BI-ISIG recommendations for cognitive rehabilitation). Clinicians working in the field of brain injury rehabilitation are referred to this manual to know which strategies to use, depending on the type of deficits experienced. For more details regarding how recommendations were developed, please refer to the Cicerone et al. [45].

Psychological Interventions (Individual and Group)

It is purported that one of the priorities of neurorehabilitation should focus on improving psychological health in those with TBI [49]. As such, various types of interventional strategies have been used in individuals with brain injury. Unfortunately, general counselors and therapists are not adequately trained to help manage the special needs of individuals with brain injury [50]. Thus, it is often the special role of a neuropsychologist or counselor with brain injury familiarity to help manage these challenges. The focus of managing emotional and behavioral challenges following BI should include addressing factors that may affect functioning such as lack of awareness versus denial and addressing defense mechanisms, coping strategies, self-esteem, self-efficacy, confidence, identity issues, and stages of grieving.

Among neuropsychological interventions, behavioral therapy (BT) has been shown to be effective in treating behavioral challenges following brain injury. These interventions primarily focus on altering unhealthy or maladaptive behaviors, coping strategies, or neurobehavioral challenges via learning theory techniques. Particularly, BT has been shown to improve problems with social skills [51], neurobehavioral disturbances [52], and depression [53] and has been used in conjunction with cognitive remediation in individuals with brain injury [54], although research is relatively scarce examining the effectiveness of pure behavioral activation treatment. Nevertheless, some research actually shows limited effectiveness of use of pure behavioral approaches in treating individuals with brain injury [55], particularly when there is an organic deficit in responsiveness to reinforcement [56, 57].

Table 30.2 BI-ISIG recommendations for cognitive rehabilitation [45, 46]

Domain	Practice standard	Practice guideline	Practice option
Executive functions	Metacognitive strategy training after TBI Components of intervention for deficits in attention, neglect, and memory	Training in systematic problem-solving techniques and their application to everyday situations after TBI during post-acute phase	Group interventions of problem-solving deficits and executive dysfunction after TBI
Memory	Memory strategy training for mild memory impairments (including internal and external aids) from TBI	Use external compensatory strategies, such as a memory notebook, with direct application to functioning for severe memory deficits following TBI and stroke	Use of group-based interventions for memory deficits following TBI Errorless learning techniques for use in TBI individuals with severe memory deficits
Attention	Remediation of attention during the post-acute rehabilitation phase after TBI *is* recommended. This includes direct attention training and metacognitive training		Computer-based interventions may be considered, but sole reliance on computer-based tasks without intervention by therapist was not recommended
Hemi-spatial functions and praxis	Visual scanning training for left visual neglect after right hemisphere stroke Specific gestural or strategy training for apraxia during acute rehabilitation for left hemisphere stroke	Isolated microcomputer exercises for left neglect has not shown to be effective and *is not* recommended	Limb activation or electronic technologies for visual scanning for neglect after right hemisphere stroke Systematic training of visuospatial deficits and visual organizational skills for visual perceptual deficits, without visual neglect, after right hemisphere stroke during acute rehabilitation Computer-based interventions to produce extension of defective visual fields after TBI or stroke
Language	Cognitive-linguistic treatment recommended during both acute and post-acute rehabilitation phases after stroke Pragmatic conversational skills for social communication deficits after TBI	Cognitive interventions for reading comprehension and language expression after stroke or TBI Treatment intensity should be considered key factor after left hemisphere stroke	Group-based interventions for language deficits and social communication deficits after TBI including the Group Interactive Structured Treatment (GIST): for Social Competence [47, 48] Computer-based interventions as adjunct to clinician-oriented cognitive linguistic therapy after left hemisphere stroke or TBI. Sole reliance on computer not recommended with therapist intervention

Specifically, these types of interventions are particularly good for managing neurobehavioral excesses in behaviors (e.g., aggression, impulsivity, agitated and combative behaviors, etc.), as well as "inexcesses" (lack of initiation, lethargy, lack of decision-making, etc.). Different behaviors may arise during different stages of recovery. During inpatient stages, behaviors most often seen include agitation, restlessness, and combativeness. These behaviors are often seen during the stages of post-traumatic confusion or disorientation, as well as when medical issues contribute to the maintenance of these behaviors. Neuropsychologists are often called upon to suggest behavioral management strategies to the staff working with the patient, so as to optimize recovery and reduce therapy-interfering behaviors. As the patient progresses to the outpatient setting, they are less likely to demonstrate these behaviors and less likely to be confused. However, they may still exhibit other neurobehavioral challenges. Influential factors to these behaviors may include family or caregiver interactions, environment, fear, and other significant emotional experiences (depression, anxiety, mania). The neuropsychologist typically provides psychoeducation to the patient and family, helps them identify antecedents for the behaviors and goals, and helps them create strategies to manage these behaviors either by manipulating their environment, educating caregivers, or teaching both the caregiver and patient behavioral strategies. As recovery and awareness occur, it is expected that the individual with the BI will hopefully develop some self-regulatory and metacognitive strategies to eventually manage the challenge themselves [40].

Cognitive behavioral therapy (CBT; [58]) is a very frequent type of neuropsychological intervention used to help the individual adjust to and cope with the effects of a BI. It is based on the premise that individuals make attributions or form opinions about themselves, the world, and/or their future. The development of these attributions is based on early experiences as well as significant events encountered in their lives. Attributional styles develop without full awareness and become automatic, occurring without knowledge, yet we react to these automatic thoughts as if they are always true or valid. The purpose of CBT is to help individuals identify any maladaptive thoughts or perceptions they have regarding certain triggers or events, develop more reassuring thoughts or restructure those perceptions (aka cognitive restructuring), and respond in with a positive problem-solving orientation to realistic challenges, while developing more healthy or positive behavioral coping strategies (the behavioral part of CBT).

For example, "Tom" suffered an ischemic stroke at the age of 42. Over the course of the year following his stroke, Tom starts feeling intense anxiety every time he experiences any physical symptom of his stroke that reminds him of having another stroke. So every time Tom gets a headache or feels dizzy, he immediately feels anxious. In examining Tom's attributions, he realizes that he is afraid of having another stroke and has been telling himself, without consciously being aware, "This headache must mean I am having another stroke, or I'm doomed to have another stroke." Tom realizes that he is experiencing catastrophic thoughts to his variations in physical functioning. He works with his therapist to examine the evidence behind those thoughts, "I have had headaches for the past 6 months and have not had another stroke," or "My dizziness is not a sign I am having another stroke, it is just a physical consequence of the injury." However, Tom is faced with the realism that anyone can have a stroke and there is no guarantee that he won't have another stroke. Thus, in order to become effective in his interpersonal and professional life, so as not to allow himself to be "paralyzed" by these fears, he learns that he must develop a positive problem-solving orientation and use effective problem-solving strategies. Subsequently, he learns to tell himself that he made it through this stroke and can deal with it again, if or when it happens. He tells himself that he is otherwise healthy and has to learn to let go of things he cannot control. Tom develops a positive plan to reduce his other stroke risk factors such as eating healthy, start using his CPAP machine to address the sleep apnea, and take his medications in a timely and routine manner. From a behavioral perspective, Tom also develops a plan to use specific strategies when he starts to feel anxious, such as engage in deep breathing, use reassuring self-talk, or examine the evidence for the validity of his distressing thoughts. This illustration demonstrates how CBT is used to improve mood and self-efficacy regarding ability to deal with brain injury-related consequences and generate a positive problem-solving orientation to BI (or even life-related) challenges.

CBT has been used in individuals, families, and couples to promote effective coping strategies and changes in perceptions and misattributions and improve psychological well-being overall. It has been criticized for its use in individuals with severe brain injuries, as those individuals may have difficulty remembering pertinent information, gaining insight into their own perceptions, and having difficulty with abstract concepts. However, there has been some research supporting the use of CBT in some individuals with brain injury [21], particularly when specific accommodations can be made based on the individual's strengths and challenges. Such accommodations may include use of memory compensatory strategies, altering the length of the session, increasing frequency of sessions, utilizing various modalities of learning such as verbal and visual aids, and including family members or significant others in the session to promote generalization of strategies.

Several studies have demonstrated the efficacy of CBT in individuals with different types of brain injuries [59–61]. In one study, when comparing CBT to antidepressant treatment and supportive-expressive group therapy in those with multiple sclerosis, all groups showed improvements in depression, with CBT and antidepressant treatment somewhat greater [62]. Anson and Ponsford [63] developed a coping skills group aimed at improving coping strategies and emotional functioning post brain injury. A total of 31 subjects with BI participated in a 10-session, 5-week program. Subjects who participated in this program showed an increase in adaptive coping immediately following the intervention, but the level of adaptive coping was then fluctuated at follow-ups. It was suggested that perhaps coping skills may stabilize better if family members participated in the group as well.

Backhaus et al. [64] found that when comparing the effects of a skills-based group CBT manualized 12-week program to those that received treatment as usual (TAU; comprehensive outpatient neurorehabilitation treatments with no CBT training), both groups showed significant improvements in mood initially, but at follow-up, the group that had not learned CBT showed significant decline in mood. The group that received CBT showed significantly improved perceived self-efficacy (PSE) when compared to the group that received no treatment. In 2012, Backhaus and colleagues repeated this study only comparing a 16-session CBT group to a 16-session support group [65]. Both groups showed significantly improved perceived self-efficacy as well as improvements in mood, but the group that received CBT showed significantly more PSE at 3- and 6-month follow-up than the support group. Additionally, the group that received CBT showed significantly better ability to manage emotional and behavioral challenges such as impulsivity and disinhibition, anger dyscontrol, irritability, and episodes of emotional lability (as rated by the caregiver) when compared to the support group. This suggests that CBT is effective in improving PSE and reducing emotional distress when compared to peer support groups.

Ming-Yun Hsieh and colleagues [66] suggest that although CBT is typically the treatment of choice for individuals with anxiety disorders, its delivery requires adaptation for those with TBI. Likewise, while pharmacotherapy can also be of help, this population is specifically vulnerable to the detrimental side effects which can cause cognitive impediments and further exacerbate TBI-related cognitive deficits [67]. Thus, Ming-Yun Hsieh and colleagues examined the effectiveness of combining motivational interviewing (MI) techniques with CBT in individuals with moderate-to-severe TBI who experience anxiety. Twenty-seven subjects were randomly assigned into an MI + CBT group, nondirective counseling + CBT group, and TAU group. Results showed that both MI + CBT and nondirective counseling + CBT showed significant reductions in anxiety when compared to the TAU group. Those in the MI group showed greater response to CBT, in terms of reduced anxiety, stress, and poor coping skills when compared to the nondirective counseling group. These results suggest that CBT intervention can be helpful in reducing anxiety, but MI+ CBT shows a good potential to help even further augment the positive benefits of CBT.

Family Interventions for Brain Injury: A Special Focus

Attention of the medical community, including rehabilitation clinicians and researchers, is often focused on the condition and functioning of the identified patient with brain injury. Interventions are designed, and outcomes are measured regarding how best to help these individuals achieve the most optimal recovery possible. All too often as the patient becomes medically stabilized and rehabilitation therapies have tapered off, the primary responsibilities of continued care needs are transferred to the family. However, unfortunately, the family typically does not have the appropriate preparation and/or training in being able to manage some of the demanding medical needs, persistent cognitive and emotional difficulties, and financial burden that may be present. As family members step up as primary caregivers, research has shown that their risk for developing their own physical and emotional problems increases [68]. Furthermore, this increase in distress would appear to become cumulative in some circumstances and may endure for years after their injured loved one has returned home [69]. Not only does it begin to become clear that brain injury affects the family as well as the survivor, but it inevitably alters the family system [70]. A bi-directional, influential relationship also begins to emerge. That is, the greater the needs for care from the survivor, the more assistance a caregiver must provide, thereby leading to increased caregiver burden [71]. Other factors that have been found to add to caregiver burden and that negatively impact family functioning include neurobehavioral and personality changes such as irritability, impulsivity, and lack of awareness of other's feelings/egocentric views [72]. These emotional and behavioral challenges have been consistently noted by family members as the most distressing changes following injury [70, 72]. It can be particularly anxiety-provoking when the survivor acts in ways that are distinct from previous functioning and is perhaps out of line with social norms. The greater the caregiver's burden becomes, the less likely he or she may be to continue to put forth effort in meeting the survivor's needs. Finally, as the survivor's needs may begin to go unmet, the relative impact of their brain injury is likely to be magnified as symptoms worsen in the absence of adequate support (see Fig. 30.1).

Research supports the notion that a survivor's potential for success in rehabilitation is influenced by the family/caregiver's ability to effectively cope with and manage the care of their loved one [73, 74]. In one study, level of caregiver burden was found to predict survivors' objective neuropsychological functioning, even after controlling for other survivor and injury variables [75]. More specifically, higher burden was associated with poorer neuropsychological functioning. Although the authors of this study note that it is quite possible that caregiver burden was higher for those providing care for more severely impaired survivors with increased care needs, the relationship is nonetheless likely reciprocal and cyclical. In a similar vein, Sander et al. [76] found family functioning to be significantly related to survivor outcome following participation in a post-acute rehabilitation program. Above and beyond the influence of disability ratings upon admit and injury severity, those survivors whose families displayed greater levels of unhealthy communication/interactions were less likely to show improvement following discharge from the program. Thus, without prompt intervention, one might assume that each individuals' (i.e., survivor and caregiver) health and psychological functioning will potentially further deteriorate.

Emotional Functioning in Caregivers

In one of the largest multicentered prospective studies to date on caregiver functioning and needs, researchers found that roughly one-third reported experiencing clinically significant psychological distress, including depression, anxiety, and somatic symptomology [77, 78]. Other studies have suggested the range of caregiver distress and family dysfunction is between 25% and 49% [76, 79]. Emotional and behavioral changes in the survivor have been found to significantly predict poor family functioning as well as symptoms of anxiety and depression at 2 and 5 years post-injury in family members [72]. Understanding that varying levels of care are inevitably based on individual needs, some of the tasks a family/caregiver may become involved with can include assistance with activities of daily living (e.g., feeding, dressing, bathing), attending to instrumental activities of daily living (e.g., household chores, shopping, transportation), providing emotional and social support, as well as management of medical, financial, and legal affairs [80]. Not surprisingly, the increased task demands can lead to greater needs in caregivers as well. Results of six focus groups revealed five interrelated themes related to caregiver needs, including (1) coping, (2) barriers, (3) supports needed, (4) supports that worked, and (5) "ideal world" recommendations [81]. Although across the groups coping was found to range widely from impaired to optimal levels, caregivers' concerns tended to be characterized by an overwhelming sense of chronic mental and sometimes physical exhaustion of caring for their loved ones' multidimensional needs. Practical barriers to caregiving were identified as balancing work, childcare, and respite needs. On a broader, systematic level, issues such as inadequate services for caregivers and lack of age-appropriate services were noted. In the "supports that are needed" category, caregivers reported a desire for more specialized knowledge of ABI among general medical providers as well as increased access to peer or professional support networks for family even via telephone or Internet formats. Caregivers also emphasized the need for greater availability of individual, couple, and family counseling to help them adjust and cope with their new challenges in the caregiving role. The needs for education on various aspects related to their loved one's injury, expectations for recovery, and specific strategies for coping with the effects of the injury were also stressed. Finally, caregivers also identified the need for a continuum of care that would extend far beyond the acute care setting with routine long-term follow-up in the community.

Impact of Coping Styles

In a study of 123 family members of individuals with brain injury, researchers found that those with higher levels of adaptive coping were significantly less distressed and reported better overall family functioning [70]. Other studies have suggested that approaching the caregiving role with a negative, avoidant, and/or impulsive problem-solving style has been found to be associated with increased depression among caregivers [74], while those who exhibited an emotion-focused coping style perceived greater burden in caring for the survivor [82]. Utilizing a task-oriented coping style as compared to an emotion-focused coping approach would appear to be helpful in mitigating one's satisfaction with the caregiving relationship [82]. One study found that family members who were experiencing more symptoms of anxiety, as compared to those with more depressive symptoms or no report of symptoms, tended to seek out emotional support from staff on an inpatient subacute brain injury unit [83]. The authors suggested that this is not to say those with primarily depressive symptoms were less distressed, but rather may have had less energy or motivation to actively seek help. Thus, it is important to be aware of each family's emotional functioning via proactive assessment and to offer emotional support early to families who may not actively seek such services on their own. In fact, when caregivers perceive that they have adequate social support, it has been shown to help buffer their experience of stress associated with the caregiving role [82]. Increases in self-efficacy, particularly in one's knowledge of coping skills and confidence in one's ability to effectively utilize the strategies, have been found to lead to increased positive regard toward the caregiving role [82].

State of the Evidence for Family and Caregiver Interventions Following Brain Injury

Unfortunately, despite the increased understanding of the potential negative impact of a brain injury on caregiver and family functioning, few interventions exist that directly address the needs of spouses and parents, and even fewer are available for siblings and children of those with an injury [80, 83, 84]. More specifically, in a critical review of the evidence base for family/caregiver interventions following ABI, Boschen et al. [84] found only four randomized controlled trials (RCTs), all of which were limited by small sample sizes. In 2010, however, Ramkumar and Elliott reported that though still limited, there appears to be a growing consensus that interventions geared toward skill building and coping with the caregiver role is superior to "treatment as usual." They suggested that interventions for caregivers should be theory-driven but may be delivered in a variety of modalities (e.g., individual, group, telephone, Internet), based on caregiver preference and needs.

Within the past 5–6 years, a few additional studies have offered some promising results on family and caregiver interventions. Kreutzer and colleagues [77, 78] investigated the efficacy of the Brain Injury Family Intervention (BIFI) program designed specifically to address the needs of families of persons with acquired brain injury. The program was delivered in a five 2-h sessions across 10 weeks and incorporated theoretical foundations in family systems theory and cognitive behavioral therapy. Areas of focus included several topics such as education on the typical effects of brain injury, coping with change, managing stress, effective problem-solving, and goal setting. Results of the intervention indicated that the program was successful in meeting many of the families' identified needs and leads to fewer perceived obstacles in obtaining various services. The intervention was not found to significantly improve psychological distress, family functioning, or overall life satisfaction, however. As mentioned earlier, Backhaus et al. [64] evaluated the efficacy of a 12-week intervention of education, coping, and problem-solving following brain injury. Findings from this study revealed significant improvements in perceived self-efficacy among the participants of the treatment group as compared to those in the control group. The effects of the intervention were maintained at 3-month post-intervention completion, and while no significant changes on emotional functioning were found between groups, the participants in the control demonstrated significantly more emotional distress at 3-month follow-up. This finding suggests that those in the treatment group may have learned to better manage and cope with the effects of the injury, thereby buffering some of the emotional difficulties. Sander [84] developed a coping skills program for caregivers that is six sessions long and occurs weekly for 2 h each. The author designed a three-centered pilot study to examine the effects of this group on coping. This CBT group focuses on teaching caregivers information about TBI effects on the family, general education and management of TBI-related problems, relationships and sexuality, stress management and coping skills, problem-solving strategies, and accessing community and national resources. Preliminary results revealed a significant reduction in anxiety and escape-avoidance coping pretest to posttest. There was also a high satisfaction with the group.

Despite the above noted evidence of some interventions in improving limited aspects of functioning among families and caregivers, the state of the evidence for such approaches remains equivocal with respect to altering emotional and family functioning. This area of research is likely plagued by the vast multidimensional nature of family and caregiver functioning and needs and limitations of measurement devices. Other types of interventions for families and caregivers have included peer support groups, which have shown some promising results in reducing caregiver stress and emotional difficulties, and respite services for family and caregivers [84]. However, much like the general literature on interventions noted above, there is a lack of rigorous effectiveness evidence for these types of interventions [84].

Summary and Recommendations for Future Interventions and Research

Clearly, the area rehabilitation and treatment after brain injury has grown tremendously. Consequences to the individual with BI have included detrimental effects on physical, emotional, behavioral, and cognitive functions, often affecting the person as a whole. These consequences have resulted in long-term challenges influencing the person's ability to function in their personal, home, work, social, and school environments. Unfortunately, these challenges are not guaranteed to continue to improve and may, in fact, worsen over time in a proportion of individuals [22]. Likewise, challenges are not specific to just the individual who sustained the brain injury, but also strongly affect the family or significant other of the person with brain injury. When the family system is disrupted following this event, this, in turn, further precipitates worsening of functioning for the BI-affected person. Thus, there is a strong need for neuropsychological follow-up and services for the person with brain injury and their family [70, 84].

The neuropsychologist is trained in understanding the brain-behavioral relationship and how disrupted neurological functions from the injury can affect the person's ability to function in their everyday environment. Depending on the background of the neuropsychologist, they are likely able to properly evaluate and diagnose, provide appropriate pharmacological and rehabilitation treatment recommendations, as well as possibly provide psychological, cognitive, and neurobehavioral treatments. Most often, neuropsychologists will work in conjunction with a treatment team to provide a comprehensive treatment milieu, when appropriate. This often starts with a comprehensive neuropsychological evaluation but can go on to include providing cognitive rehabilitation alone or within a holistic neurorehabilitation post-acute setting, individual psychotherapy via various modalities and conceptualized treatments, group treatments, and family interventions.

Implications for future interventions include a continued focus on developing specific coping skills strategies for managing the more challenging emotional and behavioral difficulties that arise in the survivor as well as promotion of active use of task-oriented problem-solving strategies [82]. Research supports the need for interventions aimed at not only helping the family system adjust to the neurobehavioral effects of the injury but also geared toward more individualized support for those family members who are experiencing significant symptoms of anxiety and depression [72]. As well, given the frequency of enduring difficulties, follow-up with not only the survivor but the family too should continue regularly for several years post-injury [72].

Recommendations for future research include (1) further clarification of the reciprocal relationship between family/caregiver and survivor functioning and long-term outcome; (2) development of more prospective, methodologically rigorous longitudinal studies of family, caregiver, and survivor persistent challenges; and (3) investigation into matching interventions with unique needs of the caregivers and family systems [84]. Other important areas for investigation may include further exploration of the impact of brain injury on siblings and children of the survivor, determination of factors contributing to survivor and family resilience and use of positive, adaptive coping skills [86], as well as the examination of treatments to improve the quality of marriage and intimate relationships after a brain injury.

Chapter Review Questions

1. Following a brain injury, the risk for developing depression is elevated:
   A. Only in the first 3 months after the injury.
   B. Only if the person is not married.
   C. At any time after the brain injury.
   D. Never. People with brain injury are not at risk for depression. Only their caregivers are.

2. According to Trexler [25], which of the following statements are true?
   A. An individual's personality traits and style of coping can influence how they recover from an injury.
   B. The most important variable that predicts recovery after brain injury is the actual medically defined severity of the injury, with the single largest factor being the Glasgow Coma Scale at the time of the accident.

   C. Having an emotional reaction to the brain injury, such as grief, is an unhealthy response that can lead to detrimental consequences to rehabilitation outcome.
   D. A and C.
   E. B and C.
   F. None of the above.

3. Which of the following statements are not true about cognitive behavioral therapy?
   A. This therapy is often used to help individual identify when they are perceiving or thinking about a situation or themselves in an unhealthy way and then teach the individual how to cope and adjust to their current circumstances.
   B. This is a treatment that includes use of electrodes to measure brain activity while the individual completes a cognitive task.
   C. Research studies have demonstrated efficacy of using this treatment in individuals with brain injury.
   D. This therapy can be used with individuals with brain injury but hopefully with accommodations or modifications to compensate for cognitive deficits.

4. Review of the evidence-based studies completed on family and caregiver interventions following a brain injury has found that:
   A. There are a plethora of studies and at this point, the field of investigating the efficacy of caregiver interventions is saturated. No more studies are needed.
   B. Neuropsychological interventions for treatment of brain injury should only be focused on the person that actually experienced the injury.
   C. Of the few interventions that have been developed and studied, results show that families and caregivers can benefit from receiving skilled interventions to help them better understand the effects of the injury and learn coping strategies.
   D. None of the above.

References

1. Jorge RE, Starkstein SE. Pathophysiologic aspects of major depression following traumatic brain injury. J Head Trauma Rehabil. 2005;20(6):475–87.
2. American Heart Association. Stroke statistics. Dallas, TX: American Heart Association; 2000.
3. Goldstein LB, Adams R, Becker K, Furberg CD, Gorelick PB, Hademenos G, Hill M, Howard G, Howard VJ, Jacobs B, Levine SR, Mosca L, Sacco RL, Sherman DG, Wolf PA, del Zoppo GJ. Primary prevention of ischemic stroke: a statement for healthcare professionals from the stroke council of the American Heart Association. Stroke. 2001;32(1):280–99.
4. Rotundi AJ, Sinkule J, Spring M. An interactive web-based intervention for persons with TBI and their families. J Head Trauma Rehabil. 2005;20(2):173–85.
5. Brooks DM, McKinlay W. Personality and behavioral change after severe blunt head injury—a relative's view. J Neurol Neurosurg Psychiatry. 1983;46:336–44.

6. Seel RT, Kreutzer JS, Rosenthal M, Hammond FM, Corrigan JD, Black K. Depression after traumatic brain injury: a national institute on disability and rehabilitation research model systems multicenter investigation. Arch Phys Med Rehabil. 2003;84:177–84.
7. Deb S, Lyons I, Koutzoukis C, Ali I, McCarthy G. Rate of psychiatric illness 1 year after traumatic brain injury. Am J Psychiatr. 1999;156:374–8.
8. Guth PE. The effects of depression in head injured adults as related to educational level, gender, and activity level. In: Dissertation abstracts international: section B: the sciences & engineering, vol. 61. US: University Microfilms International; 2000. p. 1803.
9. Kreutzer JS, Seel RT, Gourley E. The prevalence and symptom rates of depression after traumatic brain injury: a comprehensive examination. Brain Inj. 2005;15(7):563–76.
10. Lezak M. Relationship between personality disorders, social disturbances, and physical disability following traumatic brain injury. J Head Trauma Rehabil. 1987;2(1):57–69.
11. Varney NR, Martzke JS, Roberts RJ. Major depression in patients with closed head injury. Neuropsychology. 1987;1(1):7–9.
12. Dickmen SS, Bombardier CH, Machamer JE, Fann JR, Temkin NR. Natural history of depression in traumatic brain injury. Arch Phys Med Rehabil. 2004;85(9):1457–64.
13. Khan-Bourne J, Brown RG. Cognitive behaviour therapy for the treatment of depression in individuals with brain injury. Neuropsychol Rehabil. 2003;13(1/2):89–107.
14. Sandin KJ, Cifu DX, Noll SF. Stroke rehabilitation: IV. Psychological and social implications. Arch Phys Med Rehabil. 1994;75:52–5.
15. Wallace CA. Unawareness of deficits: emotional implications for patients and significant others. In: Dissertation abstracts international: section B: the sciences & engineering, vol. 60. US: University Microfilms International; 2000. p. 4257.
16. Cicerone KD, Mott T, Azulay JA, Friel J. Community integration and satisfaction with functioning after intensive cognitive rehabilitation for traumatic brain injury. Arch Phys Med Rehabil. 2004;85:943–50.
17. Dickmen SS, Ross BL, Machamer JE, Temkin NR. One year psychosocial outcome in head injury. J Int Neuropsychol Soc. 1995;1:67–77.
18. National Institutes of Health Consensus Developmental Panel on Rehabilitation of Persons with Traumatic Brain Injury. Rehabilitation of personal with traumatic brain injury. J Am Med Assoc. 1999;282:974–81.
19. US National Institutes of Health. Rehabilitation of persons with traumatic brain injury. NIH Consensus Statement. October 26-28th; 1998.
20. Klonoff PS, Lamb DG, Henderson SW. Outcomes from milieu-based neurorehabilitation at up to 11 years post-discharge. Brain Inj. 2001;15(5):413–28.
21. Ponsford JL, Sloan SS, Snow P. Traumatic brain injury. Rehabilitation for everyday adaptive living. Hove, UK: Psychology Press; 1995.
22. Corrigan JD, Hammond FM. Traumatic brain injury as a chronic health condition. Arch Phys Med Rehabil. 2013;94:1199–201.
23. Hammond FM, Malec JF. Rethinking brain injury. Brain injury professional; 2013. p. 10.
24. Sarajuuri JM, Kaipio J-L, Koskinen SK, Niemela MR, Servo AR, Vilkki JS. Outcome of a comprehensive neurorehabilitation program for patients with traumatic brain injury. Arch Phys Med Rehabil. 2005;86:2296–302.
25. Trexler LE, Trexler LC, Malec JF, Klyce D, Parrot D. Prospective randomized controlled trial of resource facilitation on community participation and vocational outcome following brain injury. J Head Trauma Rehabil. 2010;26(6):440–6.
26. Wilson B. Recovery and compensatory strategies in head injured memory impaired people several years after insult. J Neurol Neurosurg Psychiatry. 1992;55:177–80.
27. Bergquist TF, Malec JF. Neuropsychological assessment for treatment planning and research. In: Eslinger PJ, editor. Neuropsychological interventions: clinical research and practice. New York: The Guilford Press; 2002.
28. Ben-Yishay Y, Diller L. Handbook of holistic neuropsychological rehabilitation: outpatient rehabilitation of traumatic brain injury. New York: Oxford University Press; 2011.
29. Trexler LE. Rehabilitation continuum in persons with brain injury; 2014.

30. Zasler ND, Katz DI, Zafonte RD. Brain injury medicine. 2nd ed. New York: Demos; 2006.
31. Malec JF. Post-hospital rehabilitation. In: Zasler ND, Katz DI, Zafonte RD, editors. Brain injury medicine. 2nd ed. New York: Demos; 2012.
32. Ben-Yishay Y, Rattok J, Lakin P, et al. Neuropsychologic rehabilitation: quest for a holistic approach. Semin Neurol. 1985;5:252–9.
33. Prigatano GP, Fordyce DJ, Zeiner HK, Roueche JR, Pepping M, Wood BC. Neuropsychological rehabilitation after brain injury. Baltimore: Johns Hopkins University Press; 1986.
34. Christensen AL, Pinner EM, Moller PP, Teasdale TW, Trexler LE. Psychosocial outcome following individualized neuropsychological rehabilitation of brain damage. Acta Neurol Scand. 1992;85:32–8.
35. Malec JF. Impact of comprehensive day treatment on societal participation for persons with acquired brain injury. Arch Phys Med Rehabil. 2001;82:885–95.
36. Malec JF, Moessner AM, Kragness M, Lezak MD. Refining a measure of brain injury sequelae to predict post-acute rehabilitation outcome; rating scale analysis of the Mayo-Portland adaptability inventory. J Head Trauma Rehabil. 2000;15:670–82.
37. Sohlberg MM, Mateer CA. Introduction to cognitive rehabilitation. New York: The Guildford Press; 1989.
38. Mazmanian PE, Kreutzer JS, Devany CW, Martin KO. A survey of accredited and other rehabilitation facilities: education, training and cognitive rehabilitation in brain-injury programmes. Brain Inj. 1993;7:319–31.
39. Shallice T. Cognitive neuropsychology and rehabilitation: is pessimism justified? Neuropsychol Rehabil. 2000;10(3):209–17.
40. Sohlberg MM, Mateer CA. Cognitive rehabilitation: an integrative neuropsychological approach. New York: The Guildford Press; 2001.
41. Harley JP, Allen C, Braciszeski TL, Cicerone KD, Dahlberg C, Evans S. Guidelines for cognitive rehabilitation. NeuroRehabilitation. 1992;2:62–7.
42. Cappa SF, Benke T, Blarke S, Rossi B, Stemmer B, van Heugten C. EFNS guidelines on cognitive rehabilitation: report of an EFNS taskforce. Eur J Neurol. 2005;12:665–80.
43. Cicerone KD, Dahlberg MA, Kalmar K, Langenbahn DM, Malec JF, Bergquist T, et al. Evidence-based cognitive rehabilitation: recommendations for clinical practice. Arch Phys Med Rehabil. 2000;81:1596–615.
44. Cicerone KD, Dahlberg MA, Malec JF, Langenbahn DM, Felicetti T, Kneippe S, Ellmo W, Kalmar K, Giacino JT, Harley JP, Laatsch L, Morse PA, Catanese J. Evidence-based cognitive rehabilitation: updated review of the literature from 1998 to 2002. Arch Phys Med Rehabil. 2005;86:1681–92.
45. Cicerone KD, Langenbahn DM, Braden C, Malec JF, Kalmar K, Fraas M, Felicetti T, Laatsch L, Harley JP, Berquist T, Azulay J, Cantor J, Ashman T. Evidence-based cognitive rehabilitation: updated review of the literature from 2003 to 2008. Arch Phys Med Rehabil. 2011;9:519–30.
46. Haskins EC, Cicerone K, Dams-O'Connor K, Eberle R, Langenbahn D, Shapiro-Rosenbaum A, Trexler LE. Cognitive rehabilitation manual: translating evidence-based recommendations into practice. 1st ed. Reston: ACRM Publishing; 2012.
47. Hawley L, Newman J. Social skills and traumatic brain injury: a workbook for group treatment; Authors; 2006. www.brainjurysocialcompetence.com.
48. Hawley L, Newman J. Group Interactive Structured Treatment—GIST: For Social Competence. Denver, CO 2006; updated 2008 (originally titled Social Skills and Traumatic Brain Injury: A Workbook for Group Treatment; and Social Problem-solving Group, 2003). www.brainjurysocialcompetence.com.
49. Morton MV, Wehman P. Psychosocial and emotional sequelae of individuals with traumatic brain injury: a literature review and recommendations. Brain Inj. 1995;9:81–92.
50. Butler RW, Satz D. Individual psychotherapy with head injured adults: clinical note for the practitioner. Prof Psychol Res Pract. 1988;19(5):536–41.
51. Brotherton FA, Thomas LL, Wisotzek IE, Milan MA. Social skills training in the rehabilitation in patients with traumatic closed head injury. Arch Phys Med Rehabil. 1988;69:827–32.

52. Schlund MW, Pace G. Relationship between traumatic brain injury and the environment: feedback reduces maladaptive behavior by three persons with traumatic brain injury. Brain Inj. 1999;13:889–97.
53. Lewinsohn PM. A behavioral approach to depression. In: Friedman RJ, Katz MM, editors. The psychology of depression: contemporary theory of research. Washington DC: Winston; 1974.
54. Bellus SB, Kost PP, Vergo JG, Dinezza GJ. Improvements in cognitive functioning following intensive behavioral rehabilitation. Brain Inj. 1998;12:139–45.
55. Drummond A, Walker M. Generalisation of the effects of leisure rehabilitation for stroke patients. Br J Occup Ther. 1996;59:330–4.
56. al-Adawi S, Powell JH, Greenwood RJ. Motivational deficits after brain injury: a neuropsychological approach using new assessment techniques. Neuropsychology. 1998;12:115–24.
57. Wood RL, McMillan T. Neurobehavioural disabilities and social handicap following traumatic brain injury. Hove, UK: Psychology Press; 2000.
58. Beck AT. Cognitive therapy: nature and relation to behavior therapy. Behav Ther. 1970;1:184–200.
59. Larcombe NA, Wilson PH. An evaluation of cognitive behavior therapy for depression in patients with multiple sclerosis. Br J Psychiatry. 1984;145:366–71.
60. Lincoln NB, Flannaghan T, Surcliff L, Rother L. Evaluation of cognitive behavioural treatment for depression after stroke: a pilot study. Clin Rehabil. 1997;11:114–22.
61. Montgomery GK. A multi-factor account of disability after brain injury: implications for neuropsychological counseling. Brain Inj. 1995;9:453–69.
62. Mohr DC, Boudewyn AC, Goodkin DE, Bostrom A, Epsteain L. Comparative outcomes for individual cognitive-behavioral therapy, supportive-expressive group psychotherapy, and sertraline for the treatment of depression in multiple sclerosis. J Consult Clin Psychol. 2001;69:942–9.
63. Anson K, Ponsford J. Evaluation of a coping skills group following traumatic brain injury. Brain Inj. 2006;20:167–78.
64. Backhaus SL, Ibarra SL, Klyce D, Trexler LE, Malec JF. Brain injury coping skills group: a preventative intervention for patients with brain injury and the caregivers. Arch Phys Med Rehabil. 2010;91:840–8.
65. Backhaus SL, Ibarra SL, Parrot D, Malec JF. Comparison of cognitive-behavioral treatment versus peer support in individuals with brain injury. Arch Phys Med Rehabil. 2016;97(2):281–91.
66. Ming-Yun H, Ponsford J, Wong D, Schonberger M, Taffe J, Mckay A. Motivational interviewing and cognitive behavior therapy for anxiety following traumatic brain injury: a pilot randomized controlled trial. Neuropsychol Rehabil. 2012;22(4):585–608.
67. Fann JR, Hart T, Schomer KG. Treatment for depression after traumatic brain injury: a systematic review. J Neurotrauma. 2009;26(12):2383–402. https://doi.org/10.1089/neu.2009.1091.
68. Harris JKJ, Godfrey HPD, Partridge FM, Knight RG. Caregiver depression following traumatic brain injury (TBI): a consequence of adverse effects on family members? Brain Inj. 2001;15:223–38.
69. Sander A. Introduction to the special issue: brain injury and the family. NeuroRehabilitation. 2007a;22:1–2.
70. Carnes SL, Quinn WH. Family adaptation to brain injury: coping and psychological distress. Fam Syst Health. 2005;23:186–203.
71. Reinhard SC, Horwitz AV. Caregiver burden: differentiating the content and consequences of family caregiving. J Marriage Fam. 1995;57:741–50.
72. Schonberger M, Ponsford J, Olver J, Ponsford M. A longitudinal study of family functioning after TBI and relatives' emotional status. Neuropsychol Rehabil. 2010;20:813–29.
73. Anderson MI, Parmenter TR, Mok M. The relationship between neurobehavioral problems of severe traumatic brain injury (TBI), family functioning and the psychological well-being of the spouse/caregiver: path model analysis. Brain Inj. 2002;16:743–57.
74. Rivera P, Elliott TR, Berry JW, Grant JS, Oswald K. Predictors of caregiver depression among community-residing families living with traumatic brain injury. NeuroRehabilitation. 2007;22:3–8.

75. Lehan T, Arango-Lasprilla JC, de los CJ, Quijano MC. The ties that bind: the relationship between caregiver burden and uropsychological functioning of TBI survivors. NeuroRehabilitation. 2012;30:87–95.
76. Sander A, Caroselli JS, High WM, Becke Neese L, Scheibel R. Relationship of family functioning to progress in a post-acute reh ation programme following traumatic brain injury. Brain Inj. 2002;16:649–57.
77. Kreutzer JS, Rapport LJ, Marwitz JH, Ha -Felix C, Hart T, Glenn M, Hammond F. Caregivers' well-being after traumatic brain : a multicenter prospective investigation. Arch Phys Med Rehabil. 2009a;90:934–46.
78. Kreutzer JS, Stejskal TM, Ketchum JM, Marwitz Taylor LA, Menzel JC. A preliminary investigation of the brain injury family interventio pact on family members. Brain Inj. 2009b;23:535–47.
79. Kreutzer JS, Gervaio AH, Camplair PS. Primary careg ' psychological status and family functioning after traumatic brain injury. Brain Inj. 1994a; 7–210.
80. Ramkumar NA, Elliott TR. Family caregiving of persons lowing neurotrauma: issues in research, service and policy. NeuroRehabilitation. 2010;27:1 12.
81. Gan C, Gargaro J, Brandys C, Gerber G, Boschen K. Fa caregivers' support needs after brain injury: a synthesis of perspectives from caregiver rograms, and researchers. NeuroRehabilitation. 2010;27:5–18.
82. Hanks RA, Rapport LJ, Vangel S. Caregiving appraisal after trauma brain injury: the effects of functional status, coping style, social support and family functioni NeuroRehabilitation. 2007;22:43–52.
83. Norup A, Kristensen KS, Siert L, Poulsen I, Mortensen L. Neuropsyc ological support to relatives of patients with severe traumatic brain injury in the sub-acute p se. Neuropsychol Rehabil. 2011;21:306–21.
84. Boschen K, Gargaro J, Gan C, Gerber G, Brandys C. Family interventions after acquired brain injury and other chronic conditions: a critical appraisal of the quality of the evidence. NeuroRehabilitation. 2007;22:19–41.
85. Sander AM. A cognitive-behavioral intervention for family member of personals with TBI. In: Zafonte RD, Katz DI, Zasler ND, editors. Brain injury medicine: principles and practice. New York: Demos; 2007b.
86. Perlesz A, Kinsella G, Crowe S. Impact of traumatic brain injury on the family: a critical review. Rehabil Psychol. 1999;44:6–35.

Chapter 31
A Perspective on Vocational Rehabilitation for the Physician

Robert T. Fraser, Erica K. Johnson, and David Strand

Introduction

The profession of vocational rehabilitation counseling, or rehabilitation counseling, began in the early 1920s but gained crucial momentum in the United States after World War II as an effort to help veterans with disabilities access employment or return to work after disabling injury [1]. In 1954, the Vocational Rehabilitation Amendments [2] established funding through the Rehabilitation Services Administration (RSA) for the development of master's-level counselor education programs, and accreditation standards for these programs emerged in 1972. As of this writing, there are approximately 93 programs in 44 US states and territories [3]. Typical coursework encompasses medical and psychosocial aspects of disability, diverse counseling approaches, vocational assessment, disability evaluation, career development and assessment, job placement and case management strategies, legal and legislative foundations, and ethics [4]. For the past 40 years, the Commission on Rehabilitation Counselor Certification (CRCC) has regulated professional practice. The associated credential (CRC) is available and awarded to those who complete qualifying graduate training, including a supervised practicum and internship, and pass a national exam [1].

For the physician seeking vocational rehabilitation consultation, rehabilitation counselors can be found within larger medical centers, especially those with

R. T. Fraser (✉)
Neurological Vocational Services Unit, Harborview Medical Center, Rehabilitation Medicine, University of Washington School of Medicine, Seattle, WA, USA

D. Strand
Neurological Vocational Services Unit, Department of Rehabilitation Medicine, Harborview Medical Center, University of Washington, Seattle, WA, USA
e-mail: rfraser@uw.edu

E. K. Johnson
Health Promotion Research Center, University of Washington, Lynnwood, WA, USA

K. M. Sanders (ed.), *Physician's Field Guide to Neuropsychology*,
https://doi.org/10.1007/978-1-4939-8722-1_31

comprehensive medical/psychological rehabilitation programs. In other cases, they are agency- or self-employed in the community and can be referred based upon the patient's financial means, including availability of private insurance or liability benefits (e.g., worker's compensation). Credentialed vocational rehabilitation counselors can be identified through the website http://www.crccertification.com, which includes a search function specific to geographic location. For many patients, the best resource is the state vocational rehabilitation office nearest their home. A directory of these state agencies, including their website addresses, can be found at http://www.fda.gov/downloads/AboutFDA/WorkingatFDA/UCM277757.pdf.

Range of Services Offered by the Vocational Rehabilitation Counselor

There are specific knowledge and skill sets that are critical to successful vocational rehabilitation counseling practice [5]. It is important that the physician or a staff person explore some of the following qualifications to be more adept in referral to a specific counselor or counselors. Competencies below are among those that are the most relevant to a medical setting:

1. Medical and psychosocial knowledge of diverse disabilities and disability management systems, along with experience working with members of the medical rehabilitation team to include the physician, neuropsychologist, speech and language pathologist, physical and occupational therapists, and other rehabilitation therapists (viz., recreation therapist and social work), with a focus on work access/return.
2. Experience in vocational evaluation to include interest and work values assessment, personality assessment, academic abilities clarification, integration of psychological and neuropsychological information, and other relevant clinical and psychometric assessment. The most important aspect of the evaluation is that the vocational rehabilitation counselor can offer not only vocational options but also a potential gradient of work access activities and other resources (viz., accessibility or accommodation) that could be assistive in succeeding in these options.
3. Ability to skillfully use federal and state career and employment information (c.f., The Dictionary of Occupational Titles) [6], as well as integrating current labor market information (c.f., the information amalgamator http://indeed.com and other job search-based websites) to advise a client. Similarly, the rehabilitation counselor should be able to advise and train the client in job search and interviewing strategies, as well as benefits analysis relative to work return after obtaining Social Security Disability Insurance (SSDI) benefits.
4. Ability to conduct job analyses and make procedural, workstation, or assistive technology (AT) recommendations for reasonable disability accommodation purposes. If additional accommodation resources are needed, the rehabilitation counselor should have access to assistive technology consultants and resources (described in depth later in this chapter).

5. Experience arranging community-based assessments or nonpaid tryouts for the patient, either at a prior job or a new job, using either a volunteer program/status or the Department of Labor [7] waiver for unpaid work (viz., up to 215 h) to provide the patient a graduated approach to work return (e.g., part-time moving to full-time) and opportunity to assess recommended job site accommodations.
6. Significant experience engaging businesses and hiring professionals for purposes of client job placement and employer advising to assist the patient with a disability to employment access. In addition to the nonpaid tryout, resources can include tax incentives for the employer, a supported employment job coach or natural support approach (i.e., trained co-worker), and provision of client placement follow-up counseling. Depending upon the disability and associated functional concerns and environmental barriers, employers can be cautious and often intimidated about bringing a patient into the workforce due to unfamiliarity with accommodations and associated costs [8]. The presence of an experienced vocational rehabilitation counselor can be informative and reassuring to the employer in need of pertinent advisement.

Rehabilitation Counselor's Partnership with the Psychologist/ Neuropsychologist

The successful vocational rehabilitation counselor will be experienced and able to establish working relationships with diverse rehabilitation professionals—important information can come from specific therapists, but psychological status information can be particularly important. For example, emotional/characterological functioning within the context of a disability and cognitive sequelae resulting from head trauma or other neurological insult are vital considerations for successful vocational services. The following details, provided by the neuropsychologist, can significantly aid the vocational rehabilitation counselor:

1. The range of specific cognitive strengths and concerns across the domains of functioning to include verbal and perceptual intelligence, memory, attention, speed of information processing, executive functioning, expressive and receptive speech, motor and visual functioning, and other discrete data.
2. Suggestions for specific accommodation issues and/or strategies related to areas of a job's essential functions and required abilities.
3. Descriptions of a client's test engagement, motivation, behavior, and endurance/ fatigue over the assessment period.
4. Descriptions of relevant psychosocial issues and emotional/personality functioning that may have to be taken into consideration relative to a client's job goals and current life status.
5. Other vocationally relevant recommendations based upon discussion with the rehabilitation counselor, job description/analysis, and other employment/educational data collected.

The Value of Neuropsychological Testing in Predicting Successful Employment

There are several studies that support the value of neuropsychological test results as being a driver in capitalizing on a patient's cognitive strengths and allowing the identification of weaknesses and concerns for accommodation consideration. In the field of epilepsy vocational rehabilitation, Fraser et al. [9] identified that motor speed and cognitive efficiency measures were most significant in predicting job retention 1 year from placement within an epilepsy vocational rehabilitation program. In a similar study in the field of traumatic brain injury vocational rehabilitation, Machamer et al. [10] assessed the association between employment stability and cognitive functioning at 3–5 years post-injury. Results indicated the best predictors of job stability were not only motor speed and general cognitive efficiency but also visual-spatial intelligence and memory for items without context. In the field of multiple sclerosis vocational rehabilitation, Fraser et al. [11] found that a measure of verbal fluency and executive functioning were the most significant predictors of employment stability at 14 months from placement. Among demographic and other psychosocial variables, the number of months employed in the 2 years pre-injury or prevocational rehabilitation program entrance is also generally a potent employment outcome predictor (although this was not the case in the multiple sclerosis study). *Nevertheless, these studies indicate that especially in the domain of neurological vocational rehabilitation, attention to neuropsychological test results is critical, particularly in anticipating challenges that can occur in work access and work return.*

As discussed by both Barisa and Barisa [12] and Uomoto [13], neuropsychological evaluations can, at times, overestimate or underestimate an individual's actual functional capability, and this must be kept in mind. Test results may overestimate workplace performance because the evaluation occurs in a relatively quiet and controlled environment, one-on-one with the neuropsychologist or test administrator vs. a busy, stimulating, and time-pressured work setting. Underestimation of functional ability may also occur due to the absence or inhibition of valuable environmental cues and aids (e.g., reminders, helpful co-workers) and overlearning of specific information or tasks that occur with applied experience vs. the novel demands of the testing environment. Neuropsychological test results still, however, provide a strong template from which work challenges and accommodation recommendations can be anticipated.

Exchange Dynamics between the Rehabilitation Counselor and the Neuropsychologist

In order to develop an effective relationship that benefits vocational rehabilitation for a patient, the rehabilitation counselor and neuropsychologist truly need to work collaboratively in a dynamic exchange of information. The neuropsychologist needs to have all relevant educational and employee records/evaluations, existing job description or job analysis information (specifying essential job functions), listing of the referred person's problems, and the specific employment-related functional or rehabilitation-oriented information being sought. With this type of specificity, the neuropsychologist may be deterred from a more traditional technical report or pattern analysis and move toward more utilitarian employment recommendations.

With this information provided by the neuropsychologist, the vocational rehabilitation counselor should receive very careful delineation of the patient's cognitive assets and deficits. Areas of concern that are unlikely to change over time might be underscored. These areas of challenge are likely to require a compensatory approach that can be undertaken during vocational planning. The rehabilitation counselor may often also factor in a period of nonpaid work trial to allow for a period of potential cognitive improvement or accommodation attempts and refinement. It is also extremely helpful if the client's potential strengths and deficits are presented within the context of the job description as it is understood by the neuropsychologist. For example, if there is only limited speed of information processing involved in the work tasks, this capacity may not be a concern. Conversely, if a person has impaired verbal memory, this is a noteworthy concern if there are substantive verbal interactions related to essential job activities.

One of the venues that highlights the importance of neuropsychologist-rehabilitation counselor collaboration is the evaluation feedback session. When possible, including the patient, their significant other/family member/designated representative and the rehabilitation counselor in the feedback session can be extremely helpful. The rehabilitation counselor and patient may have different concerns and questions related to the information presented in the report, and inviting both parties to participate in a feedback session allows both to ask clarifying questions about cognitive strengths and weaknesses in the context of work. Inviting multiple stakeholders to the feedback session can also enhance interpretation and understanding of information contained in the neuropsychological report. This may be particularly salient in complex cases and/or when concerns related to memory or comprehension have been noted.

Reasonable Accommodations: A Primer for Health Professionals

The reasonable accommodation area is one in which most physicians, and often neuropsychologists or other members of the rehabilitation team, either have limited experience or defer to those with legal or human resources expertise. Rules and instances of reasonable accommodations as provided within the Americans With Disabilities Act of [14] (ADA) and ADA Amendments Act of [15] (ADAAA) can be somewhat overwhelming. Yet, one of the most important functions of the vocational rehabilitation counselor is to assist in determining reasonable workplace accommodations, and the value of medical information in this process is certain. *It is of critical importance to successful work return that these professionals collaborate in return to work planning with a certified rehabilitation counselor who truly understands a job's essential functions.*

Of central import is the question of whether an individual can return to work and perform the essential functions of his/her job with some type of reasonable modification to the job or other aspects of the work environment. To optimize planning in this area, the rehabilitation counselor can explore and determine accommodation considerations in a categorical manner: procedural accommodations, physical modifications to the workstation, or some type of assistive equipment or technology [16]. Recommendations can subsequently be made in one category or, in some cases, two or all three.

Procedural Accommodations

Procedural accommodations basically involve a change in how something is done. This can involve routinizing work tasks; dividing multistep procedures into smaller work segments and steps; minimizing distractions with uninterrupted periods of focused activity (e.g., no phone contact or emailing during these periods); or using sticky notes, lists, or other organizational aids for reminders. The involvement of a job coach funded by the state vocational rehabilitation agency or a paid co-worker providing periods of coaching to the individual are other examples of procedural accommodations that are very frequently utilized.

Workstation Modification

Examples under this category of accommodation often relate to change in an individual's work module location (e.g., away from office traffic or the center of activity), the sequential organization of work equipment or tools, organization of work site materials and reduction of clutter, physical risk reduction relating to the workstation or equipment, and other changes (often minor) relating to lighting, temperature regulation, seating, and dexterity demands.

Assistive Technology

Assistive technology (AT) covers a range of aids and equipment that can compensate for cognitive, sensory, or physical impairments. AT can involve commonly available marketplace tools such as email platforms, voice mail programs, cell phone (smartphone) reminders/alarms, digital applications (apps), and other kinds of software-based implements (e.g., Outlook, OneNote, Evernote, Dragon Naturally Speaking) or specialty engineered systems/devices. Often, mainstream technologies make for efficient and relatively unobtrusive compensation of memory and mild motor-language impairments. Additional AT may be a consideration when more mainstream tools do not suffice, which is more often the case with salient sensory or mobility impairments.

Resources related to accommodations in this area can be available through AT specialists as provided through comprehensive vocational rehabilitation programs or rehabilitation centers. Publicly available resources include the Job Accommodation Network (JAN), a consultation service funded by the US Department of Labor's Office of Disability Employment. Individuals can access this service by phone (toll free at 1-800-526-7234) and the Internet (http://www.askjan.org). JAN includes the Searchable Online Accommodation Resource (SOAR), an AT-based source of accommodation resources. AbleData (http://abledata.com) is another searchable database of assistive technology products and is funded through the US National Institute on Disability, Independent Living, and Rehabilitation Research (NIDILRR). In the absence of formal vocational rehabilitation partnership, AT professionals can be identified through the Rehabilitation Engineering and Assistive Technology Society of North America (RESNA; http://www.resna.org/about/consumer-and-public-information).

Comparison of Patient Work Return with and without Rehabilitation Counselor Intervention

Case of Terry: A Physician-Guided Work Return

Terry is a 56-year-old female who experienced a left MCA stroke in April 2016. At the time, she worked as a staffing and nurse scheduling coordinator at a mental health center. The stroke required neurosurgical intervention followed by residential rehabilitation treatment, but she did not undergo neuropsychological evaluation during this time. Terry desired to return to work and in discussion with her doctor, was cleared for part-time work return with transition to full-time based upon her progress. In practice, there was no actual monitoring of her progress—her increase to full-time work was principally at her own discretion with some loose agreement on her supervisor's part. By July, only a few months after her stroke, she had increased her hours to full-time. However, after a period of only a few weeks, her supervisor professed exasperation with the number of scheduling errors that she was making. In addition to putting a poor supervisory evaluation in her personnel record, the employer dismissed her from work and urged her to seek additional consultation.

Emotionally distraught, Terry was then sent for an overly delayed comprehensive neuropsychological evaluation which revealed diverse and marked neuropsychological concerns, particularly in relation to verbal memory. The neuropsychologist referred Terry for rehabilitation counseling services. The state vocational rehabilitation agency expedited its determination of eligibility for services, which included rehabilitation counseling and assistive technology consultation with the supervisor in hopes that reasonable accommodations could be made and her job retained. Unfortunately, if the referral to neuropsychology and vocational rehabilitation counseling and neuropsychological evaluation had been made earlier, a more resourced and monitored transition could have been made, and the risk to Terry's economic and vocational adjustment would likely have been considerably diminished. Terry was terminated from the position.

Case of Brandy: Work Return Guided by a Rehabilitation Counselor

Brandy is a 29-year-old female who worked as a customer service representative for a company owning numerous parking lots in a major metropolitan area. She sustained a severe traumatic brain injury secondary to a motor vehicle accident. Subsequent to hospitalization, her neurologist referred her for neuropsychological evaluation, which resulted in the identification of significant cognitive impairments, most notably in the areas of verbal memory and speed of information processing. Both the neuropsychologist and neurologist concurred that Brandy would benefit from vocational rehabilitation counseling intervention. While she previously had been quite proficient as a customer service representative, the significant cognitive challenges identified in her neuropsychological evaluation carried significant implications for return to work.

At 6 months post-injury, the rehabilitation counselor contacted Brandy's employer to begin transition to work. The counselor and Brandy's supervisor agreed on an unpaid 215 h work trial [7], in order to observe Brandy's work behavior and establish specific accommodations. Brandy initially started working 20 h per week, and after 2 weeks on the job, it became apparent that Brandy had significant difficulty sequencing and prioritizing concerns during verbal interactions with customers. She also omitted securing critical information that was necessary for specific customer service requests on several occasions. An additional issue arose from the fact that the supervisor, although committed to Brandy, was curt in interactions with her and provided information in a rapid, staccato format. Brandy, due to her memory and speed of information processing issues, missed much of this information.

After making these observations, the rehabilitation counselor facilitated several procedural and workstation accommodations. The counselor provided Brandy with a phone script and a sequence of activities for specific problems called in by parking lot lessees. She visited Brandy at scheduled times and cued her during phone calls when responses were inaccurate. She also reviewed the company's operations manual and bookmarked critical information necessary based upon a specific lessee's request. This included flagging the important pages and highlighting critical information with a colored pen. Additionally, the rehabilitation counselor worked with the supervisor to install a "tell, show, watch, and provide feedback" sequence in providing instructions to Brandy. Brandy greatly profited from the employment specialist intervention. By the end of the nonpaid tryout, approximately 9 months post-injury, she returned to full-time paid employment. The intervention involved approximately 32 h of the counselor's time over several weeks, and later follow-up was minimal (e.g., brief tutorial phone calls in the early weeks of her full-time employment). The intervention likely assisted Brandy with saving her job and yielded a relatively smooth transition.

The comparison between these two cases illustrates the benefit of the rehabilitation counselor's knowledge, skills, and timing of transition services to full-time employment, utilizing the Department of Labor non-paid job try out benefit. Had it been relevant, the rehabilitation counselor would have also been able to guide and supervise a part-time return to work for a patient receiving SSDI benefits and capable of limited employment activity. In addition to leveraging these benefits, the rehabilitation counselor also monitors and supervises the work return, to be able to anticipate and address rehabilitation-related challenges as they arise. The physician and neuropsychologist rarely have the time or expertise in monitoring efforts of this nature [17]. Referral to a skilled rehabilitation counselor is the ideal services option.

Conclusion

The purpose of this chapter is to illuminate the professional preparation, roles, and functions of the vocational rehabilitation counselor as a professional extension of the medical team. Return to work after onset or exacerbation of a disability, particularly a traumatic one, is often challenging and should not be abandoned by either the medical team or the patient until the question can be more thoroughly addressed with vocational rehabilitation expertise. This is perhaps even more the case in the domain of neurological disabilities which can be quite complex. Appendix A contains a rehabilitation counselor information sheet for the physician to use when concerned about a client's initial work access or ability to return to work. The availability of a rehabilitation counselor is often invaluable information for the patient, the patient's relatives, and significant others. Rehabilitation counselors can play a very critical role in a successful work life for individuals who have incurred a disability.

Chapter Review Questions

1. What information is critical for the neuropsychologist to be most helpful in evaluating an individual and providing helpful information to the vocational rehabilitation counselor?
   A. Neurological history.
   B. A medication list.
   C. A detailed job description.
   D. Psychosocial history.

2. What transition mechanism can be very helpful in an individual's successful work return?
   A. Selective placement.
   B. Clearance to return by human resources.
   C. Medical team discussion.
   D. US Department of Labor waiver for nonpaid work.

3. What can be said about reasonable accommodation and work access/return?
   A. Reasonable accommodations are procedural in nature.
   B. Reasonable accommodations involve workstation modifications.
   C. Reasonable accommodations utilize assistive technology.
   D. Reasonable accommodations can involve several (or all) of the above.

Appendix A
Certified Rehabilitation Counselor (CRC) Information Sheet

What is a Certified Rehabilitation Counselor (CRC)?	The professional CRC has expertise in vocational evaluation assessing transferable skills, knowledge of the medical aspects of disability and relationship to working, job analysis, job placement, the legal rights of individuals with disabilities as related to employment, and similar knowledge and skills useful in assisting qualified workers with disabilities to access or return to employment
What specific services would the CRC provide?	The CRC can provide relevant vocational rehabilitation services depending upon your needs. Examples include: • Vocational evaluation • Graduated work return or nonpaid tryout on a former job or a new job in the public or private sector (up to 215 h) • Employment search and benefits (SSDI) advisement • Job placement assistance • Job retention assistance to include accommodation consultation with an employer, job coaching, or engaging a co-worker as your mentor/trainer • Work with your physician, psychologist, neuropsychologist, and other members of your rehabilitation team to optimize your work adjustment
How can I access a rehabilitation counselor?	In your case, you are being referred directly to the following RC provider: Name: ________________________________ Contact at: _____________________________ _________________________________ It is best to contact the following state vocational rehabilitation agency for an appointment: _________________________________ _________________________________

References

1. Leahy MJ, Szymanski EM. Rehabilitation counseling: evolution and current status. J Couns Dev. 1995;74:163–6.
2. Vocational Rehabilitation Amendments of 1954, Pub. L. No. 83-565. 1954.
3. Council on Rehabilitation Education (CORE). CORE Master's programs in rehabilitation counselor education 2014–15 academic year. Schaumberg, IL: CORE; 2015.
4. Riggar TF, Maki DR, editors. Handbook of rehabilitation counseling. New York: Springer; 2004.
5. Leahy MJ, Muenzen P, Saunders JL, Strauser D. Essential knowledge domains underlying effective rehabilitation counseling practice. Rehabil Couns Bull. 2009;52:95–106.
6. U.S. Department of Labor. Dictionary of occupational titles. 4th ed. Washington, DC: Author; 1991.
7. U.S. Department of Labor. Individual vocational rehabilitation programs: transition of persons with disability into employment. Washington, DC: Author; 1993.
8. Kaye HS, Jans LH, Jones EC. Why don't employers hire and retain workers with disabilities? J Occup Rehabil. 2011;21:526–36.
9. Fraser RT, Clemmons DC, Dodrill CB, Trejo WR, Freelove C. The difficult to employ in epilepsy rehabilitation: predictions of response to an intensive intervention. Epilepsia. 1986;27:220–4.
10. Machamer J, Temkin N, Fraser R, Doctor JN. Stability of employment after traumatic brain injury. J Int Neuropsychol Soc. 2005;11:807–16.
11. Fraser RT, Clemmons D, Gibbons L, Koepnik D, Getter A, Johnson EK. Predictors of vocational stability in multiple sclerosis. J Vocat Rehabil. 2009;31:129–35.
12. Barisa MT, Barisa MW. Neuropsychological evaluation applied to vocational rehabilitation. NeuroRehabilitation. 2001;16:289–93.
13. Uomoto JM. Application of the neuropsychological evaluation in vocational planning after brain injury. In: Fraser RT, Clemmons DC, editors. Traumatic brain injury rehabilitation: practical vocational, neuropsychological, and psychotherapy interventions. Boca Raton, FL: CRC Press; 2000.
14. Americans with Disabilities Act of 1990, Pub. L. No. 101-336, 104 Stat. 328. 1990.
15. ADA Amendments Act of 2008, Pub. L. No. 110-325, 122 Stat 3406. 2008.
16. Fraser RT, Johnson EK, Uomoto JM. Using neuropsychological information in vocational rehabilitation planning: perspectives for clinical practice. In: Arzubi E, Mambrino E, editors. A practical guide to neuropsychological testing for patients, practitioners and other professionals. New York: Springer; 2009. p. 395–413.
17. Edlund C, Dahlgren L. The physician's role in the vocational rehabilitation process. Disabil Rehabil. 2002;24:727–33.

Chapter 32
Psychotherapy and Neuropsychotherapy

Michael B. Warren and Tedd Judd

Introduction

The management of problem emotions, behaviors, and thoughts as well as personality changes in people with neurological dysfunction is distinctly different from management of the same issues in patients with psychological disorders. This is because much of the time, in patients who happen to have brain conditions, these are not simply psychological disorders but rather they are distinct syndromes due to disruption of the neural substrate of those functions. Unfortunately, it was not long ago that patients with neurological dysfunction, particularly those patients with brain injuries, were perceived as incapable of recovering from the sequelae of their injuries, often including changes in personality and emotional dysregulation [1–3].

The use of psychotherapy as a rehabilitation strategy following neurological dysfunction has a relatively short history—half a century or so—that has primarily focused on the cognitive aspects of healing. Although psychotherapeutic interventions have attempted to treat the various problem emotions, behaviors, and thoughts following neurological dysfunction, these have routinely fallen short of producing desirable outcomes due to the lack of a core theoretical model [4]. More recently—over the last two decades or so—neuropsychologists have synergistically integrated an approach more commonly referred to as *neuropsychotherapy*, which is starting to show improved outcomes [4, 5]. Although few authors have outlined such a core theoretical model, many more research outcomes are uniting professionals from each corner of the globe.

Today, neuropsychotherapy is an approach that aims to treat the affective, behavioral, cognitive, and social aspects of the whole person following neurological dysfunction by integrating psychotherapeutic interventions, comprehensive assessments, psychopharmacology, neurotechnology, and advances in neuroscientific

M. B. Warren (✉) · T. Judd
Independent Practice, Bellingham, WA, USA

K. M. Sanders (ed.), *Physician's Field Guide to Neuropsychology*,
https://doi.org/10.1007/978-1-4939-8722-1_32

knowledge [4–6]. Neuropsychotherapy takes into account a person's pre-dysfunction personality and other conditions (e.g., cognitive disorders, sensory-perceptual disorders, motor disorders, pain issues, fatigue, and other medical conditions) and focuses on improving psychological function, well-being, and community reintegration [2, 7]. Neuropsychological assessments are not only used at the outset but also to adjust the course of treatment in a dynamic process during the course of the rehabilitation process. As with traditional psychotherapeutic approaches where use of psychopharmacological interventions can improve the outcomes of therapies, neuropsychotherapy takes that another step further, making use of both on-label and off-label pharmacological interventions. Neuroimaging and neuroscience continue to influence therapies, both pharmacologically and psychologically. These aspects of neuropsychotherapy require the mental health professional to collaborate with other mental health and medical professionals and integrate other resources, such as empirically supported treatments, illustrating a final unique aspect of neuropsychotherapy: the multidisciplinary team that relies on the support and care of the patient's family.

This chapter discusses the core elements of neuropsychotherapy and important questions commonly asked by physicians, such as when to refer for psychotherapy versus neuropsychotherapy; what patterns of neural substrate dysfunction affect behavior, emotional, cognitive, and social functions; what on-label and off-label drug therapies are effective or, more importantly, should be avoided; and how does the collaboration between mental health, medical, and other multidisciplinary team members influence treatment outcomes? This chapter concludes with a clinical case example that demonstrates the use and effectiveness of the neuropsychotherapeutic approach for improving the quality of life of the patient following neurological dysfunction.

Neural Substrate

Suchy [8] describes five components of emotional processing: reflexive reactions, triggered responses, communication, regulation, and awareness. Each of these has a complex of brain structures, pathways, and processes primarily involved in their manifestations. In turn, there are also a variety of ways in which disruptions in these systems may be clinically manifest.

Reflexive reactions include the functions of flight, fight, and freeze responses, appetitive behaviors, arousal, and involuntary emotional expressions. These are mediated by the autonomic nervous system, endocrine systems, and their cortical control networks.

Triggered responses include fear, anger, disgust, and various forms of attraction, of which the most widely studied is fear. The fear reaction appears to be generated primarily in the amygdala. There is a "fast route" to fear from sensory stimuli via the thalamus and primary sensory cortex in which stimuli are not carefully evaluated, but rapid arousal allows for more rapid responses. The "slow routes" are via secondary and tertiary sensory cortex and the hippocampus, modulated by frontal systems. These slow routes allow for the evaluation of object, meaning, and context in the environment. There are many triggered responses that are learned although some are present genetically. Disruptions to these systems can include reduced reactions, overreactions, and changes to learning processes. Triggered responses can lead to a cascade of cognitive, behavioral, and physiological processes discussed next.

Emotional communication includes both perception and expression. The cortex of the right hemisphere largely mediates perception. Disruptions to these perceptual systems can result in misinterpretation or failure to notice the emotional content of tone of voice, facial expressions, and body language of others. Emotional expression has both volitional components, associated primarily with the frontal lobes and basal ganglia, and non-volitional components, associated with subcortical structures, such as the pons and mesencephalon. Disruptions can produce aprosodia, "masked facies," and misperceptions of the patient's emotional state by others. Disinhibition of non-volitional emotional communication can result in pseudobulbar affect, such as reflexive crying and/or laughing.

Emotional regulation involves much of the brain, with the posterior cortex participating in the evaluation of situations and the frontal lobes and basal ganglia involved in the generation and inhibition of responses. Disruptions to frontal lobe functions can lead to abulia, or lack of emotional responsiveness, labile emotions, obsessions, compulsions, and addictive behaviors.

Emotional awareness involves both awareness of emotions in one's self and awareness of emotions in others. Awareness of self is at several levels and concerns the ability to detect and interpret one's own emotional and physiological reactions. Many parts of the brain are involved, and the neural substrates of emotional awareness are only beginning to be understood. Lack of awareness of neurological impairments is called anosognosia and may take a variety of forms from a variety of lesions. Overreactions to neurological impairments contribute to catastrophic reactions and other emotional dysregulation. Poor emotional self-awareness has been labeled "alexithymia" and is seen in the general population and in persons with various psychoneurological conditions, such as autism spectrum disorders (ASD) where it affects approximately 50% of that population [9].

The major construct concerning emotional awareness of others is empathy, and this can be seen as having cognitive and emotional components that are associated with neighboring portions of the dorsolateral prefrontal cortex. Cognitive empathy is being able to understand what others are feeling and is described by the expression, "theory of mind." Emotional empathy is sharing what others are feeling and is associated with the mirror neuron system. Disorders of empathy are notable in psychopathy and autism spectrum disorders, among others.

Many of these functions have been alternately studied and described in psychology and in the popular press under concepts such as social cognition and emotional intelligence.

Both knowledge of and experience with these populations and phenomena are critical to the accurate evaluation and treatment of these disorders. There is a large collection of emotional and behavioral peculiarities that are seen almost exclusively in brain disorders. Relatively well-known and common disorders include the autism spectrum, the reduced emotional communication of Parkinson's disease, and psychopathy. The disruptions referenced above can be much more variably distributed in patients with other diagnoses such as traumatic brain injury, strokes, and dementias. There are a wide variety of rarer, less well-known, and even freakish phenomena such as Capgras syndrome (the belief that family and others have been replaced by duplicates), phantom boarder syndrome (the belief that someone else is living in the home), reduplicative paramnesia (memories of two different versions of important people and places in the patient's life), etc.

In addition to direct changes in the neural substrates of emotions and behavior that may have resulted from neurologic disorders, patients often have significant life reactions to the event of neurologic injury (e.g., distress at the experience of a stroke or posttraumatic stress disorder due to the violent experience that led to brain injury). Furthermore, they typically have significant emotional reactions to the experiences of becoming disabled and of being regarded differently by others. In addition, one must consider that these changes take place in the context of the personality, peculiarities, history, and psychiatric disorders that the patient had prior to their acquired brain disorder (or that may have developed since though not as a direct manifestation of neurologic disease). Finally, the actual behavior, emotional experiences, and problematic symptoms of the neurologic patient are not just a function of the individual and their neurologic disease but rather of how that disease and other events become manifest in the context of a larger family, community, and physical world.

Sorting out this complexity is a very important part of a neuropsychological evaluation, although it may often be overlooked when there is a greater focus on cognitive assessment (see Fig. 32.1).

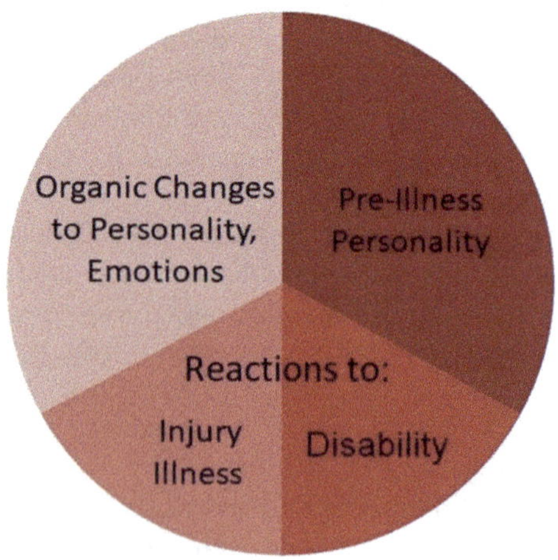

Fig. 32.1 Conceptualization of emotional problems following acquired brain disorders

Neuropsychological and Psychological Assessment

Key Point

Psychological assessment usually presumes an intact brain. It may address cognitive abilities but not always. It usually addresses cultural, social, and family context. It may focus only on personality and emotions, or even more narrowly on psychopathology and diagnoses. Most psychological tests of cognition, personality, psychopathology, and functioning exclude individuals with significant brain dysfunction from their normative groups and validations.

Neuropsychological assessment usually addresses cognitive abilities; cultural, social, and family context; personality; emotions; psychopathology; and adaptive functioning. A primary purpose of the evaluation is to determine the impact of brain dysfunction on all of those domains. Consequently, neuropsychological assessment seeks to determine premorbid functioning as well as the impact of brain dysfunction. Tests in all domains are validated on the basis of their ability to make such discriminations.

Psychological assessments of personality can be essential in the traditional psychotherapeutic setting. However, traditional personality assessments were developed for people with intact brains so when applied following neurological injury and/or impairment, they only capture a part of the whole person, which is often compromised. Understanding the functional integration of brain-behavior relationships is an essential component of a comprehensive neuropsychological evaluation and of the neuropsychotherapy process. Cognitive, behavioral, social, emotional, and adaptive functioning are also components of the neuropsychological assessment process and help to establish baselines of functions for follow-up comparisons over time and for establishing diagnosis, prognosis, and treatment recommendations.

Neuropsychological assessment often provides the first comprehensive, big picture of who a person is following neurological injury and/or impairment and covers a wide range of medical, neurological, neuropsychological, and psychological issues with detailed recommendations. As a starting place, it is essential to find out who the person was before the neurological change as well as after (for acquired conditions). Also, it is essential to seek out the knowledge of and experience with the person through the use of an informant, such as a family member or close friend. Premorbid testing is rarely available with acquired disorders. Ratings of premorbid abilities and personality functions are limited (see Braun and Schoenberg chapters), but useful, and can provide a starting place to the professional providing the neuropsychological assessment. For example, a woman who is rated by herself and her husband as moderately impulsive both before her traumatic brain injury and currently may have no active problem that needs to be addressed, but if both she and her husband rate her as not impulsive and overcontrolled prior to her injury and her husband rates her as moderately impulsive currently while she rates herself as unchanged, then she may have acquired disinhibition and anosognosia. Although test scores help to provide a clinical picture of functioning, the neuropsychologist must possess the knowledge and experience to juxtapose such cases to tease out the qualitative score differences.

The cognitive portions of a neuropsychological assessment, as elaborated in much of the rest of this book, are critical to neuropsychotherapy in order to understand what the patient and family are trying to cope with. Understanding the patient's cognitive strengths and weaknesses allows the neuropsychologist to adjust his/her psychotherapeutic technique for these. This understanding is also needed for the psychoeducation of the family and others so that they can understand and adapt to the loved one's disabilities and assist with therapy and rehabilitation.

The neuropsychological assessment of personality and emotions is distinctive. Here, the assessment requires specialized interview techniques, talking with informants, behavioral observations, and clinical experience with this population. While conventional personality tests for those with intact brains can sometimes be helpful, the interpretation of these tests for those with neurological injury has to be carried out with neuropsychological knowledge and understanding of the neurological circumstances of the individual in order to avoid major clinical errors.

There is also a growing body of specific neuropsychological personality tests and inventories such as the Frontal Systems Behavior Scale (FrSBe), Behavior Rating Inventory of Executive Functions (BRIEF-2), Neuropsychiatric Inventory, and Autism Spectrum Rating Scales. These are specifically designed as neuropsychological instruments to capture the distinctiveness of the phenomena described above. They often involve informant ratings and comparisons of pre- and post-neurologic disorder.

In addition to inventories, there is a new generation of performance tests that look at specific emotional and social perception and cognition skills. These include the Autism Diagnostic Observation Schedule (ADOS-2), the Social Perception Scale of Advanced Clinical Solutions (of the WAIS-IV and WMS-IV), and the pragmatic communication portions of the Comprehensive Assessment of Spoken Language (CASL-2).

Neuropsychological assessment can serve as a tool throughout the neuropsychotherapy process. Adapting and adjusting to life following neurological injury and/or impairment is often an intense, confusing, and debilitating experience. Although obtaining the neuropsychological assessment is helpful for other professionals providing care, it can also be an important tool for the person recovering and rehabilitating from their neurological injuries and/or impairment and their family. An essential educational piece of neuropsychotherapy integrates the assessment results into the therapy such that the person begins to understand their cognitive, behavioral, emotional, social, and/or adaptive difficulties. Assessment feedback over the course of treatment can serve as a foundation from which the therapeutic process grows. This is especially true for those with anosognosia, denial, catastrophic reactions, the lowered self-esteem of depression, and other distortions and inaccuracies of self-perception. Additionally, this feedback can facilitate the mastery of new skills through patient-centered practice and implementation. Self-efficacy then becomes a new tool, which in turn can increase good self-awareness, self-confidence, and, perhaps most importantly, hope for the future.

Neuropsychopharmacology

Key Point

Because neuropsychologists are clinical psychologists and not physicians, they cannot prescribe.* However, they often have advanced and detailed knowledge about medication use within their specialty and may have more clinical time with the client and family than physicians have to evaluate needs and medication effects. This is a key area for medicine-neuropsychology collaboration both in selecting medications and monitoring for cognitive and behavioral effects in neurologic conditions.

**Some psychologists with pharmacology training can obtain prescription privileges for a limited pharmacopeia in some jurisdictions, and this may change with time.*

The use of medications can be an important part of neuropsychotherapy, especially when these are prescribed and monitored collaboratively over the course of treatments. Neuropsychopharmacological interventions have increased over the last several decades; yet, the rate of symptom reduction and remission has not [10]. This may in part be due to the complexity of individual differences and comorbidity of many injuries, diseases, and/or disorders. This complexity necessitates the need for collaboration, identifying the best medication approach, schedule of monitoring, and the often overlooked tapering off of medications when cognitive and emotional symptoms are ameliorated or go into remission. Neuropsychologists have knowledge of medication effects and brain-related behavior to better collaborate with prescribers to find the best psychopharmacological regime for each patient. This includes the use of beta-blockers, anticonvulsants, selective serotonin reuptake inhibitors, or even stimulants for reducing the acquired impulsive anger of traumatic brain injury and similar conditions. Likewise, neuropsychologists are generally aware of the advisability of mostly avoiding benzodiazepines and phenothiazines in dementia and traumatic brain injury.

Although there are many effective *on-label* uses of neuropsychopharmacological interventions, there are also many effective *off-label* uses. Neurostimulants such as methylphenidate (Ritalin) or dextroamphetamine (Adderall) are widely known as psychopharmacological treatments for attention deficit hyperactivity disorder (ADHD). However, neurostimulants have also been demonstrated to be quite useful through off-label uses following brain conditions such as traumatic brain injury or multiple sclerosis, where improving attention, concentration, and multitasking are a focus of rehabilitation. Major depressive disorder (MDD) is often treated with different classes of medications, such as the tricyclics (amitriptyline), which are also used for the off-label use as an early intervention to slow the progression of Parkinson's disease; it is also used to manage neuropathic pain as well as sleep disturbances following brain injury. Acetylcholinesterase inhibitors such as donepezil (Aricept) or rivastigmine (Exelon) are often used on-label for treating the memory impairment of Alzheimer's disease, but they are also becoming the first choice for off-label pharmacological treatment of many of the behavioral problems of Alzheimer's disease (prior to trying selective serotonin reuptake inhibitor antidepressants, benzodiazepines, or antipsychotic medications). Furthermore, they appear to work somewhat better in Lewy body dementia than in Alzheimer's disease. Similarly, dopamine agonists such as amantadine can help improve not only motor function but also cognitive initiation in some individuals with Parkinson's disease and in other striatal and dorsomedial frontal conditions.

While exploiting demonstrated on- and off-label uses of different classes of psychotropic medications is an integral part of neuropsychotherapy, understanding which medications to avoid is also essential. For example, Lewy body dementia often includes benign visual hallucinations. It is often tempting to treat these with atypical or typical antipsychotics, but these medications are often unnecessary when the hallucinations can be managed behaviorally, and they often have consequences that tend to induce unacceptable parkinsonism. The acetylcholinesterase inhibitors, on the other hand, can be quite effective for these symptoms.

Neuropsychotherapy

Neuropsychotherapy is a term that is gaining momentum in the literature, particularly in rehabilitation medicine and in the various neuro-professions. However, some find the term a mouthful and others do not quite understand the approach and its distinction from other psychotherapies. According to Ellis [11] and Judd [6], neuropsychotherapy is psychotherapy and related interventions that are adapted to treat the emotional and behavioral disorders of brain disabilities. More recently, Grawe [12] has given the term additional meaning by adding that neuropsychotherapy, even in individuals with intact brains, is informed by professionals trained in neuroscience, especially functional imaging.

For many years cognitive rehabilitation, or the use of cognitive training exercises and compensations following neurological injury and/or impairment, has been the primary focus of neuropsychological rehabilitation. Although this approach is helpful in restoring and relearning new strategies to acquire new information or to express and comprehend language, the rehabilitation of other important functions including emotional regulation, behavioral interactions, and personality changes is often overlooked. Neuropsychotherapy aims to provide therapies for the whole person and to include the essential functions of sociability and community integration, processes that often involve family and friends [6].

Neuropsychotherapy is distinct from conventional psychotherapy in content, technique, and social context. Neuropsychotherapy is distinctive in *content* in that it takes an emotional rehabilitation approach, addressing neuroemotional dysfunction as something that can be restored through neuropsychotherapeutic exercises. That failing, compensations may be applied that may allow the person to function more normally in spite of disruption to the neuroemotional systems. That failing, the neuropsychotherapist may attempt to develop and implement accommodations applied by others in the patient's social context to allow them to function socially in spite of such problems. Neuropsychotherapy also takes account of the time-course and natural history of the specific neurologic disorder when planning interventions. In addition, changes to both cognitive and emotional learning processes are taken into account in developing interventions. Self-awareness is addressed distinctively, as called for by the patient's condition.

Neuropsychotherapy is distinctive in *technique* in the incorporation of cognitive compensations into the therapy to aid in change. This can include a therapy notebook or electronic file to help with memory for the content of therapy, cuing technologies to remind the patient to apply therapeutic techniques in their appropriate contexts, a distinctive communication style adapted to the patient's cognitive limitations, work on self-concept after disability, and presentation of the new self to others.

Neuropsychotherapy is distinctive in *social context* in that family and others are often involved as collateral to treatment to help make up for those functions that the patient may not be able to carry out effectively. Collateral helpers (rehabilitation therapists, family, friends, teachers, bosses, coworkers) are also educated about and supported in their roles. They are used to help apply therapeutic techniques in their contexts.

Neuropsychotherapy may be carried out by a neuropsychologist or by a psychotherapist or similar mental health professional who has developed such specialized skills. Such therapy will most usually be informed by a neuropsychological evaluation.

Clinical Guidance for the Physician

What to Watch for

Whenever a patient presents with unexplained emotional or behavioral changes, a neurological disorder should be considered as part of the differential diagnosis. And even for diagnosed brain disorders, it is important for physicians to take into account that most of these will have emotional/behavioral manifestations in addition to cognitive changes. Thus, when cognitive changes are reported or when there is a brain disability diagnosed, there should be an exploration of emotions and behavior, as well. Often these reports will come from family members rather than the patient, so family members should be asked. This must be done with consent, of course, and, ideally, part of this should be asked without the patient being present.

When to Refer

It is important that physicians recognize neuropsychologists as experts in emotions and behavior, not just cognition. A referral to a neuropsychologist can be considered when diagnostic and/or symptomatic clarity is needed for emotional as well as cognitive symptoms. Suspicions should rise and neuropsychology referral be considered when there are peculiar emotional or behavioral symptoms that do not fit familiar disorders such as depression, anxiety disorders, psychosis, or personality disorders, for example, especially when they have an unexplained onset. Even with a well-established diagnosis and cognitive baseline, a neuropsychological referral may be called for to assist with clarification and treatment of problematic emotions or behaviors. The neuropsychologist may be in a better position to suggest therapists they can collaborate with for ongoing neuropsychotherapy when needed.

Who to Refer to

While neuropsychologists typically develop advanced skills in cognitive assessment, it is regrettable not all are equally skilled in evaluations of emotions and behavior. Just as it can be important to know which neurologists have behavioral neurology skills, it can be important to find out which neuropsychologists in your community have a focus on emotional/behavioral disorders for the more complex and difficult cases.

How to Refer

Key Point
Referrals to neuropsychologists need to have clear referral questions and sufficient background information. Referrals may address emotional, behavioral, adaptive, and/or cognitive issues, as well as differential diagnosis of such problems where a neurologic cause is known or under consideration.

Referrals to neuropsychologists are much more useful when there are clear referral questions and expectations and when the concerning behavior is well described. Specificity is preferred ("weekly episodes of yelling and cursing at his mother without violence" is much better than "angry outbursts," "disruptive behavior," or "aggression"). It is essential to supply recent chart notes and very helpful to supply reports on brain imaging and other specialized testing, neurologic consults, mental health records, and other pertinent materials that may be available.

How to Collaborate with the Therapist

With very few exceptions, neuropsychologists are not trained to prescribe medications. When psychotropic or neurologic medications are being considered, and where cognitive and/or emotional effects may be expected, it is important to collaborate with the therapist and neuropsychologist in medication choice, treatment goals, treatment adherence, and monitoring of effects. As noted above, neuropsychologists may have specialized knowledge that can be helpful for certain symptoms and conditions. Therapists often have more frequent contact and more time with the patient for monitoring effects and for monitoring and facilitating treatment adherence.

The neuropsychotherapist often has specific goals and approaches for addressing issues of self-awareness and treatment adherence. Collaboration between physician and therapist on how symptoms, diagnoses, and treatments are presented can improve these efforts.

Case Study

SB (a pseudonym) is a 37-year-old, right-handed, married, Caucasian female with 2 years of college education who was referred by her neurologist for a neuropsychological assessment and treatment of cognitive and emotional difficulties following a severe traumatic brain injury approximately 2 years prior. She sustained her injuries from a single motor vehicle collision where she crashed into a telephone poll and rolled down a steep ravine. Although she denied drinking before the collision, she admitted to drinking heavily the night before. She was unrestrained and ejected from her vehicle. She was airlifted to a nearby trauma hospital where she was treated for her closed head injuries that included right frontal lobe subarachnoid and subdural hemorrhages. She did not remember who her four children were when they came into the hospital to visit her. She did not remember that she had gone to school to become a pharmacy technician or that she had attempted a 2-year degree at the local community college 3 years before her injury.

Following her medical treatment and stabilization, SB actively participated in rehabilitation for approximately 2 months, where she learned how to walk, talk, and essentially think again. Her primary problems during rehabilitation were:

1. *Behavioral*: crying, social isolation, avoidance, drinking, and compulsivity
2. *Cognitive*: attention and memory difficulties, visuospatial deficits, multitasking problems, impulsivity, and obsessive traits
3. *Emotional*: increased anxiety, hypervigilance, anger, irritability, frustration, and sadness
4. *Physiological*: migraine headache, sleep difficulty, daytime fatigue, vertigo, and hypertension

When SB returned home, she continued to experience cognitive, emotional, behavioral, and social difficulties. She reported increased frustration, irritability, and anger and found herself yelling at others frequently. She thought her emotional distress and cognitive difficulties were the result of her emotional trauma, yet she had no memory of the collision. She avoided driving due to the fear of being involved in another collision and reinjuring herself and had increased hyperarousal and hypervigilance coupled with an increased startle response. She had become obsessive-compulsive around the house to the extent that a bottle of wine that was opened must be finished in the same setting to avoid spoiling. She had difficulties with remembering new things and with remembering some experiences of her past. She reported constant migraine headaches and significant changes in the way she thought and felt about many things since her injury.

SB's major stressors were with emotional dysregulation and social isolation. Unfortunately, her husband, family, and friends did not fully understand the extent of her injuries or the rehabilitation process and felt like she was always faking her symptoms. Her inability to resolve anger and irritability issues with others often resulted in her social isolation, where she would retreat to her bedroom, close the door, and watch TV or read magazines for hours. Her frustration continued to get worse over time and her expression of anger more intense and disturbing to those around her and, eventually, to herself.

SB was aware of her frustration and anger as well as the need for change. However, she attributed her emotional dysregulation to psychological factors, not neurological dysfunction that likely stemmed from her injuries to the right orbito-frontal cortex—an area of the brain where a disruption of the neural substrate often results in anger and anxiety [13–16]. Additionally, it was likely that she was not able to interpret and respond to other people's needs and emotions, where subtle cues were misread and interpreted—sometimes seeing emotion when there was not, or mistaking it for another emotion. She often would project her feelings, asserting others around her felt threatened, insecure, uncomfortable, and attacked. She felt that her emotional distress developed from not recovering quickly enough or being able to return to the person she was before the injury, which triggered her and easily upset her.

Neuropsychological Testing and Recommendations

Neuropsychological testing revealed great difficulty with multitasking and her ability to learn new material and later recall it was impaired (although her recognition memory was relatively preserved). She also showed deficits in visuospatial processing, which affected her real-world navigation, as well as cognitive processing speed, where she would get hung up on mistakes under pressure. Her emotional distress was best attributed to her cognitive difficulties and frustration with her ongoing rehabilitation. She was admittedly angry and irritable, which she noticed, but others noticed more. She generally tended to pull back when cognitively challenged yet overreacted when emotionally challenged. This occurred despite her diminished cognitive functions but was clearly still intimately connected with her emotions.

SB used some coping strategies, such as walking away and returning when she was calmer, but more often she attempted to reduce her anger and irritability by drinking several glasses of wine. Unfortunately, her brain injury had seemingly changed her sensitivity to alcohol use, which was likely a contributing factor to her overall emotional dysregulation.

SB selected a goal to eliminate her current medications. This was reasonable to try provided that she used other strategies to address her symptoms, such as with attention and memory compensations (handouts provided). However, a trial of a stimulant medication, such as methylphenidate (Ritalin), for improving attention and memory was recommended, should her coping strategies alone be ineffective. Neurostimulants have been demonstrated to be quite useful following brain disorders such as traumatic brain injury, particularly for improving multitasking. Such a medication could potentially marginally improve her abilities and reduce her frustration by allowing her to concentrate better and longer, but whether and when she used a stimulant was left to be a decision between her and her physician. Additionally, a trial of a dopamine agonist such as amantadine for improving initiation following brain injury was recommended to help improve not only motor initiation but also cognitive initiation and the initiation of plans and complex activities.

SB wanted to try cannabis rather than prescription medications. In collaboration with her neurologist, a conjoint recommendation was for her to abstain at this time as it might worsen her cognitive complaints and cover up symptoms.

It was also suggested that SB would benefit from psychotherapy to help reduce the intensity of her emotional distress and improve the quality of her life and relationships. A recommendation for a program of anger and irritability management that included relaxation techniques and cognitive-behavioral modification was provided. She agreed and returned to this office occasionally with some remote (phone/video) contact sessions to begin to address these issues.

Neuropsychotherapy Approach, Sessions, and Outcome

SB's Treatment Plan

Treatment modality	Individual psychotherapy with family and friend's meetings at sessions 3, 6, and 9
Frequency	One hour per session. One week between sessions 1 and 2, and every other week until treatment success or sessions expire
Duration	12 sessions
Potential discharge plan	Support groups, cognitive rehabilitation
Problem list 1. Anger and irritability 2. Sociability 3. Anxiety and fear 4. Alcohol use	

Treatment Goals

Long-term goals: Return to school to complete her 2-year degree and work as a pharmacy technician.

Short-term goals: Recognize when getting stressed and identify the triggers of frustration and anger to better manage her emotional reactivity. Learn when to take breaks and rest. Increase independence and sociability by developing daily routines to provide structure, such as finding a hobby or skill.

Barriers/obstacles: SB was not ready to eliminate her alcoholic intake; however, she was willing to find healthy coping strategies such as reducing her consumption of alcohol.

Interventions/procedures

1. Structured problem-solving approach (e.g., problem-solving technique) for anger and irritability
2. Relaxation techniques and breathing exercises to reduce frustration and anger as well as anxiety
3. Behavioral activation therapy for anxiety and mood to increase awareness of thoughts, feelings, and behaviors that are functionally preventing her from enjoying life and being social
4. Circle of support meetings with friends and family

SB completed 8 out of 12 sessions where she worked incrementally to meet concrete and obtainable goals, but she terminated therapy after several successful sessions. She learned to recognize and control her frustration and anger through better identifying her initial feelings (e.g., overwhelmed, disrespected, misunderstood) and physical cues (e.g., blood boiling, clenched fists) through the use of cognitive-behavioral treatment that included homework assignments and a problem-solving approach. She learned to follow a plan, not her emotions. She learned to identify her problems systematically by breaking them down into smaller pieces, to monitor her mood through the use of a rating scale, and schedule both fun and pleasant activities. This, in turn, facilitated her engagement into the social world that she thought would never again be possible. Her family participated in scheduled treatments by providing other person perspectives and participated in her social activities, where they offered to take her to bowling lanes, movies, and eventually out to open markets where she shopped and negotiated with venders. She found her voice and began to teach her skills to others when she noticed they were having stress and/or expressed frustration and anger. Modeling these behaviors made her feel more confident in the work she had accomplished in therapy, which was an added bonus to her therapies and reinforced the work that she did both in office and at home. She was able to reduce her alcohol consumption, but not completely abstain. She reported less obsessive-compulsive tendencies with having to finish a bottle of wine by using smaller bottles (she would refill them and store them to prevent spoiling and for rationing her use). She was able to enroll in school but often missed classes and fell behind. She explored taking online courses, which were much better for her and her pace of learning. This was in part due to a more controlled setting that was less distracting for her (she could close her bedroom door to focus on her studying and online class participation, day or night). She participated in weekly study groups to increase her social engagement and solidify her learning.

SB chose not to use medications for her cognitive and emotional problems and was, in this case, successful with that choice. Nevertheless, the medication recommendations served at least three useful functions even though the medications were not used. First, they helped to frame her problems for her and her family as being a consequence of her brain injury, rather than an emotional reaction to it. This helped to reduce feelings of guilt and blame and provided a reason for focusing on a collaborative approach of emotional rehabilitation and skill rebuilding. Second, the recommendations served to motivate her for neuropsychotherapy so as to avoid the use of medications. Third, the recommendations served as a backup plan should neuropsychotherapy efforts prove inadequate, thereby reducing a sense of desperation and helplessness.

Chapter Review Questions

1. The contemporary relationship between referring physicians and neuropsychologists concerning medication management for neuroaffective symptoms is optimally one in which:
   A. The neuropsychologist assumes responsibility for such medications.
   B. The referring physician and neuropsychologist collaborate in medication choices, monitoring, and management, and the referring physician maintains ultimate responsibility.

C. The referring physician makes all medication decisions independently and informs the neuropsychologist of the rationale.
D. The neuropsychologist with prescription privileges only shares medication changes with the referring physician when the underlying cause is neurological.

2. Neuropsychotherapy:
A. Is distinct from conventional psychotherapy in content, technique, and social context.
B. Refers both to psychotherapy with patients with brain disorders and to psychotherapy that takes brain functioning into account.
C. Can only be performed by neuropsychologists.
D. All of the above.
E. A and B only.

3. Neuropsychotherapy:
A. Focuses primarily upon behavior management by staff and family members, since the emotional problems of brain disorders cannot be modulated.
B. Relies upon neuropsychopharmacology to change emotional states and upon behavior management and environmental manipulation to regulate behavior.
C. Integrates emotional rehabilitation strategies of restoration, compensation, and accommodation, along with medication management to address neuroaffective problems.
D. Uses individual psychotherapy approaches only, since the patient ultimately must bear responsibility for their own self-image and behavior.

4. Referrals to neuropsychologists:
A. Should contain only general questions and behavioral descriptions and few medical records so as to not prejudice the neuropsychologist's clinical judgment.
B. Need not be specific since the neuropsychologist will give a standardized battery to all patients.
C. Need not state specific referral questions since the referring physician will be making the diagnosis.
D. Should focus upon cognitive issues only, since emotional issues should be referred to psychiatrists and psychotherapists.
E. None of the above.
F. All of the above.

Definitions retrieved and amended when relevant from https://www.merriam-webster.com/medical and http://psychologydictionary.org

References

1. Coetzer R. Psychotherapy following traumatic brain injury: integrating theory and practice. J Head Trauma Rehab. 2007;22(11):39–47.
2. Klonoff PS. Psychotherapy after brain injury: principles and techniques. New York, NY: The Guilford Press; 2010.
3. Prigatano GP. Disordered mind, wounded soul: the emerging role of psychotherapy in rehabilitation after brain injury. J Head Trauma Rehab. 1991;6(4):1–10.
4. Laaksonen R, Ranta M. Introduction to neuropsychotherapy: guidelines for rehabilitation of neurological and neuropsychiatric patients throughout the lifespan. New York, NY: Psychology Press; 2013.
5. Walters H, Berger M, Schnell K. Neuropsychotherapy: conceptual, empirical, and neuroethical issues. Eur Arch Psy Clin N. 2009;259:S173–82. https://doi.org/10.1007/s00406-009-0058-5.
6. Judd T. Neuropsychotherapy and community integration: brain illness, emotions, and behavior. New York, NY: Springer/Kluwer Academic/Plenum Publishers; 1999.
7. Crowe SF. The behavioural and emotional complications of traumatic brain injury. New York, NY: Taylor & Francis; 2008.
8. Suchy Y. Clinical neuropsychology of emotion. New York, NY: Guilford Press; 2011.
9. Brewer R, Marsh AA, Catmur C, Cardinale EM, Stoycos S, Cook R, Bird G. The impact of autism spectrum disorder and alexithymia on judgments and moral acceptability. J Abnorm Psychol. 2015;124(3):589–95.
10. Hiemke C. Therapeutic drug monitoring in neuropsychopharmacology: does it hold its promises? Eur Arch Psy Clin N. 2008;258:21–7. https://doi.org/10.1007/s00406-007-1005-y.
11. Ellis DW. Neuropsychotherapy. In: Ellis DW, Christensen A-L, editors. Neuropsychotherapy. Boston, MA: Kluwer Academic Publishers; 1989.
12. Grawe K. Neuropsychotherapy: how the neurosciences inform effective psychotherapy. Mahwah, NJ: Lawrence Erlbaum Associate; 2007.
13. Bigler ED. Neuropsychology and clinical neuroscience of persistent postconcussive syndrome. J Int Neuropsychol Soc. 2008;14(1):1–22.
14. Kolb B, Wishaw IQ. Fundamentals of human neuropsychology. 6th ed. New York, NY: Worth Publishers; 2009.
15. McGoldrick M, Giordano J, Garcia-Preto N. Ethnicity & family therapy. 3rd ed. New York, NY: The Guilford Press; 2005.
16. Ogden JA. Fractured minds: a case-study approach to clinical neuropsychology. 2nd ed. New York, NY: Oxford University Press, Inc.; 2005.

Chapter 33
Medication Effects on Cognition

Jeffrey A. Sordahl, Jessica Litke, Jennifer Lewis, and Megan Dunay

Introduction

The Case of Mr. Sandy

Mr. Sandy is an 81-year-old Caucasian, Veteran, man presenting to his primary care appointment accompanied by his wife. His provider asks how he has been doing since their last visit over a year ago. Mr. Sandy reports he has noticed his memory is not what it used to be and jokingly blames it on his old age. Mrs. Sandy appears a bit more concerned about this issue than portrayed by her husband's levity. She reports that her husband's memory impairment began approximately 12 months prior to this evaluation and changes have included getting lost while driving, forgetting medications, and having difficulty paying bills. The progression is described as insidious with no specific date of onset. Mr. Sandy's medical history is significant for hypertension, hyperlipidemia, coronary artery disease, rheumatoid arthritis, benign

J. A. Sordahl (✉) · J. Litke
Boise VA Medical Center – V-IMPACT TeleHub, Boise, ID, USA

J. Lewis
Family Medicine Residency of Idaho, Geriatric Medicine, Boise, ID, USA

M. Dunay
Boise VA Medical Center, Medical Service, Geriatrics and Palliative Care Division, Boise, ID, USA

University of Washington Internal Medicine Residency, Seattle, WA, USA

K. M. Sanders (ed.), *Physician's Field Guide to Neuropsychology*,
https://doi.org/10.1007/978-1-4939-8722-1_33

prostatic hypertrophy, gastroesophageal reflux disease, and depression. He is currently prescribed the following list of medications:

Lisinopril 10 mg daily
Carvedilol 12.5 mg BID
Atorvastatin 40 mg daily
Aspirin 81 mg daily
Sulfasalazine 1000 mg BID
Prednisone 10 mg daily
Tamsulosin 0.4 mg daily
Omeprazole 40 mg daily
Ranitidine 150 mg BID
Citalopram 20 mg daily

The case above is one not uncommon to primary care providers. A patient presents to their primary care provider reporting, what could be considered, vague and subjective concerns of memory problems or general changes in cognition. While the presenting complaint is seemingly at the vanguard of the appointment, medical providers are tasked with evaluating a patient's problem within the context of their health as a greater whole. Such a task becomes increasingly complicated when conducted for patients diagnosed with chronic disease, mental health disorders, and substance use. The use of pharmacologic agents to treat acute and chronic disorders often further complicates patients' presentations to primary care, as providers must consider adverse drug effects, side effects, and drug-drug interactions.

Primary care providers are instrumental in initiating cognitive screening for patients such as Mr. Sandy. Provider observation alone, however, has been considered insufficient in assessing cognitive impairment [1]. Guidelines, algorithms, and recommended methods for screening cognitive functioning have been suggested for use in primary care settings. Initial steps in these procedures often include interviewing the patient and possible collateral informant about signs and symptoms (e.g., episodes of confusion, increased forgetfulness, failure to perform activities of daily living), as well as defining the course of the problem (e.g., rapid onset, insidious). Further evaluation may include a brief cognitive screen that may take 5–15 minutes to complete. These brief assessments typically provide a single cutoff score below which may be suggestive of cognitive impairment. However, these measures have limitations and are not independently sufficient for diagnosis. They are intended to provide a general idea of current global functioning (i.e., they do not specify domains of impairment), and the normative data collected to determine cutoff scores may not always reflect the patient population for whom they are being utilized [2]. For patients demonstrating cognitive impairment, either based on cognitive screening, observation, or clinical interview, a comprehensive neuropsychological evaluation may be warranted to better delineate domains and severity of impairment.

Cognitive Screening Measures Regularly Used in a Primary Care Setting
Mini-Mental Status Exam (MMSE)
Montreal Cognitive Assessment (MoCA)
Saint Louis University Mental Status Examination (SLUMS)

Review of current health status is also pivotal in the screening for cognitive impairment. While a patient's self-reported cognitive problem is important to consider, the primary care provider must also be sure to evaluate current physical and mental health. A patient's complaint of "memory problems" may too quickly be labeled by medical providers as resulting from possible dementia, stroke, or TBI, particularly when the patient has theorized this possible association.

Encounter Example
PCP: How are you doing today Mr. Sandy? It looks like it's been about a year since I saw you last.

Mr. Sandy: Well my memory isn't what it used to be, and I'm having trouble completing chores at home because I forget about them. I also can't remember people's names and seem to lose track of where I parked when I go to the grocery store.

Mrs. Sandy: We are concerned about dementia; his mother had dementia before she died at 94. We were wondering if there is any medication he could take to help prevent dementia.

While the above schema (i.e., cognitive problems are related to dementia, stroke, TBI, etc.) is not inaccurate, there are several other considerations that can account for changes in cognition. One such area that can be easily overlooked is medication.

Prescription medication use is nearly ubiquitous in the United States to the extent that is marketed directly to patients through television and print ads. It is not uncommon for primary care providers to be asked by patients about medications they saw in a commercial. While the accessibility of medications as treatment options has unquestionably improved care and saved lives in many instances, it would be ignorant to assume their effect has only been positive. Pharmacologic agents also convey the risk of iatrogenic effects such as damage to other bodily systems, onset of cognitive problems, mental health/behavioral changes, and addiction. Additionally, a cultural by-product of pharmaceutical advertising in modern society is the perception that there is a medication for every ailment. The general public is routinely reinforced with the idea that if you are sick, have pain, are depressed, etc., there is a medication that can remediate your problem. A patient presenting to their primary care provider with a health dilemma is now in many ways programmed to expect treatment in the modality of a prescription medication. Adding a medication or increasing a dosage can be the signal to a patient that they are receiving help from their provider; contrastingly, hearing that their medications could be the culprit of their presenting issue may not be well accepted.

This chapter will focus on medications and their side effects that impact cognition. While there are many classes of medications that have been reported to impede cognitive functioning, this chapter will review four common medication types that are regularly prescribed in a primary care setting, as well as address the issues of polypharmacy. While not directly discussed in this chapter, it should be noted that alcohol and illicit substances, including cannabis, also have significant effects on cognition, particularly when combined with medications. Furthermore, the case vignettes provided in this chapter largely focus on older adults, but this is not to dismiss the detrimental effects medications can have on the younger population. Rather, discussing medication interactions within the context of development and other factors unique to pediatrics is beyond the scope of this chapter.

- Psychotropic medications
- Sleep medications
- Anticholinergics
- Pain medications
- Polypharmacy

Psychotropic Medications

During the assessment of a patient with suspected dementia, special attention should be given to any psychotropic medications on the patient's medication list. Antipsychotics and sedative hypnotics are two common classes of psychotropics associated with the most harm when prescribed to older adults in general and to patients with cognitive impairment. Specifically, these medications can cause incident cognitive impairment and delirium, in addition to worsening dementia. Patients with dementia with Lewy bodies (LBD) are especially sensitive to cholinergic and dopaminergic deficits and often have severe reactions to neuroleptic medications [3]; the use of these agents is contraindicated in the DLB population. Dementia itself often causes sleep disturbances and delusional psychoses in addition to behaviors such as aggression and wandering, prompting psychotropic medication prescription. Treatment with these medications, however, is often associated with greater harm than efficacy. Patients with dementia are particularly susceptible to the adverse effects of sedative hypnotics and antipsychotics, yet their use remains higher in this population than in cognitively intact older adults, with prescription rates ranging from 15% to 47% of community-dwelling patients with cognitive impairment [4].

Benzodiazepines and benzodiazepine analogues not only worsen physical function and increase fall risk through impaired balance and coordination but worsen performance on cognitive assessment tools and increase the risk of developing delirium [4]. Antipsychotic use is also associated with increased falls, sedation, and cognitive impairment in older patients; and in patients with behavioral and psychological symptoms in dementia (BPSD), antipsychotics have been linked to increased all-cause mortality and stroke, prompting the FDA black box warning on the use of these medications in patients with dementia-related psychosis. Despite weak evidence for efficacy in the treatment of BPSD, these medications are still commonly prescribed in nursing homes, with about one-third of all elderly patients with dementia taking an antipsychotic in the United States, based on 2004 National Nursing Home Survey data [5].

The likelihood a patient is taking a potentially inappropriate medication, including antipsychotics, does not always appear to correlate with advanced age or gender but increases with total number of medications prescribed, often with five or more medications [4, 6]. Regular reviews of medication lists of institutionalized older patients help identify inappropriate antipsychotic use and reduce their prescription when use is not indicated. The importance of maintaining a current medication list for elderly patients cannot be overstated. Accurate medication lists make it possible to discern whether a new change in condition might be due to a medication side effect or drug-drug interaction, instead of a medical cause, and decrease the chances of starting a "prescribing cascade" [7].

Case Vignette

A 50-year-old, African American male with 13 years of education was admitted to an inpatient psychiatric unit following acute onset of confusion. The patient's medical history is significant for schizophrenia with variable adherence to medications. He had been receiving risperidone injections every 2 weeks, as well as taking oral risperidone, clonazepam, and diphenhydramine. In the week prior to the patient's admission, topiramate had been added to his medication regimen. The patient presented with complaints of feeling "foggy." His caregiver reported notable altered mental status, confusion, and word finding difficulties. Neurology workup was unremarkable for any abnormalities by head CT or EEG. A brief neuropsychological examination was conducted and results were notable for impairments in processing speed, attention, and working memory.

Digits forward < 7th percentile
Digits backward < 5th percentile
Story memory < 1st percentile
Symbol digit coding < 1st percentile

Following discontinuation of topiramate, the patient's subjective complaint of "fogginess" resolved. His alertness improved, and follow-up neuropsychological testing demonstrated cognitive functioning in domains of attention and processing speed to have returned to within normal limits.

When evaluating a patient for suspected cognitive impairment, it is important to identify the indication for all medications the patient is taking and consider stopping or tapering meds without a clear indication for use. Treatment for insomnia, wandering, aggression, and other BPSD should focus on nonpharmacologic therapies, such as activities, music, and exercise, which have greater potential efficacy and fewer adverse effects [8]. If medications are continued, shared decision-making between the prescriber and the patient or patient's caregiver ensures the risks of using such medications are understood by all parties.

Sleep Medications

Insomnia and Sedative Hypnotics

Management of insomnia and other sleep disturbances in elderly patients challenges clinicians as they endeavor to achieve adequate, restorative sleep while avoiding adverse events related to medication use. The initial approach to insomnia should emphasize nonpharmacologic interventions, examples of which include attempting to restore normal sleep wake cycles, ensuring the bedroom environment is conducive to sleep, and reducing or discontinuing maladaptive sleep behaviors. There is also strong evidence that cognitive-behavioral therapy for insomnia (CBTi) is as effective as benzodiazepine use in the short- and long-term treatment of insomnia, without the potential harms of increased sedation, falls with/without fractures, ADL impairment, cognitive impairment, and delirium [9, 10]. We believe that CBTi should be the first-line treatment for chronic insomnia, reserving the judicious use of medications for severe or refractory cases.

Melatonin and melatonin analogues (ramelteon, tasimelteon) are generally well-tolerated medications with few side effects, no abuse potential, and no residual hypnotic effects or impaired cognition. However, their efficacy is limited to sleep-onset insomnia and their effect strength is mild [11]. These agents may be an adjunct to behavioral modifications in patients with mild sleep-onset insomnia and contraindications to alternative agents described below.

The goal of sedative hypnotics in insomnia is to accelerate sleep onset and maintain sleep architecture (increase deep sleep periods and reduce nocturnal awakenings) while minimizing residual hypnotic effects during daytime. It was previously believed that the use of short-acting benzodiazepines was safer than longer-acting versions. However, studies have shown the risk of falls or other adverse events is unaffected by drug half-life [12]. Certain short-acting benzodiazepines, such as diazepam, are converted to active metabolites, the effects of which may persist longer in older patients. These medications also have increased habit-forming potential, though may have reduced residual cognitive impairment in older patients. Nevertheless, many older adults have developed a dependence on this class of medications for treatment of chronic insomnia and tapering or discontinuing use is often challenging. We recommend collaborative discussions with patients and attempt slow tapers off these medications; patient education materials such as brochures and pamphlets can also improve collaboration.

Sedating antidepressants such as trazodone or amitriptyline in the treatment for insomnia are off-label uses of these medications and are generally not recommended by the American Academy of Sleep Medicine. As previously stated, tricyclic antidepressants should be avoided in the geriatric population due to their anticholinergic activity. Low-dose trazodone, doxepin, or ramelteon is recommended by the AGS in the 2015 edition of the Beers criteria as an alternative to benzodiazepines and non-benzodiazepine receptor agonists (NBRAs). Mirtazapine in low doses is another alternative but should be used with caution in the elderly. Providers should check sodium levels when initiating or increasing mirtazapine as it can cause syndrome of inappropriate antidiuretic hormone (SIADH) [13].

There is conflicting data on the safety and efficacy of non-benzodiazepine receptor agonists (NBRAs) in older adults. In studies examining nursing home resident hospitalizations for hip fractures, the use of NBRAs was associated with increased risk of injurious falls, particularly in patients with mild or moderate cognitive impairment and those requiring partial assistance with transfers [14]. Compared to benzodiazepines, however, the use of NBRAs results in reduced frequency and severity of adverse events in older adults. Among non-benzodiazepine hypnotics, eszopiclone appears to be safer than zolpidem with reduced risk of fall-related injuries, including traumatic brain injury and hip fracture [15]. Due to concern for residual elevated drug levels and impaired driving and memory function, the FDA lowered the initial dose of zolpidem to 5 mg nightly in women in 2013. In 2014, the FDA recommended starting eszopiclone at 1 mg nightly, increasing to no more than 2 mg nightly in patients who drive or require mental alertness the following day. Regardless of the agent selected, initiation of these medications should start at the lowest possible dose and increased with caution.

Case Vignette

A 60-year-old Caucasian male with 12 years of education is admitted to an inpatient unit following several days of rectal bleeding. The patient's medical history is complicated by several years of untreated HIV. Labs indicate his CD4 count is below 35. Upon admission, the patient was alert and oriented to person, place, time, and situation. On his second night in the hospital, the patient reported problems with falling asleep and was given zolpidem to address his insomnia. The following morning he was found to be disoriented, confused, and highly distractible. A brief cognitive screen was completed using the MoCA and the patient's performance scored in the impaired range (MoCA = 15). The patient was closely monitored for 24 h and zolpidem was discontinued. The next day the patient's alertness improved and he was again fully oriented. A follow-up cognitive screen was performed and the patient's score had returned to within normal limits (MoCA = 28).

Anticholinergics

Acetylcholine is a neurotransmitter with myriad functions in the human body. It acts in the peripheral nervous system on motor neurons enabling movement of muscles. It is also found throughout the central nervous system where it is involved in functions such as arousal, learning, and memory. Numerous medications act directly and indirectly on acetylcholine pathways. Anticholinergics are a group of medications which block acetylcholine from binding its receptors. Antagonism of acetylcholine's effects can treat many common conditions such as mood disorders, motion sickness, asthma, urinary incontinence, and irritable bowel syndrome.

Common medications with anticholinergic properties	
Generic name	Brand name
Alprazolam	Xanax™
Diphenhydramine	Benadryl™
Benztropine	Cogentin™
Amitriptyline	Elavil™
Paroxetine	Paxil™
Quetiapine	Seroquel™

While anticholinergic medications are effective for treatment of various disorders and symptoms as described above, they confer a high risk of side effects including dry mouth, constipation, and sedation. Additionally, many studies have found a positive association between anticholinergic medication use and cognitive impairment, including delirium [16]. This is of particular concern in the elderly population as anticholinergic effects may be more potent due to decreases in cholinergic neurons and hepatic metabolism, as well as increases in blood-brain permeability [17]. The prevalence of anticholinergic medication use in those 65 years and older has been shown to be greater than 20% [18]. Additionally, given their efficacy treating many common ailments, as well as their availability over the counter, patients may be taking more than one as part of their regimen. Studies have indicated that the cognitive impairment associated with anticholinergic medications may not be explicitly related to dosage of a single medication, but rather a cumulative effect of taking multiple medications with anticholinergic properties as well as the underlying risk factors associated with the patient.

Anticholinergic toxidrome symptoms	
Hot as hades	Fever
Blind as a bat	Blurred vision
Dry as a bone	Dry skin
Red as a beat	Flushing
Mad as a hatter	Delirium/psychosis

Several scales have been developed to aid in the identification of patients who may be at risk of adverse events related to anticholinergic medications. These scales often employ a scoring system that weigh the number and type of anticholinergic medications an individual is taking. For instance, the anticholinergic cognitive burden (ACB) scale, published in 2008, rates different anticholinergic medications on a scale from 1 (possible anticholinergic effects) to 3 (definite anticholinergic effects) [19]. A benefit of such scales is their emphasis on the need to assess the cumulative anticholinergic burden. Additionally, research has shown an association between higher scores on anticholinergic scales and serum anticholinergic activities assay (SAA) [20]. Higher SAA values have been identified in those with delirium. Limitations to current scales exist, however, including poor consensus across the various scales regarding burden value of different anticholinergic medications [21]. Furthermore, there are hundreds of medications with anticholinergic properties, and scales must be routinely updated to stay current.

Concern for anticholinergic effects on cognitive functioning is well acknowledged among prescribing providers [22]. However, there is much that remains to be understood about this class of medications including more extensive research regarding their longitudinal effects. Additionally, studies including comprehensive neuropsychological testing would further elucidate the impact on specific domains of cognitive functioning these medications have. Currently, most research on the cognitive effects of anticholinergic medications utilizes brief screeners (e.g., MMSE) to assess functioning. While these assessment tools are practical and commonly used across settings, they are limited in their ability to assess the breadth of potential cognitive problems. Impairments in processing speed, attention, or psychomotor functioning may not be well evaluated using such brief assessment tools, leaving patients with subtle deficits unnoticed.

Pain Medications

Pain management in older adults and adults with cognitive impairment is fraught as both pain medication and pain itself can affect cognition. Uncontrolled pain can worsen cognition and even contribute to delirium. Alternately, pain medications, particularly opiates and opioids, are associated with neurologic side effects and delirium in both the inpatient and outpatient settings. A classic example is meperidine which is inadvisable in the geriatric population due to its clear correlation with impaired cognition and contribution to delirium, primarily related to its neurotoxic metabolite [23]. Numerous formal and validated neuropsychological tests exist and can be utilized to measure the impact of new or existing pain medications on an individual's cognitive functioning.

Data is mixed about the effects of opioids on cognition and function in the general population. Studies indicate likely slower reactions times and impaired memory but possibly similar global cognitive functioning [24]. It is important to find the appropriate pain medication for each patient, as sedation, mental dullness, and poor concentration caused by opiates/opioids can be severely limiting for patients working or in settings requiring fast reaction times such as machine operating. Nonnarcotic pain medications such as acetaminophen and NSAIDs should be considered when appropriate due to their low risk for cognitive side effects.

Cognitive side effects are not limited solely to narcotic pain medications. Many treatments for neuropathic pain carry central nervous system side effects. Gabapentin and pregabalin can frequently cause drowsiness as well as emotional lability and altered thinking. Tricyclic antidepressants, as previously discussed, have definite links with cognitive impairment due to their anticholinergic activity. It is important to consider medical and psychiatric comorbidities and psychosocial factors when selecting an appropriate pharmacologic pain regimen, as these medications, when appropriately selected, can be helpful to improve pain and pain's own effects on cognition. In the elderly, consider starting with lower doses or the newer serotonin norepinephrine reuptake inhibitors that have less anticholinergic burden and carefully monitor response and tolerance.

Assessment of the whole patient when choosing a pain medication is crucial as cognitive effects can frequently be due to altered pharmacokinetics or drug interactions rather than just the typical side effect profile. Renal impairment can affect medication clearance and lead to pronounced cognitive side effects of medications such as tramadol, morphine, and gabapentin. Concomitant use of opioid pain medications with sleeping medications and/or muscle relaxants compounds the potential cognitive effect risk. An individual may tolerate one or both medication classes as monotherapy, but when combined, they may observe significant cognitive and functional impairment. Careful review of a patient's current medications to assess risk for interaction is again a key step in safe medication prescribing.

Case Vignette

A 92-year-old woman with end-stage renal disease, hypertension, insomnia, pain, history of stroke, and history of breast cancer is placed on hospice. Her current medications include atenolol, diphenhydramine, and hydrocodone/acetaminophen. Once placed on hospice, her hydrocodone/acetaminophen is changed to morphine as part of the hospice standard home care protocol. Following placement on hospice, family and caregivers note a significant decline in her cognitive abilities as well as increased agitation, paranoia, and sedation. They also describe development of involuntary muscle twitching.

There are several medication concerns here related to cognition, but the most concerning cause for her recent deterioration in mental status is likely the initiation of morphine. Morphine metabolites M3G and M6G can accumulate in renal impairment and contribute to CNS stimulation and respiratory depression, respectively. Symptoms can include behavioral excitation, hallucinations, somnolence, and myoclonus among others. It is important to note that the cognitive impact of pain medications can be both a direct effect and indirect if standard pharmacokinetics are altered and care should be taken to appropriately choose specific pain medications utilized.

Polypharmacy

As demonstrated by the introductory patient case, it is common to encounter patients taking numerous medications. This scenario is often defined by the term polypharmacy, though the word does not have a standard definition. Generally, the concept is defined as the use of multiple medications, whether appropriate or inappropriate. Polypharmacy is increasingly common with one study finding the overall use of prescription drugs among US adults increased from 51% to 59% from 1999–2000 to 2011–2012, with an increased prevalence from 8.2% to 15% of using five or more drugs, increasing correspondingly with age [25]. Numerous other publications corroborate these trends. While type of medication is certainly important in potential cause of altered cognition, the number of medications alone has been linked with adverse outcomes in elderly with and without dementia [26–28].

When determining the cause of a new complaint of memory impairment or change in cognition, a crucial first step is medication review. A useful medication review requires an accurate medication history or reconciliation. The Joint Commission found this to be such a vital component of healthcare that a medication reconciliation is part of their National Patient Safety Goals relating to the safe use of medications [29]. Multiple factors contribute to the critical importance of regular medication reconciliation including increasing availability of over the counter (OTC) medications, herbal products, cannabis, and vitamins, as well as the common scenario of multiple prescribing providers per patient with each focusing on one specialized area of care. Unintentionally, individuals can find themselves taking numerous medications and vitamins per day, unaware of potential interactions and side effects. Asking about alcohol use and illicit substances, including cannabis, is another often overlooked component of a thorough medication review. These substances can have significant detrimental effects on cognition and global functioning that can be further compounded by interactions with prescribed and OTC medications. Many medications strongly associated with cognitive adverse effects (e.g., anticholinergics, sleep aids, histamine blockers, ethanol, cannabis) are available without a prescription and taken by patients without ever telling their medical provider.

Resources are available to aid in identification and substitution of potentially inappropriate medications, particularly in the elderly population, and appropriate deprescribing should always be considered. Developed in 1991 by the American Geriatric Society and updated in 2011 and 2015, the Beers Criteria provides an informative list of potentially inappropriate medications in older adults. Organized by organ system and medication class, it provides concise guidance on what medications to avoid and its reasoning [13]. The STOPP (Screening Tool of Older Persons' potentially inappropriate Prescriptions) and START (Screening Tool to Alert doctors to Right Treatment) criteria are a useful pair of tools that not only help identify what medications are potentially inappropriate in the elderly (STOPP criteria) but provide recommendations on alternative therapies (START criteria). Additional tools include the Medication Appropriateness Index (MAI), Fit for the

Aged Criteria (FORTA), and Assess, Review, Minimize, Optimize, Reassess tool (ARMOR). Each is slightly different and providers can utilize whichever they find most effective in their practice setting. These tools can aid the process of medication deprescribing, a consideration that should be given to all patients but especially those of advanced age on numerous medications. Utilizing input from the patient, family and/or caregivers, and a multidisciplinary team including palliative care and pharmacy is highly valuable to determine which medications provide substantial benefit versus those that may not but contribute to medication burden and potentially adverse effects. A useful description including a decision algorithm has been published by Scott et al. [30].

Returning to Mr. Sandy

Mr. Sandy is an 81-year-old male presenting with concerns of slow and progressive memory decline over the past 12 months. His medical history includes several vascular problems, as well as rheumatoid arthritis, benign prostatic hypertrophy, gastroesophageal reflux disease, and depression. Mr. Sandy is currently prescribed lisinopril, carvedilol, atorvastatin, aspirin, sulfasalazine, prednisone, tamsulosin, omeprazole, ranitidine, and citalopram. His primary care provider is concerned about a possible Alzheimer's or vascular dementia given the patient's age and medical history. However, there is also concern that the patient's number of medications could be contributing to this change in cognitive functioning. Older age and declines in health status increase Mr. Sandy's vulnerability to potential iatrogenic effects of polypharmacy. Taking this into account, Mr. Sandy's PCP developed the following plan of care to address the problem.

Medication evaluation	Labs	Neuropsychological evaluation
Mr. Sandy's PCP worked with clinical pharmacy to adjust/discontinue medications to reduce potential effects on cognition • Patient successfully weaned off ranitidine without significant reflux symptoms • Prednisone reduced to 1 mg daily over the course of 6 months • Trazadone reduced to 25 mg at bedtime to decrease serotoninergic burden. Melatonin 3 mg added	Labs were ordered to assess alternative factors that can produce cognitive problems such as low B12 or thyroid problems In this case, Mr. Sandy's labs returned normal	Mr. Sandy was referred for a neuropsychological evaluation. Test results demonstrated impairments in attention and short-term memory. The patient and his wife were provided with recommendations to assist with memory problems. The patient was recommended to not drive given recent episodes of getting lost

After 12 months adhering to his new medication regimen, Mr. Sandy and his wife reported perceived improvements in cognitive functioning. The patient had reportedly been managing his activities of daily living with more success and no more episodes of getting lost occurred. Repeat neuropsychological testing revealed slight improvements in both attention and memory. While the patient's cognitive problems did not fully resolve following the change in medication regimen, it was evident that polypharmacy had been exacerbating these symptoms.

Chapter Review Questions

1. What are some of the risk factors associated with the likelihood of medications having an effect on cognition?
2. What are the benefits to a medication evaluating when a patient presents with memory complaints?
3. How might an integrated care approach benefit patients presenting with cognitive problems who are also medically complex (e.g., several medical problems, prescribed >5 medications)?
4. Why are cognitive screens, observation, or clinical interview not sufficient independently for a diagnosis of dementia?

References

1. Cordell CB, Borson S, Boustani M, Chodosh J, Reuben D, Verghese J. Alzheimer's Association recommendations for operationalizing the detection of cognitive impairment during the Medicare annual wellness visit in a primary care setting. Alzheimer's Demen. 2013;9:141–50.
2. Rossetti HC, Lacritz LH, Cullum CM, Weiner MF. Normative data for the Montreal Cognitive Assessment (MoCA) in a population-based sample. Neurology. 2011;77:1272–5.
3. McKeith IG, Dickson DW, Lowe J, et al. Consensus criteria of the third report of the DLB consortium. Diagnosis and management of dementia with Lewy bodies: third report of the DLB consortium. Neurology. 2005;65:1863.
4. Patel T, Slonim K, Lee L. Use of potentially inappropriate medications among ambulatory home-dwelling elderly patients with dementia: a review of the literature. Can Pharm J (Ott). 2017;150(3):169–83.
5. Kamble P, Chen H, Sherer JT, et al. Use of antipsychotics among elderly nursing home residents with dementia in the US: an analysis of National Survey Data. Drugs Aging. 2009;26(6):483–92.
6. Lenander C, Midlov P, Viberg N, et al. Use of antipsychotic drugs by elderly primary care patients and the effects of medication reviews: a cross-sectional study in Sweden. Drugs Real World Outcomes. 2017;4(3):159–65.

7. Shrank W, Pollinski J, Avorn J. Quality indicators for medication use in vulnerable elders. J Am Geriatr Soc. 2007;55:S373–82.
8. Livingston G, Kelly L, et al. Non-pharmacological interventions for agitation in dementia: systematic review of randomised controlled trials. BJ Psych. 2014;205:436–42.
9. Alessi C, Martin JL, Fiorentino L, et al. Cognitive behavioral therapy for insomnia in older veterans using nonclinician sleep coaches: randomized controlled trial. J Am Geriatr Soc. 2016;64(9):1830–8.
10. Huedo-Medina TB, Kirsch I, Middlemass J, et al. Effectiveness of non-benzodiazepine hypnotics in treatment of adult insomnia: meta-analysis of data submitted to the Food and Drug Administration. BMJ. 2012;345:e8343.
11. Kuriyama A, Honda M, Hayashino Y. Ramelteon for the treatment of insomnia in adults: a systematic review and meta-analysis. Sleep Med. 2014;15(4):385–92. (Epub 2014 Feb 8)
12. Pierfitte C, Macouillard G, Thicoipe M, Chaslerie A, Pehourcq F, Aissou M, et al. Benzodiazepines and hip fractures in elderly people: case-control study. BMJ. 2001; 322(7288):704–8.
13. American Geriatrics Society 2015 Beers Criteria Update Expert Panel. American Geriatrics Society 2015 Updated beers criteria for potentially inappropriate medication use in older adults. J Am Geriatr Soc. 2015;63(11):2227–46.
14. Berry SD, Lee Y, Cai S, Dore DD. Nonbenzodiazepine sleep medication use and hip fractures in nursing home residents. JAMA Intern Med. 2013;173(9):754–61.
15. Tom SE, Wickwire EM, Park Y, Albrecht JS. Nonbenzodiazepine sedative hypnotics and risk of fall-related injury. Sleep. 2016;39(5):1009–14.
16. Campbell N, Boustani M, Limbil T, Ott C, Fox C, Maidment I, Gulati R. The cognitive impact of anticholinergics: a clinical review. Clin Interv Aging. 2009;4:225–33.
17. Tune LE. Anticholinergic effects of medications in elderly patients. J Clin Psychiatry. 2001;62(21):11–4.
18. Sura S, Carnahan R, Chen H, Aparasu R. Prevalence and determinants of anticholinergic medication use in elderly dementia patients. Drugs Aging. 2013;30:837–44.
19. Boustani MA, Campbell NL, Munger S, Maidment I, Fox GC. Impact of anticholinergics on the aging brain: a review and practical application. Aging Health. 2008;4(3):311–20.
20. Carnahan RM, Lund BC, Perry PJ, Pollock BG, Culp KR. The anticholinergic drug scale as a measure of drug-related anticholinergic burden: associations with serum anticholinergic activity. J Clin Pharmacol. 2006;46:1481–6.
21. Lertxundi U, Domingo-Echaburu S, Hernandez R, Peral J, Medrano J. Expert-based drug lists to measure anticholinergic burden: similar names, different results. Psychogeriatrics. 2013;13(1):17–24.
22. Winterswyk A, Hammond J, Thomas H, Wetherbee L, Sordahl J (2017) Improving screening for cognitive disorders. Improvement project presentation at the Boise VA Grand Rounds
23. Kornitzer BS, Manace LC, Fischberg DJ, Leipzig RM. Prevalence of meperidine use in older surgical patients. Arch Surg. 2006;141:76–81.
24. Ersek M, Cherrier MM, Overman SS, Irving GA. The cognitive effects of opioids. Pain Manag Nurs. 2004;5(2):75–93.
25. Kantor ED, Rehm CD, Haas JS, Chan AT, Giovannucci EL. Trends in prescription drug use among adults in the United States from 1999–2012. JAMA. 2015;314(17):1818–31.
26. Allen ME, Yanchick VA, Cook JB, Foss S. Do drugs affect social behavior in the confused elderly? J Gerentol Nurs. 1990;16:34–9.
27. Larson EB, Kukull EA, Buchner D, Reifler BV. Adverse drug reactions associated with global cognitive impairment in elderly persons. Ann Intern Med. 1987;107:169–73.
28. Moore AR, O'Keefe TO. Drug-induced cognitive impairment in the elderly. Drugs Aging. 1999;15:15–28.
29. The Joint Commission (2015) National patient safety goals. http://www.jointcommission.org/assets/1/6/2015_NPSG_HAP.pdf
30. Scott IA, et al. Reducing inappropriate polypharmacy: the process of deprescribing. JAMA Intern Med. 2015;175(5):827–34.

Chapter 34
Effective Feedback Conversations

Karen Postal

How do you tell parents that their child has autism? How do you tell a 10-year-old boy that he has attention deficit hyperactivity disorder but in a way that doesn't lead him to give up on himself as a learner? How do you tell someone with early Alzheimer's dementia that he can't drive anymore unless he passes a driving test?

The latter conversation is particularly challenging, as one of the first brain functions destroyed by Alzheimer's dementia is the ability to keep track of how well the rest of the brain is working (anosognosia, or lack of awareness of deficit). Telling patients with early Alzheimer's disease they are no longer safe on the road usually doesn't work, because they literally can't know they are unsafe on the road. To make the feedback conversation even more complicated, adult children of early dementia patients often feel like they are taking away their parent's dignity when they agree to restrict driving, so their first response to clinician feedback about driving is often, "But Dad only drives in a 5 mile radius to and from the grocery store..."

Neuropsychologists diagnose the presence of brain disorders like Alzheimer's disease and autism or the effects of known brain disorders like stroke or traumatic brain injury. We therefore share a lot of difficult news. Those conversations are particularly challenging as our patients usually have limitations in their ability to understand and remember information, and their family members are often so worried and stressed by the effects of the illness that it is hard for them to process information.

While providing effective feedback is one of the most difficult things we do as neuropsychologists, we are of course not the only medical professionals who must share difficult news with complex patients and their worried families. Understanding how neuropsychologists provide feedback is therefore useful to those in other

K. Postal (✉)
Harvard Medical School, Cambridge, MA, USA

Independent Practice, Andover, MA, USA

K. M. Sanders (ed.), *Physician's Field Guide to Neuropsychology*,
https://doi.org/10.1007/978-1-4939-8722-1_34

medical specialties who treat patients with central nervous system conditions. Why not share effective techniques across specialties to improve patient conversations in a way that not only delivers the message but also improves lives?

Why Learn to Have Effective Feedback Conversations with Patients?

Cultural shifts in healthcare have changed expectations for communication between doctors of all specialties and their patients. Patients now expect to have doctors fully explain their conditions to them. Happily, communicating effectively with patients doesn't just improve satisfaction with the medical encounter. This is not a fluffy "add on" to improve quality measures. The shift toward greater patient-doctor collaboration has been shown to produce better medical outcomes, even with complex, neurologically compromised patients [1]. For example, Phillip Pegg and his team from the Virginia Commonwealth University found direct communication of health information to cognitively impaired patients significantly improved treatment outcomes, including effort in therapy and gains in functional independence. This is an important finding. It tells us that (1) we should not assume that neurologically compromised patients couldn't understand or benefit from our direct feedback about their condition and (2) feedback conversations are not about treatment, they are part of treatment.

How Can We Learn to Have Effective, Memorable Feedback Conversations?

Historically, most graduate training in neuropsychology did not offer courses or explicit instruction on how to give feedback to patients and families. And remarkably, as the field of neuropsychology's focus has shifted to identification of ever more complex cognitive processes, there has been almost no parallel literature describing techniques for communicating the complex information. A large number of clinicians have therefore learned how to have effective feedback conversations "on the job," through watching mentors, or most typically, through trial and error. A clinician might try out a metaphor or analogy. Should patients and family members begin to smile, nod, and "light up," those analogies and metaphors are "filed" as useful feedback approaches. If the metaphor or analogy results in a patient glazing over, the approach would likely not be used again.

To address the question of how we can most effectively engage with patients in feedback conversations, my collaborator Kira Armstrong and I have conducted in-depth interviews with neuropsychologists from all over the country: training directors, members of tertiary medical teams, and private practitioners. We asked seasoned neuropsychologists to share their most effective metaphors, stories, and analogies: the literal words that facilitate "ah-ha! moments" when explaining particular disorders of the central nervous system or addressing tough issues such as driving. Like receiving the best feedback training from 100 different mentors, we gathered compelling, accessible strategies for explaining complex neuropsychological concepts. We also opened up an online data collection tool, inviting clinicians in several national neuropsychological organizations to share their favorite analogies, stories, metaphors, and feedback strategies with the idea of casting the widest possible net. This chapter shares some of the effective strategies gathered from the 3-year research project and compiled in the book *Feedback That Sticks; the Art of Effectively Communicating Neuropsychological Assessment Result*s [2].

What Are the Goals of an Effective Feedback Conversation?

Educate

Feedback sessions are not only about sharing a diagnosis with patients. In many cases, such as stroke or traumatic brain injury, the diagnosis is already known by the time patients come to our office. However, many patients have never had the opportunity to hear in detail what happened to their brain following their stroke or what the expected recovery course will look like for them following a traumatic brain injury. An effective feedback session therefore is an opportunity to educate patients and family members about their diagnosis and expected prognosis.

Of course, effective education must begin with the unique set of thinking, emotional, and cultural contexts patients bring to our examining rooms. The brothers Chip and Dan Heath, one a professor of organizational behavior at Stanford Graduate School of Business and the other an educator, bring a novel perspective to the topic of pitching our message in a manner that our listeners can understand in their compelling book, *Made to Stick: Why Some Ideas Survive and Others Die* [3]. The Heath brothers note that as professionals, we use jargon so frequently and are so familiar with the basic assumptions of our field that it is easy to forget that others have never heard our basic assumptions and cannot understand our jargon. Patients can't understand our messages because they do not understand our jargon and have never heard our basic assumptions. The Heaths refer to this as "the curse of knowledge."

Here is a very common example. While it is obvious to clinicians working in the field that thinking problems caused by a stroke or a head trauma are static or improve over time, while thinking problems associated with Alzheimer's disease get worse, many of our patients do not have this basic understanding. This "curse of knowledge" may prevent us from sharing critical information with families. We might not realize that a family is leaving our office assuming that their mother's mild stroke-related thinking problems will eventually progress to the point that she is demented like her brother who suffers from Alzheimer's dementia.

Create a Therapeutic Interaction

Seasoned clinicians frequently stop talking after providing information and invite patients and family members to share their emotional response by saying something as simple as "This is sad" or "This is hard." Effective feedback conversations may become (in some cases unique) opportunities for patients and families to enter into a discussion about their emotional experiences associated with the medical condition. For example, parents of children with developmental disorders may have spent years reassuring their child, family, neighbors, and school professionals that "everything is going to be fine. We can handle this." And while that may be true, a mother or father may have literally had no place in their lives where they can express grief for the loss of the childhood they thought their daughter would enjoy or the loss of the parenting experience they expected.

Similarly, in the weeks and months following a severe traumatic brain injury or a catastrophic injury or illness, a husband may have focused on the miracle that his spouse of 50 years survived, but never have had the opportunity to grieve the profound personality changes or thinking abilities in his loved one. As clinicians, we can give permission to patients and family members to express vulnerabilities, to grieve, to ask questions, to cry, and to consider their own needs. This is often done with a very simple question, "How is this for you?"

Create Change in a Larger System

Feedback conversations often include members of patients' extended families. With permission, school administrators, work supervisors, and other treating clinicians can join the conversation in person or via speakerphone. Feedback conversations become feedback loops where additional perspectives of various stakeholders in patients' lives can feed back information about symptoms and day-to-day difficulties that need to be addressed in order to refine treatment plans. In turn, the more stakeholders in patients' lives who directly hear about their condition and recommendation, the higher the likelihood something positive will emerge from the patient encounter.

Sharing Test Scores

For seasoned clinicians, communication of specific test scores from neuropsychological measures is typically far down on the list of goals for feedback conversations. Feedback conversations can become bogged down in numbers that mean little to individuals not trained in psychometric theory. A focus on details may also obscure the broader message and lead listeners to feel lost in the conversation. Some clinicians therefore avoid discussing specific scores altogether or discuss a score only when sharing the score helps to meets a therapeutic goal. As an example of the latter, if a patient shares during the course of the assessment that she has felt stupid her entire life because of her problem with reading, a neuropsychologist might begin the feedback conversation by sharing a high IQ score (if it exists) before discussing the diagnosis of dyslexia.

Social Pragmatics of Feedback Conversations

While the words we use to communicate with patients are important, equally important are how the conversation is set up and how the words are delivered. Who is invited to participate in the feedback conversation? Does the conversation take place in person, over the phone, or in the hallway? What social pragmatics are used, such as tone of voice and body posture?

Hallway Feedback

While feedback conversations typically occur in our consulting rooms, a critical portion of the feedback conversation may occur after the formal feedback session is over. For example, while escorting the family back to the waiting room many clinicians slow their pace so they are walking next to a family member. This allows family members to ask questions or provide additional information they felt they could not in front of the patient. Clinicians might also repeat or rephrase key information in a way that applies specifically to a family member's care giving concerns.

Props

Props are powerful tools for feedback conversations. One of the most common props for clinicians working with patients affected by central nervous system disorders is the brain model, which can be used to orient patients to various systems of the brain as findings are described. Clinicians in tertiary care centers may additionally have access to dedicated brain imaging monitors in their offices. When communicating to young adults and adolescents, a tablet with a 3D interactive brain atlas allows clinicians to communicate in a format that is familiar and compelling.

Props can also facilitate feedback conversations with interdisciplinary and educational teams. Any clinician who has attended patient's school Individual Education Plan (IEP) meetings knows that the meetings often overfocus on scores and the neurological condition of the child is lost ("Hmmm… I see in the your report Sally had a standard score of 85 on the test, but we have a standard score of 90…").

A highly effective technique to lead the team conversation toward the child's brain function is to bring a "brain in a bag." A classic brain model can be pulled out as soon as one is invited to present ones "report."

> I brought this so we can talk about what's happening in Sally's brain. (Holds up model) Here are the eyes, and this part of the brain is the frontal lobe. This is the part of the brain that brings us all of the functions we value in successful students: the ability to focus and concentrate, resist distracters, the ability to drag one's attention from the most interesting thing in the room towards work on has to do, manage time, and set goals. It's also involved in regulating mood and handling frustration. What happened with Sally's severe TBI a few months ago, is that this part of the brain stopped working as well as it used to for Sally. This is one reason that Sally is so distractible in math class. She can focus in art class really well because to her, art is the most interesting thing in the room, but in math, her frontal system isn't working well to keep her focused. It also speaks to why she is blowing up with temper so often. Let's talk about some strategies to help her frontal system do its job more efficiently.

Specific Social Pragmatics

A man is asking another man in a bar to go outside. Depending on his body language and tone of voice, the same words might mean "let's fight" or "let's leave for some air." How something is said is often as important as the words that are used when communicating with patients and their families. While clinicians might simply use the tone of voice and body language patterns they are comfortable with in day-to-day life, or what was modeled by their mentors during residency, seasoned clinicians will often intentionally regulate their use of social pragmatics as a clinical tool: titrating their degree of eye contact, choosing specific social greetings, and modulating their tone of voice to achieve specific goals. The following are some examples of conscious use of social pragmatics to further clinical goals during feedback conversations.

Greetings as Stealth Reorientations

Severely impaired memory scores forewarn us that a patient is unlikely to remember our name or even who we are to them in a broad sense. In those cases, a "reintroduction" is critical at the beginning of a feedback conversation to avoid our patients' attention becoming entirely focused on trying to figure out who we are and why she is sitting in the room with us. If a patient has just been cued by her son ["Mom, this is Dr. Postal,"] prior to sitting down in the exam room, a formal introduction, "Mrs. Peterson, I'm Dr. Postal," might be insulting or a sign that I do not recall meeting her. The dilemma can be solved by offering a brief pronouncement of one's name along with a handshake, "Dr. Postal." This quick reference to one's name might be followed by a reorientation to the situation disguised as pleasantries, "It was so nice meeting you last week. I was impressed by how patient you were with all of that memory testing we did together! Not every patient is. Wow- after three hours of testing your memory, and attention, and language, and mood, you still were a great sport. Thank you!" Now everyone is on the same page and no feelings have been hurt.

Self-Disclosure

Are we going to include personal anecdotes in our feedback conversations or be a blank screen upon which our patients project? Some clinicians are more comfortable with self-disclosure than others. Those that use self-disclosure in specific circumstances point out that it can help clinicians to connect with a patient or family in ways that may not otherwise be available. Using self-disclosure with somatoform patients is a good example.

Feedback conversations with a person who has a somatoform disorder can be like walking through a minefield. Often "good news" that test results are normal is experienced by the patient as "bad news." A patient may feel that we do not understand him or think he is crazy. As appropriate, self-disclosure of our own tendency to somaticize can be a powerful message communicating that (1) it is normal to experience stress in one's body and (2) the experience of physical symptoms can be a cue to engage in stress reduction rather than in medical procedures. Here is an example of how a clinician might share a personal experience with a somatoform patient.

> You know, I get migraines, and the first thing that I think when one hits me is "Oh! I must be stressed out!" On an everyday basis, I am not the type of person who is good at keeping track of how stressed I am. I tend to be good at ignoring my stress so I can get the stuff done that I need to get done. Of course, the more stressed I get, the more tension I hold in my muscles. I know the stress eventually triggers my migraines. Now I see a migraine as a red flag for me to think, "OK, my body is telling me I am stressed." I need to add an extra yoga class or go on another run this week.

Finding Open Channels of Communication

While clearly beneficial, communicating complex neuropsychological assessment results to patients who are cognitively impaired is a significant challenge. Having just completed a measurement of each thinking system in a patient's brain lends neuropsychologists a considerable advantage in understanding what information from the feedback conversation the patient will literally be able to hear, understand, and recall. For example, handing a dyslexic patient a brochure to read about her condition would be an obviously ineffective communication channel. Similarly, speaking slowly and, in short, grammatically simple sentences increases the likelihood that a mildly aphasic patient will understand the message. Doing so also provides a model of effective communication for family members in the room. Likewise, repeating key points several times and handing a patient a sheet with a few bullet points to take home increase the likelihood that a patient with a memory problem will retain the message.

Feedback Conversations in Our Diverse Medical Context

The days when a clinician from a specific cultural, linguistic, economic, and religious background treats only patients from the same cultural, linguistic, economic, and religious background are rapidly disappearing. The most effective feedback conversations occur in the context of a clear understanding of the differences between the cultural assumptions of the clinician and those of the patient and family. Sometimes it is clear that the clinician and patient come from different backgrounds, such as when they speak different languages. At other times, the underlying differences are not as obvious but may have similar effects of creating a barrier to effective communication. Different socioeconomic status or religious backgrounds are examples that may be harder for clinicians to initially detect. Because it is impossible to become fully "fluent" in the multiple cultures of our diversifying society, acknowledging one's limitations can be a useful way to facilitate trust and further support the feedback process.

> We don't need to walk into feedback sessions with complete a priori awareness of the cultural implications of our message: that would be impossible. Neuropsychologists are best able to pitch their message when they are open to engaging in a dialogue and asking questions about their patients' culture; it's important for someone from a different background to be ok with not knowing everything. So even if I suspect I know a different culture well, it's important to give the patient a chance to tell me. I will invite them to do so by directly asking, "How's this in your culture." Or "From your background, how do you deal with this?" When I am on their turf, I find out about their turf.—Tony Wong, Ph.D [4].

A Caution When Using Translators during Feedback Conversations

First generation immigrants may take their children to medical visits to translate. In this context, a child might walk into a feedback session ready to help his parents understand the findings. A professional translator or another adult family member is preferable as the content of the feedback session may be inappropriate for a child. It is important to clarify prior to scheduling a feedback session who will translate.

Six Principles of Effective Feedback Conversations

In their book, *Made to Stick*, the Heath brothers note that messages that are unexpected, emotional, simple, come from a credible source, trigger emotions, include stories, and are concrete tend to stick with people. As we interviewed neuropsychologists for our research about their stories, metaphors, and communication strategies, we recognized many of these principals at work. Each principal will be illustrated below with an example of a compelling feedback message useful for communicating with patients who have disorders of the central nervous system.

Unexpected

Using an unexpected or surprising metaphor or analogy grabs patients' attention. We know from basic memory research that people are better able to attend to and recall information that is novel. Here is an unexpected metaphor used to explain thinking and motor recovery after a stroke.

> It's like you have 10 men carrying a heavy log. A couple of them get injured and leave. Then you have eight men left carrying the log. At first it's hard, but eventually they get stronger and stronger and then they can carry the log. But sometimes, you get a situation in which eight of the ten men get injured and leave. Then you only have two men carrying the log. Then it takes a long time. They will eventually get stronger. As long as there are some men there, you can eventually improve. But for the duration, even when the men get as strong as they can, the log is carried more slowly. There are only two men carrying that log. And of course, in the situation in which all the men get injured - there are no men left to carry the log. In those situations, function is not going to return.—Yana Suchy, Ph.D. [5].

Emotions

Similarly, people are much better able to pay attention to and recall information that is emotional. Including an emotionally laden metaphor, story, or analogy is an effective way to ensure that the feedback message is remembered.

Most clinicians have had the experience of patients expressing that they feel more comfortable with herbal remedies than FDA-regulated medications. Here is an effective, highly emotional method of communicating the concept that just because a medication is natural, doesn't mean it is safe.

> Just because a product is "natural" doesn't mean it is safe. After all, rattlesnake toxin is "natural" too.—Kira Armstrong, Ph.D. [6]

Credibility

Establishing credibility is an important step in helping patients and families listen to the complex messages we are presenting. Sometimes, it is others in the specific disorder community that have the most credibility in the eyes of our patients. This is why patients may become convinced of a medical "fact" through a single testimonial on the internet. Communicating the message through positive experiences of other patients is therefore a powerful way to use the tool of credibility in feedback conversations. Here is an example of framing a recommendation to enter psychotherapy for a teenage girl following neurosurgery. Convincing a teenager to begin psychotherapy is always difficult; convincing a teenager who already feels different due to a seizure disorder is often particularly challenging.

> You know, I just saw a 17 year old who had the same surgery you had about a year and a half ago (temporal lobe resection). She had gotten really depressed and she went to see a psychotherapist. It was really helpful to her. She was having some trouble with her parents because they were so over protective. The therapist helped her figure out how to be more independent, how to talk to her parents about this.—Hillary Shurtleff, Ph.D. [7].

Stories

How do we communicate critical information about prognosis with families whose loved one had a severe traumatic brain injury without crushing their sense of hope? Too much focus on the typical deficit picture results in patients and families feeling hopeless. Alternatively, too much focus on positive exceptions to the rule interferes with families' ability to appropriately plan and manage their expectations. Storytelling is a unique tool that allows patients and families to imagine nuanced information in a manner that is impossible when using statistics or outcome data.

> When Dr. Joe Ricker discusses the prognosis of recently severely brain damaged individuals, he will often share the story of a teen he worked with whose clinical picture was initially so hopeless that he was almost placed in a nursing home. The teen is now in college and is doing well with the help of considerable accommodations. When told in all of its detail, it includes information that he was being assessed at the bedside for a neurovegetative state when someone noticed a slight response. The punch line of the story, "Everyone thought he would be in a nursing home, now he's a senior in college," helps families to identify and access two important threads at the same time: (1) there *is* hope for amazing gains, well beyond what we predicted; and (2) *but* he still has deficits.

Simplicity

Patients and family members can become anxious in feedback conversations when overloaded with too much information. They may have trouble processing multiple points given the newness or emotional nature of the feedback message. To avoid this seasoned clinicians often chose to present families with only 2–3 points, especially when giving difficult news.

> I know what those points are before I go in. I tell them within the first 10 minutes, and then spend the rest of the hour dealing with it.—E. Mark Mahone [8].

Concrete

Messages that address concrete, everyday concerns rather than abstract, theoretical issues are often better understood and remembered. Concrete messages have the added benefit of allowing clinicians to skip arguments with patients who are neurologically unaware (anosognosic) of their deficits. Rather than attempt to convince patients they are unable to drive, for example, clinicians might focus on legal consequences of driving without a document from a driving test showing they are safe on the road now that they have a medical condition that affects their brain.

So how do you tell a man with early Alzheimer disease he can't drive unless he passes a driving test? Concrete works beautifully.

> Mr. Smith, everyone in this country sues everyone else. If you get into a car accident, even if it's not your fault, and the other person gets the feeling you might have a memory problem because you are asking the same questions a lot at the accident scene, they could sue you. Once they see from your medical records that you have a brain condition like

Alzheimer's and don't have a driving test proving you are safe on the road, they would win that lawsuit. You could lose everything you've ever worked for. Everyone sues everyone else in this country. You've got to get a driving test to protect yourself and your family financially, and repeat it every 6 months.

When I use that particular feedback strategy with my Alzheimer patients, the first thing adult children say (rather than hedge that Dad only drives to the grocery store and back) is "Where do we get the driving test?"

It is all about how we deliver the feedback. And as clinicians in any medical specialty, it is up to us to devise understandable, memorable feedback strategies so our messages stick.

Chapter Review Questions

1. The shift toward greater patient-doctor collaboration has been shown to:
   A. Produce better medical outcomes with non-complex cases.
   B. Produce better medical outcomes even with complex, neurologically compromised patients.
   C. Have no effect on medical outcomes.
2. Patients often can't understand our messages because:
   A. They are not as educated as doctors.
   B. They do not understand our jargon and have never heard our basic assumptions.
   C. People with neurological disorders cannot truly understand their own medical issues.
3. The most effective feedback conversations occur:
   A. In the context of a clear understanding of the differences between the cultural assumptions of the clinician and those of the patient and family.
   B. Only between clinicians and patients with the same cultural backgrounds.
   C. Only between clinicians and patients of different cultural backgrounds.
4. Establishing credibility:
   A. Isn't a factor in good feedback to patients.
   B. Is out of our hands as clinicians.
   C. Is an important step in helping patients and families listen to the complex messages we are presenting.

References

1. Pegg O, et al. The impact of patient-centered information on patients' treatment satisfaction and outcomes in traumatic brain injury research. Rehabil Psychol. 2005;50(4):366–74.
2. Postal K, Armstrong K. Feedback that sticks: the art of effectively communicating neuropsychological assessment results. New York: Oxford University Press; 2013.
3. Heath C, Heath D. Made to Stick: Why Some Ideas Survive and Others Die. New York: Random House; 2007.
4. Scharre DW, Chang SI, Murden RA, et al. Self-administered Gerocognitive Examination (SAGE): a brief cognitive assessment Instrument for mild cognitive impairment (MCI) and early dementia. Alzheimer Dis Assoc Disord. 2010;24(1):64–71.
5. Ibid, p. 110.
6. Ibid, p. 130.
7. Ibid, p. 21.
8. Ibid, p. 18.

Answers for Chapter Review Questions

Chapter 1: Braun	(1B, 2C, 3D)
Chapter 2: Queally	(See text for answers*)
Chapter 3: Lanca	(1A, 2False, 3False, 4True, 5C)
Chapter 4: Schoenberg	(1A, 2B, 3D)
Chapter 5: Gerstle	(1A, 2D, 3D, 4D, 5C, 6D, 7A, 8D, 9C)
Chapter 6: Lebby	(1A, 2C, 3B, 4D, 5B)
Chapter 7: Davis	(1True, 2True, 3False: Although the American Academy of Pediatrics does recommend screening for ASD when the child exhibits delays, these children who are found to be at risk should then be referred for more extensive assessments by clinicians with experience in diagnosing autism, 4 There is no prototypical profile as children with ASD present with a broad phenotype. Language and intellectual impairments are the most common findings, but not all children with ASD exhibit this, particularly higher functioning children, 5A, 6C, 7B, 8D)
Chapter 8: Janzen	(1A, 2D, 3B, 4C)
Chapter 9: Westmacott	(1A, 2C, 3C, 4B)
Chapter 10: Williams	(1F, 2False, 3C)
Chapter 11: Warner	(1F, 2E, 3F, 4H)
Chapter 12: Trittschuh	(1B, 2B & C, 3D, 4A, 5C)
Chapter 13: Fung	(1D, 2C, 3B, 4True, 5B, 6A)
Chapter 14: Phillips-Sobal	(1D, 2E, 3D)
Chapter 15: Woolley	(1C, 2A, 3B, 4A, 5C)
Chapter 16: Goldstein	(1D, 2 see text, 3B, 4 see text, 5 see text)
Chapter 17: Sanders	(1True, 2E, 3False, 4B)

K. M. Sanders (ed.), *Physician's Field Guide to Neuropsychology*,
https://doi.org/10.1007/978-1-4939-8722-1

Chapter 18: Kubu (1C: As noted above, PD is a multisystem disorder that includes a spectrum of cognitive symptoms. The early cognitive symptoms of PD include evidence of slowed processing speed and executive cognitive deficits. Somewhat later in the course, visuospatial or visuoconstructional impairments become apparent followed by more frank memory impairments and dementia,
2E: All the above neurobehavioral symptoms can be seen in the context of PD. This highlights (once again) the fact that PD is a multisystem disorder that can present with a host of neurobehavioral symptoms, either due to the underlying pathophysiology of the disease or as a consequence of treatment side effects (e.g., dopamine dysregulation syndrome),
3A: Determination regarding candidacy for DBS is a team decision that includes input from neuropsychology, neurology, neurosurgery, and other team members. It involves a deliberative process in which all team members are provided with the relevant information from the various pre-operative consultations, and the team, as a whole, comes to a consensus decision regarding treatment. The neuropsychological data are only one set of data that figure into determinations regarding candidacy)

Chapter 19: Sanders (1D, 2D, 3A, 4D, 5True, 6D, 7D)

Chapter 20: Coppel (1E, 2D, 3C)

Chapter 21: Parsons (1D, 2D, 3A)

Chapter 22: Brandling-Bennett (See text for answers*)

Chapter 23: Alschuler (1F, 2G, 3C, 4F)

Chapter 24: Marcopulos (See text for answers*)

Chapter 25: Bigler (1D, 2D)

Chapter 26: Backhaus (See text for answers*)

Chapter 27: Lanca (1False: AD/HD is classified as a neurodevelopmental disorder with symptom onset prior to age 12,
2True: They are (1) combined presentation, (2) predominantly inattentive presentation, and (3) predominantly hyperactive/impulsive presentation,
3False: The relationship between sleep and attention is bidirectional,
4True,

	5C: A thorough clinical interview is the gold standard for diagnosing AD/HD, but neuropsychological testing, review of collateral information (academic records, caregivers), and self-report measures can be used to support the diagnosis, rule out other causes, and develop a treatment plan, 6D: All of the above)
Chapter 28: Lanca	(1A, 2C, 3D)
Chapter 29: Marcopulos	(1True, 2False, 3True, 4True, 5True, 6False)
Chapter 30: Backhaus	(1C, 2A, 3B, 4C)
Chapter 31: Fraser	(1C, 2D, 3D)
Chapter 32: Warren	(1B, 2E, 3C, 4E)
Chapter 33: Sordahl	(See text for answers*)
Chapter 34: Postal	(1B, 2B, 3A, 4C)

*See text for answers—answers to questions in the body of the chapter

Glossary of Neuropsychological and Medical Terms

Abulia An abnormal lack of ability to act or to make decisions.

Agrammatism Speech is characterized by containing mainly content words, with a lack of function words. This is typically characteristic of non-fluent aphasia.

Akathisia A movement disorder characterized by feelings of motor restlessness and an urge to be in constant motion; muscular quivering.

Akinetic mutism Inability to move or speak due to frontal lobe impairment.

Alexithymia An inability to identify and express or describe a person's feelings.

Alpha-fetoprotein (AFP) A human protein encoded by the AFP gene, located on the q arm of chromosome 4 (4q25). AFP is a major plasma protein produced by the yolk sac and liver during fetal development. An AFP test is routinely conducted during the 14th to 22nd week of pregnancy to assess for genetic birth defects, such as Down syndrome.

Anosognosia An inability to recognize a defect or disorder that is clinically evident.

Antiepileptic drugs (AEDs) The category of medications available for the treatment of seizures in patients with epilepsy. Many AEDs are tried in combination. Additionally, many AEDs are given, usually in lower doses, to treat psychiatric conditions, such as depression and bipolar mood disorder.

Anti-thrombotic therapy Medication to reduce the formation of blood clots.

Apneic events Cessation of respiratory airflow.

Aprosodia An inability to produce rhythmic and intonational aspects of language.

Area of epileptogenesis An area of the brain that has changed in such a way, either due to developmental or acquired alterations in the brain, that causes the neurons in that area of the brain to fire in a hyper-synchronous manner, known as a seizure.

Arterial ischemic stroke A disruption of arterial blood supply to the brain, causing focal injury in a vascular territory.

K. M. Sanders (ed.), *Physician's Field Guide to Neuropsychology*,
https://doi.org/10.1007/978-1-4939-8722-1

Arterial stiffness A loss of elasticity of the arteries which decreases their ability to expand and take up blood ejected from the heart. Consequently, the heart needs to exert greater force, leading to eventual cardiac damage and increased systolic blood pressure. Risk factors are advanced age and vascular comorbidities including hypertension, diabetes mellitus, hypercholesterolemia, kidney disease, and smoking.

Augmentative communication Methods used to supplement or replace speech or writing for those with impairments in the production or comprehension of spoken or written language.

Basal ganglia A group of bilateral subcortical structures in the brain, closely interconnected with the thalamus and multiple cortical networks.

Behavior intervention plan (BIP) Developed from a functional behavioral analysis, a BIP defines problematic behaviors that the child is having in class, and then determines appropriate strategies and interventions that will be used by the school staff to diminish these behaviors in the classroom.

Botox Also called botulinum toxin type A; blocks nerve activity in the muscles and can be used to treat spasticity and dystonia.

Capgras syndrome A delusional condition that is characterized by the false belief that known individuals, including family or friends, have been replaced by doubles or impostors.

CAP scores A research measure used to estimate expected motor signs in HD to understand prodromal changes in cognition and behavior. The CAP score is based on group data and should not be used for individual diagnosis.

Cerebral perfusion pressure (CPP) The difference between the mean arterial pressure and intracranial pressure, and is a measure of the pressure most closely correlated with cerebral blood flow. The normal range for adults is 70 to 100 mmHg; CPP varies according to age of a child, although should be at least 40 to 60 mmHg.

Childhood stroke A stroke with onset between 1 month and 18 years of age.

Clot lysis A treatment in which a medicine is used to break down a blood clot.

Coagulation disorders Disruptions in the body's ability to control blood clotting.

Constraint therapy Also called constraint-induced movement therapy; a type of rehabilitation to improve arm/hand function following stroke by restricting the use of the unaffected limb.

Chelation therapy A medical procedure that involves the administration of chelating agents to remove heavy metals from the body. Chelation therapy was initially developed for toxic exposure to heavy metals, and research does not support its use for anything other than that. In more recent years, it has been a controversial therapy used to treat various psychiatric and neurological disorders, including Autism Spectrum Disorder. This therapy poses various inherent risks including death.

DAN (Defeat Autism Now) doctor Defeat Autism Now (DAN!) was a project of the Autism research institute, founded by Dr. Bernard Rimland in the 1960s. DAN! Doctors have been trained in the DAN! Protocol, which believes that autism is a biomedical disorder, but uses controversial treatment approaches that have not been supported by research.

De novo mutations A gene alteration that occurs for the first time in a family line as a result of a mutation in a germ cell (egg or sperm) of one of the parents or in the fertilized egg itself.

Dystonia A movement disorder characterized by involuntary muscle contractions and limb posturing, often due to damage or dysfunction of the basal ganglia and/or cerebellum.

Endothelium A thin layer of cells lining the interior of all blood vessels. The endothelium is critical for processes such as lipid transport, platelet adhesion and aggregation, regulation of vascular tone, and vascular smooth muscle proliferation.

Epilepsy A neurological disorder marked by the recurrence of seizures, which are associated with abnormal electrical activity in the brain.

Epicanthic folds Skin folds of the inner corner of the eye.

Extubation Removal of a breathing tube previously placed in the trachea, usually due to improved respiratory condition or transition to a tracheostomy.

Functional behavioral analysis (FBA) An assessment typically conducted by the school psychologist to ascertain the triggers resulting in behavioral problems that the child is exhibiting in the classroom and to determine the outcome or consequences that may be maintaining these behaviors.

Functional MRI (fMRI) An activation technique using noninvasive magnetic resonance imaging to measure differences in activation of blood oxygen levels in brain locations for a given task. Often this is done in a block design, with blocks of time of task (cognitive, motor, sensory) compared to a contrast. It can help define a region of interest prior to brain surgery for epilepsy.

Hemiparesis Weakness on one side of the body; also called hemiplegia.

Hydrocephalus Excessive accumulation of cerebrospinal fluid in the brain causing potentially harmful pressure on the brain tissue.

Hyperadrenergic Excessively adrenergic, relating to or denoting nerve cells in which epinephrine or similar substance acts as a neurotransmitter.

Hyperbaric medicine Hyperbaric medicine typically involves hyperbaric oxygen therapy. This is a controversial therapy in which the body is placed in an oxygen chamber where the atmospheric pressure is increased and controlled. It is believed to have a healing process in inhalation of 100% oxygen in the chamber and has some clinical utility in the treatment of decompression sickness, gas gangrene, and carbon monoxide poisoning. It is also being used to treat various neurological and psychiatric conditions, including Autism Spectrum Disorder. There is no research supporting the efficacy of this treatment in these populations.

Hypercarbia Abnormally high level of carbon dioxide in the arterial blood.

Hyperemesis gravidarum A complication during pregnancy characterized by severe nausea/vomiting, which can result in dehydration and weight loss.

Hypernatremia An elevated concentration of salt in the blood.

Hypovolemia A state of decreased blood volume.

Iatrogenic Unintentional outcome secondary to a treatment or procedure.

Intrauterine growth retardation A term used if there has been fetal growth restriction such that the fetus is unable to achieve its genetically determined potential size.

Inflammatory cytokines A group of polypeptides involved in inflammation, known as inflammatory mediators.

Intracarotid amobarbital procedure (IAP or Wada test) A suppression technique used to assess cerebral language lateralization and memory functions. It involves administration by a radiologist of sodium amobarbital through the internal carotid artery, resulting in transient suppression of cortical activity of the affected hemisphere, and testing by the neuropsychologist of language, motor and memory functions during the period of drug effect.

Intracranial pressure (ICP) The pressure inside the skull relating to the brain tissue and cerebrospinal fluid (CSF) with pressures varying by age. Approximate normal ranges are 1.5 to 6 mmHg for supine infants; 3 to 10 mmHg for supine children; and <10 to 15 mmHg for supine adults.

Intraventricular hemorrhage (IVH) Bleeding into the ventricles inside the brain. One characteristic of the immature brain is a weakness of the blood vessels next to the ventricles increasing susceptibility to rupture and bleed.

Intubation Insertion of a breathing tube into the trachea to protect the airway following trauma and for mechanical ventilation.

Kangaroo care Skin-to-skin contact between mother and infant.

Leukoaraiosis Attenuation of the cerebral white matter, associated with multiple ischemic lesions, but also occurs in Alzheimer's disease and in normal aging.

Leukomalacia Bad white matter referring to evidence of an earlier stroke.

Lyme disease therapy There is significant controversy in regard to treatment of Lyme disease with two opposing medical views. The Infectious Diseases Society of America (IDSA) believes that Lyme disease is "hard to catch and easy to cure," with a short course of antibiotics being the treatment of choice. This group denies the existence of chronic Lyme disease. The other camp, the International Lyme and Associated Diseases Society (ILADS) believes Lyme disease is difficult to diagnose and treat, and results in persistent infection in many patients. ILADS recommends individualized treatment based on severity of symptom presentation, presence of tick-borne coinfections, and patient response to treatment. ILADS doctors are likely to recommend more aggressive and longer antibiotic treatment protocols.

Medically intractable epilepsy Patients are considered to have medically intractable epilepsy when they have tried two different AEDs but those have failed to result in sufficient seizure freedom or have caused the patient intolerable side effects.

Myocarditis Inflammation of the heart muscle.

Neonatal stroke A stroke diagnosed in the acute neonatal period, usually due to focal seizures in the first 12–24 hours of life.

Neuroplasticity The ability of the brain to form and reorganize synaptic connections based on experience, learning, and/or injury.

Normocapnic Normal arterial carbon dioxide pressure, usually around 40 mmHg.

Normothermic Normal body temperature.

Pathophysiology of seizures The underlying physiological process that is associated with the seizures, such as a lesion in the brain or hippocampal sclerosis of the mesial temporal lobes.

Patent ductus arteriosus The ductus arteriosus is a hole that allows fetal blood to skip circulation to the lungs. However, when the baby is born, the blood must receive oxygen in the lungs and this hole is supposed to close. If the ductus arteriosus is still open (or patent), the blood may skip this necessary step of circulation. The open hole is called the patent ductus arteriosus.

Patent foramen ovale A flap in the heart that may allow a clot from the circulation to go to the brain and produce a stroke.

Penetrance A genetic term that addresses the rate of incidence of a trait or disease in individuals who carry the gene which causes the trait or disease to occur.

Periventricular leukomalacia (PVL) Injury to cerebral white matter that consists of periventricular focal necrosis in a characteristic distribution, with subsequent cystic formation or more diffuse cerebral white matter injury.

Presumed perinatal stroke A stroke that is presumed to have occurred in the perinatal period, but is not diagnosed until later in infancy or childhood when an emerging focal neurological deficit (usually hemiparesis between 4 and 6 months of age) prompts a brain MRI to be conducted.

Psychometrist A member of a neuropsychology team who administers and scores psychological and neuropsychological tests, working under the supervision of a licensed neuropsychologist.

Psychogenic nonepileptic seizures (PNES) Seizures that do not have correlated epileptogenic changes on EEG during the behavioral manifestation of the seizure. Common etiologies for PNES include past history of abuse, particularly, sexual abuse, and trauma.

Pseudobulbar affect A condition that is marked by episodes of uncontrolled crying or laughing which is inappropriate or of disproportionate intensity and is associated with various neurological disorders (such as multiple sclerosis, traumatic brain injury, and stroke).

Reduplicative paramnesia A belief that a person or location has been duplicated, either existing in two or more locations at the same time or that it has been relocated to a different place. A delusional misidentification syndrome, it is commonly associated with brain injury, in particular, simultaneous damage to the right cerebral hemisphere and both frontal lobes.

Retinopathy of prematurity A disorder that primarily affects premature infants, where abnormal blood vessels grow in the retina of the eye.

Secondary brain injury Damage caused by pathological changes to brain tissues, vascular integrity, or cerebrospinal fluid that evolve over time following the primary brain trauma. Examples of processes causing secondary brain injury include, but are not restricted to, bleeding, swelling (edema), disruption of neurotransmitter functioning or equilibrium, electrolyte disruption, or chemical cascade effects.

Seizure A sudden surge of electrical activity in the brain that may or may not affect a person's outward behavior. Veritable seizures can only be detected with electroencephalography (EEG) monitoring that captures that electrical activity at the time it is occurring.

Subependymal hemorrhage The most common type of intracranial hemorrhage in neonates, related to a perinatal stress affecting the highly vascularized subependymal germinal matrix.

Theory of mind A person's capacity to imagine or form opinions about the cognitive states of other people.

Thrombocytopenia When the blood has a lower than normal number of platelets. In a severe degree, it may lead to neonatal intracranial hemorrhage.

Ventriculomegaly Occurs when the ventricles in the brain are dilated. In fetuses, the most common definition uses a width of the atrium of the lateral ventricle greater than 10 millimeters in size.

Wallerian degeneration The process of degeneration of an axon distal to the site of injury.

Working memory The early laying down of new information/data. Small amounts of data that need further rehearsal to lay down in permanent memory. This is the first stage of eventual memory traces and one step beyond brief awareness or focus.

Index

A

Acalculia, 284
Acculturation, 482
Acetylcholinesterase inhibitors, 550
Acquired brain injury (ABI), 507
  depression, 507
  family/caregiver interventions, 522
Acute umbilical inflammation, 173
ADA Amendments Act of 2008 (ADAAA), 535
Adjudicative competence, 500
Adjuvant craniospinal radiation, 134
Adult ADHD
  academic accommodations, 472
  collaborative discussion, 470–472
  inattention and hyperactivity, 470
  inattention and impulsivity, 464
  neuropsychological
    academic achievement, 469
    attention and executive functioning, 469
    behavioral functioning, 470
    memory and learning, 469
    mood functioning, 470
    performance validity, 466
    perspective, 462–463
    premorbid functioning and IQ, 469
    test results, 466–468
    visual spatial functioning, 470
  psychiatric interview, 463–464
  study/homework strategies, 472
Adult daily living skills (ADLs), 285
Aggressive investment strategy, 498
Alexithymia, 545
Alpha-fetoprotein (AFP) test, 48
ALS Cognitive Behavioral Screen (ALS CBS), 256
Alzheimer's disease (AD), 223, 231, 239, 240, 249, 269, 273, 575
  cognitive aging, 416
  diagnosis, 416
  economic impact, 210
  examination, 213
  family history, 213
  labs and imaging, 213–214
  memory loss, 412
  neurodegenerative diseases, 209
  neuropsychological evaluation, 211
  past medical history, 212
  pathognomonic pathology, 210
  progressive dementia, 410
  risk factors, 211
  social history, 213
Amantadine, 442
American Academy of Clinical Neuropsychology, 52, 483
American Academy of Pediatrics, 176
American Academy of Sleep Medicine, 567
American Board of Clinical Neuropsychology (ABCN), 11
American Board of Pediatric Neuropsychology (ABPdN), 11
American Board of Professional Neuropsychology (ABN), 11
American Board of Professional Psychology (ABPP), 11
American Congress of Rehabilitation Medicine (ACRM), 514
American Heart Association/American Stroke Association (AHA/ASA), 270

K. M. Sanders (ed.), *Physician's Field Guide to Neuropsychology*,
https://doi.org/10.1007/978-1-4939-8722-1

American Psychological Association (APA), 11, 488
American Psychological Association Division of Neuropsychology, 10
Americans with Disabilities Act (ADA), 498, 535
Amitriptyline, 567
Amphetamines, 460
Amyloid plaques, 210
Amyotrophic lateral sclerosis (ALS)
  apathy, 258
  behavioral observations and mental status, 260
  clinical management, 255
  clinical recommendations, 262
  cognitive and behavioral syndromes, 255
  cognitive impairment, 256
  collaborative issues, 262–263
  depression, 258
  dysarthria, 257
  executive functioning, 261
  expressive language, 260
  frontotemporal syndromes, 257
  FTD, 255, 256
  identifying information and reason for referral, 258, 259
  language-based dementia, 257
  medical history, 259
  neuropsychological assessment, 257
  neuropsychologist perspective, 260
  numerical reasoning, 261
  orientation and memory, 260
  physician perspective, 259, 260
  psychiatric care prior, 256
  psychiatric presentation, 261
  receptive language, 261
  subsequent interventions, 262
  visuospatial reasoning, 261
ANAM Readiness Evaluation System (ARES), 54
Ankle-foot orthotics (AFOs), 102
Anosognosia, 282, 545, 575
Anterior cingulate cortex (ACC), 292, 314
Anticholinergic cognitive burden (ACB), 569
Anticholinergics, 412, 568–569
Antidepressants, 225
Antiepileptic drugs (AEDs), 380, 382, 384, 386
Antipsychotics, 564
Arterial ischemic stroke (AIS), 147
Arterial stiffness, 274
Assess, Review, Minimize, Optimize, Reassess tool (ARMOR), 572
Assistive technology (AT), 536, 537
Asthma, 459
Astrocytoma, 432
Atenolol, 570
Attention-deficit/hyperactivity disorder (ADHD), 34, 64, 68, 95, 116, 154, 159, 170, 549, 575
  amphetamines, 460
  anxiety and episodic depression, 459
  comorbidity, 457, 461
  diagnosis, 459, 460, 470
  disorganization, procrastination and forgetfulness, 458
  elevated substance, 460
  heterogeneous disorder, 457
  inattention, 457, 459
  learning disorders, 460, 461
  mood disorders, 459
  neurodevelopmental disorder, 462
  neuropsychological testing, 460
  prevalence, childhood, 457
  substance use disorder, 460
  See also Adult ADHD
Atypical parkinsonian syndromes, 248
Autism Diagnostic Interview, 120
Autism Diagnostic Observational Schedule, 120
Autism Diagnostic Observation Schedule-second edition (ADOS-2), 548
Autism spectrum disorder (ASD), 545
  anxiety disorder, 123
  Asperger's disorder and pervasive developmental disorder, 120–121
  attention and executive functioning deficits, 122
  cerebral dysfunction, 118
  communication and language deficits, 121
  early intervention (EI) services, 117
  genetic disorders, 115
  genetic testing, 116
  gross motor deficits, 122
  heterogeneous disorder, 121
  hyperintensities, 116
  Lyme disease, 126
  medical/genetic condition, 121
  neurology, 115
  neuropsychology, 118, 119
  pediatric, 126
  seizure disorders, 115
  social communication and interaction, 117
  social deficits, 121
  visual memory, 122
Autism Spectrum Rating Scales, 548
Automated Neuropsychological Assessment Metrics (ANAM), 54

B

Balint's syndrome, 230
Behavior Rating Inventory of Executive Functions (BRIEF-2), 548
Behavioral and psychological symptoms in dementia (BPSD), 565
Behavioral coping strategies, 517
Behavioral therapy (BT), 515
Benign prostatic hypertrophy, 572
Benzodiazepines, 92, 564, 567
Bilateral periventricular leukomalacia (PVL), 171
Bipolar disorder, 226
Blood oxygen level-dependent (BOLD), 430
Boston naming test (BNT), 482, 485
Botox injections, 149
Brain atrophy, 297, 298
Brain-behavior relationships, 547
Brain imaging, 149
Brain injury, 575
  behavioral therapy (BT), 515
  CBT (*see* Cognitive behavioral therapy (CBT))
  challenges, 509
  consequences, 508
  depression, 507
  emotional and behavioral challenges, 515
  family interventions
    coping styles, 521–522
    emotional functioning in caregivers, 520–521
    recommendations, future interventions, 523–524
    state of evidence, 522–523
  ISIG recommendations, cognitive rehabilitation, 516
  meningioma (*see* Meningioma)
  neuropsychological interventions
    cookie-cutter approach, 512
    premorbid personality and psychosocial characteristics, 509
    psychological interventions (individual and group), 515–519
    rehabilitation, 510, 511, 513, 514
    testing, 510–511
    treatment approaches, 509
  personality and emotional functioning, 507 (*see also* Traumatic brain injury (TBI))
Brain Injury-Interdisciplinary Special Interest Group (BI-ISIG), 514
Brain injury rehabilitation, 85

C

California Verbal Learning Test, 485
Canadian Psychological Association (CPA), 11
Canadian Stroke Network (CSN), 269
Cannabis, 564
Capgras syndrome, 546
Carotid Doppler, 280
Catastrophic injury, 578
Celiac disease, 226
Centers for Disease Control and Prevention, 169
Central nervous system (CNS), 34, 401
Cerebellum, 173
Cerebral cortex, 173
Cerebral perfusion pressure (CPP), 95
Cerebrospinal fluid (CSF), 134, 401, 422
Cerebrovascular accident (CVA), 67
Cerebrovascular disease, 273
Cervical spine injury, 330
Chemotherapy, 134
Chorionic vasculitis, 173
Chronic traumatic encephalopathy (CTE), 337
Civil capacity
  brain tumor, 498
  brokerage firm, 498
  clinical contexts, 497
  competency, 497
  consent, 497
  developmental disability, 497
  ecological validity, 497
  functional parameters, 499
  legal disputes, 499
  medical disorders, 497
  mild TBI, 498
  neuropsychological testing, 497
  timing, 498
Civil competency, 497
Civil law, 496
Clonazepam, 245, 565
Clozapine, 241, 251
Cognition
  acute and chronic disorders, 562
  anticholinergics, 568–569
  global functioning, 562
  health status, 563
  iatrogenic effects, 563
  medications, 562, 564
  memory problems, 563
  pain medications, 569–571
  polypharmacy, 571–573
  prescription medication, 563
  primary care providers, 562
  psychotropic medications, 564–566
  side effects, 564, 568, 570
  sleep medications, 566–568

Cognitive behavioral therapy (CBT), 78, 517
  coping strategies, 518
  efficacy, 518
  individuals with anxiety disorders, 519
  individuals with brain injury, 518
  mood and self-efficacy, 518
  motivational interviewing (MI) techniques, 519
  neuropsychological intervention, BI, 517
  PSE, 518, 519
  teaching caregivers information, 523
Cognitive-behavioral therapy for insomnia (CBTi), 566
Cognitive decline/dementia, 240
Cognitive deficits, 441
Cognitive empathy, 545
Cognitive impairment, 226
  chronic schizophrenia, 413
  hypertension and diabetes, 414
  schizophrenia-spectrum disorder, 409, 417
Cognitive rehabilitation, 282, 405, 514–515
Color Trails Test (CTT), 487
Commission on Rehabilitation Counselor Certification (CRCC), 531
Comorbidity, 461
Comorbid psychiatric disorders, 461
Competency to stand trial, 500–501
Comprehensive Assessment of Spoken Language (CASL-2), 548
Computed tomography (CT), 86, 421–423
Coping strategies, 511
Cortical-basal ganglionic degeneration (CBD), 239
Cortical brain dysfunction, 224
Cortical stimulation mapping, 190, 192, 194
Corticobasal syndrome (CBS), 235
Craniectomy, 95
Craniospinal radiation, 134, 136
Criminal cases
  assessments, 499, 500
  competency to stand trial, 500–501
  criminal responsibility, 502
  diligence and adherence, 500
  diminished capacity, 502
  disputed confession, 500
  forensic psychiatrists, 499
  insanity, 501
  malingering, 502–503
  neuropsychologist and physician, 499
Criminal law, 496
Criminal responsibility, 502
Cross-cultural validity, 486
Cultural variables, 480, 490
Culture-fair tests, 487
Curse of knowledge, 577
Cytosine-adenine-guanine (CAG), 310

D

DaTscan, 251
Daubert criteria, 500
Day-of-injury (DOI) CT scan, 425–428
Deep brain stimulation (DBS)
  anxiety, 298
  bilateral surgery, 298
  blood pressure, 298
  brain atrophy, 298
  cognitive and neurobehavioral function, 291
  dyskinesia, 300
  infection, 298
  interdisciplinary evaluation, 297
  lesion procedures, 291
  motor symptoms of PD, 291
  neuropsychiatric symptoms, 294
  neuropsychological evaluation, 299, 300
  neuropsychologists, 294
  non-motor symptoms, 292
  preoperative neuropsychological assessment, 294
Defendants, 501, 502
Dementia, 54, 294
  Alzheimer's disease, 410
  cognitive change, 410
  degenerative, 413
  neuropsychological testing, 416
  risk, 413
Dementia with Lewy bodies (DLB), 564
  anticholinesterase inhibitors, 241
  cognitive functioning, 245
  dopaminergic medications, 241
  mild bilateral action tremor, 246
  movement disorder specialists, 251
  neurobehavioral exam and behavioral observations, 248
  neurodegenerative syndromes, 245
  neuropsychological assessment (*see* Neuropsychology)
  neurotransmitters, 240
  non-dopaminergic medications, 241
  Parkinson's Plus disorders, 239
  pathology, 240
  PD, 239
  personality and emotional functioning, 247
  REM behavior disorder, 247
  test selection, 248
  typical/atypical neuroleptic, 248
  visual hallucinations, 240, 247

visuoconstructional tasks, 241
visuoperceptual processing, 252
Department of Defense (DoD), 54
Depression, 293, 507, 572
Diagnostic and Statistical Manual-IV (DSM-IV), 449
Diazepam, 566
Diffuse axonal injury (DAI), 426
Diffusion tensor imaging (DTI), 240, 423
Diminished capacity, 502
Diphenhydramine, 565, 570
Disease-modifying therapies (DMT), 405
Disputed confession, 500
Diversity, 480
Donepezil (Aricept), 550
Dopamine agonist, 555
Dopamine transporter scan (DaT scan), 241
Dorsolateral frontal issues, 314
Dorsolateral prefrontal cortex (DLPFC), 292
Drug-drug interaction, 565
Dyskinesias, 297, 300
Dyssomnias, 439
Dysthymia, 293

E

Eighth Joint National Committee (JNC-8), 273
Electromyography, 259
Eloquent cortex, 194, 199
Emergency department (ED), 83
Emotional and behavioral challenges, 520
Emotional and behavioral changes, 520
Emotional awareness, 545
Emotional communication, 545
Emotional dysregulation, 554
Emotional empathy, 545
Emotional functioning, 273
Emotional processing
awareness, 545
communication, 545
reflexive reactions, 544
regulation, 545
triggered responses, 544, 545
Emotional regulation, 545
Employment law applications, 498
Endocrine abnormalities, 439
Endothelial dysfunction, 274
Endotracheal tube (ETT), 96
Epilepsy
comprehensive neuropsychological evaluations, 380
etiologies, 380
heterogeneity, 379
medically intractable seizures (*see* Medically intractable seizures)
mesial temporal lobe (*see* Mesial temporal lobe epilepsy)
neurological diseases, 379
neurologist perspective, 380–381
neuropsychological evaluation, 388–392
neuropsychologist perspective, 381–383
recurrent seizures, 379
seizures (*see* Seizures)
syndromes, 379
Essential tremor (ET), 247
Ethnicity, 480
Evidence-based medicine (EBM), 282
Executive functioning (EF), 272, 316
abstract reasoning, 285
ADLs, 285
emotional regulation and synthesis, 286
frontal lobe issues, 286
multitasking, organization, planning, sequencing and problem-solving, 285
natural environment, 285
Expert testimony, 500

F

Fatigue, 438
Federal Aviation Agency, 54
Feedback conversations
cultural shifts, 576
education, 577
functional independence, 576
hallway, 579
metaphor/analogy, 576–577
online data collection tool, 577
patient-doctor collaboration, 576
patient's extended families, 578
principals
concrete, 584–585
credibility, 583–584
emotions, 583
simplicity, 584
stories, 584
unexpected, 583
props
central nervous system disorders, 579
interdisciplinary and educational teams, 579
social pragmatics, 580
sharing test scores, 578–579
stakeholders, 578
stealth reorientations, 580–582
therapeutic interaction, 578
Fit for the Aged Criteria (FORTA), 571–572

Fluid-attenuated inversion recovery (FLAIR), 269, 423
Fluid Reasoning Index, 123
Forced vital capacity (FVC), 259
Forensic psychiatry, 500, 502
Frontal Assessment Battery (FAB), 286
Frontal Systems Behavior Scale (FrSBe), 548
Frontotemporal dementia (FTD), 245, 247
Functional impairment, 281
Functional magnetic resonance imaging (fMRI), 52, 190–192, 194, 195, 201, 385
Functional neuroimaging, 430–433

G
Gabapentin, 570
Gastroesophageal reflux disease, 572
Generalized tonic-clonic (GTC) seizure, 383, 386
Genome-wide association studies (GWAS), 211
Geriatric Research Education and Clinical Center, 211
Gestational Lyme disease, 116
Glasgow Coma Scale (GCS), 95, 437
Globus pallidus internus (GPi), 291, 301
Gradient-recalled echo (GRE), 423

H
Headaches, 438
Hemicraniectomy, 95
Hemidystonia, 149
Hemiparesis/hemianopsia, 270
Hemorrhagic lesions, 427
HIPAA privacy rules, 489
Holistic day treatment program (DTP), 513
Holistic neuropsychologically oriented post-acute rehabilitation programs, 513
Huntington's disease (HD)
  autosomal dominant heredodegenerative disease, 308
  cognitive and psychiatric symptoms, 309, 321
  genetics, 309–319
  imaging, 310–311
  language functioning, 318
  memory deficit, 317
  motor abnormality in adult-onset, 309
  motor signs, 309
  motor symptoms, 306, 312, 319
  neurological evaluation, 306
  neurological exams and findings, 307–308
  neuropsychiatric symptoms, 309
  neuropsychological assessment, 306, 311
  neuropsychological testing
    cognitive screens, 312–314
    cognitive symptoms, 321
    complex attention, 314–315
    depression, 311
    evidence-based research, cognitive domain, 312
    executive functioning (EF), 311, 314–315
    functional domain, 312
    functional evaluation, 319
    general ability/cognitive reserve, 312–314
    medical treatment, 321
    psychological, 319
    treatment and recommendations, 320
    validity indicators, 319
  neuropsychology evaluations, 306
  neuropsychology research, 306
  obsessive-compulsive psychological symptoms, 312
  prodromal, 309, 311, 312, 314
  serial neuropsychological (NP), 305
  signs and symptoms, 310
  visuospatial functioning, 318–319
Hydrocodone/acetaminophen, 570
Hyperarousal, 554
Hypercarbia, 173
Hyperemesis gravidarum, 116
Hypervigilance, 554
Hypometabolism, 224
Hypopituitarism, 439
Hypothyroidism, 116
Hypovolemia, 173

I
Inattention, 457, 458, 469
Individual education plan (IEP), 74, 137, 138, 170, 579
Individuals with Disabilities Education Act (IDEA), 69
Inflammatory cytokines, 173
Insanity, 501
Insomnia, 566–568
Instrumental activities of daily living (IADLs), 53, 270
Intellectual functioning, 248, 445
Interdisciplinary collaboration, 504
Intracarotid amobarbital procedure (Wada test), 197

Intracranial pressure (ICP) monitoring, 95
Intraventricular hemorrhage (IVH), 173
Ischemic perinatal stroke (IPS), 150

K
Kaufman Brief Intelligence Scale, 2nd Edition (KBIT-2), 152
Kaufman Brief Intelligence Test (K-BIT), 200

L
Learning disorders, 34, 461
Lebby-Asbell Neurocognitive Screening Examination for Adolescents (LANSE-A), 103
Lebby-Asbell Neurocognitive Screening Examination for Children (LANSE-C), 103
Left mesial temporal lobe epilepsy
- AEDs, 386
- cognitive complaints, 387
- collaborative process, 395
- GTC seizure, 386
- impressions, 395
- neuropsychological evaluation, 386
- neuropsychological test results, 387, 392–394
- video-EEG monitoring, 386
- Wada test, 394

Leukoaraiosis, 269
Litigation, 496, 499
Lyme disease, 226

M
Magnetic resonance (MR), 423
Magnetic resonance imaging (MRI), 150, 421–423
Major depressive disorder (MDD), 550
Malingering, 502–503
Mayo's Older African Americans Normative Studies (MOANS), 486
Medial temporal lobes (MTL), 210, 216
Medical care, 490
Medical interpreters
- bilingual/bicultural neuropsychologist, 488
- college education and facility, 488
- cultural community, 489
- culturally diverse populations, 488
- examiner-patient relationship, 489
- formal translation procedures, 489
- hidden patient, 489
- neuropsychological assessment, 488
- out-group, 489
- positive triadic relationship, 489
- pressures and constraints, 489

Medically intractable epilepsy, 380
Medically intractable seizures
- focal epilepsy, 380
- mesial temporal lobe epilepsy (*see* Mesial temporal lobe epilepsy)
- scalp video-EEG monitoring, 380

Medically refractory seizures, 395
Medical management, 19, 21, 90, 95, 405
Medical professionals, 496, 575
Medical rehabilitation, 532, 543, 544, 550, 554
Medication Appropriateness Index (MAI), 571
Medication consultation, 78
Medulloblastoma, 134
Melatonin, 566
Memory Disorders Clinic, 212
Memory problems, 240
Meningioma
- cognitive deficits, 370, 374
- cognitive impairment, 374
- cognitive outcome, 372, 375
- cognitive symptoms, 363, 364, 366, 367, 369, 373–374
- decision-making process, 375
- medical comorbidities
  - neuropsychological evaluations, 364–365
  - neuropsychologist's perspective, 366
  - neurosurgeon's perspective, 365–366
- multiple sclerosis
  - follow-up, 372–373
  - neuropsychological evaluation, 370
  - neuropsychologist's perspective, 371–372
  - neurosurgeon's perspective, 372
- neuropsychology and neurosurgery, 374–375
- orbital groove
  - neuropsychologist's perspective, 369
  - neuropsychology follow-up, 368
  - neurosurgeon's perspective, 368–369
- radiation therapy, 367, 369

Mesial temporal lobe epilepsy
- AEDs, 384
- comprehensive neuropsychological evaluation, 385
- comprehensive presurgical evaluation, 385
- electrophysiological and neuroimaging findings, 385
- epileptogenic focus, 383
- fMRI, 385
- hippocampus, 383

Mesial temporal lobe epilepsy (*cont.*)
intracranial EEG monitoring, 384
medically intractable epilepsy, 385
memory tests, 385
mesial temporal sclerosis, 384
neuropsychological evaluations, 384
neurosurgical resection, anteromesial temporal structures, 384
status epilepticus, 383
Wada test, 385
Methylphenidate, 438, 442, 453, 555
Microvascular ischemic disease, 226
Middle cerebral artery (MCA), 427, 428
Mild cognitive impairment (MCI), 53, 54, 270
Mild traumatic brain injury (mTBI), 84, 496
Mini Mental Status Examination (MMSE), 14, 47, 268, 441, 563
Mirtazapine, 567
Modified Assessment for Cognitive Functioning in MS (MACFIMS), 400, 403
Montreal Cognitive Assessment (MoCA), 38, 213, 244, 245, 269, 441, 486, 563
Mood impairments, 439, 440
Morphine, 570
Motor vehicle accident (MVA), 437
Multicultural assessment tools
case preparation, 483–484
clinical interview, 484–485
cultural factors
acculturation, 482
bilingual individuals, 482
culturally informed approaches, 480
education and schooling, 482
literacy and education, 481
medical care, 480
monolingual English-speaking individuals, 482
neurologic disorder, 480
neuropsychological measures, 481
operational thinking, 482
preliteracy skills, 481
psychiatric disorders, 480
race, ethnicity and diversity, 480
task completion, 481
world illiteracy levels, 481
culturally informed assessments, 479
neuropsychological assessment, 479
test interpretation, 487–488
test selection, 485–487
US immigrant population, 479
Multiculturalism, 480
Multicultural neuropsychological assessment, 479, 490
Multicultural testing, 483, 490
Multiple sclerosis (MS), 423
assessment methods, 400
central nervous system, 399, 401
cognitive changes, 399, 404
cognitive evaluation, 402–404
cognitive impairment, 400
cognitive problems, 399
diagnosis, 401
MACFIMS, 400, 403
MRIs, 402
neurocognitive impairments, 402
recommendations, 404–406
rehabilitation therapies, 405
specialist, 401
symptoms, 402
Multiple system atrophy (MSA), 239
Multi-trial verbal learning, 385

N

National Institutes of Health (NIH), 514
National Nursing Home Survey data (2004), 565
National Research Council Committee on Educational Interventions for Children with Autism, 120
Neonatal arterial ischemic stroke (NAIS), 150
Neonatal cerebral sinovenous ischemic stroke (NCSVT), 150
Neonatal pain, 174
Neural substrate, 544
Neurobehavioral symptoms, 295
Neurocognitive dysfunction, 69
Neurodevelopmental disorder, 462
Neurofibrillary tangles, 210, 216
Neuroimaging, 502
brain metabolism, 421
critical brain regions, 433
CT and MRI, 422–423
DOI CT scan, 425–428
FLAIR images, 425
functional, 430–433
and neuropsychology, 423–425
principles, 421
psychometric technique, 421
quantitative, 428–430
Neuroleptic malignant syndrome, 251
Neurological Disorders and Stroke (NINDS), 269
Neurology
case presentation, 242–244
examination, 244
labs and imaging, 244

Neuronal activation, 430
Neuroplasticity, 194, 199, 204
Neuro-professions, 550
Neuropsychiatric Inventory, 548
Neuropsychological assessment, 416
Neuropsychological domains
  academic achievement, 125
  attention and executive functioning, 124
  autistic spectrum behavior, 125
  language and social cognition, 123
  memory and learning, 124
  social-emotional ratings, 125
  visual motor functioning, 124
Neuropsychological evaluation, 68
  anatomy, 6–9
  behavioral observations, 215
  cerebrospinal fluid and urine, 4
  cognitive and behavioral domains, 8
  cognitive dysfunction, 3
  cognitive screening devices, 13
  cognitive screening tools, 4, 12
  contextual factors, 4
  cost-effectiveness, 13–14
  diagnostic tool, 3
  electronic medical record, 214
  episodic memory, 216
  indications, 5
  medical methods, 13
  medical/psychiatric/neurological history, 215
  neurocognitive measures, 5
  neurocognitive syndromes, 4, 12
  neurodiagnostic tests, 4
  neurofibrillary tangles, 216
  neuroimaging techniques, 3–4
  patients, 10
  test data, 12
  training, 11
  value of, 10
Neuropsychological screening, 68
Neuropsychological testing, 70, 555
  attention/executive functioning, 70
  clinical findings and history, 70
  cognitive domains, 71
  effort/validity, 71
  visual-spatial/visual-motor, 71
Neuropsychologists administer tests, 497
Neuropsychology
  brain-behavior relationships, 45
  cognitive deficits/dementia, 249
  cognitive functioning, 241
  cognitive screening, 47
  complaints and interview information, 246
  computerized neurocognitive testing, 54–55
  etiology, 242
  feedback (*see* Feedback conversations)
  guiding patient care, 45
  impressions, 250
  in-depth interview, 242
  interpretive and psychometric issues, 51
  memory-based dementia, 241
  memory deficits, 249
  neuroradiology, 52–53
  nomothetic and idiographic deficit measurements, 46
  normative comparison standards, 48–49
  patient care, 46
  physician's impression, 244, 245
  population-based norms, 48–49
  premorbid ability estimates, 49–50
  PVTs, 50–51
  referral, 242
  verbal memory testing, 249
  visuoconstructional deficits, 249
Neuropsychopharmacology, 549
Neuropsychotherapy, 543, 544, 550, 551
Neurorehabilitation, 453, 511, 513, 514
Neurostimulants, 555
Newborn Individualized Developmental Care and Assessment Program, 174–175
Non-benzodiazepine receptor agonists (NBRAs), 567
Nontraditional assessment techniques, 485
Norepinephrine (NE), 95
Not otherwise specified (NOS), 116

O

Obstructive sleep apnea (OSA), 439
Occupational therapists (OT), 514
Oppositional Defiant Disorder (ODD), 116
Orbitofrontal cortex (OFC), 292
Orbitofrontal decline, 314
Other Health Impairment (OHI), 117
Over the counter (OTC) medications, 571

P

Paediatric brain tumours
  assessment process and objectives, 137–138
  assessment results, 139–142
  brain radiation, 133
  chemotherapy treatment, 138
  cognitive functioning, 133, 136, 137, 139
  diagnosis of exclusion, 219

Paediatric brain tumours (*cont.*)
medulloblastoma, 134
multidisciplinary teams, 144
neuroimaging, 138
neuropsychological impact, 136–137
neuropsychological impairment, 133
neuropsychologist's feedback session and recommendations, 218–219
neuropsychologist's impression, formal testing, 217–218
nystagmus, 138
patient, 135–136, 138–139
PFS, 134
recommendations, 143
standard-risk medulloblastoma, 133
Pain medications, 569–571
Parkinson's disease (PD), 239–241, 249
anxiety, 293
cognitive and behavioral symptoms, 292 (*see also* Deep brain stimulation (DBS))
dopamine dysregulation syndrome, 293
dysfunction, 292
forgetfulness and occasional nocturia, 297
hallucinations and delusions, 293
left-leg tremor, 300
levodopa-carbidopa, 297
neurocognitive and neurobehavioral symptoms, 292
neuropathology, 292
neuropsychiatric symptoms, 293
neuropsychological assessments, 293
neuropsychological evaluation, 294, 295
neuropsychological test scores, 296
neuropsychologist's perspective, 295, 300
symptoms, 291, 292
Parkinson's disease with dementia (PDD), 240, 249, 250
Parkinson's Plus disorders, 239
Patient-doctor collaboration, 576
Peabody Picture Vocabulary Test (PPVT), 485
Pediatric brain injury, 92
Pediatric care teams
changing expectations, 19
children and young adults, 24
chronic conditions, 24
communication, medical providers, 27
consultation to medical team, 22–24
cystic fibrosis, 25
decisionmaking supports, 26
in-depth assessment, 25
integrated team care models, 21–22
integration, 17
intervention/treatment-related effects, 19
localization/disease process, 18
management, 26–28
managing access, 28
medical care, 26
medical conditions, 24
neurocognitive functioning, 23, 24, 28
neuropsychological assessment, 19, 26
neuropsychological care, 20–22
pediatric medical model, 22
referral model, 20
symptoms and medical conditions, 27
timing/developmental status, 18
Pediatric epilepsy surgery team
cognitive assessment, 190
cognitive functioning, 191
cortical stimulation mapping, 190
eloquent brain cortex, 190
focal seizures, 191
left mesial temporal lobe
EEG monitoring to confirm, 197
eloquent cortex, 199
fMRI language paradigms, 196
fMRI memory paradigms, 196
left hemisphere cortical activation, 195
neuropsychological test scores, 198
physician perspective, 199
rheumatology service, 195
verbal memory skills, 195
Wada test, 197
magnetic resonance imaging (MRI), 191
neuropsychological evaluation, 191
neuropsychological test scores, 193
occipital lobe
abnormal visual and secondary ocular motility deficits, 200
epilepsy, 200
functional MRI, 201
K-BIT, 200
neuropsychological evaluation, 200, 202
neuropsychological test scores, 203
physician perspective, 204
postsurgical re-evaluation, 202
preoperative axial FLAIR MRI, 201
presurgical intracranial EEG grid monitoring, 201
pediatric psychology, 190
positron emission tomography (PET), 191
posterior frontal lesion and cortical location, 191
radiology image processing, 192
Seattle Children's Hospital, 190
subdural intracranial electrode grid, 192
Pediatric intensive care unit (PICU), 83

Pediatric stroke
acute neonatal stroke, 147
brain development, 148
case presentation
family and medical history, 148, 149
poststroke recovery and development, 149
reason for referral, 148
cognitive and psychosocial difficulties, 148
collaborative discussion
academic skills, 159–160
attention and executive functioning, 159
focal lesions, 158
impact of dystonia, 158
intellectual ability, 158
language, 158
psychosocial outcomes, 160
role of neuropsychologist, 160–162
definitions and epidemiology, 150
early brain injury, 161
heterogeneity, 148
management, 150
neuropsychological assessment, 155–157
outcomes, 151
rehabilitation strategies, 151, 152
Sarah's neurological outcome and dystonia, 151
tracking development, 152–158
Pediatric Stroke Outcome Measure (PSOM), 151
Performance validity tests (PVTs), 13, 50, 56, 272
Perinatal brain injury, 200
Periventricular leukomalacia (PVL), 172
Personal digital assistants (PDAs), 54
Personality Assessment Inventory, 449
Phantom boarder syndrome, 546
Physicians
clinical care environment, 495
cognitive assessment, 552
emotional/behavioral changes, 551
fact/expert witness, 496
neuropsychologists, 495, 552, 553
psychotropic/neurologic medications, 553
sexual consent, 495
Pimavanserin, 241, 251
Polypharmacy, 564, 571–573
Posterior cortical atrophy (PCA)
acetylcholinesterase inhibitor, 225
atrophy, 224
awareness, 231
classification, 224
clinico-radiological syndrome, 233–234
cognitive dysfunction, 224
differential diagnosis, 223
genetic testing, 225
neurofibrillary tangles and neuritic plaques, 225
neurologic disorders, 225
neuropsychiatric disturbance, 225
neuropsychological evaluation
behavioral observations, 228
formal testing, 229–230
interview data, 227, 228
patient, 230
test results, 229
test selection, 228
PCA-AD, 235
PCA-CBD, 236
PCA-LBD, 235
PCA-plus, 234–235
PCA-prior, 236
PCA-pure, 234
physician's impression, neuropsychological testing, 227
post-assessment, 230–231
visuoperceptual and visuospatial functioning, 223
visuospatial skills, 225
Posterior Cortical Atrophy Professional Interest Area Group, 224
Posterior fossa syndrome (PFS), 133, 134
Post-traumatic stress disorder (PTSD), 212
Pregabalin, 570
Premorbid functioning, 484, 485
Premorbid testing, 547
Presumed perinatal ischemic stroke (PPIS), 150
Presurgical neuropsychological evaluation, 384, 395
Preterm birth
additional speech and language support, 180
attention and behavioral regulation, 179
brain injury, 172–173
clinical neuropsychological assessment, 181
definitions, 172
early school-age assessments, 176
educational planning and school support, 179
environmental risk factors, 174–175
family support, 180
global *vs.* selective vulnerability
academic skills, 178
adaptive functions, 178
attention and executive functioning, 177
diagnosis, 179
intellectual outcomes, 177
language, 177
memory and learning, 178

Preterm birth (*cont.*)
neuropsychological outcomes, 176
psychosocial health, 178
specific/selective cognitive impairment, 176
visual perceptual and motor skills, 178
hypotonia and spasticity, 170
lateral ventricles, 171
medical and psychosocial interventions, 181
neonatal care, 180
neurological exam, 171
neuropsychology, 175
reassessment, 180
social skills, 180
Primary care neuropsychology
acute and chronic liver diseases, 34
Bayesian principles, 35
behavioral health integration, 37
biologic disease and psychiatric disorders, 42
brain metabolism, 34
brief neuropsychological assessments, 39
chronic diseases, 42
CNS conditions, 40
cognitive abilities and emotional functioning, 39
cognitive assessments and interventions, 41
cognitive dysfunction, 31, 40
cognitive functioning, 37
cognitive remediation, 40
cognitive screens, 38
cognitive symptoms, 38
cognitive testing and neuropsychological assessment, 39
complex psychiatric and neurological disorders, 36
gastroesophageal reflux disease, 35
individualized and evidence-based treatments, 38
integration and efficiency, 38
medical diseases, 34
Mini-Cog test, 39
mood and biopsychosocial information, 40
neuropsychological contributions, 37
neuropsychological integration, 37
neuropsychologists, 32
neurotransmitter dysregulation, 34
nutritional deficiencies, 34
patients' cognitive functioning, 31
patient's neuropsychological testing, 32–33
pretest probability, 35
psychiatric and neurological diagnoses, 36
psychiatric diseases, 37
psychiatry, 36
routine drug and alcohol, 39
stepped model of care, 39
Primary care providers (PCPs), 31, 562
Problem-solving strategies, 518
Procedural accommodations, 536
Progressive non-fluent aphasia (PNFA), 256
Progressive supranuclear palsy (PSP), 239
Pseudobulbar affect, 545
Pseudodementia, 252
Psychopharmacological management, 454
Psychotherapy
emotional dysregulation, 543
neurological dysfunction, 543
neuropsychological assessment, 547, 548
personality changes, 543
psychological assessment, 547
Psychotropic medications, 412, 564–566
Pulse sequence, 423

Q

Quantitative neuroimaging, 428–430
Quetiapine, 241

R

Race, 480
Radiation therapy, 136, 367–369
Rancho Los Amigos Levels of Cognitive Functioning, 97
Randomized controlled trials (RCTs), 522
Rectal bleeding, 567
Reduplicative paramnesia, 546
Reflexive reactions, 544
Region of interest (ROI), 429
Rehabilitation Services Administration (RSA), 531
Rehabilitation therapies, 405
REM behavioral disorder (RBD), 240, 249, 301
Repetitive motor, 293
Residual thought disorder, 409, 417
Retentive memory loss, 217
Rey Complex Figure Test (RCFT), 314
Reynolds Intelligence Assessment Scales—2nd Edition (RIAS-2), 152
Rey-Osterrieth Complex Figure Test, 485
Rheumatoid arthritis, 572
Right middle cerebral artery stroke
anosognosia, 282
attention/speed of processing, 287
diagnosis and pattern of thinking, 279, 280
EF, 284–286
emotional functioning, 287

epidemiology and demographics, 278–279
evidenced-based citations, 288
general ability, 283
language, 286
learning and memory, 284
neurocognitive testing, 278
neuropsychological evaluation, 280–281
neuropsychological testing, 277, 281–282
recovery course, 280
visuospatial ability, 284
Risperidone, 92, 565
Rivastigmine, 251, 550
RMCA neurocognitive disability, 278

S
Saint Louis University Mental Status Examination (SLUMS), 563
Schizophrenia
and aging, 410
chronic mental illness, 410
cognitive deficits, 410
neuropsychological evaluation
testing, dementia detection, 416
test results, 414
test validity, 414
neuropsychological test data, 415
psychiatry
anticholinergic drugs and cognition, 412
cognitive effects, metabolic syndrome, 413
differential diagnosis, 413
mental status exam, 412–413
psychotropic drugs and cognition, 412
residual thought disorder, 409
Schizophrenia-spectrum disorder, 409
Screening Tool of Older Persons' potentially inappropriate Prescriptions (STOPP), 571
Screening Tool to Alert doctors to Right Treatment (START), 571
Second impact syndrome (SIS), 336
Sedative hypnotics, 564, 566–568
Seizures
AEDs, 380, 383
focal, 380, 386
frequency, 385
localization, 384
medically intractable (*see* Medically intractable seizures)
neurosurgical treatment, 384
psychogenic nonepileptic, 380
Self-Administered Gerocognitive Examination (SAGE), 47
Self-disclosure, 581
Self-efficacy, 549
Sensory Processing Disorder, and Anxiety Disorder, 116
Sensory stimulation, 99
Serum anticholinergic activities assay (SAA), 569
Sickle cell disease (SCD)
autosomal recessive or codominant genetic disorders, 65
brain dysfunction, 73
capacity/competency, 76–77
central nervous system, 66
cerebral arterial vasculopathy, 66
chronic erythrocytapheresis therapy, 64
chronic transfusion therapy, 67
educational and vocational planning, 75
fibroid tumors, 64
focal neurologic deficits, 67
hemoglobin C/β-thalassemia, 65
hemoglobin S (Hb S), 65
neurological complications, 63
neuropsychological evaluations, 64
organization and time management strategies, 74
pediatric considerations, 69–70
preliminary impressions, 65–70
RBC, 66
role of neuropsychology, 67–69
SCI, 67
screening *vs.* comprehensive evaluation, 74
sickle-hemoglobin C disease, 74
supportive healthcare tools, 76
transition to adulthood, 77–78
Silent cerebral infarction (SCI), 67
Single-family rooms (SFR), 174
Sleep medications, 566–568
Social Communication Questionnaire (SCQ), 120
Social context, 551
Social isolation, 554
Social Perception Scale of Advanced Clinical Solutions, 548
Socioeconomic status (SES), 174
Spanish Multicenter Normative Studies (NEURONORMA), 486
Specific language impairments, 121
Speech and language pathologists, 514

Sports concussion
case study, 338–341
CTE, 337
definition, 328
diagnosis
baseline computerized testing, 332
biopsychosocial model, 331
cervical spine injury, 330
headache, 330
neurocognitive testing, 331
neuropsychological testing, 331, 333
structured approach, 329
symptoms suggestive, 330
traumatic brain injury, 331
epidemiology, 328–329
graduated return-to-school strategy, 337
graduated return-to-sport strategy, 334
long-term consequences, 336–342
management, 333–335
pathophysiology, 329
premature return to play, 336
return-to-learn protocol, 336
risk factors, 333
Stealth reorientations
diverse medical context, 582–585
impaired memory scores, 580
open channels of communication, 581
self-disclosure, 581
translators, 582
Subcortical ischemic vascular disease (SIVD), 269
Subthalamic nucleus (STN), 291, 301
Susceptibility-weighted imaging (SWI), 423, 426
Syndrome of inappropriate antidiuretic hormone (SIADH), 567
Systolic Blood Pressure Intervention Trial (SPRINT), 273

T

Tertiary care center, 230
Test of Nonverbal Intelligence, Fourth Edition (TONI-4), 487
Thalamocortical fibers, 173
Thalamus, 173
Theory of mind, 545
Thought disorder, 410
Thrombocytopenia, 173
Tonic-clonic seizures, 200
Trail Making Test (TMT), 430, 431
Tramadol, 570
Transcranial Doppler (TCD), 64, 280
Traumatic brain injury (TBI), 425, 507, 553, 577, 578
anterior and medial temporal lobes, 86
axonal shear injury, 87
bifrontal and bitemporal contusions, 95
bradycardia and facial trauma, 95
child mortality and morbidity, 85
cognitive deficits, 441
cognitive functioning, 93
cognitive, motor/sensory skills, 86
cognitive rehabilitation, 514
collaboration considerations, 451–452
collaborative care
cognitive abilities, 89
cortical and/or subcortical structures, 87
medication issues, 89
physician's assessment, 88
secondary brain injury, 89
concussion, 84–85
depression, 507
dyssomnias, 439
effects of damage, 93
endocrine abnormalities, 439
family-centered care, 94
fatigue, 438
focal injuries, 86
functional assessment, 453
goals, 437
headaches, 438
MD impressions, 102
medical and health-related consequences, 436
medical treatments and concerns, 437–442
medication alterations, 453
medication management post-PICU, 91–92
moderate-to-severe, 509, 514, 519
mood impairments, 439, 440
neurobehavioral consequences, 436
neuropathological processes, 99
neuropsychological impressions, 103–105
neuropsychological testing, 452
attention, 446
brain injury rehabilitation care, 442
emotional functions, 448, 449
executive functions, 448
higher-level attentional abilities, 449

intellectual functions, 449
intelligence, 445
language functions, 447
medication management, 451
memory, 446
neurobehavioral functioning, 450
nonstructured environments, 450
observations, 445
occupational therapy, 450
personality testing, 450
psychoeducation training, 450
rationale, 443
retrograde amnesia, 442
sensory motor functions, 447
test battery approach and selection, 443, 444
transitional rehabilitation, 450
and treatment, 435
visual spatial functions, 447
neuropsychology follow-ups, 453
neuropsychology impressions, 96–97, 100–101
orbital and inferior medial frontal contusions, 86
outpatient follow-up examinations, 106–110
pathophysiological effects, 83
pediatric intensive care, 95–96
pediatric rehabilitation, 92
periorbital and frontal edema, 95
petechial hemorrhages, 87
physician impressions, 105
primary clinical considerations, 97–100, 103
problems, 523
related cognitive deficits, 519
return to work, 443, 451, 452
sports concussion (*see* Sports concussion)
subdural/subarachnoid bleeds, 87
visual deficits, 438, 439
Trazodone, 453, 567
Treatment goals
barriers/obstacles, 556
cognitive-behavioral treatment, 556
emotional rehabilitation, 557
interventions/procedures, 556
long-term, 556
obsessive-compulsive tendencies, 557
short-term, 556
skill rebuilding, 557
social activities, 557
Tricyclic antidepressants, 570
Tricyclics (amitriptyline), 550
Triggered responses, 544
T2-weighted MRI, 269

U
US Armed Services, 211
US Department of Health and Human Services, 274
US National Institute on Disability, Independent Living, and Rehabilitation Research (NIDILRR), 537

V
Vascular cognitive impairment (VCI)
cognitive screening instruments, 268
description, 267, 269
diagnosis, 270–271
emotional stress, 273
etiology, 273
IADLs, 273
magnetic resonance imaging, 269
MCI and dementia, 274
neurological exam and findings, 268
neuropsychological evaluation, 271
neuropsychological testing
effort testing, 272
emotional functioning, 273
executive functioning, 272
information processing speed, 272
memory, 272
referral, 267
vascular comorbidities, 273
Vascular cognitive impairment-no dementia (VCIND), 269
Vascular dementia (VaD), 239, 269
Vascular depression, 273
Ventral intermediate (VIM), 291
Ventriculomegaly, 173
Verbal Comprehension Index, 123
Verbal memory, 403
Veterans Affairs Puget Sound Health Care System, 211
Virginia Commonwealth University, 576
Visual deficits, 438, 439
Vocational rehabilitation, 287, 288
consultation, 531
counseling, 531
physician-guided work return, 537–538
work return, 538–539

Vocational rehabilitation (*cont.*)
counselor's partnership, neuropsychologist, 533
exchange dynamics, 534–535
neuropsychological test results, 534
range of services, 532–533
reasonable accommodation
assistive technology, 536, 537
procedural, 536
workstation modification, 536

W
Wada test, 384–386, 394, 395
Wechsler Adult Intelligence Scale-Fourth Edition (WAIS-IV), 486
Wechsler Intelligence Scale for Children, 104

Y
Yalom's group therapy, 451

CPSIA information can be obtained
at www.ICGtesting.com
Printed in the USA
LVHW080028180619
621551LV00001B/2/P

9 781493 987207